CONTROL OF
COMMUNICABLE
DISEASES

CLINICAL PRACTICE

For access to digital chapters,
visit the CCDM website (https://ccdm.aphapublications.org);
free access to CCDM's "Explanation of Terms" also available on the site
(https://ccdm.aphapublications.org/doi/10.2105/CCDM.2745.156).

CONTROL OF
COMMUNICABLE
DISEASES
CLINICAL PRACTICE

Editors
Omar A. Khan, MD
David L. Heymann, MD

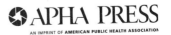

APHA PRESS
AN IMPRINT OF AMERICAN PUBLIC HEALTH ASSOCIATION

American Public Health Association
800 I Street, NW
Washington, DC 20001-3710
www.apha.org

Georges C. Benjamin, MD, Executive Director

Printed and bound in the United States of America
Book Production Editor: Maya Ribault
Typesetting: The Charlesworth Group
Cover Design: Alan Giarcanella
Printing and Binding: Sheridan Books

Library of Congress Cataloging-in-Publication Data

Names: Khan, Omar A., 1973- editor. | Heymann, David L., editor. | American Public Health Association, issuing body.
Title: Control of communicable diseases. Clinical practice / editors, Omar A. Khan, David L. Heymann.
Other titles: Clinical practice | Control of communicable diseases manual.
Description: Washington, DC : American Public Health Association, [2019] | Includes index. | Summary: "This manual provides clinicians working in varied settings and locations with the means to review what their capability and capacity should be with respect to specific communicable diseases. It also provides them with the tools to determine what type of response is warranted"-- Provided by publisher.
Identifiers: LCCN 2019037411 (print) | LCCN 2019037412 (ebook) | ISBN 9780875533070 (paperback) | ISBN 9780875533087 (adobe pdf)
Subjects: MESH: Communicable Disease Control--methods | Communicable Diseases
Classification: LCC RA643 (print) | LCC RA643 (ebook) | NLM WA 110 | DDC 616.9--dc23
LC record available at https://lccn.loc.gov/2019037411
LC ebook record available at https://lccn.loc.gov/2019037412

EDITORS

Omar A. Khan, MD
Christiana Care Health System/Delaware Health Sciences Alliance
United States

David L. Heymann, MD
London School of Hygiene & Tropical Medicine
United Kingdom

MANAGING EDITOR

Elizabeth Healy, MPH
Delaware Public Health Association/Academy of Medicine United States

EDITORIAL BOARD

Mary Kamb, MD, MPH
Centers for Disease Control
United States

Jilllian Laude, PharmD, BCPS
Christiana Care Health System
United States

Yee-Sin Leo, MBBS, M Med, MPH, MRCP, FRCP, FAMS
National Centre for Infectious Diseases
Singapore

Thomas Peterman, MD, MSc
Centers for Disease Control
United States

REVIEWERS

Jon Andrus, MD
University of Colorado
George Washington University
United States

Hishamuddin Badaruddin, BMBS, MPH, FAMS
Duke-NUS Medical School
Singapore

Georges C. Benjamin, MD
American Public Health Association
United States

Carlos Castillo-Salgado, MD, JD, DrPH
Johns Hopkins Bloomberg School of Public Health
United States

John Clemens, MD
International Centre for Diarrhoeal Disease Research
Bangladesh

Johan Giesecke, MD
Karolinska Institute
Sweden

Eduardo Gotuzzo, MD
Alexander von Humboldt Institute of Tropical Medicine and Infectious Diseases
Peru

Duane J. Gubler, ScD, MS
Duke-NUS Graduate Medical School
Singapore

Peter Hotez, MD
National School of Tropical Medicine
United States

James M. Hughes, MD
Emory University School of Medicine
United States

Rima F. Khabbaz, MD
Centers for Diseases Control and Prevention
United States

Peter Kilmarx, MD
National Institutes of Health
United States

James W. LeDuc, PhD
University of Texas Medical Branch
United States

Thomas Quinn, MD
National Institutes of Health
United States

AUTHORS

Centers for Disease Control and Prevention
United States
http://www.cdc.gov

Anyalechi G.
Appiah G.
Armstrong P.
Backer L.
Beer K.
Belay E.
Benedict K.
Blaney D.
Bruce B. B.
Caceres D.
Chancey R.
Chatham-Stephens K.
Cherry C. C.
Cherry-Brown D.
Chow N.
Cope J.
Crowe S.
Dasch G. A.
Fischer M.
Francois Watkins L. K.
Friedman C.
Furness B.
Gould C.
Gray E.
Griffin P. M.
Guagliardo S.
Healy J. M.
Herwaldt B.
Hills S.
Hughes M.
Jackson B.
Kamb M.
Kato C.
Kersh G. J.

Kirkcaldy B.
Laughlin M. E.
Llata L.
Markowitz L.
Martin S.
Marx G.
McCotter O. Z.
Mead P.
Medalla F.
Meites E.
Montgomery S.
Nichols Heitman K.
Nicholson W. L.
Peterson A. E.
Pillay A.
Plumb I. D.
Powers A.
Rabe I.
Ridpath A.
Roellig D.
Roy S.
Sapp S. G. H.
Schillinger J.
Staples E.
St. Cyr S.
Straily A.
Strockbine N. A.
Tack D. M.
Taylor M.
Toda M.
Tsay S.
Vallabhaneni S.
Winstead A.
Workowski K.

Other Organizations

Abel M.
Abel Jr R.
Adams L.
Amare M.
Andrus J.
Archuleta S.
Aronson N.
Azhar E.
Badaruddin H.
Berk J.
Berk S.
Blanton L.
Bowen A.
Bradbury R. S.
Brett-Major D.
Bruschi F.
Cabada M. M.
Carapetis J.
Chow N.
Chuang I.
Cohen D.
Davis A.
Decker C. F.
de Gijsel D.
Donahue M. L.
Donovan P.
Doshi R.
Eppes S.
Ewers E.
Gilani M.
Gilbert L. J.
Haque R.
Harrison C.
Healy E.
Ho Z. J. M.
Hoff N.
Hughes J.
Hui D. S.
Jones J.
Khan O. A.

Klausner J.
Lee V.
Longworth D.
Maguire M.
Marimuthu K.
Mate S.
Mertz G.
Modjarrad K.
Molnar M.
Montgomery S.
Muth E.
Panwalker A.
Parikh A.
Pust R.
Ressner R. A.
Rimoin A.
Robben P.
Robinson S. L.
Ronald A. R.
Ruiz-Tiben E.
Scollard D.
Scott P.
Siddiqui A.
Smith D.
Storme C.
Strebel P.
Talbot E.
Tanabe M.
Vasoo S.
Vilcins I.-M.
von Seidlein L.
Walker D.
Webb C. M.
Wong C. S.
Wright S.
Yee-Sin L.
Yeoh D.
Young B.
Zaman K.
Zumia A.

CONTENTS

FOREWORD

The clinical component of communicable disease control requires a sound understanding of the scientific basis of infectious diseases and of the core principles of prevention, which comprise personal and environmental hygiene; personal protective barriers such as condoms, gloves, and masks; and appropriate immunizations. Once infected, the rapid and correct identification of the infectious agent(s) through screening and diagnostic testing is the required next step followed by sound medical and nursing care.

Medical care is often described as both a science and an art. It begins with observing the patient, taking a history of the chief complaint, doing an appropriate physical exam, and conducting the correct tests needed to confirm the diagnosis. Therapy commonly includes supportive therapy to control fever, fluid rehydration, and medications such as antibiotics or antivirals targeted to the presumed pathogen. Therapeutic success is often based on a sound understanding of the scientific basis of disease, a full comprehension of the clinical and diagnostic findings, good nursing, and skilled application of the art of medicine.

Control of Communicable Diseases: Clinical Practice (*Clinical Practice*) comes at a time of incredible progress in preventive medicine, diagnostic testing, and clinical treatment. Because of these profound advancements, there is a need for an up-to-date, authoritative reference for the practicing communicable disease control clinician. *Clinical Practice* provides timely information in a portable format, one that's well suited to the rapid clinical decision-making often required in managing communicable diseases.

This first edition of *Clinical Practice* provides an overview of the latest clinical information for each pathogen and disease, including causative agents, diagnosis, treatment, and prevention. This manual balances detail with efficiency and features writing by top experts from the world's leading health agencies. *Clinical Practice* is designed to serve as a complement to *Control of Communicable Diseases Manual* (*CCDM*), which has been the primary reference source for disease control specialists for over 100 years. Along with *Control of Communicable Diseases: Laboratory Practice*, its laboratory diagnostic companion for laboratory scientists, *Clinical Practice* completes the trilogy of essential *CCDM* references aiding health practitioners in their disease control efforts. Taken together, these 3 manuals provide a comprehensive resource for practitioners tasked with controlling communicable diseases.

The 21st century public health and clinical landscapes are rapidly evolving. Emerging and re-emerging infectious diseases are on the rise while outstanding advances in therapeutics and scientific knowledge are transpiring as we speak. *Clinical Practice* is a world-class resource for our times. It is an essential resource for all clinicians tasked with controlling communicable diseases.

Georges C. Benjamin, MD
Executive Director
American Public Health Association

PREFACE

We are pleased to present the first clinical companion to the *Control of Communicable Diseases Manual* (*CCDM*), published by the American Public Health Association (APHA). The work herein captures thousands of hours of painstaking work by authors, editors, and advisors. The editorial board is a true working body of globally renowned professionals, many of whom are also chapter authors and all of whom have contributed immensely to this undertaking. We appreciate each author's tremendous effort in updating the chapters for clinicians' use, adding information that the editor himself would find useful (and who, despite all advice to the contrary, continues to add to his overcommitted schedule by seeing patients).

The support provided by APHA, in particular from our editorial liaison, Richard Lampert, has been outstanding. Our administrative and editorial team at APHA, including Maya Ribault, Ashell R. Alston, and David Hartogs, has been helpful at all phases of this work. Several years ago, when the editor chaired the APHA publications board, he was fortunate enough to get to know Dr. Georges C. Benjamin, executive director of APHA. Over the years, Dr. Benjamin has been a friend and colleague of the highest caliber. His leadership of APHA and his unwavering support for *CCDM* are 2 big reasons why this work is continuing to flourish in the 21st century.

Several aspects of *CCDM: Clinical Practice* deserve mention. A major innovation of this companion volume is the addition of expert pharmacist review of clinical recommendations. This has allowed us to dig deeper in select chapters, particularly those with complex regimens, in order to provide readers with the best knowledge available. This book, however useful, is not intended as a substitute for medical advice from a trained professional. It should also be pointed out that the findings and conclusions in these chapters are those of the authors and do not necessarily represent the official position of their employers, government entities, or anyone else except the authors.

We have derived tremendous satisfaction in working with our colleagues and supporters. We have relied on reference texts, experts, coffee makers, and each other, perhaps all in equal measure, as we helped construct this volume. We are grateful to you, our readers, for the opportunity to serve a need in public health and clinical medicine.

Omar A. Khan, MD
Elizabeth Healy, MPH

READER'S GUIDE

Each disease chapter in *Control of Communicable Diseases: Clinical Practice* is presented in a standardized format that includes the following information:

Disease name: each disease is identified by the numeric code assigned by WHO's *International Statistical Classification of Diseases and Related Health Problems*, 10th Revision (ICD-10). Common names are also listed and can be matched to the ICD names using the index.

1. **Clinical features:** presents the main signs and symptoms of the disease and differentiates the disease from others that may have a similar clinical picture. Case-fatality rates may also be included.
2. **Risk groups:** describes human population groups at increased risk of infection or development of diseases or that are resistant to either infection or disease. Information on immunity subsequent to infection may also be given.
3. **Causative agents:** identifies the specific agent(s) that cause the disease; classifies the agent(s); describes variations, subtypes, and strains; and may indicate important characteristics.
4. **Diagnosis:** describes methods most commonly used to diagnose the disease and provides information on how results should be interpreted.
5. **Occurrence:** provides information on where the disease is known to occur and the magnitude of its burden. Information on past and current outbreaks may also be included.
6. **Reservoirs:** describes any person, animal, arthropod, plant, or substance—or combination of these—in which an infectious agent normally lives and reproduces itself in such a manner that it can be transmitted to a susceptible host. Intermediate hosts and animal populations at risk are described in this section.
7. **Incubation period:** describes the interval between infection and the first appearance of symptoms associated with the infection.
8. **Transmission:** provides information on the mechanisms by which the infectious agent is spread to or among humans; the period of time during which it may be transferred to humans from an infected human, reservoir, or vector; and the factors that influence transmissibility.
9. **Treatment:** usually in table format, unless treatment is supportive or otherwise not applicable. Will usually include drug, dose, route, alternative drugs (if relevant), recommended duration of treatment, and special considerations. As always, this is not intended as medical advice substituting for a physician. Local expertise and consultation are recommended for diagnosis and treatment. This information is intended as an aid, developed through expert guidance.

10. **Prevention:** describes measures that can be used to prevent infection of individuals and/or groups.
11. **Special considerations:** describes any special considerations relevant for the disease. For instance, when applicable it notes reporting requirements, whether free drugs are available through WHO or CDC, and what measures are recommended for public health workers in case of deliberate use of biologic agents to cause harm. Disaster implications or special epidemic measures are also described, if applicable.

READER'S GUIDE: PHARMACOLOGY

Antimicrobial Therapy Basics

When determining how to effectively manage patients with infectious diseases, it is critical to assess patient, pathogen, and antimicrobial factors in order to ensure successful outcomes. The purpose of this guide is to give a general overview of some of the key antimicrobial features that can be used in the management of infectious diseases.

There are 3 different types of antimicrobial therapy: prophylactic, empiric, and definitive therapy.[1,2]

- **Prophylactic therapy**: refers to the use of an antimicrobial agent to prevent the development of an infection that has not yet occurred. For example, patients with human immunodeficiency virus with low cluster of differentiation 4 counts will be on trimethoprim-sulfamethoxazole prophylaxis to prevent the development of *Pneumocystis jiroveci* pneumonia.

- **Empiric therapy**: refers to treating a suspected or confirmed infection with an antimicrobial agent before the susceptibility data are known. For example, cefepime would be considered empiric therapy in a patient being treated for a Gram-negative rod bacteremia before knowing the pathogen identification or susceptibility profile. When initiating empiric therapy, it is important to consider regional- or institution-based susceptibility data, if available, to help determine the best empiric antimicrobial that would provide appropriate coverage against the suspected pathogen.

- **Definitive therapy**: refers therefore the use of an antimicrobial agent once the definitive susceptibility information is known. We therefore definitively know which antimicrobial agent will work against the identified pathogen. Ideally, the antimicrobial agent used for definitive therapy should be as narrow in spectrum as possible in order to maximize efficacy while minimizing cost and toxicity. An example of definitive therapy would be transitioning from cefepime (a broad spectrum cephalosporin) to cephalexin (a much more narrow spectrum cephalosporin) to treat an *Escherichia coli* urinary tract infection that is found to be susceptible to cephalexin.

When selecting antimicrobial therapy, it is important to understand the pharmacokinetics of the drug. Pharmacokinetics refer to how a drug moves through the body; this is important when determining how much of a drug will reach the active site of infection and how the drug is eliminated from the body. The key components of pharmacokinetics are absorption, distribution, metabolism, and excretion.[1,2]

- **Absorption:** refers to the ability of a drug to enter the bloodstream after oral administration. Related to absorption, the bioavailability of an orally administered drug is the amount of the drug that actually enters the bloodstream and therefore has the ability to exert a therapeutic effect. Different oral antimicrobials have different bioavailabilities. Table 1 lists common antimicrobials and their bioavailability.[1-3]

Table 1. Antimicrobial Bioavailability

Antimicrobial Agent	Bioavailability
Doxycycline	95%–100%
Fluconazole	95%–100%
Levofloxacin	95%–100%
Linezolid	95%–100%
Metronidazole	95%–100%
Trimethoprim-sulfamethoxazole	90%–100%
Cephalexin, cefadroxil	~90%
Amoxicillin	~90%
Clindamycin	~90%
Ciprofloxacin	~80%
Cefuroxime	40%
Acyclovir	25%

- **Distribution:** the movement of a drug from the bloodstream to body tissues. The concentration of a particular drug in a particular tissue can vary depending on a drug's properties, including the size of the drug and the amount of free drug circulating in the bloodstream. Distribution is therefore an important step in ensuring that a drug is able to reach its targeted site of action.[1,2]
- **Metabolism:** drugs are typically eliminated from the body via 2 main mechanisms: metabolism or excretion. Metabolism refers to the process by which a drug is transformed into metabolites that are more easily eliminated from the body than the parent drug compound. The majority of metabolism takes place in the liver as many of the enzymes responsible for metabolism can be found there. One of the major groups of metabolizing enzymes are the cytochrome P450 enzymes. There are many different antimicrobial agents that are metabolized by these cytochrome P450 enzymes; additionally, many antimicrobials also serve as potent inhibitors or potent inducers of these enzymes. When an antimicrobial acts as a potent inhibitor of cytochrome P450 enzymes and the antimicrobial is given in combination with another drug that is typically broken down by these enzymes, it can lead to elevated concentrations of the latter drug and

potentially lead to toxicity. Alternatively, when an antimicrobial agent acts as an inducer of the cytochrome P450 enzymes and is given in combination with another drug that is metabolized via these enzymes, it can lead to a subtherapeutic concentration of the latter drug. It is therefore critical to review a patient's medication list to screen for drug-drug interactions.[1,2]

- **Excretion:** the other main mechanism of drug elimination is via excretion through the kidneys. It is important to remember whether a drug is eliminated via the kidneys as these drugs will require dose adjustment in patients with renal dysfunction.[1,2]

Antimicrobial Properties

One of the important characteristics of an antimicrobial agent is whether the agent is bactericidal or bacteriostatic in nature. Bactericidal means that the drug kills the bacterium. Bacteriostatic, on the other hand, means that the drug inhibits the growth of the bacterium but does not actively kill the pathogen. For most indications, either a bacteriostatic or bactericidal agent could be used to achieve similar outcomes; however, bactericidal agents would be preferred for certain indications, such as meningitis and endocarditis, to ensure that the pathogen is fully eradicated. With either bactericidal or bacteriostatic activity, there will always be a minimum inhibitory concentration (MIC) associated with the pathogen; the MIC is the minimum concentration of an antibiotic that will visibly inhibit the growth of the bacterium.

Another important property is related to *how* an antimicrobial agent exhibits its activity. There are 2 main types of activity that will be discussed: concentration-dependent and time-dependent activity. Some antibiotics are most effective when the antibiotic concentration is maintained about the organism's MIC for a maximal period of time; this type of property is described as time-dependent activity. Other antibiotics are most effective when the antibiotic concentration reaches a very high peak level relative to the MIC of the organism; this is referred to as concentration-dependent activity. The type of activity that an antimicrobial agent displays is often taken into account when designing a drug's dosing regimen. For example, aminoglycoside agents are often given as a large once-daily dose to maximize concentration-dependent activity; however, an agent such as cephalexin is given in smaller doses more frequently throughout the day to maximize its time-dependent activity.[2,3]

Unfortunately, antimicrobial agents differ in their ability to withstand heat and light and a universal statement cannot be made for all antimicrobials; therefore, we recommend utilizing the individual antimicrobial's product labeling for the most accurate stability information.

Pediatrics

Antimicrobial dosing in pediatrics is often weight-based and can be age-dependent. Supplementary recommendations for the management of infectious diseases in the pediatric population can be found in *Red Book: 2018—2021*

Report of the Committee on Infectious Diseases. Refer to local weight-based dosing practices. The definitions of pediatric terms are given in Table 2.

Table 2. Pediatric Definitions

Term	Definition
Premature	Newborn infants born at < 37 weeks of gestational age
Neonate	Between 1 day and 1 month old
Infant	Between 1 month and 1 year old
Child	Between 1 and 11 years old
Adolescent	Between 12 and 16 years old

Pregnancy

Physiologic changes occur during pregnancy that may impact the pharmacokinetics of antimicrobials. These changes typically begin during the first trimester and peak during the second trimester. In addition, data on the safety and efficacy of select agents in pregnancy may be limited. Refer to local package labeling for specific details. Supplementary information may be found in *Drugs in Pregnancy and Lactation: A Reference Guide to Fetal and Neonatal Risk.* Further details are given in Tables 3 and 4.

Table 3. Pharmacokinetic Changes in Pregnancy

Pharmacokinetic Parameter	Physiologic Change	Pharmacokinetic Implication
Absorption	Nausea and vomiting	↓ absorption of oral antimicrobials
	Delayed gastric emptying	↑ absorption of oral antimicrobials
Distribution	↑ body fat	↑ volume of distribution (↓ serum concentration) of lipid-soluble antimicrobials
	↓ plasma albumin	↑ volume of distribution (↓ serum concentration) of highly protein-bound antimicrobials; however, unbound drugs may clear more rapidly via the liver and kidneys during pregnancy
Elimination	↑ maternal plasma volume ↑ cardiac output ↑ glomerular filtration by 30%–50%	↑ clearance of renally eliminated antimicrobials

Table 4. Medications Generally Considered Safe in Pregnancy

Acetaminophen
Azithromycin
Beta lactams (penicillin, amoxicillin)
Carbapenems
Cephalosporins

Lactation

Most medications can transfer into breast milk with variable effects on the child. Drug factors impacting transfer from maternal circulation into breast milk include protein binding, molecular weight, lipid solubility, maternal plasma concentration, drug half-life, and drug pH. Supplementary information may be found in *Drugs in Pregnancy and Lactation: A Reference Guide to Fetal and Neonatal Risk* or the National Library of Medicine's Drugs and Lactation Database.

Geriatrics

Geriatric patients are at an increased risk of antimicrobial complications due to physiologic and pharmacokinetic changes. Understanding these principles may help minimize the risk for adverse drug reactions. Refer to Table 5 and to local dosing protocols.[4]

Table 5. Pharmacokinetic Changes in Geriatrics

Pharmacokinetic Parameter	Physiologic Change	Pharmacokinetic Implication
Absorption	Increased gastric pH	↓ absorption of pH-dependent agents ↑ absorption of acid-labile agents
	Decreased small-bowel surface area	↓ absorption
	Decreased blood flow to small bowel	↓ absorption
	Decreased gastric emptying and gastro-intestinal motility	↓ delayed absorption

(Continued)

Table 5. Pharmacokinetic Changes in Geriatrics (Continued)

Pharmacokinetic Parameter	Physiologic Change	Pharmacokinetic Implication
Distribution	Increase in adipose tissue	↑ half-life of lipid-soluble antimicrobials
	Decrease in total body water	↑ concentration of water-soluble antimicrobials (e.g., aminoglycosides)
	Decrease in plasma albumin	↑ free concentration of acidic antimicrobials (e.g., penicillins, ceftriaxone, sulfonamides, and clindamycin)
	Increased plasma α_1-acid glycoprotein level	↓ free concentration of basic antimicrobials (e.g., macrolides)
Metabolism	Decreased CYP450 activity	↑ half-life of antimicrobials metabolized via CYP450 pathway-soluble antimicrobials
	Decreased hepatic blood flow	↓ first pass metabolism
Elimination	Decreased renal blood flow and glomerular filtration rate	↑ half-life of renally eliminated antimicrobials

Guidelines for Treatment of Fever

Fever occurs as a physiologic response to an underlying condition, most often an infection, and can provide beneficial effects in fighting that infection. It is uncertain if treatment of fever can increase the risk of complications of infection. Antipyretics are often given for the benefits of relieving pain and discomfort as well as reducing insensible water loss, therefore reducing the risk of dehydration.

Physicians commonly recommend treating children with a fever of higher than 38.8°C (101°F) with antipyretics; however, there are no consensus recommendations. Although there is no evidence of adverse effects such as brain damage due to high fever, these concerns may begin when the fever reaches 40°C (104°F) or higher. Table 6 provides recommended antipyretic agents and dosing for adults and children.[3,5,6]

Table 6. Acetaminophen and Ibuprofen Dosing for Fever[a]

	Pediatric Dosing	Maximum Pediatric Dose	Adult Dosing	Maximum Adult Dose
Acetaminophen	10–15 mg/kg every 4–6 hours	75–90 mg/kg/day[b] (≤ 4 g/day)	650 mg every 4–6 hours	4 g/day[c]

(Continued)

Table 6. Acetaminophen and Ibuprofen Dosing for Fever[a] (Continued)

	Pediatric Dosing	Maximum Pediatric Dose	Adult Dosing	Maximum Adult Dose
Ibuprofen	5–10 mg/kg every 6–8 hours[d]	40 mg/kg/day (≤ 400 mg/ dose)	200–400 mg every 4–6 hours	2.4 g/day

[a]Dose adjustments may be required for renal or hepatic dysfunction.
[b]90 mg/kg/day should be limited to < 3 consecutive days.
[c]Some products have lower maximum doses in an attempt to protect against inadvertent overdoses.
[d]Limited data are available in infants < 6 months.

Alternating or combining acetaminophen with ibuprofen is a common practice to control fever. Although there is no consensus on dosing intervals, alternating agents every 2, 3, 4, and 6 hours has been reported. Although this practice has been studied, there is no consensus on its efficacy, safety, or impact on other clinical outcomes besides fever reduction.[5,6]

Antimicrobial Stewardship Statement

Antimicrobial stewardship refers to coordinated multidisciplinary efforts to improve antimicrobial use, resulting in optimized treatment of infections while reducing adverse events. Antimicrobial stewardship practices have become increasingly important in the current age of rising global rates of antibiotic resistance, *Clostridium difficile* infection, and emerging research on potential negative downstream effects of altering the gut microbiome with the use of antibiotics.

In general, reviewing the "5 Ds of stewardship" (drug, dose, de-escalation, duration, and discernment) can be applied to optimize any antimicrobial regimen. Table 7 illustrates the 5 Ds of stewardship along with an example of each scenario.

Table 7. The 5 Ds of Stewardship

D of Stewardship	Example
Drug	Selecting the appropriate antimalarial treatment regimen based on the geographic area of exposure and drug resistance patterns.
Dose	Reducing the dose of fluconazole by 50% in patients with renal impairment (CrCl < 50 mL/min).
De-escalation	Changing from a broad spectrum agent (e.g., levofloxacin) to a narrow spectrum agent (e.g., cephalexin) for the treatment of a UTI based on the susceptibility profile of the urine culture isolate.

(Continued)

Table 7. The 5 Ds of Stewardship (Continued)

D of Stewardship	Example
Duration	Prescribing a short course (i.e., 5–7 days) of therapy for pneumonia in a patient who is responding appropriately to therapy.
Discernment	Not prescribing antibiotics for acute rhinosinusitis as 98% of cases are caused by a viral infection and will not respond to antibiotics.

Note: CrCl = creatinine clearance; UTI = urinary tract infection.

References

1. Leekha S, Terrell CL, Edson RS. General principles of antimicrobial therapy. *Mayo Clin Proc.* 2011;86:156–167.
2. Eliopoulos GM, Moellering RC. Principles of anti-infective therapy. In: Bennett JE, Dolin R, Blaser MJ, eds. *Mandell, Douglas, and Bennett's Principles and Practice of Infectious Diseases.* Philadelphia, PA: Elsevier Saunders; 2014:224–234.
3. Wolters Kluwer. Lexicomp. Available at: https://www.wolterskluwercdi.com/lex-icomp-online. Accessed July 23, 2020.
4. Faulkner CM, Cox HL, Williamson JC. Unique aspects of antimicrobial use in older adults. *Clin Infect Dis.* 2005;40:997–1004.
5. Sullivan JE, Farrar HC, the Section on Clinical Pharmacology and Therapeutics, Committee on Drugs. Fever and antipyretic use in children. *Pediatrics.* 2011;127:580–587.
6. Hoover L. AAP reports on the use of antipyretics for fever in children. *Am Fam Physician.* 2012;85:518–519.

Bibliography

AAP Committee on Infectious Diseases; Kimberlin DW, Brady MT, Jackson MA, eds. *Red Book: 2018—2021 Report of the Committee on Infectious Diseases.* 31st ed. Elk Grove Village, IL: American Academy of Pediatrics; 2018.

Briggs GC, Freeman RK, Towers CV, Forinash AB. *Drugs in Pregnancy and Lactation: A Reference Guide to Fetal and Neonatal Risk.* 11th ed. Philadelphia, PA: Wolters Kluwer; 2017.

National Library of Medicine. Drugs and lactation database. Available at: https://toxnet.nlm.nih.gov/newtoxnet/lactmed.htm. Accessed June 17, 2020.

[J. Dougherty, J. Gardner, N. Harrington]

ACTINOMYCOSIS

DISEASE	ICD-10 CODE
ACTINOMYCOSIS	ICD-10 A42

1. Clinical features—Actinomycosis is a chronic bacterial disease, most frequently localized in the orocervicofacial (55%), abdominopelvic (20%), or thoracic regions (15%), but the organism may cause endocarditis, osteo-myelitis, or disseminated disease. The lesions, firmly indurated areas of purulence and fibrosis, spread slowly to contiguous tissues with no respect for anatomic barriers. Eventually, draining sinuses or fistulas may appear and surface on the skin. Symptoms may include low-grade fever, weight loss, malaise, neck swelling, cough, abdominal pain, and drainage from cutaneous surfaces. Severe pain is rather uncommon. Lesions may mimic tuberculosis, fungal infections, mycetomas caused by *Nocardia* spp., or cancer. In infected tissue, the organism grows in clusters, called sulfur granules.

2. Risk groups—Mucosal barrier disruptions are caused by poor oral hygiene, trauma, surgery, irradiation, and immunocompromising conditions such as malnutrition, diabetes, steroid use, and human immunodeficiency virus. They enable the entry of organisms into contiguous tissues. Prolonged use of intrauterine devices (IUDs) may cause pelvic infections. Prior infection does not confer immunity.

3. Causative agents—*Actinomyces israelii* is the most common human pathogen and, with several other actinomycete species, is part of the normal human flora. *Propionibacterium propionicus* has been reported to cause an actinomycosis-like disease. All species are non–spore-forming, Gram-positive, non–acid-fast, slow-growing strict or facultative anaerobes and need incubation in special media with 6% to 10% CO_2. Plates should be held for 10 to 21 days. Actinomycotic infections are typically associated with oral anaerobes and other commensals.

4. Diagnosis—Actinomycosis is an uncommon disease that often masquerades as cancer, tuberculosis, or mycetoma. Thus a high index of suspicion is required to avoid diagnostic delays. The demonstration of typical organisms from tissue or pus uncontaminated by oral flora, evidence of sulfur granules, and growth on an appropriate medium establishes the diagnosis. Monoclonal antibody staining and 16S ribosomal ribonucleic acid gene probes may be needed to confirm the diagnosis when conventional methods are not diagnostic. Serologic tests are not useful.

On pathology, the hallmarks are fibrosis, acute or chronic granulation, infiltration with polymorphonuclear cells, macrophages, and the presence of sulfur granules.

5. Occurrence—Actinomycosis is an infrequent infection, occurring sporadically worldwide. It is most commonly seen in the age group 20 to 60 years, with a male-to-female ratio of 3:1. There is no racial predilection.

6. Reservoirs—Humans are the natural reservoir of *A. israelii* and other agents. The organisms reside in gingival and periodontal spaces, in dental plaque, on carious teeth, and in tonsillar crypts. Oral cavity colonization with *Actinomyces* is nearly 100% by 2 years old. *A. israelii* has been found in vaginal secretions of approximately 10% of women using IUDs. There are no known external environmental reservoirs.

7. Incubation period—Variable, depending on the clinical presentation and underlying host factors.

8. Transmission—Except for rare instances of human bite, there is no evidence for human-to-human disease transmission. The source of clinical disease for most patients is endogenous. The organism may be aspirated into the lung from the oral cavity or introduced into jaw tissues through injury, extraction of teeth, or mucosal abrasion. Abdominal disease also results from introduction through breaks in the mucosal barrier. Pelvic disease is most often associated with the presence of an IUD.

9. Treatment—There are no randomized controlled trials to determine the ideal drug, dose, or duration of antibiotics for actinomycosis. However, most experts agree that oral drugs should be prescribed for prolonged periods after initial intravenous treatment. Penicillin G has been the drug of choice for many years and remains so (see later table). Prolonged therapy is recommended because of the fibrotic, "woody," and chronic nature of the infection and the disruption of lymphatics and the arterial blood supply. Surgical excision of necrotic tissue, fibrous tracks, and infected bone is often necessary. Close follow-up is necessary to prevent a recurrence. However, treatment decisions may be individualized based on the clinical circumstances. There is no need to prescribe cephalosporins, broad-spectrum penicillins and carbapenems, aminoglycosides, or quinolones.

Preferred therapy	Initial IV therapy:
	• Penicillin G 10–24 MU/day IV in divided doses every 4–6 hours for 2–6 weeks OR • Ampicillin 200 mg/kg/day IV in divided doses every 6–8 hours for 2–6 weeks
	Subsequent PO therapy:
	• Penicillin VK 2–4 g/day PO for 6–12 months OR • Amoxicillin 500 mg PO TID for 6–12 months

(Continued)

(Continued)

Alternative therapy options	For patients with a penicillin allergy, desensitization to penicillin is preferred. • Doxycycline 100 mg IV BID for 2–6 weeks followed by doxycycline 100 mg PO BID for 6–12 months OR • Ceftriaxone 2 g IV once daily for 2–6 weeks followed by PO antibiotic therapy for 6–12 months OR • Clindamycin 600–900 mg IV every 8 hours for 2–6 weeks followed by 300 mg PO TID for 6–12 months
Special considerations and comments	• Metronidazole is not active. • Surgical drainage of abscesses or removal of IUD is often necessary. • Antibiotic doses and duration of therapy should ultimately be based on the location, severity, and extent of disease.

Note: BID = twice daily; IUD = intrauterine device; IV = intravenous(ly); PO = oral(ly); MU = million units; TID = thrice daily.

10. Prevention—Good oral hygiene and removal of dental plaque.

11. Special considerations—None.

[A. Panwalker]

AMEBIC INFECTIONS

DISEASE	ICD-10 CODE
AMEBIASIS	ICD-10 A06
INFECTIONS WITH FREE-LIVING AMEBAE	ICD-10 B60.2, B60.1

I. AMEBIASIS (amoebiasis)

1. Clinical features—Most infections are asymptomatic and commensal, but some may be invasive and give rise to intestinal or extraintestinal disease. Intestinal disease varies from acute or fulminating dysentery with fever, chills, and bloody or mucoid diarrhea (amebic dysentery) to mild abdominal discomfort with diarrhea containing blood or mucus, alternating with periods of constipation or remission.

Amebic granulomas (ameboma), sometimes mistaken for carcinoma, may occur in the wall of the large intestine in patients with intermittent dysentery or colitis of long duration. Dissemination through the bloodstream may occur and produce abscesses of the liver and, less commonly, of the lung or brain. Painful ulceration of the skin is a rare manifestation that can occur anywhere but most commonly in the perianal and genital regions, usually in association with amebic dysentery. Penile lesions may result from anal intercourse. Amebae reach the skin either directly through contact with contaminated feces or indirectly through hematogenous spread. Amebic colitis is often confused with forms of inflammatory bowel disease, such as ulcerative colitis; care should be taken to distinguish the two because corticosteroids may exacerbate amebic colitis.

Amebiasis can also mimic numerous noninfectious and infectious diseases. Conversely, the presence of amebae may be misinterpreted as the cause of diarrhea in a person whose primary enteric illness is the result of another condition.

2. Risk groups—Those at greatest risk live in areas of poor sanitation, crowding, and unsafe drinking water or where unsafe water or human fecal fertilizer ("night soil") is used in agriculture. Other risk groups include immigrants from or travelers to endemic areas and persons engaging in oral-anal sexual contact.

3. Causative agents—*Entamoeba histolytica*, a parasitic organism. Other similar organisms are *Entamoeba dispar*, *Entamoeba moshkovskii*, *Entamoeba bangladeshi*, or other intestinal protozoa. Not all *E. histolytica* strains are equally virulent. Additionally, the morphologically identical *E. dispar*, present in many asymptomatic cyst passers and once thought to be nonpathogenic, has recently been associated with cases of amebic colitis and amebic liver abscess, putting into question its avirulent status. Immunologic differences, isoenzyme patterns, and polymerase chain reaction (PCR) permit differentiation between *E. histolytica* and *E. dispar*.

4. Diagnosis—By microscopic demonstration of trophozoites or cysts in fresh or suitably preserved fecal specimens, smears of aspirates, scrapings obtained by proctoscopy, or aspirates of abscesses or sections of tissue. The presence of trophozoites containing red blood cells is indicative of invasive amebiasis. Examination should be done on fresh fecal specimens by a trained microscopist, as the organism must be differentiated from macrophages. However, even trained microscopists cannot differentiate *E. histolytica* from the morphologically identical *E. dispar* and *E. moshkovskii*. In patients with intestinal disease, examination of at least 3 specimens collected on 3 separate days will increase the yield of organisms from approximately 50% in a single specimen to 75% to 95%, but the yield in stool from patients with amebic liver abscesses is only 8% to 44%, even with repeated stool examinations. Only one commercially available stool antigen-detection test distinguishes *E. histolytica* from *E. dispar*. Other available assays specific for *E. histolytica*, such as enzyme immunoassay and PCR, may require reference laboratory services.

Serologic tests, particularly immunodiffusion and enzyme-linked immunosorbent assay, are very useful in diagnosis of invasive disease in persons living in nonendemic areas. Ultrasonography and computerized axial tomography scanning are helpful in revealing the presence and location of an amebic liver abscess and can be considered diagnostic when associated with a specific antibody response to *E. histolytica* in persons from a nonendemic area.

5. Occurrence—Amebiasis is distributed globally. Persons of all ages are susceptible, but infection is less common in infants and young children. Females and males are equally likely to be infected, but invasive disease is more common in males. For example, liver abscesses occur predominantly in adult males. Asymptomatic carriers are common in endemic areas. The proportion of cyst passers who have clinical disease is usually low. Published prevalence rates of cyst passage, usually based on cyst morphology, vary from place to place, with rates generally higher in areas with poor sanitation and crowding, in mental institutions, and among men who have sex with men. In areas with good sanitation, amebic infections tend to cluster in households and institutions.

6. Reservoirs—Humans, usually a chronically ill or asymptomatic cyst passer.

7. Incubation period—Variable, from a few days to several months or years; commonly 2 to 4 weeks.

8. Transmission—Either person to person or through ingestion of fecally contaminated food or water containing amebic cysts, which are relatively chlorine resistant. Cysts can survive in moist environmental conditions for weeks to months. Transmission may occur sexually by oral–anal contact with a chronically ill or asymptomatic cyst passer. The period of communicability lasts as long as cysts are passed, which may be for months or years. Patients with acute amebic dysentery probably pose only limited danger to others because of the absence of cysts in dysenteric stools and the fragility of trophozoites.

9. Treatment—

Symptomatic Intestinal or Extraintestinal Disease

Drug	Metronidazole
Dose	500–750 mg TID
Route	PO
Alternative drug	Tinidazole 2 g once daily
Duration	7–10 days
Special considerations and comments	<ul><li>Treatment should be followed by either iodoquinol 650 mg PO TID for 20 days OR</li><li>Paromomycin 25–35 mg/kg/day PO in 3 doses for 7 days to eliminate luminal cysts</li></ul>

Note: PO = oral(ly); TID = thrice daily.

Patients with asymptomatic disease (asymptomatic cyst passer) should be treated with iodoquinol 650 mg orally 3 times daily for 20 days or paromomycin 25 to 35 mg/kg orally in 3 doses daily for 7 days.

10. Prevention—

1) Educate the general public and asymptomatic carriers on personal hygiene, particularly the sanitary disposal of feces, handwashing after defecation, and handwashing before preparing or eating food. Disseminate information regarding the risks involved in eating unwashed or uncooked fruits and vegetables and in drinking water of unknown quality.

2) Dispose of human feces in a sanitary manner and do not use as fertilizer.

3) Protect public water supplies from fecal contamination. Water of unknown quality can be made safe by boiling for 1 minute (at altitudes greater than 6,562 ft or 2,000 m, water should be boiled for 3 minutes). Small quantities of water can be treated with prescribed concentrations of iodine, either liquid or crystalline, or with water purification tablets (tetraglycine hydroperiodide), allowing for at least 30 minutes of contact time and longer for colder water. The most effective treatment of small quantities of water is achieved through the use of portable filters with a pore size of 1.0 μm or less.

4) Treat asymptomatic carriers with a luminal amebicide to reduce the risk of transmission and to protect the patient from symptomatic amebiasis. Common luminal amebicides are paromomycin and iodoquinol.

5) Educate high-risk groups about washing hands, anus, and genitals before and after sex, use of barriers when engaging in anilingus, and avoiding sex while symptomatic.

6) Health agencies should regulate the sanitary practices of people who prepare and serve food in public eating places and the general cleanliness of the premises involved. Routine stool examination of food handlers as a control measure is impractical.

7) Disinfectant dips for fruits and vegetables are of unproven value in preventing transmission of *E. histolytica*. Thorough washing with potable water and keeping fruits and vegetables dry might help; cysts are killed by desiccation, by temperatures above 50°C (122°F), and by irradiation.

8) Chemoprophylaxis is not advised.

11. Special considerations—Disruption of normal sanitary facilities and food management will favor an outbreak of amebiasis, especially in populations that include large numbers of cyst passers.

II. INFECTIONS WITH FREE-LIVING AMEBAE (naegleriasis, acanthamoebiasis, balamuthiasis)

1. Clinical features—Naegleriasis causes a typical syndrome of fulminating pyogenic meningoencephalitis (primary amebic meningoencephalitis [PAM]) with headache, nausea, vomiting, fever, nuchal rigidity, and somnolence; death occurs within an average of 5 days (range, 1–18 days) of symptom onset. The mortality rate of PAM in the USA is 97%. Acanthamoebiasis causes a granulomatous disease (granulomatous amebic encephalitis [GAE]) of insidious onset that lasts from weeks to several months. Balamuthiasis also causes GAE. The mortality rate from GAE in the USA is greater than 90%. In addition to causing GAE, *Acanthamoeba* can cause skin lesions, sinusitis, and osteomyelitis, with or without central nervous system (CNS) disease. *Balamuthia mandrillaris* has also been associated with skin lesions preceding CNS infections in some cases. Infections of the cornea (keratitis due to *Acanthamoeba*) can result in blindness.

2. Risk groups—Naegleriasis occurs mainly in active immunocompetent children and young adults who have had recent contact with warm freshwater. Immunodeficient individuals have increased susceptibility to infection with *Acanthamoeba* and probably *Balamuthia*, although balamuthiasis occurs in immunocompetent persons as well and appears to occur more frequently in persons of Hispanic ethnicity. Eye infections associated with *Acanthamoeba* have occurred primarily in contact lens wearers.

3. Causative agents—*Naegleria fowleri*, several species of *Acanthamoeba* (*A. culbertsoni*, *A. polyphaga*, *A. castellanii*, *A. astronyxis*, *A. hatchetti*, *A. rhysodes*, and *A. lenticulata*), and *B. mandrillaris*.

4. Diagnosis—Although free-living amebae (*N. fowleri*, *Acanthamoeba* spp., and *Balamuthia*) have sometimes been misidentified as macrophages, they can be differentiated morphologically and through immunohistochemical staining and PCR testing of brain tissue in cases of PAM and GAE. *N. fowleri* and *Acanthamoeba* spp. can be cultured on nonnutrient agar seeded with *Escherichia coli*, *Enterobacter aerogenes*, or other suitable *Enterobacter* spp.; *Balamuthia* require mammalian cell cultures for isolation. These techniques can also be used with skin biopsy specimens in suspected *Acanthamoeba* and *Balamuthia* infections involving the skin. Likewise, suspected *Acanthameoba* eye infections can be diagnosed by histology, PCR, or culture of corneal scrapings; confocal microscopy can also be used. In addition, a preliminary diagnosis of PAM can be made through microscopic examination of wet-mount preparations of fresh cerebrospinal fluid (CSF) showing motile amebae and of stained smears of CSF.

5. Occurrence—The organisms are thought to be ubiquitous in the environment. Cases have been diagnosed in many countries on all continents except Antarctica.

6. Reservoirs—*Acanthamoeba* and *Naegleria* are free living in aquatic and soil habitats. Less is known about the reservoir of *Balamuthia*, but it has also been identified in soil and water.

7. Incubation period—From 1 to 9 days (mean 5 days) in documented US cases of *Naegleria* infection; mostly unknown but probably weeks to months for infections with *Acanthamoeba* and *Balamuthia*.

8. Transmission—Naegleriasis occurs through exposure of the nasal passages to water, most commonly by diving or swimming in warm freshwater, especially ponds or lakes in warm climate areas or during summer months; thermal springs or bodies of water warmed by the effluent of industrial plants; or inadequately maintained swimming pools. Naegleriasis has also occurred following direct nasal irrigation with tap water or with solutions made from tap water containing the ameba. After entering the sinuses, *Naegleria* trophozoites invade brain and meninges by extension along the olfactory nerves. *Acanthamoeba* and *Balamuthia* trophozoites reach the CNS through hematogenous spread, probably from a skin break or other site of primary colonization, such as the respiratory tract. Acanthamoebiasis frequently occurs in chronically ill or immunosuppressed patients with no history of swimming or known source of infection. Balamuthiasis also occurs in such patients but develops in immunocompetent patients as well. Additionally, transmission of *Balamuthia* through solid organ transplantation has been documented in the USA on 3 separate occasions since 2009. Contact lens use, contact lens exposure to water, and poor contact lens hygiene habits have been implicated as risk factors for corneal *Acanthamoeba* infection. Other than solid organ transplant transmission, no person-to-person transmission has been observed with any of the free-living amebae.

9. Treatment—

Drug	Dose	Route	Maximum Dose	Duration	Comments
Amphotericin B	1.5 mg/kg/day in 2 divided doses	IV	1.5 mg/kg/day	3 days	
THEN	1 mg/kg/day once daily	IV		11 days	14-day course

(Continued)

(Continued)

Drug	Dose	Route	Maximum Dose	Duration	Comments
Amphotericin B[1]	1.5 mg once daily	Intrathecal	1.5 mg/day	2 days	
THEN	1 mg/day every other day	Intrathecal		8 days	10-day course
Azithromycin[2,3]	10 mg/kg/day once daily	IV/PO	500 mg/day	28 days	
Fluconazole	10 mg/kg/day once daily	IV/PO	600 mg/day	28 days	
Rifampin[1]	10 mg/kg/day once daily	IV/PO	600 mg/day	28 days	
Miltefosine	• < 45 kg: 50 mg BID • > 45 kg: 50 mg TID	PO	2.5 mg/kg/day	28 days	50 mg tablets
Dexamethasone	0.6 mg/kg/day in 4 divided doses	IV	0.6 mg/kg/day	4 days	

Note: BID = twice daily; IV = intravenous(ly); PO = oral(ly); TID = thrice daily.

Conventional amphotericin (AMB) is preferred. When AMB was compared with liposomal AMB against *N. fowleri*, the minimum inhibitory concentration for AMB was 0.1 μg/mL, while that of liposomal AMB was 10-fold higher at 1 μg/mL. Liposomal AMB was found to be less effective in the mouse model and in in vitro testing than the more toxic form of AMB.

Effective treatment for infections caused by *B. mandrillaris* or *Acanthamoeba* spp. has not been established.

Several patients with *Acanthamoeba* GAE and *Acanthamoeba* cutaneous infections without CNS involvement have been successfully treated with a multidrug regimen consisting of various combinations of pentamidine, sulfadiazine, flucytosine, either fluconazole or itraconazole, trimethoprim-sulfamethoxazole, and topical application of chlorhexidine gluconate and ketoconazole for skin lesions. Voriconazole, miltefosine, and azithromycin might also be of some value in treating *Acanthamoeba* infections.

A few patients have survived *Balamuthia* GAE following treatment with multidrug combinations of pentamidine, sulfadiazine, flucytosine, fluconazole, and either azithromycin or clarithromycin, in addition to surgical resection of the CNS lesions. Miltefosine might also be of some value in treating *Balamuthia* infections.

Clinicians who suspect they have a patient with a free-living ameba infection are encouraged to contact CDC 24/7 by phone (770-488-7100) to discuss diagnostic and treatment recommendations with a subject matter expert.

10. Prevention—

1) PAM and swimming or diving: the only sure way to prevent swimming- or diving-associated PAM is to refrain from swimming, diving, and other water-related activities in warm freshwater. Infections may be reduced by educating the public about the risks of swimming or diving in lakes and ponds during periods of warm water temperatures (particularly when infection has occurred before or is presumed to have been acquired) and of allowing such water to go up the nose through diving or underwater swimming. Protect the nasopharynx from exposure to water likely to contain *N. fowleri* (e.g., through the use of a nose clip). In practice, this is difficult, since the amebae may occur in a wide variety of aquatic bodies, including inadequately treated swimming pools. Swimming pools containing residual free chlorine of 1 to 2 ppm are considered safe. No infection is known to have been acquired in a well-maintained chlorinated swimming pool.

2) PAM and nasal irrigation: solutions used for nasal irrigation should be made with boiled, distilled, or sterile water.

3) *Acanthamoeba* keratitis: contact lens wearers should not wear lenses while bathing, showering, swimming, or using hot tubs. They should follow strictly the wear and care procedures recommended by lens manufacturers and health care professionals.

11. Special considerations—None.

[J. Cope, S. Roy]

ANGIOSTRONGYLIASIS

DISEASE	ICD-10 CODE
ANGIOSTRONGYLIASIS	ICD-10 B83.2
INTESTINAL ANGIOSTRONGYLIASIS	ICD-10 B81.3

I. ANGIOSTRONGYLIASIS (eosinophilic meningoencephalitis, eosinophilic meningitis)

1. Clinical features—Angiostrongyliasis affecting the central nervous system (CNS), also known as eosinophilic meningitis, may be asymptomatic or symptomatic; it is commonly characterized by severe headache, neck and back stiffness, and paresthesias. Low-grade fever may be present, especially in children. Illness is thought to be usually self-limiting and may last a few days to several months, although complications may occur related to focal neurologic damage. Deaths have rarely been reported. Differential diagnosis includes cerebral cysticercosis; paragonimiasis; echinococcosis; gnathostomiasis; tuberculous, coccidioidal, or aseptic meningitis; and neurosyphilis.

2. Risk groups—Malnutrition and debilitating diseases may contribute to an increase in severity, and even (rarely), in the case of CNS disease, to a fatal outcome.

3. Causative agents—*Angiostrongylus (Parastrongylus) cantonensis*, a zoonotic nematode (lungworm of rats). The third-stage larvae in the intermediate host (terrestrial or marine mollusks) are infective for humans.

4. Diagnosis—Cerebrospinal fluid (CSF) usually exhibits pleocytosis with more than 10% eosinophils; blood eosinophilia is not always present but can be quite elevated. Presence of eosinophils in the CSF and a history of eating raw mollusks or eating raw foods (such as leafy greens) that may be contaminated by snails or slugs suggest the diagnosis, especially in endemic areas. Immunodiagnostic tests have limited use because of poor specificity as a result of cross-reactivity. In rare cases, the worm has been found in the CSF, lung, and eye. Some public health laboratories have developed diagnostic polymerase chain reaction tests for use with CSF and tissue.

5. Occurrence—Widely distributed, reported as far north as Japan; as far south as Brisbane, Australia; in Africa as far west as Côte d'Ivoire; and also in Egypt, Madagascar, the USA, and Puerto Rico. Most cases of infection are diagnosed in China (including Taiwan), Cuba, Indonesia, Malaysia, the Philippines, Thailand, Vietnam, Pacific islands including Hawaii and Tahiti, and much of the Caribbean.

6. Reservoirs—The rat (*Rattus* and *Bandicota* spp.).

7. Incubation period—Usually 1 to 3 weeks.

8. Transmission—Ingestion of raw or insufficiently cooked mollusks (snails, slugs), which are intermediate hosts or transport hosts (land planarians, freshwater prawns, or land crabs) harboring infective larvae. The mollusks are infected by first-stage larvae excreted by an infected rodent; when third-stage larvae have developed in the mollusks, rodents (and people) ingesting the mollusks are infected. Land planarians, prawns, fish, and land crabs that have ingested snails or slugs may also transport infective larvae as paratenic hosts. Lettuce and other leafy vegetables contaminated by small mollusks may serve as a source of infection. In the rat, larvae migrate to the brain and mature to the adult stage; young adults migrate to the surface of the brain and through the venous system to reach their final site in the pulmonary arteries, where they become sexually mature and mate. After mating, the female worm deposits eggs that hatch in terminal branches of the pulmonary arteries; first-stage larvae enter the bronchial system, pass up the trachea, are swallowed, and are passed in the feces. In humans, young adult worms are not able to leave the brain, do not reach maturity, and do not complete the life cycle. Angiostrongyliasis is not transmitted from person to person, and humans are a dead-end host.

9. Treatment—

Drug	Prednisolone
Dose	60 mg/day in 3 divided doses
Route	PO
Alternative drug	Not applicable
Duration	2 weeks
Special considerations and comments	• Treatment is usually supportive with corticosteroids to control inflammation. • There is concern that anthelmintics could exacerbate neurologic symptoms due to a systemic response to dying worms. • In small studies, clinical outcomes were not improved with the addition of anthelmintics (albendazole or mebendazole) to corticosteroid therapy.

10. Prevention—

1) Avoid eating raw or undercooked snails, slugs, and possible paratenic hosts such as freshwater prawns, fish, and land crabs.
2) Control rats.

3) Boil or cook snails, slugs, prawns, fish, and crabs for 3 to 5 minutes or freeze at −15°C (5°F) for 24 hours.
4) Avoid eating raw foods that may be contaminated by snails or slugs; thoroughly clean lettuce and other greens to remove snails or slugs.
5) Wear gloves (and wash hands) if snails or slugs are handled.

11. Special considerations—Report cases of angiostrongyliasis to public health authorities. Any grouping of cases in a particular geographic area or institution warrants prompt epidemiologic investigation and appropriate control measures.

II. INTESTINAL ANGIOSTRONGYLIASIS

1. Clinical features—Common findings of the intestinal form of angiostrongyliasis include abdominal pain and tenderness in the right iliac fossa and flank, fever, anorexia, vomiting, abdominal rigidity, a tumor-like mass in the right lower quadrant, and pain on rectal examination. Fever, anorexia, vomiting, constipation, or diarrhea are frequent in children. Leukocytosis is usually present, with eosinophils ranging from 20% to 60%. Adult worms and eggs in the mesenteric arteries damage the endothelium, causing inflammation, thrombosis, and necrosis. On surgery, the whole wall of the intestine is thickened and hardened, with yellow granulations in the subserosa of the intestinal wall; adult worms are found in the small arteries, generally in the ileocecal area, while eggs and larvae are found in lymph nodes, the intestinal wall, and omentum. Intestinal obstruction and perforation can occur. Differential diagnosis includes malignant tumors, appendicitis, Crohn's disease, and Meckel's diverticulum.

2. Risk groups—Risk groups are not well established but are likely to include those who ingest infected slugs or raw vegetables contaminated with slugs or their slime, which contains larvae. Some reports have shown higher case rates in children aged 6 to 12 years and in males.

3. Causative agents—*Parastrongylus* (*Angiostrongylus*) *costaricensis*, a nematode worm. The third-stage larvae in the intermediate host (slugs) are infective for humans.

4. Diagnosis—High eosinophilia suggests the diagnosis, especially in children living in endemic areas. Clinical diagnosis may be aided by X-ray. Serologic diagnostic techniques are also available. Parasitologic diagnosis by biopsy or resective surgery is confirmative. In humans, eggs are not found in feces.

5. Occurrence—Reported in Argentina, Brazil, Colombia, Costa Rica, Dominican Republic, Ecuador, El Salvador, Guadeloupe, Guatemala,

Honduras, Martinique, Nicaragua, Panama, Peru, USA, and Venezuela. It is not known if transmission occurs outside the Caribbean and Americas.

6. Reservoirs—The cotton rat (*Sigmodon hispidus*). Several species of other rodents and mammals, such as marmosets, dogs, and coatimundis, can be final hosts, like humans.

7. Incubation period—Usually 2 to 4 weeks, although can be months.

8. Transmission—Ingestion of raw or insufficiently cooked slugs, which are intermediate or transport hosts harboring infective larvae; also accidental ingestion of slugs in lettuce or other leafy vegetables, or following playing with slugs (in children). Slugs are infected when they ingest first-stage larvae excreted with feces by an infected rodent; when third-stage larvae have developed in the slugs, rodents (and humans) ingesting the slugs are infected. In the cotton rat, larvae penetrate the intestinal wall and migrate to the lymphatics of the intestinal wall and mesentery. After molting into young adults, they migrate to the mesenteric arteries, where they mature and release eggs that hatch and are excreted with feces by 24 days after infection. In humans, adult worms release eggs into the intestinal tissues. The eggs and larvae degenerate and cause intense local inflammatory reactions and do not appear to be shed in the stool.

9. Treatment—There is no proven treatment for illness caused by *A. costaricensis*.

10. Prevention—

1) Avoid eating raw or undercooked snails, slugs, and other possible hosts.
2) Control rats.
3) Boil snails and slugs for 3 to 5 minutes or freeze at -15°C (5°F) for 24 hours; this effectively kills the larvae.
4) Avoid eating raw foods that may be contaminated by snails or slugs; thoroughly cleaning lettuce and other greens does not always eliminate infective larvae.
5) Wear gloves (and wash hands) if snails or slugs are handled.

11. Special considerations—Any grouping of cases in a particular geographic area or institution warrants prompt epidemiologic investigation and appropriate control measures.

[M. Kamb]

ANISAKIASIS

DISEASE	ICD-10 CODE
ANISAKIASIS	ICD-10 B81.0

1. Clinical features—Symptoms vary according to the site of *Anisakis* larval invasion into the gastrointestinal mucosa. After eating uncooked or undercooked seafood, abdominal pain, nausea, and vomiting—and occasionally hematemesis—starting within several hours result from invasion in gastric mucosa (gastric anisakiasis). Subsequently, or alternatively, abdominal pain, distension, diarrhea (often with blood/mucus), and mild fever may occur about 1 to 2 weeks after eating seafood and persist (granulomatous enteritis; also called enteric anisakiasis). In heavy infestation, larvae may lodge in the esophagus, causing esophagitis with pain and difficulty in swallowing. In some, allergic symptoms such as skin rash including urticaria, itching, and, rarely, anaphylaxis may develop. Occasionally, only the allergic manifestations occur without larval infestation. Rarely, submucosal granulomas can cause intestinal obstruction; intestinal perforation may also occur, leading to peritonitis. Clinically, anisakiasis can be confused with peptic ulcer, acute abdominal neoplasm, appendicitis, and ileitis.

2. Risk groups—Persons eating uncooked, undercooked, or inadequately treated marine fish and squid.

3. Causative agents—Human anisakiasis is caused by nematode parasites of marine mammals through tissue invasion by the third-stage larvae of *Anisakis simplex* (and other *Anisakis* spp.) or *Pseudoterranova decipiens*. Although the adult worms are in marine mammals, the third-stage larvae are found in fish and squid. Larvae do not develop further in humans. The larvae are 2- to 5-cm long, either coiled on a mucosal surface or embedded in tissue in both fish and humans.

4. Diagnosis—Requires clinical suspicion based on a history of eating seafood. Endoscopic detection of larvae confirms diagnosis. Embedded dead larvae within granulomas are recovered by surgery or endoscopy. A skin-prick test with *A. simplex* antigen and a serologic test for immunoglobulin class E antibody against *A. simplex* are available; both are helpful in diagnosis.

5. Occurrence—The disease occurs in individuals who eat uncooked, undercooked, and inadequately treated (refrigerated, frozen for a brief period, salted, marinated, or smoked) saltwater fish or squid. Anisakiasis has been diagnosed most frequently in Japan, where thousands of cases have been described (after eating sushi and sashimi). Cases have also been detected in Scandinavian countries (after eating gravlax); on the Pacific coast of Latin America (ceviche); in the Netherlands (herring); and in Spain (anchovies). Cases are seen with increasing frequency because of the rising consumption of raw fish.

6. Reservoirs—*Anisakis* spp. are widely distributed in all oceans and many sea mammals. The natural life cycle involves transmission of larvae through predation from small crustaceans to squid, or fish, then to sea mammals, the definitive hosts. In fish and squid, the third-stage larvae migrate to fleshy body tissues; humans become infected when they eat these tissues. As accidental and dead-end hosts, humans do not contribute to the nematode's life cycle. Herring, cod, mackerel, tuna, salmon, and squid are sources of infection by *A. simplex*. Cod, halibut, flatfish, and red snapper are sources of infection by *P. decipiens*.

7. Incubation period—Gastric symptoms may develop within a few hours of ingestion. Symptoms referable to the small intestine occur within a few days or weeks, depending on the number of ingested larvae. Allergic reactions may occur within hours or take more time—days to weeks. Even dead larvae in raw or undercooked fish can elicit allergic reactions without larval infestation.

8. Transmission—Through ingestion of uncooked, undercooked, or inadequately treated marine fish and squid containing nematode larvae. The larvae may remain in the gastrointestinal tract of the fish and migrate into the internal organs or flesh (muscles) even after the fish dies. When ingested by humans and liberated through digestion in the stomach, they may penetrate the gastric or intestinal mucosa. There is no human-to-human transmission.

9. Treatment—No medical treatment. Removal of worms by endoscopy or surgery if there is a large worm burden. Worms are eventually destroyed by host reaction.

10. Prevention—

1) Avoid ingestion of inadequately cooked marine fish and squid. Larvae are killed by heating to 60°C (140°F) for 10 minutes; blast-freezing to -35°C (-31°F) or below for 15 hours; freezing to -35°C (-31°F) or below until solid and storing at -20°C (-4°F) for 24 hours; or freezing at -20°C (-4°F) for 7 days. Irradiation also kills the larvae.

2) Cleaning (evisceration) of fish and squid as soon as possible after they are caught reduces the number of larvae penetrating into the muscles from the mesenteries.

3) Candling (exposure to a light source) is useful for fishery products when parasites can be visualized.

11. Special considerations—Reporting: report to the local health authority, if required.

[I. Chuang]

ANTHRAX
(malignant pustule, malignant edema, woolsorter disease, ragpicker disease)

DISEASE	ICD-10 CODE
ANTHRAX	ICD-10 A22

1. Clinical features—An acute bacterial zoonotic disease that historically has been described as occurring in 3 forms—cutaneous, inhalation, and gastrointestinal—depending on the route of exposure. A fourth form, injection anthrax, has been described in recent outbreaks among heroin users in northern Europe. Systemic illness, including fever, shock, and dissemination to other organs, can occur with any form of anthrax and may include meningitis, which is usually fatal.

1) Cutaneous: more than 95% of naturally acquired human cases are cutaneous anthrax. This manifests as initial itching of the affected site, followed by a lesion that becomes papular and then vesicular; in 2 to 6 days the lesion develops into a depressed black eschar. Moderate-to-severe edema usually surrounds the eschar, sometimes with small secondary vesicles. Pain is unusual; if present, it is due to edema or secondary infection. The head, neck, forearms, and hands (i.e., exposed areas of the body) are the most common sites of infection. Differential diagnoses include arachnid bites (e.g., *Loxosceles reclusa* in North America) and a variety of other infections (e.g., staphylococcal or streptococcal cellulitis, dermatomycoses, rickettsial pox, orf virus, varicella zoster, herpes simplex, vaccinia). Untreated infections may spread to regional lymph nodes and the bloodstream with overwhelming septicemia. Edema associated with cutaneous lesions involving the head and neck can result in respiratory compromise due to compression of the trachea and patients may require intubation. Untreated cutaneous anthrax has a case-fatality rate between 5% and 20%;

however, with effective treatment deaths from cutaneous anthrax are very rare. The lesion evolves through typical local changes even after the initiation of antimicrobial therapy.

2) Inhalation: initial symptoms of inhalation (also referred to as pulmonary) anthrax are mild and nonspecific and may include fever, malaise, and mild cough or chest pain. Symptoms progress to include respiratory distress, stridor, severe dyspnea, hypoxemia, diaphoresis, shock, and cyanosis over 3 to 4 days. X-ray evidence of mediastinal widening is present in the majority of patients and pulmonary infiltrates or pleural effusions are usually observed. The maximum case-fatality rate is estimated to be greater than 85%; however, early diagnosis and initiation of aggressive combination antimicrobial therapy and supportive care may considerably reduce mortality.

3) Gastrointestinal: gastrointestinal anthrax is rare and difficult to recognize. It tends to occur in outbreaks following consumption of contaminated meat from anthrax-infected animals. Symptoms include abdominal distress, which is characterized by pain, nausea, and vomiting, followed by fever, signs of septicemia, and death in typical cases. The case-fatality rate of gastrointestinal anthrax is estimated to be 40%. A rare oropharyngeal form of primary disease, characterized by edematous lesions, necrotic ulcers, and swelling in the oropharynx and neck, has been described.

4) Injection: this new form of anthrax was first identified in 2000 in Norway. The largest outbreak occurred in 2010 in Scotland (~119 cases), England (5 cases), and Germany (2 cases) among heroin users. Presentation has been varied. Most patients have serious localized soft-tissue infections in the deeper layers of the skin accompanied by significant soft-tissue edema without a raised border with a black center as in cutaneous anthrax. Fever is not a prominent feature, and pain is less severe than with other serious soft-tissue infections. Compartment syndrome may be present. Not all patients have localized injection-related lesions; some present with features more typical of systemic anthrax infection, including hemorrhagic meningitis and multiorgan failure. Differential diagnoses include necrotizing fasciitis, cellulitis, and abscess. Injection anthrax has a case-fatality rate of 21% to 35% in confirmed and probable cases despite treatment. No injection anthrax has been found in the USA to date.

2. Risk groups—Workers involved in industrial processing of hides, wool, or bone; veterinarians; agricultural and wildlife workers in areas with a high incidence of epizootic anthrax; and workers who repeatedly enter potentially contaminated areas as part of emergency response activities, such as environmental investigators, remediation workers, and laboratory workers who routinely work with *Bacillus anthracis*. Cases of cutaneous, gastrointestinal, and inhalation anthrax have been reported among persons making or playing drums consisting of contaminated goatskin or among those participating in events where such drums were played. Heroin injection drug users in northern Europe are the only population of drug users thus far in whom cases of injection anthrax have been reported.

3. Causative agents—*B. anthracis*, a Gram-positive, encapsulated, spore-forming, nonmotile rod. Specifically, the spores of *B. anthracis* are the infectious form; vegetative forms of *B. anthracis* rarely transmit disease. *B. anthracis* has 3 main virulence factors: a poly-D-glutamic acid capsule and 2 protein exotoxins—edema toxin and lethal toxin.

4. Diagnosis—Laboratory confirmation is through demonstration of the causative bacilli in blood, lesion exudates or smears, or discharges by direct polychrome methylene blue (McFadyean)-stained smears; or through culture on sheep blood agar or selective media; or through detection of the bacterial deoxyribonucleic acid, antigens, toxins, or host antibody. Standard diagnosis remains culture of the organism from clinical specimens, but this may be difficult to achieve after antimicrobial treatment is initiated. Rapid detection methods include polymerase chain reaction (PCR), antigen-detection methods including direct fluorescent antibody test and immunohistochemistry, and anthrax lethal toxin detection in serum by mass spectrometry. The sensitivity of these methods may also decline after antimicrobial treatment has been initiated. Serologic assays may be available at sentinel, reference (often state), and national laboratories; a commercial enzyme-linked immunosorbent assay test is available for antibody testing. Rapid assays such as real-time PCR are only available at reference laboratories and laboratories participating in the laboratory response network.

5. Occurrence—In most developed countries, anthrax is an infrequent and sporadic human infection and is primarily an occupational hazard of veterinarians, agriculture and wildlife workers, or workers who butcher animals or process meat, hides, hair, wool, or bone. Human anthrax is endemic in the agricultural regions of the world where anthrax in animals is common, such as sub-Saharan Africa, Asia, South and Central America, and southern and eastern Europe. Outbreaks related to handling and consuming meat from infected livestock have been reported in Africa, Asia, and eastern Europe.

Examples of laboratory-acquired infection exist, and an extensive outbreak occurred in the former USSR in 1979 as the result of an accidental release from a military research institute. Anthrax may also occur through deliberate release of spores. In 2001, spores deliberately released via the postal system in the USA resulted in 11 cutaneous and 11 inhalation cases, including 5 deaths. The remoteness of some of the cases to the original source suggests that disease resulted from exposure to low concentrations of spores through cross-contaminated mail.

6. Reservoirs—Animals (normally herbivores, both livestock and wild-life) shed the bacilli in terminal hemorrhages at death. On exposure to the air, vegetative cells sporulate, and the *B. anthracis* spores, which resist adverse environmental conditions and disinfection, contaminate the under-lying soil and may remain viable for years. Skins, hides, hair, and other pro-ducts from infected animals may pose a risk to those coming into contact with them. The disease spreads among herbivorous animals through ingestion of spore-contaminated feed or water, and omnivorous and carnivorous animals may become infected through eating meat from infected carcasses. Environmental events such as floods, disruption of soil over pre-vious burial sites of infected carcasses, or scavengers feeding on infected carcasses may provoke epizootics or may redistribute spores.

7. Incubation period—The incubation period for cutaneous anthrax is generally 5 to 7 days, with a range of 1 to 12 days. The incubation period for inhalation anthrax reported for humans ranges from 1 to 43 days, although incubation periods of up to 60 days may be possible based on studies in animal models. The incubation period for gastrointestinal anthrax is estimated to range from 1 to 6 days. The incubation period for injection anthrax reportedly ranges from 1 to 10 days or more.

8. Transmission—Anthrax infection can be transmitted through contact with infected livestock or wild animals or with skins, hides, hair, carcasses, or tissues of the animals; it is also possibly transmitted by biting flies that have fed on infected animals. Contact with soil contaminated by infected animals is rare; so is reinfection following recovery from a prior infection. There is limited evidence that seroconversion occurs among people with frequent occupational exposures. Person-to-person transmission has rarely been reported for cutaneous anthrax via direct contact with skin lesions. Dried or otherwise processed skins, hides, bones, bonemeal, and wool from infected animals may harbor spores for years; they can serve as fomites, resulting in the introduction of novel strains or the introduction of anthrax into regions where it was not previously reported.

Cutaneous infection almost always occurs at the site of a preexisting lesion, mostly on exposed areas of the body (hands, wrists, neck, face). Inhalation anthrax results from inhalation of *B. anthracis* spores, mainly in risky industrial processes (e.g., tanning hides, processing wool or bone) in which spore-containing dust or aerosols are generated in an enclosed poorly ventilated area. The risk of inhalation anthrax is determined not only by bacillary virulence factors but also by infectious aerosol production, removal rates, and host factors. Intestinal and oropharyngeal anthrax may arise from ingestion of inadequately cooked meat from such animals; little evidence exists for transmission through milk. Injection anthrax has been associated with the use of heroin by any route. Strains isolated from infections in 2 separate outbreaks in northern Europe are closely related; they are also genetically related to strains from infected animals in Turkey. The means by which heroin was contaminated with spores remains unknown.

9. **Treatment—**

1) For patients with systemic anthrax with suspected or proven meningitis and normal renal function treatment should include the antibiotics listed in the first table plus raxibacumab.

Drug, dose, route	• Ciprofloxacin: ○ Adults: 400 mg IV every 8 hours ○ Children: 30 mg/kg/day IV divided every 8 hours ($\leq$ 400 mg/dose) PLUS • Meropenem: ○ Adults: 2 g IV every 8 hours ○ Children: 120 mg/kg/day IV divided every 8 hours ($\leq$ 2 g/dose) PLUS • Linezolid: ○ Adults: 600 mg IV every 12 hours ○ Children < 12 years: 30 mg/kg/day IV divided every 8 hours ($\leq$ 600 mg/dose) ○ Children $\geq$ 12 years: 30 mg/kg/day IV divided every 12 hours ($\leq$ 600 mg/dose)
Alternative drug	Not applicable
Duration	10–14 days
Special considerations and comments	Not applicable

Note: IV = intravenous(ly).

2) Antitoxin for systemic or inhalation anthrax: raxibacumab, a human immunoglobulin class G1-γ monoclonal antibody directed against protective antigen, was approved in 2012 by FDA for the treatment of inhalation anthrax.

Drug, dose, route	Raxibacumab (premedication with diphenhydramine needed): • > 50 kg: 40 mg/kg IV • 15–50 kg: 60 mg/kg IV • $\leq$ 15 kg: 80 mg/kg IV
Alternative drug	Not applicable

(Continued)

(Continued)

Duration	Single dose
Special considerations and comments	Not applicable

Note: IV = intravenous(ly).

Obiltoxaximab, a monoclonal antibody directed against the protective antigen of *B. anthracis*, was approved in 2016 by FDA for the treatment of inhalation anthrax (in combination with antimicrobial therapy). It does not cross the blood-brain barrier and does not treat anthrax meningitis.

Drug, dose, route	Obiltoxaximab (premedication with diphenhydramine needed): • > 40 kg: 16 mg/kg IV • 15–40 kg: 24 mg/kg IV • ≤ 15 kg: 32 mg/kg IV
Alternative drug	Not applicable
Duration	Single dose
Special considerations and comments	Not applicable

Note: IV = intravenous(ly).

3) For adults with systemic anthrax in whom meningitis has been ruled out:

Drug, dose, route	• Ciprofloxacin 400 mg IV every 8 hours PLUS • Clindamycin 900 mg IV every 8 hours OR linezolid 600 mg IV every 12 hours
Alternative drug	Not applicable
Duration	10–14 days
Special considerations and comments	Not applicable

4) For children with systemic anthrax in whom meningitis has been ruled out:

Drug, dose, route	Ciprofloxacin 30 mg/kg/day IV divided every 8 hours (≤ 400 mg/dose)
	For penicillin-susceptible strains (MIC ≤ 0.5 μg/mL): • Penicillin G 400,000 units/kg/day IV divided every 4 hours (≤ 4 MU/dose) PLUS • Clindamycin 40 mg/kg/day IV divided every 8 hours (≤ 900 mg/dose)
Alternative drug	Not applicable
Duration	10–14 days
Special considerations and comments	Not applicable

Note: MIC = minimum inhibitory concentration; MU = million units.

5) Cutaneous anthrax without systemic involvement—adults:

Drug, dose, route	Nonpregnant adults, PO therapy with: • Ciprofloxacin 500 mg every 12 hours OR • Doxycycline 100 mg every 12 hours OR • Levofloxacin 750 mg every 12 hours OR • Moxifloxacin 400 mg every 24 hours
	Pregnant, lactating, and postpartum women: • The agent of choice is ciprofloxacin 500 mg PO every 12 hours. • If ciprofloxacin is unavailable, alternative agents that are likely to cross the placenta adequately include levofloxacin, amoxicillin, and penicillin; amoxicillin or penicillin can be used for penicillin-susceptible strains. Clindamycin and doxycycline are also likely to cross the placenta, but data are limited.
Alternative drug	Clindamycin 600 mg PO every 8 hours
	For penicillin-susceptible strains (MIC ≤ 0.5 μg/mL): • Amoxicillin 1 g PO every 8 hours or penicillin VK 500 mg PO every 6 hours
Duration	3–7 days

Note: MIC = minimum inhibitory concentration; PO = oral(ly).

6) Cutaneous anthrax without systemic involvement—children:

Drug, dose, route	Ciprofloxacin 30 mg/kg/day PO divided every 12 hours ($\leq$ 500 mg/dose)
	For penicillin-susceptible strains (MIC $\leq$ 0.5 μg/mL): • Amoxicillin 75 mg/kg/day PO divided every 8 hours ($\leq$ 1 g/dose)

Alternative drug	• Doxycycline:
	   ○ < 45 kg: 4.4 mg/kg/day PO divided every 12 hours ($\leq$ 100 mg/dose)
	   ○ $\geq$ 45 kg: 100 mg PO every 12 hours
	OR
	• Clindamycin 30 mg/kg/day PO divided every 8 hours ($\leq$ 600 mg/dose)
	OR
	• Levofloxacin:
	   ○ < 50 kg: 16 mg/kg/day PO divided every 12 hours ($\leq$ 250 mg/dose)
	   ○ $\geq$ 50 kg: 500 mg PO every 24 hours

	For penicillin-susceptible strains (MIC $\leq$ 0.5 μg/mL): • Penicillin VK 50–75 mg/kg/day PO divided every 6–8 hours
Duration	3–7 days

Note: MIC = minimum inhibitory concentration; PO = oral(ly).

10. Prevention—

1) Prevention of naturally acquired human anthrax begins with prevention and control in animals. Effective control centers around vaccination of livestock in endemic regions and appropriate procedures in the event of outbreaks of anthrax in livestock (correct disposal of carcasses); decontamination of carcass sites and items in contact with the carcasses or sites; vaccination of unvaccinated animals in the affected herd; treatment of symptomatic animals in such herds with penicillin or other suitable antibiotic; and quarantine. (Note that, because the animal vaccine is a live vaccine, antibiotics and the vaccine should not be administered simultaneously.)

2) Preexposure prophylaxis with anthrax vaccines: immunize high-risk persons with a cell-free vaccine prepared from a culture filtrate containing the protective antigen. This vaccine is effective in preventing cutaneous and inhalation anthrax. It is recommended for laboratory workers who routinely work with *B. anthracis* and for workers who handle potentially contaminated industrial raw materials or engage in activities with high potential for production of, or exposure to, *B. anthracis* spore-containing aerosols. It may also be used to protect military personnel against potential exposure to anthrax used as a biologic warfare agent. Vaccination may be indicated for veterinarians and

other persons handling potentially infected animals in areas with a high incidence of enzootic anthrax. Under certain conditions when the threat of deliberate use of anthrax to cause harm is a concern, first-responder organizations may consider vaccination on a voluntary basis. Annual booster injections are recommended if the risk of exposure continues. Vaccines for administration to humans are produced in the USA and UK (protein-based nonliving vaccines) and in China and Russia (live-spore vaccines); availability is limited outside these countries.

Preexposure prophylaxis for adults older than 65 years:

- Intramuscular (IM), preferred:

  - Primary immunization: 3 injections of 0.5 mL each given at day 0 and then at 1 month and 6 months.
  - Booster injections: 0.5 mL each should be given 6 and 12 months after completion of the primary series and at 1-year intervals thereafter for persons who remain at risk.

- Subcutaneous (SubQ):

  - Primary immunization: 4 injections of 0.5 mL each given at day 0 and then at 2 weeks, 4 weeks, and 6 months.
  - Booster injections: 0.5 mL each should be given 6 and 12 months after completion of the primary series and at 1-year intervals thereafter for persons who remain at risk.
    Note that SubQ administration is only to be used for primary immunization in persons who are at risk for hematoma formation following IM injection.

3) Postexposure prophylaxis (PEP): PEP of asymptomatic individuals should start as soon as possible after exposure and ideally within 48 hours because its effectiveness decreases with delay in administration. Clinicians should seek advice from public health officials to determine which individuals should receive PEP. When selecting a PEP regimen, the potential for antimicrobial drug resistance and the presence of latent spores must be taken into account. Individuals exposed to aerosolized *B. anthracis* are presumed to be at prolonged risk for inhalation anthrax from unsporulated spores retained in their lungs following the initial exposure. The presence of *B. anthracis* spores requires prolonged antimicrobial prophylaxis (60 days). Clinicians should remain alert to the possibility of nonadherence to prescribed regimens, which can be very high in this setting.

The PEP regimens include both (a) antimicrobial drug prophylaxis for 60 days and (b) a 3-dose series of anthrax vaccines adsorbed, SubQ, 0.5 mL each given at day 0 and then at 2 weeks and 4 weeks post exposure.

Drug, dose, route	Nonpregnant adults:
	• Ciprofloxacin 500 mg PO every 12 hours OR • Doxycycline 100 mg PO every 12 hours
	Pregnant women and nursing mothers: • Ciprofloxacin 500 mg PO every 12 hours is considered the first-line drug for PEP, but clindamycin 600 mg PO every 8 hours or doxycycline 100 mg PO every 12 hours may be given if ciprofloxacin is unavailable.

	Children:
	
	 • Ciprofloxacin 30 mg/kg/day PO divided every 12 hours ($\leq$ 500 mg/dose)
	 OR
	 • Doxycycline:
	    ○ < 45 kg: 4.4 mg/kg/day PO divided every 12 hours (< 100 mg/dose)
	    ○ $\geq$ 45 kg: 100 mg PO every 12 hours

	Penicillin-susceptible strains (MIC $\leq$ 0.5 µg/mL): • Amoxicillin 75 mg/kg/day PO divided every 8 hours ($\leq$ 1 g/dose) for all adults and children
Alternative drug	Not applicable
Duration	60 days

Note: MIC = minimum inhibitory concentration; PEP = postexposure prophylaxis; PO = oral(ly).

- Anthrax vaccine for PEP: anthrax vaccine adsorbed (AVA) was approved by FDA in 2015 and is recommended by CDC as part of the PEP regimen for inhalation anthrax exposure. Clinicians in the USA seeking AVA for anthrax PEP should notify CDC or their state or local health department for suspicion of exposure to anthrax and for any requests for anthrax vaccine. Alternatively, AVA can be obtained directly from the manufacturer (Emergent BioSolutions, Rockville, MD).

- In the postexposure setting, CDC recommends that anthrax vaccine be administered, within 10 days of exposure, to exposed adults and children older than 6 weeks in 3 SubQ doses (at 0, 2, and 4 weeks) in conjunction with a 60-day course of antimicrobial therapy. CDC recommends the use of AVA for both pregnant and lactating women exposed to aerosolized *B. anthracis* spores. Exposed infants younger than 6 weeks should be given antimicrobial PEP immediately but should receive the first dose of the AVA series when they reach 6 weeks old. For exposed children, AVA should be given priority over routine childhood immunizations; administration of routine immunizations should be delayed until 4 weeks after the last AVA dose.

4) Educate employees who handle potentially contaminated animal products about modes of anthrax transmission, signs and symptoms of anthrax, care of skin abrasions, and personal cleanliness. If anthrax is suspected in an animal, do not necropsy the animal; instead, aseptically collect a blood sample for smear and/or culture. Avoid contamination of the area. If a necropsy is inadvertently performed, autoclave, incinerate, or chemically disinfect/fumigate all instruments or materials used.

Because anthrax spores may survive for years in the soil if carcasses are buried and be a source for new outbreaks—there are many instances on record of outbreaks following disturbance of old burial sites—the preferred disposal techniques for carcasses of animals that die of anthrax and for bedding straw and other contaminated materials are incineration at the site of death or removal to an incinerator or rendering plant, taking care to ensure that no contamination occurs en route to the plant. Should these methods prove impossible, after disinfection, such as with formalin, bury carcasses at the site of death as deeply as possible without digging below the local water table level.

Promptly immunize, and annually reimmunize, all domestic animals at risk. Treat symptomatic animals with penicillin or tetracyclines; immunize them after cessation of treatment. These animals should not be used for food until quarantine and drug clearance times have passed. Treatment in lieu of immunization may be used for animals exposed to a discrete source of infection, such as contaminated commercial feed.

The affected herd or flock should be quarantined for at least 14 days, preferably 20 days, after the last case is diagnosed.

Do not sell the hides or other parts of animals infected with anthrax or sell their carcasses as food or feed supplements (bonemeal or blood meal).

Control dust and properly ventilate work areas in hazardous industries, especially those handling raw animal materials. Maintain continued medical supervision of employees and provide prompt medical care for all suspicious skin lesions. Workers must wear protective clothing (e.g., gloves, boots, impermeable gowns); adequate facilities must be provided for washing and changing clothes after work. Where possible, workers in at-risk occupations should be vaccinated. Locate eating facilities away from places of work. Vaporized formaldehyde has been used for disinfection of workplaces contaminated with *B. anthracis*. Fumigation with chlorine dioxide or vaporized hydrogen peroxide is also effective.

Thoroughly wash, disinfect, or sterilize animal hair, wool, and bonemeal—or other feed of animal origin—prior to processing, using disinfecting protocols demonstrated as being effective against *B. anthracis* spores, such as the Duckering process or irradiation.

Control effluents and wastes from rendering plants that handle potentially infected animals and from factories that manufacture products from animal hair, wool, bones, or hides likely to be contaminated. If appropriate, decontaminate.

Detailed guidance on prevention, treatment, and control of anthrax in animals and in humans and on procedures for disinfection and decontamination is provided in the WHO anthrax guidelines (http://www.who.int/csr/resources/publications/AnthraxGuidelines2008/en/index.html).

11. Special considerations—

1) Reporting: case reporting is obligatory in many countries. Even a single case of human anthrax, especially of the inhalation variety, is so unusual in industrialized countries and urban centers that it warrants immediate reporting to public health and law enforcement authorities. When naturally occurring, it should also be reported to agricultural or wildlife authorities.

2) Floods in previously infected areas may increase the risk of new cases occurring in livestock.

3) In accordance with the *Terrestrial Animal Health Code*,[1] imported animals or animal products should be accompanied by international veterinary certificates that the animals involved are free from anthrax and were not on premises quarantined for anthrax at the time of harvesting. Imported bonemeal should be sterilized if used as animal feed. Disinfect wool, hair, and hides when indicated and feasible.

4) Measures in case of deliberate use: anthrax has been associated with biologic weapons programs and bioterrorism. The general procedures for dealing with deliberate civilian release include the following:

   - Anyone who receives a threat about dissemination of anthrax organisms or a suspicious package or envelope should immediately notify the relevant local law enforcement authorities and/or those with responsibility for the investigation of deliberately caused biologic threats.
   - Local and state health departments should also be notified and be ready to provide public health management and follow-up as needed.
   - If the threat of exposure to deliberately aerosolized anthrax is credible or confirmed, persons at risk should promptly begin PEP as described earlier.

- Primary responders should use an approved pressure-demand self-contained breathing apparatus, in conjunction with a level A protective suit, in responding to a suspected biologic incident when any of the following information is unknown or the event is uncontrolled: the type(s) of airborne agent(s); the dissemination method; whether aerosol dissemination is still occurring or it has stopped, but there is no information on the duration of dissemination; or what the exposure concentration might be. Guidance for protective actions for responders in the event of a wide-area anthrax release has been published by various governments. The US guidance can be found at: http://www.phe.gov/Preparedness/responders/Pages/anthraxguidance.aspx.

- Responders may use a level B protective suit with an exposed or enclosed approved pressure-demand self-contained breathing apparatus when the suspected biologic aerosol is no longer being generated or when other conditions may present a splash hazard.

- Responders may use a full-face respirator with a P100 filter or a powered air-purifying respirator with high-efficiency filters when the following can be determined: an aerosol-generating device was not used to create high airborne concentration or dissemination was by a letter or package that can be easily bagged.

- Quarantine is not appropriate. Persons who may have been exposed and who may be contaminated should be decontaminated with soap and copious amounts of water in a shower.

- All persons who are to be decontaminated should remove clothing and personal effects and place all items in plastic bags clearly labeled with the owner's name, telephone number, and inventory of contents. Personal items that are contaminated should be disposed of following local regulations. Personal items may be kept as evidence in a criminal trial or returned to the owner if the threat is unsubstantiated.

- If the suspect item associated with an anthrax threat remains sealed (e.g., an unopened envelope), first responders should not take any action other than to notify the relevant authority and safely package the evidence. Evacuation, decontamination, and chemoprophylaxis will be dictated by subsequent epidemiologic and environmental investigation.

References

1. World Organisation for Animal Health (OIE). *Terrestrial Animal Health Code.* 28th ed. Paris, France: OIE; 2019.

[I. Chuang]

ARBOVIRAL DISEASES
(arthropod-borne viral diseases)

Arboviruses are transmitted to humans primarily through the bites of infected arthropods (i.e., mosquitoes, ticks, sandflies, and biting midges). The virus families responsible for most arboviral infections in humans are Flaviviridae, Peribunyaviridae, Phenuiviridae, Togaviridae, and Reoviridae. More than 100 arboviruses are known to cause human disease. Although most infections are subclinical, symptomatic illness usually manifests as 1 of 4 primary clinical syndromes: systemic febrile illness, polyarthritis and rash, acute central nervous system disease, or hemorrhagic fever. Some of the arboviruses are covered in separate chapters because of their international public health importance (e.g., dengue, Japanese encephalitis, Rift Valley fever, West Nile, yellow fever, and Zika viruses). Many arboviral infections can have more than 1 primary clinical syndrome. However, the arboviruses in this chapter are organized in sections according to their currently understood most severe clinical presentation.

Most arboviruses are maintained in zoonotic cycles between birds or small mammals and arthropod vectors. Humans are infected incidentally and usually do not develop a sustained or high enough level of viremia to infect arthropod vectors. In a small number of important exceptions (e.g., chikungunya, dengue, yellow fever, and Zika viruses), humans can be the primary source of virus amplification and arthropod infection, and the virus can be spread from person to arthropod to person (anthroponotic transmission). Direct person-to-person spread of arboviruses is rare but has been documented for some arboviruses through blood transfusion, organ transplantation, intrauterine and intrapartum transmission, breastfeeding, or sexual transmission. Percutaneous and aerosol transmission of arboviruses can occur in the laboratory setting.

The arboviruses are listed in the tables that accompany each section with the type of vector and geographic distribution. In some instances, observed cases of disease due to particular viruses have been too few to be certain of the usual clinical course. Viruses recognized to cause human disease only through laboratory exposure or when the only evidence of human infection is based solely on serologic surveys are not included.

[S. Hills, M. Fischer]

I. ARBOVIRAL FEVERS

VIRUS	ICD-10 CODE	VECTOR	OCCURRENCE
BANZI	ICD-10 A92.8	Mosquito: *Culex* spp.	Africa
BHANJA	ICD-10 A93.8	Tick: *Haemaphysalis intermedia* in Asia *Hyalomma* spp. in Africa *Dermacentor* spp. in Europe	Africa, Asia, Europe
BOURBON	ICD-10 A93.8	Tick: Likely *Amblyomma americanum*	North America
BUNYAMWERA	ICD-10 A92.8	Mosquito: *Aedes* spp.	Africa
BWAMBA	ICD-10 A92.8	Mosquito: Primarily *Anopheles* spp. but also *Aedes* spp.	Africa
CHANDIPURA	ICD-10 A93.8	Sandfly: *Phlebotomus* and *Sergentomyia* spp. Mosquito: *Aedes* spp., *Anopheles stephensi*, and *Culex tritaeniorhynchus*	Africa, India
CHANGUINOLA	ICD-10 A93.8	Sandfly: *Lutzomyia* spp.	Central and South America
COLORADO TICK FEVER	ICD-10 A93.2	Tick: *Dermacentor andersoni*	Western parts of USA and Canada

(Continued)

(Continued)

VIRUS	ICD-10 CODE	VECTOR	OCCURRENCE
DUGBE	ICD-10 A93.8	Tick: *Amblyomma* spp.	Africa
GROUP C VIRUSES (Apeu, Caraparu, Itaqui, Madrid, Marituba, Murutucu, Nepuyo, Oriboca, Ossa, and Restan)	ICD-10 A92.8	Mosquito: *Culex* spp.	South America, Panama, Trinidad, Mexico
HEARTLAND	ICD-10 A93.8	Tick: *A. americanum*	North America
IQUITOS	ICD-10 A93.8	Biting midge: Primary vector unknown	South America
NAIROBI SHEEP DISEASE	ICD-10 A93.8	Tick: primarily *Rhipicephalus appendiculatus* (Africa) *H. intermedia* (India)	Africa, India
OROPOUCHE	ICD-10 A93.0	Biting midge: *Culicoides paraensis*	South America, Panama, Trinidad
QUARANFIL	ICD-10 A93.8	Tick: *Argas* spp.	Africa, Middle East
SANDFLY FEVER NAPLES, SICILIAN (phlebotomus fever, papatasi fever)	ICD-10 A93.1	Sandfly: *Phlebotomus perniciosus, Phlebotomus perfiliewi*, and *Phlebotomus papatasi*	Europe, Asia, Africa
SEMLIKI FOREST	ICD-10 A92.8	Mosquito: *Aedes* spp.	Africa, Asia
SEPIK	ICD-10 A92.8	Mosquito: *Mansonia* spp., *Ficalbia* spp., and *Culex sitiens*	Papua New Guinea
SEVERE FEVER WITH THROMBOCYTOPENIA SYNDROME (Huaiyangshan)	ICD-10 A93.8	Tick: *Haemaphysalis* spp.	Eastern Asia
SPONDWENI	ICD-10 A92.8	Mosquito: Various species	Africa
TAHYNA	ICD-10 B33.8	Mosquito: *Aedes* and *Culex* spp.	Europe, Africa, Asia

(Continued)

(Continued)

VIRUS	ICD-10 CODE	VECTOR	OCCURRENCE
THOGOTO	ICD-10 A93.8	Tick: *Amblyomma, Boophilus, Hyalomma,* and *Rhipicephalus* spp.	Africa, Europe
VESICULAR STOMATITIS	ICD-10 A93.8	Sandfly: *Lutzomyia* spp.	Americas
WESSELSBRON	ICD-10 A92.8	Mosquito: *Aedes* spp.	Africa

Arboviruses (arthropod-borne viruses) are members of different taxonomic families and are transmitted from infected to susceptible vertebrates by arthropod vectors (e.g., mosquitoes, ticks, sandflies, biting midges). In accordance with vector and host activity, arboviral diseases often follow distinct seasonal patterns. The arboviral diseases described here are typically characterized by febrile illnesses usually lasting a week or less and are seldom fatal. Certain clinical features may occur more frequently during infection with specific arboviruses; however, they are not typically specific enough to obviate the need for laboratory confirmation. Diagnosis is confirmed most frequently by measurement of virus-specific antibodies in serum; for some viruses, ribonucleic acid (RNA) may be detected or, rarely, the virus may be isolated from acute samples collected soon after illness onset. Symptomatic management is indicated, but there is no specific treatment. Standard precautions are recommended for prevention of health care-associated transmission.

1. Clinical features—Febrile illnesses usually lasting a week or less. Initial symptoms include fever, headache, malaise, arthralgia, or myalgia. Occasional symptoms include nausea and vomiting, conjunctivitis, photophobia, or rash. Symptoms usually resolve within a week but may be markedly incapacitating for that time. For most of these viruses, fatalities are rare.

Certain clinical features may occur more frequently during infection with specific arboviruses. Sandfly-borne viral fevers often include retro-orbital pain, injected sclerae, and pain in the limbs and back. Severe fever with thrombocytopenia syndrome and Heartland virus infection are characterized by fever, headache, fatigue, leukopenia, and thrombocytopenia. Several viruses (e.g., Colorado tick fever, Bhanja, Thogoto) may occasionally cause central nervous system infection. In vesicular stomatitis, patients typically have pharyngitis, oral mucosal vesicular lesions, and cervical adenopathy.

2. Risk groups—Risk of infection is generally determined by exposure to infected vectors and is dependent on many factors, including environmental conditions, season, and human activities. In highly endemic areas, adults have often acquired natural immunity following subclinical or mild infection in childhood; illness occurs mainly in children, visitors, or people new to the area. Patients with immunocompromising conditions may be more susceptible to severe disease. Infection is generally thought to result in lifelong immunity.

3. Causative agents—Single-stranded RNA viruses of various families, primarily Flaviviridae, Peribunyaviridae, Phenuiviridae, and Togaviridae, or double-stranded RNA viruses of the family Reoviridae (see earlier table).

4. Diagnosis—Arboviral infections that cause a febrile syndrome are confirmed most frequently by measurement of virus-specific antibody in serum. Acute-phase specimens should be tested for virus-specific immunoglobulin (Ig) M antibodies. For most arboviral infections, IgM is detectable within the first week after onset of illness and persists for several months, but longer persistence (i.e., years) has been documented. Therefore, a positive IgM test result may reflect a past infection. Serum IgG antibodies generally are detectable shortly after IgM antibodies and persist for years. Plaque-reduction neutralization tests can be performed to measure virus-specific neutralizing antibodies, which are predominantly IgG. A 4-fold or greater rise in virus-specific neutralizing antibodies between acute- and convalescent-phase serum specimens collected 2 to 3 weeks apart may be used to confirm recent infection or discriminate between cross-reacting antibodies in primary arboviral infections. In patients who have been infected with another arbovirus from the same virus family in the past (i.e., who have secondary arboviral infections), cross-reactive IgM and IgG antibodies may make it difficult to identify which arbovirus, particularly among flaviviruses, is causing the patient's current illness. Immunization history, date of symptom onset, and information regarding other arboviruses known to circulate in the geographic area that may cross-react in serologic assays should be considered when interpreting results. For Colorado tick fever virus infections, antibody development may be delayed; approximately 50% of patients only have detectable antibodies 2 to 4 weeks after illness onset. Diagnosis can also be made for some viruses (e.g., Colorado tick fever or severe fever with thrombocytopenia syndrome viruses) by testing of serum using molecular methods such as reverse transcription polymerase chain reaction (RT-PCR) or by virus isolation. For most arboviral infections, however, humans usually have low levels of transient viremia and neutralizing antibodies are present by the time of clinically apparent infection, so viral culture and testing for nucleic acids are less sensitive for detecting recent infections. Immunohistochemical staining can detect specific viral antigens in fixed tissue.

5. Occurrence—The occurrence of specific arboviruses is dependent on many factors, including climate and the presence and relative abundance of competent vectors and susceptible hosts. A number of these viruses are extremely rare and seldom encountered. Marked seasonality is often observed with arboviral diseases (see earlier table).

6. Reservoirs—Reservoirs for many of the arboviruses listed have not been identified. Some of these viruses are maintained in a continuous cycle between invertebrate vectors and vertebrate amplifying hosts. Identified vertebrate amplifying hosts include rodents for group C viruses, small mammals for Colorado tick fever, rodents for the sandfly-borne viral fevers, and primates, sloths, and birds for the sylvatic cycle of Oropouche virus. Humans are not usually involved in the maintenance and spread of these arboviruses; however, humans are an amplifying host for the urban cycle of Oropouche virus, and reports have suggested that severe fever with thrombocytopenia virus can be transmitted from human to human.

7. Incubation period—Usually 2 to 14 days for mosquito-borne viruses; 3 to 4 days for tickborne viruses; and 3 to 6 days for sandfly-borne viruses.

8. Transmission—By mosquitoes, ticks, biting midges, or sandflies (see earlier table). Mosquitoes become infected either when feeding on viremic animals or vertically through infected eggs. Infected mosquitoes transmit the virus to humans during subsequent feeds and typically remain infectious throughout their life. Tickborne arboviruses are typically acquired by immature ticks feeding on viremic animals; they retain the viruses from one life stage to the next and transmit viruses to humans during subsequent feeds. For some viruses the cycle is entirely maintained by ticks. Sandfly-borne arboviruses are transmitted transovarially by infected sandflies but may also be acquired by adult sandflies when they feed on infected humans and other animals. They become infective about 7 days after blood feeding and remain so for their normal life span of about 1 month.

Humans may be directly infected with vesicular stomatitis virus through handling of infected animals or their tissues. Rare cases of human-to-human transmission of certain arboviruses have occurred through blood transfusions, transplanted organs, breastfeeding, and the transplacental route. Percutaneous and aerosol transmission of arboviruses can occur in the laboratory setting.

9. Treatment—There is no specific treatment for infection with any of the arboviruses mentioned. Management is supportive and directed at the predominant clinical features. In the acute phase, fever and pain can be managed with antipyretics and analgesics; if the patient may have dengue, nonsteroidal anti-inflammatory medications should be avoided until dengue virus infection is ruled out. Although various antiviral and immunologic therapies have been evaluated for several arboviral diseases, none has shown clear benefit.

Standard precautions are sufficient for infection control. As a precaution to prevent further transmission of viruses that typically produce a high level of viremia (e.g., Oropouche virus), patients should be advised during the first few days after onset of symptoms to avoid further mosquito or sandfly exposure, either by staying in places with screens or by using mosquito nets and other personal protective measures. In particular for sandflies, very fine screening or mosquito bed nets (10–12 mesh/cm or 25–30 mesh/inch, aperture size 0.085 cm or 0.035 inches) should be used, and any sandflies in the residence should be destroyed. To prevent transfusion-associated transmission, blood donations (especially from patients infected with Colorado tick fever virus) should be deferred for 6 months.

10. Prevention—Primary prevention of arboviral diseases involves both vector control and personal protective measures.

1) Epidemic measures: eliminate or treat all potential mosquito breeding sites with larvicides. Spraying the inside of all houses in the community with insecticides has shown promise for controlling urban epidemics of some mosquito-borne viruses. Use approved insect repellents for people exposed to bites by vectors. For Nairobi sheep disease, consider immunizing sheep and goats where vaccines are available; use acaricides prior to moving potentially exposed animals. Tick-infested locations and breeding areas of sandflies around dwellings should be identified and eradicated.

2) Other prevention measures: for vesicular stomatitis viruses, precautions in care and handling of infected animals and their tissues are important. For severe fever with thrombocytopenia syndrome virus, precautions should be taken in the care and handling of human acute-phase blood. To prevent laboratory infections, precautions should be taken when handling viruses in the laboratory at the appropriate biosafety level. For further information, see section VIII-F in the following: https://www.cdc.gov/labs/BMBL.html.

11. Special considerations—

1) Reporting: local health authorities may be required to report cases in selected endemic areas or in areas where the virus has not been previously reported. For vesicular stomatitis and Nairobi sheep disease, notify the World Organisation for Animal Health.

2) Management of contacts and the immediate environment: a search for unreported or undiagnosed cases wherever the patient lived during the 2 weeks prior to the onset of symptoms should be considered for sporadic or travel-associated cases with exposures in unexpected locations.

3) International measures: for vesicular stomatitis and Nairobi sheep disease, restrict the movement of infected animals; for others, none except enforcement of international agreements designed to prevent transfer of mosquitoes and infected vertebrates by ships, airplanes, and land transport.

[C. Gould, I. Rabe]

II. ARBOVIRAL ARTHRITIS AND RASH

VIRUS	ICD-10 CODE	VECTOR	OCCURRENCE
BARMAH FOREST	ICD-10 A92.8	Mosquito: *Culex annulirostris, Aedes vigilax,* and other *Aedes* spp.	Australia
CHIKUNGUNYA	ICD-10 A92.0	Mosquito: *Aedes aegypti, Aedes albopictus,* and other *Aedes* spp.	Africa, Americas, Asia, Pacific Islands, southern Europe, Middle East
MAYARO	ICD-10 A92.8	Mosquito: *Haemagogus* spp. and possibly other species	Central America, northern South America, Caribbean
O'NYONG-NYONG	ICD-10 A92.1	Mosquito: *Anopheles* spp.	Africa
ROSS RIVER	ICD-10 B33.1	Mosquito: *Culex annulirostris, Aedes vigilax, Aedes camptorhynchus, Aedes polynesiensis, Aedes pseudoscutellaris,* and other *Aedes* spp.	Australia; sporadic in Papua New Guinea, Pacific Islands
SINDBIS	ICD-10 A92.8	Mosquito: *Aedes* spp., *Culex* spp., and *Culiseta morsitans*	Africa, northern Europe, Asia, Australia, eastern Europe

Most arboviruses are capable of causing a systemic febrile illness that often includes headache, arthralgia, myalgia, and rash. Some alphaviruses can also cause a more characteristic clinical manifestation with severe polyarthralgia or arthritis, lasting days to months. These viruses are found throughout much of the world, including parts of Africa, Asia, Australia, Europe, the Americas, and the Western Pacific, and have the potential to cause large disease outbreaks (e.g., chikungunya virus in the Americas and Ross River virus in Australia). The viruses are typically maintained in transmission cycles involving mosquito vectors and birds, small mammals, or nonhuman primates. Infection can be confirmed through molecular or serologic testing. Treatment for both acute and more chronic symptoms is supportive. Personal protective measures, such as using insect repellent or staying in screened accommodation, can help to decrease the risk of human infection.

1. Clinical features—Febrile disease characterized by mild-to-severe arthralgia or arthritis, primarily in the wrist, knee, ankle, and small joints of the extremities. A maculopapular rash often occurs 1 to 10 days into the illness. The rash affects mainly the trunk and limbs and may be pruritic with certain viruses (e.g., O'nyong-nyong virus). In infants, chikungunya viral infections can cause vesiculobullous lesions. Buccal and palatal enanthema may occur. Rashes typically resolve within 7 to 10 days and can be followed by a fine desquamation. Myalgia, fatigue, headache, and lymphadenopathy are often reported. Conjunctivitis, paresthesias, and tenderness of palms and soles occur in a small proportion of cases. With chikungunya, severe perinatal infections, mild hemorrhagic manifestations, and rare deaths can occur. Mild hemorrhagic disease symptoms can occur with Mayaro fever. Chikungunya virus has a similar clinical presentation to these alphaviruses. Varying proportions (10%–70%) of persons infected with these viruses have reported persistent arthralgia or arthritis for several months to years following their acute infection.

2. Risk groups—Risk of infection is generally determined by exposure to infected vectors and is dependent on many factors, including environmental conditions, season, and human activities. In highly endemic areas, adults have often acquired natural immunity following subclinical or mild infection in childhood; illness occurs mainly in children, visitors, or people new to the area. Underlying medical conditions have been identified as a risk factor for poor disease outcome.

3. Causative agents—RNA viruses of the family Togaviridae, genus *Alphavirus* (see earlier table).

4. Diagnosis—Diagnosis can be made for most viruses (i.e., chikungunya, Mayaro, O'nyong-nyong, and Ross River viruses) by molecular methods such as real-time RT-PCR on serum or by virus isolation from blood in the first few days of illness. Serologic testing shows IgM antibodies in acute serum samples beginning approximately 1 week after onset of illness and a rise in virus-specific titers between acute and convalescent samples. IgM antibodies commonly persist for weeks to months. Infection generally results in lifelong immunity.

5. Occurrence—Outbreaks of disease occur during warm and wet conditions that favor proliferation of the mosquito vectors. However, dry conditions can be associated with outbreaks if human behaviors are adapted to bring mosquitoes into close proximity to humans.

Chikungunya virus caused a major epidemic throughout the Indian Ocean region starting in 2004 and spread to temperate areas of Europe, where autochthonous transmission was found to occur. In late 2013, the first autochthonous transmission of chikungunya virus in the Americas was identified in Caribbean countries and territories. The virus subsequently spread to 45 countries or territories throughout the Americas with more than 1.7 million suspected cases reported within 2 years.

Thousands of cases of Ross River virus disease are reported in Australia every year. Transmission of the virus has also been previously documented in the South Pacific with large outbreaks occurring in several Pacific islands, including American Samoa, the Cook Islands, and New Caledonia in 1979-1981. Outbreaks of Sindbis virus disease occur in summer and autumn in Europe and South Africa; in Finland epidemic disease is seen in 7-year cycles. Epidemics of O'nyong-nyong virus disease in 1959-1963 and 1996-1997 involved millions of cases throughout eastern Africa; cases and clusters of sporadic disease continue to be detected in the region. Outbreaks of Mayaro virus disease traditionally have been relatively small and focal to the Amazon River Basin, but seroprevalence studies suggest widespread human exposure in South America; 1 case of locally acquired human disease was reported in Haiti in 2015.

6. Reservoirs—Vertebrate amplification hosts linked to arthralgic arboviruses include

1) Ross River virus: marsupials, especially kangaroos, wallabies
2) Barmah Forest virus: natural amplification host is unverified but possums and other marsupials are suspected
3) Chikungunya virus: primates and possible rodents
4) Sindbis virus: birds
5) Mayaro virus: unverified, though nonhuman primates and humans are suspected
6) O'nyong-nyong virus: unknown.

7. Incubation period—From 1 to 12 days.

8. Transmission—By mosquito (see earlier table). Health care and laboratory workers have become infected with chikungunya virus mostly through exposure to infected blood, and neonates have become infected during the intrapartum period. Experimental data also suggest that chikungunya virus may be transmitted by infected organs and tissues. One case of transfusion-transmitted Ross River virus infection has been reported.

Other modes of transmission, such as through respiratory droplets or sexual contact, have not been documented.

9. Treatment—Symptomatic management with analgesics, antipyretics, and antipruritics. Persistent joint pain might require long-term management with anti-inflammatory agents. For patients with disabling peripheral arthritis lasting several months following a confirmed infection, short-term corticosteroids or methotrexate have been reported to provide some benefit in small, uncontrolled case series. A careful risk-benefit assessment should be performed before considering treatment with immunosuppressive agents.

To prevent further transmission for most of these viruses, patients should be advised to avoid further mosquito exposure during the first few days after the onset of symptoms by staying in places with screens, by using mosquito nets, or by using other personal protective measures.

10. Prevention—

1) General measures applicable to vectors and other prevention measures: see "III. Arboviral Encephalitides."
2) Management of contacts and the immediate environment: a search for unreported or undiagnosed cases wherever the patient lived during the 2 weeks prior to onset should be considered for sporadic or travel-associated cases with exposures in unexpected locations. This is particularly important for those regions with competent mosquito vectors (e.g., mosquitoes able to acquire the virus and transmit it).

11. Special considerations—

1) Reporting: the local health authority may be required to report cases in selected endemic areas or in areas where the virus has not been previously reported.
2) Epidemic measures: eliminate or treat all potential mosquito breeding places with larvicides. Spraying the inside of all houses in the community with insecticides has shown promise for controlling urban epidemics of some mosquito-borne viruses.

[E. Staples, A. Powers]

III. ARBOVIRAL ENCEPHALITIDES

VIRUS	ICD-10 CODE	VECTOR	OCCURRENCE
BANNA	ICD-10 A83.8	Mosquito: primary vector unknown	Southeast Asia, China
CACHE VALLEY	ICD-10 A83.8	Mosquito: *Anopheles*, *Culiseta*, and *Aedes* spp.	North America
CALIFORNIA ENCEPHALITIS	ICD-10 A83.5	Mosquito: *Aedes* spp., primarily *Aedes melanimon*	USA, Canada
EASTERN EQUINE ENCEPHALITIS	ICD-10 A83.2	Mosquito: *Culiseta melanura* (zoonotic cycle); some *Aedes*, *Coquillettidia*, and *Culex* spp. (human transmission)	North America
EYACH	ICD-10 A84.8	Tick: *Ixodes* spp.	Europe
ILHÉUS	ICD-10 A83.8	Mosquito: primary vector unknown	Central and South America
JAMESTOWN CANYON	ICD-10 A83.8	Mosquito: *Aedes* and *Culiseta* spp.	North America
KEMEROVO	ICD-10 A84.8	Tick: *Ixodes persulcatus*	Russia
LA CROSSE	ICD-10 A83.5	Mosquito: *Aedes triseriatus*	USA
LIPOVNIK	ICD-10 A93.8	Tick: *Ixodes ricinus*	Russia
LOUPING ILL	ICD-10 A84.8	Tick: *I. ricinus*	UK, Ireland, Norway, Spain
MURRAY VALLEY ENCEPHALITIS	ICD-10 A83.4	Mosquito: *Culex annulirostris*	Australia, Papua New Guinea, Indonesia
POWASSAN	ICD-10 A84.8	Tick: *Ixodes* spp.; primarily *Ixodes cookei* and *Ixodes scapularis* in North America; *Ixodes persulcatus* and *Haemaphysalis longicornis* in Russia	Canada, USA, Russia
ROCIO	ICD-10 A83.6	Mosquito: primary vector unknown	Brazil

(Continued)

(Continued)

VIRUS	ICD-10 CODE	VECTOR	OCCURRENCE
SNOWSHOE HARE	ICD-10 A83.8	Mosquito: *Aedes* and *Culiseta* spp.	USA, Canada, China, Russia
ST. LOUIS ENCEPHALITIS	ICD-10 A83.3	Mosquito: *Culex* spp.	Americas
TICKBORNE ENCEPHALITIS (including European, Far Eastern, and Siberian subtypes)	ICD-10 A84.1 ICD-10 A84.0 ICD-10 A84.8	Tick: *Ixodes ricinus* (European subtype); *Ixodes persulcatus* (Far Eastern and Siberian subtypes)	From Scandinavia down to the Adriatic region and east to the Urals, Korea (European subtype) Russia, China, northern Japan (Far Eastern subtype) Siberia and the Baltic region (Siberian subtype)
TOSCANA	ICD-10 A93.8	Sandfly: *Phlebotomus* spp.	Southern Europe
TRIVITTATUS	ICD-10 A83.8	Mosquito: *Aedes* spp.	North America
USUTU	ICD-10 A92.8	Mosquito: *Culex* spp.	Africa, Europe
VENEZUELAN EQUINE ENCEPHALITIS	ICD-10 A92.2	Mosquito: primarily *Culex (Melanoconion)* spp. (enzootic cycle); *Aedes* and *Psorophora* spp. (epizootic cycle)	Americas
WESTERN EQUINE ENCEPHALITIS	ICD-10 A83.1	Mosquito: *Culex tarsalis*	Americas
Japanese encephalitis virus (see "Japanese Encephalitis")			

The arboviral encephalitides are caused by arboviruses that belong to various families, primarily Flaviviridae, Togaviridae, Peribunyaviridae, Phenuiviridae, and Reoviridae. Primary neurologic manifestations of infection include encephalitis, meningitis, or myelitis. The causative agents are found worldwide, with the distribution of specific arboviruses dependent on factors such as climate, ecology, and the presence and abundance of competent vectors and susceptible hosts. Diagnosis of infection is primarily by serologic methods. Transmission is mainly by mosquitoes, ticks, or sandflies, with a variety of birds and mammals acting as vertebrate amplification hosts. Humans usually are not involved in the maintenance and spread of arboviral encephalitides. Prevention primarily focuses on vector control methods, although vaccines are available to prevent some arboviral encephalitides (e.g., tickborne encephalitis, Japanese encephalitis).

1. Clinical features—Most arboviral infections are asymptomatic or result in undifferentiated febrile illness. When neurologic disease occurs, the main presentations are meningitis, encephalitis, or myelitis. The clinical manifestations of meningitis are similar to those of other viral meningitides and include fever, headache, meningeal signs, and photophobia. Encephalitis ranges in severity from mild altered mental status to severe encephalopathy, coma, and death. Extrapyramidal signs can occur, including a coarse tremor, myoclonus, rigidity, postural instability, and bradykinesia. Neuroimaging may display lesions in brain parenchyma on computed tomography or magnetic resonance imaging, but there are no pathognomonic features. If myelitis occurs, it can result in acute flaccid paralysis. Patients present with asymmetric weakness of the limbs that develops rapidly after symptom onset. Symptoms can occur with or without meningitis or encephalitis. Cranial nerve palsies and other neurologic manifestations of arboviral infections can occur but are uncommon.

The severity and long-term outcome of illness vary by virus, syndrome, and patient characteristics, such as age and underlying medical conditions. Case-fatality rates vary widely. Among the mosquito-borne viral encephalitides, case-fatality rates for encephalitis caused by eastern equine encephalitis, Japanese encephalitis (see "Japanese Encephalitis"), and Murray Valley encephalitis viruses are among the highest, with rates often greater than 25%. By contrast, among patients with La Crosse virus encephalitis, fatal cases are rare (<1%). Among the tickborne encephalitis virus subtypes, the Far Eastern subtype causes the most severe disease with a case-fatality rate of 20% to 40%. Neurologic sequelae following arboviral encephalitis can occur in up to 50% of survivors and may vary from mild peripheral or cranial nerve palsies to spastic quadriparesis. Neuropsychiatric illness or cognitive problems can also occur.

The differential diagnosis of arboviral central nervous system disease is broad and includes many infectious (e.g., viral, bacterial, mycoplasmal, protozoal, or mycotic) and noninfectious (e.g., autoimmune, toxic, metabolic, or postinfectious) causes. Other viral causes of acute neurologic illness include herpes simplex, enterovirus, rabies, measles, mumps, Epstein-Barr, varicella zoster, and influenza viruses.

2. Risk groups—Risk of infection generally results from exposure to infected vectors and is dependent on many factors, including environmental conditions, season, and human activities. In highly endemic areas, adults often acquire natural immunity following subclinical or mild infection in childhood; illness occurs mainly in children, visitors, or people new to the area. Risk of neurologic illness is generally related to age, with the risk for more severe disease usually greater in older adults. However, risk varies by virus, and clinical illness may be seen more often in children (e.g., La Crosse virus disease). Other factors such as immunosuppression and other underlying medical conditions (e.g., chronic renal failure, hypertension) have been associated with risk for severe disease for some arboviruses. Infection generally results in lifelong immunity.

3. Causative agents—Single-stranded RNA viruses of various families, primarily Flaviviridae, Peribunyaviridae, Phenuiviridae, and Togaviridae, or double-stranded RNA viruses of the family Reoviridae (see earlier table).

4. Diagnosis—Routine clinical laboratory studies done on peripheral blood samples do not distinguish arboviral infections from other viral infections. Cerebrospinal fluid (CSF) usually demonstrates an elevated protein and moderate pleocytosis with a predominance of lymphocytes. However, neutrophils may predominate in early infection.

Neuroinvasive arboviral infections are confirmed most frequently by measurement of virus-specific antibody in serum or CSF. Acute-phase specimens should be tested for virus-specific IgM antibodies. IgM in CSF is more specific for diagnosing neurologic disease than IgM in serum. For most arboviral infections, IgM is detectable within the first week after onset of illness and persists for several months, but longer persistence has been documented. Therefore, a positive IgM test result occasionally may reflect a past infection. Serum IgG antibodies generally are detectable shortly after IgM antibodies and persist for years.

Plaque-reduction neutralization tests can be performed to measure virus-specific neutralizing antibodies. A 4-fold or greater rise in virus-specific neutralizing antibodies between acute- and convalescent-phase serum specimens collected 2 to 3 weeks apart may be used to confirm recent infection or discriminate between cross-reacting antibodies in primary arboviral infections. In patients who have been immunized against, or infected with, another arbovirus from the same virus family in the past (i.e., those who have a secondary arboviral infection), cross-reactive antibodies may make it difficult to identify which arbovirus, particularly among flaviviruses, is causing the patient's illness. Immunization history, date of symptom onset, and information regarding other arboviruses known to circulate in the geographic area that may cross-react in serologic assays should be considered when interpreting results.

Diagnosis can also be made for some viruses by testing of serum or CSF in the first few days of illness by molecular methods such as RT-PCR or by virus isolation. For most arboviral infections, however, humans usually have low levels of transient viremia and have neutralizing antibodies by the time they have clinically apparent infection, so viral culture and testing for nucleic acids are less sensitive for detecting infections. Molecular testing is more likely to be successful in immunocompromised patients. Immunohistochemical staining can detect specific viral antigen in fixed tissue.

5. Occurrence—The occurrence of specific arboviruses is dependent on many factors, including climate, ecology, and the presence and abundance of competent vectors and susceptible hosts. Marked seasonality is often observed with arboviral diseases.

6. Reservoirs—A variety of bird and mammal species act as amplifying hosts in transmission cycles; several different vertebrate species may be involved in each cycle. Some arboviruses are maintained in a continuous cycle between invertebrate vectors and vertebrate hosts. Humans are usually not involved in the maintenance and spread of most arboviral encephalitides.

7. Incubation period—Usually 3 to 14 days. Longer incubation periods can occur for tickborne viruses and in immunocompromised people.

8. Transmission—By mosquitoes, ticks, or sandflies (see earlier table). Mosquitoes become infected either when feeding on viremic animals or vertically through infected eggs. Infected mosquitoes transmit virus to humans during subsequent feeds and typically remain infectious throughout their life. Tickborne arboviruses are typically acquired by immature ticks feeding on viremic vertebrate hosts; they retain the virus transstadially and transmit virus to humans during subsequent feeds.

Human infection with tickborne encephalitis virus has occurred following consumption of unpasteurized dairy products, such as milk and cheese from infected goats, sheep, or cows. Rare cases of human-to-human transmission of certain arboviruses have occurred through blood transfusions, transplanted organs, sexual transmission, breastfeeding, and intrauterine and intrapartum transmission. Percutaneous and aerosol transmission of arboviruses can occur in the laboratory setting.

9. Treatment—There is no specific treatment for infection with any of the arboviruses mentioned. Management is supportive and directed at the predominant clinical features. In the acute phase, fever and pain can be managed with antipyretics and analgesics. For patients with neurologic disease, attention should be given to possible complications of recurrent seizures, cerebral edema, and syndrome of inappropriate antidiuretic hormone secretion. Long-term neurologic and psychiatric sequelae may occur and require continued monitoring and supportive care. Although various antiviral and immunologic therapies have been evaluated for several arboviral diseases, none has shown clear benefit. Standard blood and body substance precautions are sufficient.

10. Prevention—

1) Personal protective measures and vector control:

   - Avoid exposure to mosquitoes during peak biting hours if possible, or use personal protective measures to decrease exposure to mosquitoes and ticks (e.g., use insect repellent, wear permethrin-impregnated clothing, and cover up with long sleeves and pants while outdoors; see "Lyme Disease" and "Malaria").

- Screen sleeping and living quarters, use air-conditioning if available, or use bed nets. Insecticide-treated bed nets are preferable. In addition, spraying sleeping quarters with an effective insecticide may help to lower risk.
- Educate the public about modes of spread and control, including household efforts to reduce vector densities (e.g., eliminating mosquito breeding sites around the home).
- Implement an integrated vector management program, which should include control of larval mosquitoes through source reduction and larvicide application and reducing adult mosquitoes through space and residual spraying of appropriate insecticides.

2) Vaccines: 2 safe, effective, inactivated tickborne encephalitis virus vaccines are available in Europe, in adult and pediatric formulations. Inactivated tickborne encephalitis vaccines are also produced in Russia and China. See "Japanese Encephalitis" for information on Japanese encephalitis vaccines.

3) Other prevention measures:

- In areas where tickborne encephalitis virus occurs, boil or pasteurize milk of susceptible animals and use protection when slaughtering animals.
- Screening blood and organ donations may be useful in certain settings.
- To prevent laboratory infections, precautions for the appropriate biosafety level should be taken when handling viruses in the laboratory. See: https://www.cdc.gov/labs/BMBL.html.
- Although some arboviruses can be transmitted through human milk, transmission is rare; because the benefits of breastfeeding likely outweigh the risk of illness in breastfeeding infants, mothers should be encouraged to breastfeed even in areas of ongoing arboviral transmission.

4) Management of contacts and the immediate environment: a search for unreported or undiagnosed cases around the patient's residence or place of work during the 2 weeks prior to onset of symptoms should be considered for sporadic or travel-associated cases with exposures in unexpected locations. If transmission through unpasteurized dairy products is a possibility, search for animals excreting tickborne encephalitis virus in milk.

11. Special considerations—

1) Reporting: local health authority may be required to report cases in selected endemic areas or in areas where the virus has not been previously reported.

2) Epidemic measures:

- Use personal protective measures, including mosquito repellents.
- Eliminate or treat all potential mosquito breeding places. Consider adult mosquito control measures.
- Specific measures suggested for Venezuelan equine encephalitis virus epidemics include identifying infected horses to determine the extent of the outbreak, immunizing all horses in and surrounding the affected areas, and restricting the movement of horses from the affected areas.

[S. Hills, M. Fischer]

ARENAVIRAL HEMORRHAGIC FEVERS, NEW WORLD

DISEASE	ICD-10 CODE
JUNIN (ARGENTINE) HEMORRHAGIC FEVER	ICD-10 A96.0
MACHUPO (BOLIVIAN) HEMORRHAGIC FEVER	ICD-10 A96.1
GUANARITO (VENEZUELAN) HEMORRHAGIC FEVER	ICD-10 A96.8
SABIA (BRAZILIAN) HEMORRHAGIC FEVER	ICD-10 A96.8
CHAPARE HEMORRHAGIC FEVER	NONE

While lessons from Old World arenavirus infections are commonly invoked in characterizing New World disease, increasingly differences in virus-cell interactions, resulting cytokine responses in patients, host tropism, and geography by newly identified members of the viral group, such as discovery in rodents, bats, and ticks in North America and rodents in Asia, all highlight the merit of being careful of historical presumptions across the genus.

1. Clinical features—Most of the clinical experience with New World arenaviral hemorrhagic fevers is from Argentine hemorrhagic fever (AHF). Limited experience with the others has been similar, and so AHF provides the prototypical syndrome. The contemporary experience with New World arenaviral disease is colored by identification bias for severe, sporadically presenting cases, although historically Argentina, in particular, has identified sustained case presentations of both mild and severe disease. The disease begins with an influenza-like illness 6 to 14 days after exposure, often marked by fever, malaise, headache, retro-orbital pain, myalgias (notably of the lower back), and conjunctival injection. Facial flushing, palatal petechiae, and cervical lymphadenopathy may also be noted. Faget sign (relative bradycardia) is commonly observed. Up to 20% to 30% of AHF infections may advance to a more severe neurologic-hemorrhagic syndrome typically 1 to 2 weeks after the onset of symptoms, which may include epistaxis, hematemesis, melena, hematuria, gingival hemorrhage, or neurologic manifestations (confusion, ataxia, intention tremors and convulsions, and coma). Vasodilatory shock may ensue; however, when the patient does not have shock, pulmonary signs and symptoms, hepatosplenomegaly, and manifestations of liver failure may be notably absent. Case-fatality rates range from 15% to 30%. Convalescence from moderate and severe disease may last for several months and include minor personality and memory changes. Ten percent of patients treated with immune plasma (see Treatment in this chapter) develop a late neurologic syndrome, including fever, cranial nerve palsies, and cerebellar abnormalities.

Hematologic findings are notable for leukopenia and thrombocytopenia, which are often accompanied by mild elevations in aspartate aminotransferase, lactate dehydrogenase, and creatine kinase, consistent with mild myositis. Azotemia and renal failure may be present in more severe cases. By contrast, proteinuria has been observed in the prodromal phase. Like Old World arenaviruses, subclinical infections occur. Because of the very limited number of cases described, the full clinical spectrum of Sabia and Chapare infections is unknown.

2. Risk groups—All age groups are susceptible. In endemic areas, agriculture workers, especially young males, represent most cases. Additional risk groups include laboratory workers processing clinical specimens or working in research laboratories; people in contact, or working, with rodents in endemic areas; and those caring for infected patients or who encounter infected bodily fluids, especially in cases of Bolivian hemorrhagic fever and potentially for the other related viruses.

3. Causative agents—New World arenaviruses (enveloped ambisense ribonucleic acid [RNA] virus in the genus *Mammarenavirus*, family Arenaviridae) belong predominantly to the Tacaribe complex. Of the 25 New World arenaviruses, 5 have been associated with naturally occurring hemorrhagic fever in humans: Junin virus in Argentina (AHF), Machupo and Chapare viruses in Bolivia (Bolivian and Chapare hemorrhagic fevers), Guanarito virus in Venezuela (Venezuelan hemorrhagic fever), and Sabia virus in Brazil (Brazilian hemorrhagic fever). However, their geographic ranges are likely broader than the specific areas where they have been identified to date. These viruses are related to the Old World arenaviruses, which include lymphocytic choriomeningitis, Lassa, and Lujo viruses.

4. Diagnosis—During the acute phase of disease, specific diagnosis is mostly done by virus isolation, RNA detection (conventional or real-time polymerase chain reaction), or antigen detection in blood or organs (Machupo infections). Serologic diagnosis by detection of immunoglobulin (Ig) class M and detection of IgG by enzyme-linked immunosorbent assay can help to confirm a suspected infection if nucleic acid testing is not feasible. Laboratory studies for virus isolation and neutralizing antibody tests require biosafety level 4 conditions. In the USA, testing should be coordinated with the state health department in conjunction with CDC's Special Pathogens Branch.

5. Occurrence—AHF is endemic in certain heavily populated areas of the Argentine Pampas. Cases are identified seasonally from February through October, with some years having caseloads of up to 4,000 cases. There were a few substantial outbreaks of Bolivian hemorrhagic fever reported between 1959 and 1964, although since that time cases have been more scattered. Infections with Guanarito virus (Venezuelan hemorrhagic fever) occurred in outbreaks in 1989, 1990, and 1991, but few cases have been reported subsequently. Sabia virus has caused very few natural infections, although a laboratory infection occurred in 1994. Chepare virus was isolated from a small cluster of cases of hemorrhagic fever in Bolivia in 2003–2004, with no further infections reported in the literature.

6. Reservoirs—The naturally occurring reservoirs for arenaviruses causing human disease are rodents, though, more broadly, arenaviruses have been observed in some bats and, in Florida, *Amblyomma americanum* ticks. The full breadth of tropism is not known. Reservoir associations with human disease include the following:

1) In Argentina, wild rodents of the Pampas (*Calomys musculinus* and *Calomys laucha*) are the hosts for Junin virus.
2) In Bolivia, *Calomys callosus* is the reservoir animal.
3) In Venezuela, cane rats (*Zygodontomys brevicauda*) have been shown to be the main reservoir of Guanarito virus.

7. Incubation period—Usually 6 to 14 days (rarely 5 to 21 days).

8. Transmission—Much like early experience with Lassa fever virus, transmission to humans is thought to occur primarily by inhalation of small-particle aerosols from rodent excreta containing virus, from saliva, or from rodents disrupted by mechanical harvesters. Viruses deposited in the environment may also be infective when secondary aerosols are generated by farming and grain processing, when ingested, or by contact with cuts or abrasions. However, like the Lassa fever virus experience, it is possible that eventually more mundane routes such as oral intake of contaminated foodstuffs may become understood to dominate epizootic crossover events. While uncommon, person-to-person transmission of Machupo virus has been documented in health care and family settings. Fatal scalpel accidents during necropsy, without further person-to-person transmission, have been described. Laboratory infections are described with Junin and Sabia viruses.

9. Treatment—The treatment of New World arenaviruses focuses on managing the physiologic, hematologic, and coagulopathic complications that arise during the course of disease, for which general viral hemorrhagic fever and Ebola virus disease guidelines provide useful reference. Severe neurologic sequelae may require additional long-term management.

Convalescent immune plasma has been employed as a therapeutic option against AHF, with 1 randomized clinical trial demonstrating a reduction in case fatality: 16.5% in control subjects compared with 1.1% in those receiving Junin virus-specific immune plasma. This led to the development of standardized dosing for immune plasma, as outlined in this chapter.

The role of ribavirin in the treatment of New World arenaviruses is even less established than it is in Lassa fever. In AHF, the overall case-fatality rate for those treated with ribavirin has been 28.7%, but in a randomized clinical trial a case-fatality rate of only 12.5% was observed. Unfortunately, the sample size is too small to draw significant conclusions. There is a lack of data for the use of ribavirin in Guanarito, Chepare, or Machupo virus infections. The patient with laboratory-acquired Sabia virus survived, having been treated with ribavirin using a protocol adapted from one for Lassa fever. Treatment with ribavirin is a reasonable consideration in suspected cases of New World arenaviral diseases. Preclinical data exist for favipiravir against Junin virus, as well as potential synergy with ribavirin.

Direct Acting Therapeutic Options Against New World Arenaviral Disease

Parenteral Dose	Frequency
Immune plasma[a]	
3,000–4,000 TU/kg neutralizing antibody	Once
Ribavirin[b]	
30 mg/kg (≤ 2 g)	First, a single loading dose
15 mg/kg (≤ 1 g/dose)	THEN every 6 hours for 4 days
7.5 mg/kg (≤ 500 mg/dose)	THEN every 8 hours for 6 days

Note: TU = therapeutic units.
[a]Efficacy signal when administered within first 8 days of illness.
[b]As recommended by WHO for therapy of Lassa fever.

10. Prevention—Limiting exposure to the known or suspected vectors through rodent control programs and limiting contact with rodents have proven effective in both Bolivia and Argentina. Importantly, an effective live attenuated Junin vaccine, called Candid #1, has been administered to high-risk groups in Argentina through government-assisted programs, although this is not commercially available in the USA. A recent study has indicated potential cross-reactivity with Machupo virus in immunized humans. Education campaigns to avoid rodents and appropriately store food could favorably impact risk.

11. Special considerations—

1) Reporting: individual cases should be reported to the local health authority and are notifiable at the national level in several countries. While not expressly listed in the International Health Regulations' algorithm for mandatory reporting, any VHF illness should be reported to biosecurity agencies and considered by an affected country's national focal point as a potential reportable event.

2) Epidemic measures: rodent control, storing of grains and other food in rodent-proof containers, adequate infection control and barrier nursing measures in hospitals and health facilities, identification of convalescent immune sera and ribavirin sources, and contact tracing and follow-up.

3) During flooding seasons, *Calomys* and other rodent vectors may become more numerous in homes and food storage areas and increase the risk of human exposures across the class.

4) Notify the source country and receiving countries of possible exposure by infected travelers.

Bibliography

CDC. Old World/New World Arenaviruses. 2013. Available at: https://www.cdc.gov/vhf/virus-families/arenaviruses.html. Accessed January 17, 2019.

Lamontagne F, Fowler RA, Adhikari NK, et al. Evidence-based guidelines for supportive care of patients with Ebola virus disease. *Lancet.* 2018;391(10121):700–708.

Maiztegui JI, Fernandez NJ, de Damilano AJ. Efficacy of immune plasma in treatment of Argentine haemorrhagic fever and association between treatment and a late neurological syndrome. *Lancet.* 1979;2(8154):1216–1217.

WHO. *Clinical Management of Patients with Viral Haemorrhagic Fever: A Pocket Guide for the Front-Line Health Worker.* 2016. Available at: https://www.who.int/csr/resources/publications/clinical-management-patients/en. Accessed January 15, 2019.

[D. Brett-Major, E. Ewers]

ARENAVIRAL HEMORRHAGIC FEVERS, OLD WORLD

DISEASE	ICD-10 CODE
LASSA FEVER	ICD-10 A96.2
LUJO DISEASE	NONE
Lymphocytic choriomeningitis (see "Lymphocytic Choriomeningitis")	

1. Clinical features—

1) Lassa fever: up to 4 out of 5 patients infected with Lassa fever virus (LFV) may experience asymptomatic disease or have only mild symptoms. Among those patients who are ill, fever is almost always present, often accompanied by malaise, headache, nausea, vomiting, diarrhea that may be profound, myalgias, sore throat, and abdominal pain. Chest pain and cough may also occur but can be from a concomitant bacterial pneumonia. Pharyngeal exudates and conjunctivitis are common. Severe illness is a multisystem disease marked by distributive shock with accompanying hypotension, ascites, pleural effusions, azotemia, and albuminuria. Severe hemorrhage is rare, though observed in larger outbreaks; in some series coagulopathy with mucosal bleeding is present in fewer than 20% of cases. Central nervous system (CNS) involvement can include encephalopathy, encephalitis, or cerebral edema and cases of fatal brain herniation have been reported. Laboratory derangements in severe cases are similar to other hemorrhagic fevers: lymphopenia and thrombocytopenia can be seen in early illness and can rebound after several days, similar to Ebola virus disease. Renal dysfunction occurs. Liver enzyme abnormalities are often seen with severe disease, with aspartate aminotransferase (AST) levels disproportionately elevated compared with other liver-associated enzymes. In early studies, elevated AST (> 150 U/L) and high viremia have been correlated with fatal outcomes, although a recent study from Nigeria found that CNS abnormalities, bleeding, jaundice, and elevated AST, creatinine, and potassium were predictive of fatal outcome in a multivariate logistic regression model.

Convalescent symptoms are frequently reported in patients with Lassa fever. Transient alopecia and ataxia may occur during convalescence, and sensorineural hearing loss occurs in 25% of patients; of these, only half recover some function after

1 to 3 months. The overall case-fatality rate is about 1%, but can be as high as 15% among hospitalized patients and even higher in some epidemics. Disease is more severe in pregnancy. Fetal loss occurs in more than 80% of cases; maternal death is frequent, particularly in the third trimester of pregnancy.

2) Lujo hemorrhagic fever: in a small series of 5 patients in South Africa, 4 of whom died, the clinical description is similar to that of severe Lassa fever. Initial signs and symptoms included fever, headache, and myalgias. These then progressed rapidly, becoming more severe with a maculopapular rash on the face and trunk, soft-tissue edema, pharyngitis, and diarrhea. Bleeding was not a prominent feature except in 1 case. In the fatal cases, a transient improvement was followed by a rapid deterioration with respiratory distress, neurologic signs, and circulatory collapse. Death occurred 10 to 13 days after onset. Similar to Lassa fever, hematologic abnormalities, including lymphopenia and thrombocytopenia, as well as elevated liver-associated enzymes were seen.

2. Risk groups—All ages are susceptible. The main human groups at risk are health care providers, family members, and other close associates handling infected patients, their secretions, or their excretions; laboratory workers processing clinical specimens or working in research laboratories; and people in contact, or working, with the rodent reservoir in endemic areas.

3. Causative agents—LFV and Lujo fever virus are enveloped ambisense ribonucleic acid viruses of the family Arenaviridae, genus *Mammarenavirus*. Lassa and Lujo viruses are the only Old World arenaviruses known to cause hemorrhagic fever in humans. Lymphocytic choriomeningitis virus is the other Old World arenavirus of pathogenic concern to humans.

4. Diagnosis—Lassa fever infections are rare outside of West Africa, and diagnostic reagents are available only at select reference laboratories with biosafety level 4 (BSL-4) capabilities. Lassa fever can be confirmed by direct detection of virus in blood or tissue samples by virus isolation, conventional or real-time polymerase chain reaction, antigen-detection enzyme-linked immunosorbent assay, immunohistochemistry on formalin-fixed tissues, or by detection of virus-specific immunoglobulin (IG) class M antibodies or rising IgG antibody titers. Although a combination of laboratory techniques is recommended, in some instances, such as an individual with a documented clinically compatible illness in an outbreak setting, infection may be confirmed by the presence of IgG reactive antibodies in a single convalescent sample. The diagnosis of Lujo hemorrhagic fever is similar, although this is limited to the novel arenavirus detected in the aforementioned 5 cases. Rapid diagnostics for Lassa fever are in development.

5. Occurrence—LFV is endemic in Guinea, Liberia, Sierra Leone, Mali, and Nigeria, and possibly other countries across West and Central Africa. Recurrent outbreaks occur in these areas. The index case of the Lujo outbreak acquired the illness while in Zambia.

6. Reservoirs—Rodents in the genus *Mastomys* are the reservoir of LFV. The reservoir of Lujo virus is unknown, but likely a rodent, as is the case for other arenaviruses.

7. Incubation period—From 7 to 21 days for Lassa fever. In the South African Lujo hemorrhagic fever outbreak, the incubation period ranged from 7 to 13 days.

8. Transmission—Primarily occurs through direct contact with excreta of infected rodents deposited on surfaces or in food and water and, in some cases, through aerosols. Person-to-person spread may occur early in the course of illness when patients have only fever and virus is present in secretions; person-to-person transmission may also occur throughout illness and in death when unsafe burial practices are performed. Nosocomial transmission is well documented via either inoculation with contaminated needles or unprotected contact with the patient's bodily fluids. The virus may be excreted in urine for 3 to 9 weeks from the onset of illness. Infection can also spread from person to person by sexual contact through semen for up to 3 months after infection.

9. Treatment—The treatment of viral hemorrhagic fevers such as Lassa fever and Lujo requires an aggressive approach to managing the consequences of infection, such as proactive fluid resuscitation, electrolyte monitoring and repletion, and, as appropriate to each case, critical care support such as the use of vasopressors and renal replacement therapy. Judicious use of antibiotics or antimalarial agents should be employed if coinfection is suspected or confirmed. Supplemental oxygenation and mechanical ventilation might be required. Currently, ribavirin is the only recognized antiviral therapy for Lassa fever, although it is not approved by FDA for this indication. Data in support of use of this drug are mixed, and parenteral formulations are often difficult to obtain. Optimal use of the oral formulation is unclear. The results of a study conducted in Sierra Leone in the 1980s strongly favored parenteral ribavirin therapy to no ribavirin, and earlier treatment yielded better results. However, subsequent careful study has not occurred. Generally, ribavirin is contraindicated in pregnancy because of teratogenicity and in patients with renal failure and creatinine clearance less than 50 mL/min. However, these patients carry a higher risk of poor outcomes from LFV infection. Careful, frequent monitoring is required when using this medication—to include hematology and serum chemistry studies—with a reduction in the dose or termination of the medication in the setting of adverse events, which include anemia, hemolysis, and worsened renal function.

Parenteral Dosing of Ribavirin for Lassa Fever Recommended by WHO

Parenteral Dose[a]	Frequency
30 mg/kg (≤ 2 g)	Onetime loading dose
15 mg/kg (≤ 1 g/dose)	THEN every 6 hours for 4 days
7.5 mg/kg (≤ 500 mg/dose)	THEN every 8 hours for 6 days

[a]Ribavirin should be administered with 0.9% normal saline.

10. Prevention—There are no vaccines currently available for human use. Prevention measures during outbreaks should include identifying cases and close contacts and controlling the multimammate mice (*Mastomys*) that serve as the primary vector.

In the health care setting, patient isolation and personal protective measures are imperative and should follow procedures recommended for other viral hemorrhagic fevers. LFV is considered a category A pathogen; ideally infected materials should be handled under BSL-4 conditions when possible. Clinical laboratory tests should be employed via point-of-care devices or in a laboratory setting equipped for the pathogen.

Postexposure chemoprophylaxis with ribavirin can be considered for those with intimate contact (household members, sexual contacts during the infectious period) without contraindications to the medication. It can also be considered for health care workers with exposure to bodily fluids or respiratory secretions without appropriate infection prevention and control practice, such as inappropriate or absent personal protective equipment. Bausch et al. recommended oral ribavirin at a loading dose of 35 mg/kg (dose ≤ 2.5 g), followed by 15 mg/kg (dose ≤ 1 g) every 8 hours for 10 days.[1]

11. Special considerations—

1) Reporting: Lassa virus is listed as an agent that must be assessed in terms of the potential to cause public health emergencies of international concern under the International Health Regulations. Individual cases should be reported to the local or national health authority. The same approach should be taken with Lujo virus reporting.

2) Epidemic measures: rodent control; storing of grains and other food in rodent-proof containers; infection prevention and control to include barrier nursing measures in hospitals and health facilities; active case finding and contact tracing and following; availability of ribavirin.

3) During disasters, *Mastomys* may become more numerous in homes and food storage areas and increase the risk of human exposures.

4) Notify the source country and receiving countries of possible exposures by infected travelers.

References

1. Bausch DG, Hadi CM, Khan SH, Lertora JJ. Review of the literature and proposed guidelines for the use of oral ribavirin as postexposure prophylaxis for Lassa fever. *Clin Infect Dis*. 2010;51(12):1436–1441.

Bibliography

Lamontagne F, Fowler RA, Adhikari NK, et al. Evidence-based guidelines for supportive care of patients with Ebola virus disease. *Lancet*. 2018;391(10121):700–708.

WHO. *Clinical Management of Patients with Viral Haemorrhagic Fever: A Pocket Guide for the Front-Line Health Worker*. 2016. Available at: https://www.who.int/ csr/resources/publications/clinical-management-patients/en. Accessed January 15, 2019.

[D. Brett-Major, E. Ewers]

ASCARIASIS
(roundworm infection, ascaridiasis)

DISEASE	ICD-10 CODE
ASCARIASIS	ICD-10 B77

1. Clinical features—Infection with the intestinal helminth *Ascaris lumbricoides* is often asymptomatic. If clinical symptoms do occur, the most frequent complaint is vague abdominal pain. Pulmonary symptoms that may occur during the lung phase of larval migration include cough, dyspnea, hemoptysis, or eosinophilic pneumonitis (Loeffler's syndrome). The first overt sign of infection may be passage of 1 or more live worms in stools or occasionally from the mouth, anus, or nose. Worm migration may be stimulated by anesthetic agents, fever, or subtherapeutic anthelmintic treatment. Heavy parasite burden may aggravate existing nutritional deficiencies and, if chronic, may affect work and school performance. Serious complications include bowel obstruction by a bolus of worms, particularly in children, or obstruction of bile duct, pancreatic duct, or appendix by 1 or more adult worms.

2. Risk groups—People (especially children) living in warm moist climates where personal hygiene and sanitation are poor or where human feces are used as fertilizer. People who raise pigs or use raw pig manure as fertilizer may also be at risk for ascariasis.

3. Causative agents—*A. lumbricoides,* a large intestinal roundworm of humans. Based on molecular studies, *Ascaris suum,* the cause of ascariasis in pigs, is now thought to be the same species.

4. Diagnosis—The most common method of diagnosis is through microscopic identification of eggs during fecal examination. The use of concentration methods in the laboratory may enhance the recovery of eggs in fecal samples submitted for analysis. Adult worms passed from the anus, mouth, or nose are recognizable based on their macroscopic characteristics. Fecal polymerase chain reaction testing is increasingly used for surveillance studies. Intestinal worms may be visualized by radiologic and sonographic techniques; more rarely, pulmonary involvement may be confirmed by identifying ascarid larvae in sputum or gastric washings.

5. Occurrence—Common and worldwide, with greatest frequency in countries or regions with moist tropical climates, where prevalence often exceeds 50%. Prevalence and intensity of infection are usually highest in children aged 3 to 8 years. Frequently, family members may be infected and reinfected because of shared food, water sources, and hygiene practices.

6. Reservoirs—Humans, pigs; ascarid eggs in soil.

7. Incubation period—The life cycle from time of infection (ingestion) to adult intestinal stage requires between 2 and 3 months for completion. Adult worms can live 1 to 2 years.

8. Transmission—Eggs, living in warm moist soil where infected humans have defecated, undergo development (embryonation) and become infective after 2 to 3 weeks; they may remain infective in soil for several months or years in favorable conditions. Human infection occurs when eggs from contaminated soil are ingested, either directly or from uncooked produce that is contaminated with soil containing infective eggs; infection does not occur directly from person to person or from fresh feces. Most transmission occurs near homes where children defecate outside in the absence of sanitary facilities, and heavy infections in children are frequently the result of ingesting soil. After ingestion by a human host, embryonated eggs hatch in the intestinal lumen, where the female worm may produce more than 200,000 eggs per day. Larvae penetrate the intestinal mucosa and are carried via the portal then systemic circulatory systems to the lungs. Larvae grow and develop in the lungs (10–14 days), pass into the alveoli, ascend the trachea, and are swallowed. Upon reaching the small intestine they grow to maturity, mate, and begin laying eggs. Between 2 and 3 months are required from initial ingestion to oviposition by the adult female. Eggs passed by gravid females are discharged in feces. The period of communicability lasts as long as mature fertile worms continue to live in the intestine.

9. Treatment—

Drug	Albendazole or mebendazole
Dose	• Albendazole 400 mg as a single dose OR • Mebendazole 100 mg BID for 3 days or 500 mg as a single dose
Route	PO
Alternative drug	Ivermectin 150–200 μg/kg PO as a single dose
Special considerations and comments	• Available evidence suggests that these drugs are safe for use among women during the second and third trimesters of pregnancy or among those who are lactating. Evidence also suggests that these drugs are safe among children ≥ 2 years. • Although these drugs are generally considered safe, limited data exist on the risk of treatment in pregnant women during the first trimester or in children < 2 years; thus risk of treatment needs to be balanced with the risk of disease progression in the absence of treatment. If very young children (1–2 years) are treated, they should be given tablets that are crushed and mixed with water; treatment should be supervised by trained personnel. • Mebendazole is available in the USA only through compounding pharmacies.

Note: BID = twice daily; PO = oral(ly).

10. Prevention—

1) Encourage good hygiene habits in children; in particular, train them to wash hands before eating and handling food. Supervise children around pigs, ensuring that they do not put unwashed hands in their mouths.

2) Provide adequate facilities for proper disposal of feces and prevent soil contamination in areas immediately adjacent to houses, particularly children's play areas.

3) Construct latrines that prevent dissemination of ascarid eggs through overflow, drainage, or otherwise. Treating human feces by composting for later use as fertilizer may not kill all eggs. Human feces, pig feces, and sewage effluents are hazardous, especially when used as fertilizer.

4) In endemic areas, avoid ingesting soil or food contaminated with human or pig feces, including where fecal matter ("night soil"), wastewater, or pig manure is used to fertilize crops. Wash, peel, or cook all raw vegetables and fruits before eating, particularly those that have been grown in soil that has been fertilized with

manure. In endemic areas, food that has been dropped on the floor should not be eaten unless washed or reheated.

5) In endemic areas, WHO recommends periodic treatment with anthelmintic drugs (mebendazole, albendazole) for all preschool- and school-aged children (including adolescents who are not in school) and women of childbearing age (15–49 years) in order to control morbidity due to the soil-transmitted helminths causing ascariasis, trichuriasis, and hookworm disease (https://www.who.int/intestinal_worms/en). WHO guidance recommends that treatment be given once a year when the prevalence of soil-transmitted helminth infections in the community is greater than 20% and twice a year when the prevalence exceeds 50%. The global target is to eliminate morbidity due to soil-transmitted helminthiases in children by 2020 by regularly treating at least 75% of children in endemic areas (estimated total number, 873 million).

11. Special considerations—None.

[R. S. Bradbury, M. Kamb]

ASPERGILLOSIS

DISEASE	ICD-10 CODE
ASPERGILLOSIS	ICD-10 B44

1. Clinical features—An opportunistic fungal disease that may present with a wide spectrum of clinical syndromes in the human host, ranging from hypersensitivity reactions to direct angioinvasion. It primarily affects the lungs and is thought to cause several distinct syndromes: (a) allergic bronchopulmonary aspergillosis (ABPA), (b) chronic pulmonary aspergillosis, which includes aspergilloma and chronic necrotizing pulmonary aspergillosis, and (c) invasive aspergillosis.

ABPA is a hypersensitivity reaction to *Aspergillus* spp. colonization of the tracheobronchial tree that occurs in conjunction with asthma or cystic fibrosis. Up to 5% of adults with asthma may develop ABPA at some time; increasing evidence suggests that fungal allergy is associated with increasing severity of asthma. It is also estimated that 2% to 7% of patients with cystic fibrosis reaching adolescence and adulthood develop ABPA. It can lead to permanent lung damage (fibrosis) if untreated. Allergic fungal sinusitis may also occur.

Aspergilloma is a noninvasive form of aspergillosis in which the fungus grows inside a cavity, typically in a previously damaged area of the lung (such as those damaged by tuberculosis, sarcoidosis, or other cavity-causing lung diseases), forming a fungal ball. Aspergillomas may be asymptomatic or may lead to hemoptysis. In other forms of chronic aspergillosis such as chronic necrotizing pulmonary aspergillosis, symptoms such as weight loss, chronic cough, and fatigue may be slowly progressive over months to years.

Acute invasive aspergillosis usually occurs in persons with significant immunosuppression (e.g., due to hematopoietic stem cell transplant, neutropenia, therapy with corticosteroids and/or other immunosuppressive medications, solid organ transplantation, and advanced acquired immunodeficiency syndrome [AIDS]). A rare inherited immunodeficiency, chronic granulomatous disease (CGD), also confers moderate risk. Invasive aspergillosis primarily involves the lungs and/or sinuses; however, hematogenous dissemination occurs. Symptoms of invasive pulmonary aspergillosis usually include fever, cough, chest pain, and/or breathlessness that do not respond to standard antibiotics. In up to 40% of such cases hematogenous dissemination occurs to the brain or to other organs—including, in particular, the eye, heart, kidneys, and skin—with worsening of the prognosis. *Aspergillus* spp. may cause keratitis after minor injury to the cornea, often leading to unilateral corneal opacity and blindness. The organisms may infect the implantation site of a cardiac prosthetic valve or other surgical sites.

Several species of *Aspergillus* produce aflatoxins (mycotoxins); high levels of exposure cause liver necrosis and are associated with hepatic cancer.

2. Risk groups—*Aspergillus* spp. thrive in the environment and exposure is common, but most individuals with healthy immune systems do not develop disease. Immunosuppressive therapy or cytotoxic therapy increase susceptibility, and invasive disease is seen primarily in those with prolonged neutropenia or corticosteroid treatment. Transplant recipients (especially hematopoietic stem cell transplants) and those with advanced AIDS or CGD are also susceptible.

3. Causative agents—Of the approximately 180 species of *Aspergillus*, about 40 have been reported to cause disease in humans. Those most commonly causing invasive infection in humans include *Aspergillus flavus*, *Aspergillus fumigatus*, *Aspergillus nidulans*, *Aspergillus niger*, and *Aspergillus terreus*. Common allergenic species include *A. fumigatus*, *Aspergillus clavatus*, and *Aspergillus versicolor*. The most common species implicated in aspergilloma is *A. fumigatus*; *A. niger* is the most common fungal cause of external otitis. *A. flavus* and *Aspergillus parasiticus* produce aflatoxin most commonly.

4. Diagnosis—Diagnosis of ABPA is based on a combination of radiographic, clinical, and laboratory findings. In patients with asthma, these include the presence of eosinophilia, a positive skin test result for *Aspergillus*, elevated serum immunoglobulin class E level, positive tests for *Aspergillus* precipitins, and radiographic abnormalities that include infiltrates on radiographs or central bronchiectasis on computed tomography (CT) scans. In patients with cystic fibrosis, the diagnosis of ABPA is challenging and consensus criteria have been developed. The diagnosis of an aspergilloma is most readily made on imaging; a CT scan may show a mass within a cavity or characteristic crescent sign. In invasive pulmonary (or disseminated) aspergillosis, histopathology and culture examination together with bronchoscopy may confirm the diagnosis. Sputum cultures have low sensitivity and specificity. The *Aspergillus* galactomannan antigen assay, performed in blood and bronchoalveolar lavage fluid, may help to confirm the diagnosis, especially in patients with hematologic malignancies. Weekly monitoring of serum levels of galactomannan can be used to screen patients at high risk to help facilitate early diagnosis.

Antifungal susceptibility testing, when available, may help detect azole antifungal-resistant strains, although no susceptibility breakpoints exist.

5. Occurrence—Worldwide; uncommon and sporadic; occasional clusters recognized in health care settings that may be related to concurrent construction or remediation activities. No distinctive differences in incidence by race or gender. Outbreaks of acute aflatoxicosis (liver necrosis with ascites) have been described in humans in India and Kenya and in animals; an association between high aflatoxin levels in foods and hepatocellular cancer has been noted in Africa and Southeast Asia.

6. Reservoirs—*Aspergillus* spp. are common in nature, particularly in decaying vegetation, such as piles of leaves or compost piles. Conidia are commonly present in the air, both outdoors and indoors and during all seasons of the year. Water and foods may also be contaminated.

7. Incubation period—Variable, but probably between 2 days and 3 months.

8. Transmission—By inhalation of airborne conidia. No person-to-person transmission. Rare instances of transmission through contaminated water/spray/aerosols have been documented. People are exposed to aflatoxins by consuming contaminated food.

9. Treatment—

Preferred therapy	ABPA:
	• Corticosteroids 0.5–2 mg/kg/day PO prednisone equivalent (≤ 60 mg/day) for 1–2 weeks and tapered over 2–3 months
	Invasive pulmonary aspergillosis:
	• Voriconazole 6 mg/kg IV every 12 hours for 1 day, followed by 4 mg/kg IV every 12 hours[a]
	• Treatment duration: ≥ 6–12 weeks (largely dependent on the degree and duration of immunosuppression, site of disease, and evidence of disease improvement [strong recommendation, low-quality evidence])

(Continued)

(Continued)

Alternative therapy options	ABPA: • Itraconazole 5 mg/kg/day (≤ 400 mg/kg/day) PO, but solution route preferred for cystic fibrosis because of low absorption of capsules • Voriconazole or posaconazole PO possibly also effective but not extensively studied • Treatment duration is 3–6 months
	Invasive pulmonary aspergillosis: • Liposomal AMB 3–5 mg/kg/day IV PLUS • Isavuconazole 200 mg every 8 hours for 6 doses, THEN 200 mg daily for 6–12 weeks

Salvage therapy 6–12 weeks	Salvage therapy for invasive pulmonary aspergillosis:
	
	• AMB liposomal complex 5 mg/kg/day PLUS caspofungin 70 mg/kg IV as a single dose, THEN 50 mg/kg IV thereafter
	OR
	• Micafungin 100–150 mg/day IV
	OR
	• Posaconazole:
	  ○ PO suspension: 200 mg TID on day 1, THEN 300 mg daily
	  ○ PO tablet: 300 mg BID on day 1, THEN 300 mg daily
	  ○ IV: 300 mg BID on day 1, THEN 300 mg daily
	OR
	• Itraconazole suspension 300 mg PO every 12 hours
	• Treatment duration: 6–12 weeks

Special considerations and comments	• Corticosteroids are the preferred agent for the treatment of exacerbations of ABPA. In patients who are symptomatic despite receiving steroids, itraconazole is recommended. It is recommended to add itraconazole for patients with cystic fibrosis who have frequent exacerbations. The addition of itraconazole can minimize the use of steroids. Therapeutic drug monitoring is recommended where possible when using azoles. • Surgical resection, if possible, is the treatment of choice for patients with aspergilloma who cough blood, but it is best reserved for single cavities. • Asymptomatic patients may not require treatment; antifungal agents will not kill fungi within the cavity. • Immunosuppressive therapy should be discontinued or reduced as much as possible. Endobronchial colonization should be treated by measures to improve bronchopulmonary drainage. In sinusitis, surgery may be of help, although relapse is common. • Inhaled corticosteroids, bronchodilators, and environmental manipulation may be useful in asthma.

Note: ABPA = allergic bronchopulmonary aspergillosis; AMB = amphotericin B; BID = twice daily; IV = intravenous(ly); PO = oral(ly); TID = thrice daily.
^aCan use 200–300 mg PO every 12 hours or weight-based dosing.

10. Prevention—High-efficiency particulate air filtration and other air quality improvement measures may decrease the incidence of invasive aspergillosis in hospitalized patients with profound and prolonged neutropenia. Antifungal prophylaxis might be considered for high-risk conditions, such as construction sites in health care settings. Special caution (properly fitted filtering facepiece mask, also known as N-95) should be taken during transport of high-risk patients.

11. Special considerations—

1) Azole-resistant *Aspergillus* spp. have been recently identified and pose a challenge to treatment.
2) Aflatoxins, which are produced by several *Aspergillus* spp. and are highly carcinogenic, could be used deliberately to cause harm through contamination of water and/or food.

Bibliography

Patterson TF, Thompson GR 3rd, Denning DW, et al. Practice Guidelines for the Management of Aspergillosis: 2016 update by the Infectious Diseases Society of America. *Clin. Infect Dis.* 2016;63(4):e1–e60.

[K. Beer, S. Tsay]

BABESIOSIS

DISEASE	ICD-10 CODE
BABESIOSIS	ICD-10 B60.0

1. Clinical features—The clinical spectrum ranges from asymptomatic to life-threatening. Common manifestations include fever, other nonspecific influenza-like symptoms (e.g., chills, sweats, myalgia, fatigue), and hemolytic anemia; thrombocytopenia is also common. Severe cases can be associated with hemodynamic instability, acute respiratory distress, renal failure, hepatic compromise, disseminated intravascular coagulation, altered mental status, and death. Even persons with asymptomatic infection may have low-level parasitemia for months—sometimes for longer than a year—making transmission via blood transfusion a year-round concern.

2. Risk groups—Persons who are asplenic, immunocompromised, elderly, born prematurely, or otherwise debilitated are at increased risk for symptomatic infection, which can be severe.

3. Causative agents—Intraerythrocytic protozoan parasites of the *Babesia* genus. In the USA, the identified zoonotic agents include, predominantly, *Babesia microti*; also, *Babesia duncani* (formerly, the WA1-type parasite) and related organisms, as well as *Babesia divergens*-like parasites. In Europe, the identified agents include *B. divergens* and the EU1 agent (*Babesia venatorum*); also, *B. microti*. In other regions of the world, various *Babesia* spp. and strains have been identified.

4. Diagnosis—Acute cases with patent parasitemia may be diagnosed through identification with a light microscope of intraerythrocytic *Babesia* parasites on Wright- or Giemsa-stained blood smears. In some circumstances, morphologically distinguishing *Babesia* spp. from *Plasmodium* (malaria) spp., especially *Plasmodium falciparum*, can be difficult. Some *Babesia* spp. (e.g., *B. microti* and *B. duncani*) are morphologically indistinguishable from one another. Confirmation of the diagnosis/species by a reference laboratory should be considered; adjunctive molecular and serologic testing should be tailored to the setting and *Babesia* spp. If indicated by the epidemiologic and clinical context, the possibility of coinfection with *Borrelia burgdorferi* (Lyme disease) or *Anaplasma phagocytophilum* (human granulocytic anaplasmosis) should be considered.

5. Occurrence—Overall, most of the documented zoonotic cases in the world have occurred in the USA, some have occurred in Europe, and relatively few have occurred in various other regions. However, the geographic distribution of zoonotic transmission of *Babesia* parasites (in general and for particular species) is inadequately understood; underrecognition, misdiagnosis (e.g., as malaria), and underreporting of cases are common. Increased awareness among clinicians and laboratorians is needed. In the USA, most documented cases have been acquired in the Northeast (particularly, but not exclusively, in parts of New England, New Jersey, and New York) and the upper Midwest (Minnesota and Wisconsin).

6. Reservoirs—White-footed mice (*Peromyscus leucopus*) and other small mammals for *B. microti* in the USA; cattle for *B. divergens* in Europe; not definitively established for some zoonotic *Babesia* spp.

7. Incubation period—Variable; in part dependent on host, parasite, and epidemiologic factors. Around 1 to 3 weeks or longer for tickborne transmission, and from weeks to months for transfusion-associated transmission. Symptoms may appear or recrudesce many months (even > 1 year) after initial exposure, particularly in the context of immunosuppression or surgical splenectomy.

8. Transmission—Tickborne in nature, although the tick bite often is not noticed, and the tick vector has not been identified for some *Babesia* spp. The vectors include *Ixodes scapularis* for *B. microti* in the USA (typically, the nymphal stage, during warm spring/summer months) and *Ixodes ricinus* for *B. divergens* and the EU1 agent (*B. venatorum*) in Europe. Nymphal *I. scapularis* ticks become infected by feeding on infected white-footed mice

(*P. leucopus*) or other small mammals (e.g., voles [*Microtus pennsylvanicus*]). Adult *I. scapularis* ticks typically feed on white-tailed deer (*Odocoileus virginianus*), which are not infected with *B. microti*.

Person-to-person transmission may occur via blood transfusion (documented for *B. microti* and *B. duncani*), even months to more than 1 year after the donor became infected; asymptomatic, undiagnosed parasitemia may be protracted. Transfusion-associated transmission is not inherently restricted by season or geographic region. Rare instances of congenital/perinatal transmission have been reported.

9. Treatment—

Drug	Combination therapy is recommended: • Atovaquone PLUS azithromycin OR • Clindamycin PLUS quinine (this drug combination is the standard of care for severely ill patients).
Dose	The typical daily doses for adults are • Atovaquone 750 mg PO BID PLUS • Azithromycin: on the first day, a total dose in the range of 500–1,000 mg PO; on subsequent days, a total daily dose in the range of 250–1,000 mg. The upper end of the dosage range (600–1,000 mg/day) has been used for immunosuppressed adults. OR • Clindamycin 600 mg PO TID OR 300–600 mg IV QID PLUS quinine 650 mg PO TID
Route	PO for atovaquone, azithromycin, and quinine; PO or IV for clindamycin
Alternative drug	• Only 1 randomized controlled clinical trial has been conducted. In that trial, only the drug combinations mentioned earlier were studied. However, some anecdotal data are available for various other drugs and drug combinations. • Although substitution of IV quinidine for PO quinine may be a consideration for severely ill patients without adequate absorption of PO quinine, availability of IV quinidine in the USA may be limited.
Duration	The typical duration of treatment is 7–10 days. However, a longer course of therapy may be indicated for patients who have or are at risk for severe, persistent, or relapsing infection.

(Continued)

(Continued)

Special considerations and comments	Treatment decisions should be individualized, with expert consultation, if indicated. Antimicrobial therapy typically is reserved for infected persons who are symptomatic or have other clinical manifestations (e.g., hemolytic anemia). Patients with severe babesiosis (e.g., with parasitemia levels ≥ 10% and/or organ-system dysfunction) might benefit from exchange transfusions, vasopressor therapy, mechanical ventilation, or dialysis.

Note: BID = twice daily; IV = intravenous(ly); PO = oral(ly); QID = 4 times a day; TID = thrice daily.

10. Prevention—

1) Educate the public about personal protective measures to reduce the risk for tick exposures/bites. Control rodents around human habitation and use tick repellents. See "Lyme Disease" and Tickborne Spotted Fevers in "Rickettsioses."

2) In March 2018, FDA approved 2 *Babesia* tests for screening blood donors in the USA. In May 2019, FDA issued guidance for blood collection agencies that included a recommendation for year-round molecular testing of blood donations in 14 US states and the District of Columbia.

11. Special considerations—Reporting: reporting requirements/criteria vary by country and local jurisdiction.

[E. Gray, M. Kamb, B. Herwaldt]

BALANTIDIASIS
(balantidiosis, balantidial dysentery)

DISEASE	ICD-10 CODE
BALANTIDIASIS	ICD-10 A07.0

1. Clinical features—An infection of the colon that may produce diarrhea or dysentery, accompanied by abdominal colic, tenesmus, nausea, and vomiting. Occasionally the dysentery resembles that due to amebiasis, with stools containing much blood and mucus. Peritoneal or urogenital invasion and infections in other sites (e.g., lungs) are rare. Infection can be asymptomatic.

2. Risk groups—Individuals debilitated by other diseases—especially those associated with immunosuppression—may have serious, and even fatal, infections.

3. Causative agents—*Balantidium coli*, a large ciliated protozoan. With advances in molecular epidemiology, other related species of ciliated protozoa have been defined but their role as human pathogens is unknown.

4. Diagnosis—Identification of trophozoites or cysts of *B. coli* in fresh feces or trophozoites in material obtained by sigmoidoscopy.

5. Occurrence—Worldwide, with higher risk in tropical and subtropical areas where pigs and humans are in proximity and water and sanitation safety are suboptimal. The incidence of human disease is low and epidemics have rarely been identified. Occasional waterborne epidemics have occurred in areas of poor sanitation where infected pigs are present. Environmental contamination with swine feces may result in higher incidence.

6. Reservoirs—Swine and possibly nonhuman primates. Laboratory pigs may carry this parasite.

7. Incubation period—Unknown; may be only a few days.

8. Transmission—Through ingestion of contaminated food or water containing cysts from feces of infected hosts; in epidemics, mainly through fecally contaminated water. Sporadic transmission by transfer of feces to mouth via hands or contaminated water or food. Transmissible for as long as infection persists.

9. Treatment—

Drug	Tetracycline
Dose	• Adults: 500 mg QID • Children ≥ 8 years: 40 mg/kg/day (≤ 2 g) PO in 4 doses
Route	PO
Alternative drug	• Metronidazole[a]: o Adults: 500–750 mg PO TID for 5 days o Children: 35–50 mg/kg/day PO in 3 doses for 5 days OR • Iodoquinol[a] (should be taken after meals): o Adults: 650 mg PO TID for 20 days o Children: 30–40 mg/kg/day (≤ 2 g) PO in 3 doses for 20 days • Nitazoxanide[a,b]: o Adults: 500 mg PO BID for 3 days o Children 4–11 years: 200 mg PO BID for 3 days o Children 1–3 years: 100 mg PO BID for 3 days
Duration	10 days
Special considerations and comments	Tetracycline should not be used in pregnant women owing to positive evidence of maternal and fetal risk. Use during pregnancy should be limited to instances when there are contraindications to the use of other appropriate antibiotics and the potential benefit justifies the known risk.

Note: BID = twice daily; PO = oral(ly); QID = 4 times daily; TID = thrice daily.
[a]Not FDA-approved for this indication.
[b]Tried in small studies that suggest some therapeutic benefit.

10. Prevention—

1) Educate the general public in personal hygiene, especially on the need for handwashing before handling food, before eating, and after toilet use.
2) Educate and supervise food handlers through health agencies.
3) Dispose of feces in a sanitary manner.
4) Minimize contact with swine feces.
5) Protect public water supplies against contamination with swine feces. Given the large size of the cysts, water filtration systems that are effective for removal of smaller protozoan cysts such as *Cryptosporidium* likely would also remove *B. coli*. Levels of chlorination typically used for water treatment do not destroy cysts. Small quantities of water are best treated by boiling.

11. Special considerations—None.

[M. Kamb]

BARTONELLOSIS
(Oroya fever, verruga peruana, Carrión's disease)

DISEASE	ICD-10 CODE
OROYA FEVER	ICD-10 A44.0
VERRUGA PERUANA	ICD-10 A44.1

1. Clinical features—A bacterial infection with 2 clinical forms: a life-threatening febrile illness with anemia (Oroya fever) and a benign dermal eruption (verruga peruana). Asymptomatic infection and a carrier state may both occur. Oroya fever is characterized by irregular fever, headache, myalgia, arthralgia, pallor, severe hemolytic anemia (macrocytic or normocytic, usually hypochromic), and generalized nontender lymphadenopathy. Verruga peruana occurs weeks to months after untreated acute infection. It has a pre-eruptive stage characterized by arthralgias and myalgias. The dermal eruption may occur as the following: miliary with widely disseminated small hemangioma-like papules occurring in crops, highly vascular bulbous nodules (mular lesions) with a tendency to bleed and ulcerate, or nontender wart-like lesions. Atypical cases with milder manifestations (prolonged splenomegaly and mild anemia) may occur. The case-fatality rate of Oroya fever is up to 90% in the untreated and less than 10% in those receiving treatment. Opportunistic infections (e.g., salmonellosis and toxoplasmosis) occur in as many as 70% of those with Oroya fever. Verruga peruana has a prolonged course but seldom results in death.

2. Risk groups—The disease is milder in children than in adults. Oroya fever is most common in immunologically naive persons, such as tourists, and verruga peruana usually occurs in those from the endemic zone.

3. Causative agents—*Bartonella bacilliformis.*

4. Diagnosis—Visualization of *B. bacilliformis* on Giemsa-stained blood smears can establish the diagnosis (the organism infects erythrocytes), but sensitivity is poor. Isolation of the organisms from blood is usually achieved through bacteriologic culture of blood using specific agar medium enriched with rabbit or sheep blood. Culture may require up to 14 days. An application of cell culture-based techniques and specifically designed liquid media can improve the cultivation of the bacteria from clinical specimens. Molecular techniques, particularly conventional and real-time polymerase chain reaction assays, have been successfully used for detection and identification of *Bartonella* deoxyribonucleic acid in most types of clinical materials (blood, tissues, and bodily fluids) but are often not available in endemic areas. Nonspecific histologic stains (e.g., Warthin-Starry) may provide presumptive evidence of infection. Serologic methods for the detection of *Bartonella* antibodies include the indirect immunofluorescence assay and an immunoblot test, which are the most common and convenient diagnostic methods.

5. Occurrence—Historically limited to mountain valleys of southwestern Colombia, Ecuador, and Peru at altitudes between 600 and 2,800 m (2,000-9,200 ft), where the sandfly vector is present. In Peru, outbreaks have been documented at lower altitudes between highlands and jungle, while coastal lowlands in Ecuador have become endemic.

6. Reservoirs—Humans. In endemic areas, the asymptomatic carrier rate may reach 5%. There is no known animal reservoir.

7. Incubation period—Usually 16 to 22 days; occasionally 3 to 4 months.

8. Transmission—Through the bite of sandflies of the genus *Lutzomyia* (subfamily Phlebotomidae). Species are not identified for all areas; *Lutzomyia verrucarum* is important in Peru. These insects feed only from dusk to dawn. Blood transfusion, particularly during the Oroya fever stage, may transmit infection. Recovery from untreated Oroya fever almost invariably gives permanent immunity to this form but the verruga stage may recur. After human infection following the sandfly bite, the agent may be present in blood for a long period of time (weeks before and up to several years after clinical illness). Duration of infectivity of the sandfly is unknown.

9. Treatment—

Oroya Fever

Preferred therapy	Ciprofloxacin 500 mg PO BID for 14 days
Alternative therapy options	• Chloramphenicol 50–75 mg/kg/day IV in divided doses every 6 hours for 14 days PLUS • Ceftriaxone 1 g IV once daily for 10–14 days
Special considerations and comments	• Amoxicillin/clavulanic acid should be used in children (40 mg/kg PO in 3 divided doses ≤ 2 g/day for 14 days) and during pregnancy (1 g PO BID for 14 days). • In severe disease, ceftriaxone can be administered with ciprofloxacin.

Note: BID = twice daily; IV = intravenous(ly); PO = oral(ly).

Verruga Peruana

Preferred therapy	Azithromycin 500 mg PO/IV daily for 7 days
Alternative therapy options	• Ciprofloxacin 500 mg PO/IV BID for 7–10 days OR • Rifampin 10 mg/kg/day PO (max. total daily dose = 600 mg/day) for 14 days
Special considerations and comments	• Chloramphenicol is not as effective for verruga peruana as it is for Oroya fever. • Azithromycin is safe in children and during pregnancy.

Note: BID = twice daily; IV = intravenous(ly); PO = oral(ly).

10. Prevention—

1) Control sandflies (see Prevention under Cutaneous and Mucosal Leishmaniasis in "Leishmaniasis").
2) Avoid known endemic areas after sundown; apply insect repellent (e.g., N,N-diethyl-meta-toluamide) to exposed parts of the body; and use fine-mesh bed nets, preferably treated with insecticide. For more information on insecticide-treated mosquito nets, see "Malaria." Further information on WHO-recommended bed nets can be found at: https://www.who.int/malaria/publications/atoz/use-of-pbo-treated-llins/en.
3) Blood from residents of endemic areas should not be used for transfusions until it has tested negative.

11. Special considerations—Reporting to local health authority is required in some countries, such as Peru.

Bibliography

Rolain JM, Brouqui P, Koehler JE, Maguina C, Dolan MJ, Raoult D. Recommendations for treatment of human infections caused by *Bartonella* species. *Antimicrob Agents Chemother*. 2004;48(6):1921–1933.

[L. Blanton, D. Walker]

BEJEL
(njovera, nonvenereal endemic syphilis)

DISEASE	ICD-10 CODE
BEJEL	ICD-10 A65

1. Clinical features—Bejel is a chronic, nonvenereal infection characterized by lesions that initially involve the mouth and the skin and later the bones. It usually occurs without an evident primary sore, as seen in yaws. Like other pathogenic treponemal diseases, bejel is characterized by distinct early and late stages.

The infection first appears as 1 or several tiny, painless papules or ulcers on mucous membranes within the mouth or on the skin around the mouth and lips. The initial lesions may resolve or may progress to involve the trunk and extremities. Secondary lesions are characterized by shallow, painless mucous patches in the oropharyngeal mucosa and on the lips and by bony lesions. Secondary symptoms may include hoarseness; stomatitis of the labial commissures; alopecia and patchy skin depigmentation or hyperpigmentation; macular-papular rashes involving intertriginous areas; plantar and palmar hyperkeratosis; or condyloma lata (wart-like lesions on the external genitalia) that may resemble the lesions of venereal syphilis. Bony involvement and pain due to periostitis favor the long bones of the leg. Left untreated, late complications can include juxta-articular nodules and late destructive lesions of the skin, long bones, and nasopharynx, especially the nasal septum and soft palate (similar to yaws). Unlike venereal syphilis, bejel rarely shows neurologic or cardiovascular involvement. The case-fatality rate is low.

2. Risk groups—Bejel typically occurs in children aged 2 to 15 years (peak, 5-10 years) living in endemic areas, primarily in the hot, dry regions of the Middle East and North Africa, particularly Sudan. Cases may occur in adults who are in close contact with infected children, typically in impoverished or unsanitary environments with poor hygiene.

3. Causative agents—*Treponema pallidum* subsp. *endemicum*, a Gram-negative spirochete bacterium in the genus *Treponema* and closely related to the pathogenic treponemal strains causing syphilis, yaws, and pinta. The organism multiplies very slowly in humans and has not been cultured.

4. Diagnosis—See "Yaws." The bacterium causing bejel is morphologically and serologically indistinguishable from other pathogenic treponemes; thus, diagnosis is based on geography and clinical and epidemiologic suspicion in concert with laboratory findings. Pathogenic treponemal diseases are confirmed on the basis of darkfield or direct fluorescent antibody microscopic examination of lesion exudate during early disease. Serologic assays include nontreponemal tests that are reactive in early stages and gradually wane, while treponemal tests remain positive regardless of treatment. Rapid point-of-care tests are increasingly available; most are treponemal tests. Molecular methods using polymerase chain reaction and deoxyribonucleic acid sequencing have been developed that can detect *T. pallidum* subsp. *endemicum*-specific sequences in lesion exudate. In advanced infections, radiographic imaging may show typical bone deformities (e.g., marked cortical thickening).

5. Occurrence—Can be a common disease of childhood in endemic areas where socioeconomic conditions are poor. Low-level transmission occurs in a few areas in the eastern Mediterranean and the Middle East, while major foci exist in the Sahel region (southern border of the Sahara desert). Bejel should be considered in the evaluation of a reactive syphilis serology in any person who has emigrated from an endemic area.

6. Reservoirs—Humans.

7. Incubation period—From 2 weeks to 3 months.

8. Transmission—Infection is spread from person to person (typically from child to child) through direct or indirect contact with infectious early lesions of skin and mucous membranes (e.g., through kissing or the shared use of eating and drinking utensils). Infected individuals are contagious until the moist skin eruptions and mucous patches disappear, which can be several weeks or months. Unlike syphilis, bejel is not transmitted from mother to child during pregnancy. Although believed to be rare, sexual transmission has been reported in bejel cases involving primary genital lesions.

9. Treatment—

Preferred therapy	Benzathine penicillin G:
	• Adults or children ≥ 10 years: 2.4 MU IM as a single dose
	• Children < 10 years: 1.2 MU as a single dose
Alternative therapy options	Azithromycin 20 mg/kg PO (≤ 2 g) as a single dose

(Continued)

(Continued)

Special considerations and comments	<ul><li>Close contacts of those with bejel should receive empiric treatment.</li><li>Skin lesions become noninfectious within 24 hours of treatment; lesions complete healing within 2–4 weeks in most cases.</li><li>Resistance to azithromycin has been reported in yaws and syphilis; however, no data are available for bejel.</li></ul>

Note: IM = intramuscular(ly); MU = million units; PO = oral(ly).

10. Prevention—See "Yaws." Measures apply to all nonvenereal treponematoses. Mass treatment campaigns led by WHO and UNICEF in the 1950s and 1960s greatly reduced endemic treponematoses and bejel was eliminated in some regions (e.g., Bosnia). These campaigns have not been prioritized for many years and epidemiologic data suggest that endemic treponematoses have begun to reemerge in some regions.

11. Special considerations—

1) Reporting: Bejel cases should be reported to the local health authority.

2) For disaster implications and international measures, see "Yaws."

[M. Kamb]

BLASTOMYCOSIS
(North American blastomycosis, Gilchrist's disease)

DISEASE	ICD-10 CODE
BLASTOMYCOSIS	ICD-10 B40

1. Clinical features—A granulomatous systemic mycosis that primarily affects the lungs but with manifestations ranging from subclinical infection to severe and disseminated disease. Pulmonary blastomycosis may be acute or chronic. Acute infection, which often goes unrecognized as blastomycosis, produces symptoms similar to viral and bacterial pneumonia, usually involving cough, fatigue, and frequently fever and chest pain. Chest X-ray often reveals pulmonary infiltrates. The acute disease usually resolves spontaneously after 1 to 3 weeks of illness; however, severe respiratory disease, sometimes involving acute respiratory distress syndrome, can occur even in young previously healthy patients. Chronic pulmonary disease occurs as well; this may last for months and may sometimes be mistaken for malignancy, tuberculosis, or histoplasmosis. Some patients exhibit extrapulmonary infection during or after the resolution of pneumonia. Disseminated disease is more common in the immunocompromised. Cough and chest pain may be mild or absent, and patients may present with infection already spread to other sites, particularly the skin, and less often to bone, prostate, or epididymis. Cutaneous lesions begin as erythematous papules that become verrucous, crusted, or ulcerated and that spread slowly. Untreated disseminated or chronic pulmonary blastomycosis can eventually progress to death.

2. Risk groups—Classically reported to be most common among middle-aged men with outdoor occupations, but also occurs in a wide range of the population, including children. Exposure to soil and waterways is common in outbreak-associated cases.

3. Causative agents—Most disease in North America is caused by *Blastomyces dermatitidis* (teleomorph *Ajellomyces dermatitidis*) and the more recently described *Blastomyces gilchristii*. Both are dimorphic fungi and produce similar clinical manifestations. Other *Blastomyces* spp. have been described and *Emmonsia* spp. may be confused with *Blastomyces*; taxonomy of these organisms is in flux.

4. Diagnosis—Blastomycosis is likely widely underdiagnosed. Patients who receive the diagnosis often receive multiple courses of empiric antibacterial medications, which are ineffective against this fungal disease. When detected, it is commonly diagnosed by culture of respiratory specimens or of body sites (e.g., skin scrapings, joint fluid, cerebrospinal fluid) where disseminated disease manifestations occur. Histopathologic and cytopathologic examination can allow identification of the fungus; polymerase chain reaction (PCR) testing is also used, although PCR methods differ across laboratories. An enzyme immunoassay test is commercially available for detection of antigen in urine, serum, or broncho-alveolar lavage, although sensitivity is low in some populations and cross-reactions with other fungi, particularly *Histoplasma*, can occur. Serologic antibody tests have some limitations as sensitivity and specificity vary with the test employed and antibodies also cross-react with *Histoplasma*. The immunodiffusion test is more sensitive and specific than the complement fixation test and antibodies against A antigen have been reported in 52% to 80% of patients with blastomycosis. No commercially available skin test exists for blastomycosis.

5. Occurrence—Endemic to parts of central and eastern North America. Maps of estimated endemic areas are based on reports of human and animal cases and new cases occur routinely outside of these areas.

Parts of Wisconsin, Minnesota, and Michigan as well as western Ontario have high rates of blastomycosis, although lack of mandatory disease reporting in most of North America limits geographic comparisons. The disease is also known to occur in areas bordering the Mississippi and Ohio river basins and in midwestern states and Canadian provinces that border the Great Lakes and the St. Lawrence River seaway. Autochthonous blastomycosis cases have also been reported in western North America and outside the continent; however, some of these cases have since been identified as fungi other than the 2 *Blastomyces* spp. described earlier and involve a wide range of clinical manifestations.

6. Reservoirs—Moist soil and decomposing matter such as wood and leaves, particularly in wooded areas along waterways and in undisturbed places, such as under porches or sheds. However, much remains unknown about the habitat of these organisms, in part because it is difficult to isolate *Blastomyces* spp. from the environment. Disease is common in dogs and has also been reported in cats and other animals, but animals do not appear to directly transmit the disease to humans.

7. Incubation period—For symptomatic infections, typically reported as 3 to 6 months.

8. Transmission—Inhalation of conidia in spore-laden dust, typically of the mold or saprophytic growth forms. No person-to-person transmission with the exception of rare pregnancy-associated transmission from mother to neonate.

9. Treatment—

Preferred therapy	Mild-to-moderate pulmonary/disseminated disease: • Itraconazole 200 mg PO TID for 3 days THEN • Itraconazole 200 mg PO once daily or BID for 6–12 months[a]
	Moderately severe to severe pulmonary/disseminated disease: • Lipid AMB 3–5 mg/kg/day IV OR • Deoxycholate AMB 0.7–1 mg/kg/day IV for 1–2 weeks, THEN itraconazole 200 mg PO TID for 3 days, THEN 200 mg BID for 6–12 months[b]

	CNS disease:
	• Lipid AMB 5 mg/kg/day IV for 4–6 weeks, THEN 1 of the following for ≥ 1 year:
	  o Fluconazole 800 mg PO daily
	  o Itraconazole 200 mg PO BID or TID
	  o Voriconazole 200–400 mg BID

(Continued)

(Continued)

	Immunosuppressed patients: • Lipid AMB 3–5 mg/kg/day IV OR • Deoxycholate AMB 0.7–1 mg/kg/day IV for 1–2 weeks, THEN itraconazole 200 mg PO TID for 3 days, and THEN itraconazole 200 mg PO BID for at least a total of 12 months
	Pregnant women[c]: • Lipid AMB 3–5 mg/kg/day IV
	Newborns showing evidence of infection: • Deoxycholate AMB 1 mg/kg/day IV
	Children with mild-to-moderate disease: • Itraconazole 10 mg/kg/day PO for 6–12 months
	Children with moderately severe to severe disease: • Deoxycholate AMB 0.7–1 mg/kg/day IV OR • Lipid AMB 3–5 mg/kg/day IV for 1–2 weeks, THEN itraconazole 10 mg/kg/day PO for a total of 12 months
Alternative therapy options	Alternative but less effective therapy options for mild or moderate pulmonary disease: • Fluconazole 400 or 800 mg PO daily • Ketoconazole 400 or 800 mg PO daily (greater potential for toxicity)
Special considerations and comments	• Immunosuppressed patients may need lifelong suppressive treatment if the immunosuppression cannot be reversed. • Itraconazole should be avoided in pregnancy. • The maximum daily dose of itraconazole in children is 400 mg. • Serum levels of itraconazole should be obtained when possible after 2 weeks of therapy to ensure adequate drug exposure.

Note: AMB = amphotericin B; BID = twice daily; CNS = central nervous system; IV = intravenous(ly); PO = oral(ly); TID = thrice daily.

[a] Treat osteoarticular disease for 12 months.
[b] Treat disseminated disease for 12 months.
[c] Duration of treatment in pregnant women has not been studied, and IDSA guidelines do not include a recommended treatment duration.

10. Prevention—There is no vaccine to prevent blastomycosis and it may not be possible to completely avoid being exposed to *Blastomyces* spp. in areas where it is common in the environment. People who have weakened immune systems may want to consider avoiding activities that involve disrupting soil in these areas.

11. Special considerations—Immunocompromised persons are more likely to develop disseminated disease.

Bibliography

Brown EM, McTaggart LR, Zhang SX, Low DE, Stevens DA, Richardson SE. Phylogenetic analysis reveals a cryptic species Blastomyces gilchristii, sp. nov. within the human pathogenic fungus Blastomyces dermatitidis. *PLoS One.* 2013;8(3):e59237.

Castillo CG, Kauffman CA, Miceli MH. Blastomycosis. *Infect Dis Clin N Am.* 2016;30(1): 247-264.

Chapman SW. Clinical practice guidelines for the management of blastomycosis: 2008 update by the Infectious Diseases Society of America. *Clin Infect Dis.* 2008;46(12): 1801-1812.

McDonald R, Dufort E, Jackson BR, et al. Notes from the field: blastomycosis cases occurring outside of regions with known endemicity—New York, 2007-2017. *MMWR Morb Mortal Wkly Rep.* 2018;67(38):1077-1078.

Schwartz IS, Govender NP, Sigler L, et al. *Emergomyces:* the global rise of new dimorphic fungal pathogens. *PLoS Pathog.* 2019;15(9):e1007977.

Schwartz IS, Wiederhold NP, Hanson KE, Patterson TF, Sigler L. Blastomyces helicus, a new dimorphic fungus causing fatal pulmonary and systemic disease in humans and animals in Western Canada and the United States. *Clin Infect Dis.* 2019;68(2):188-195.

[M. Toda, B. Jackson]

BOTULISM

DISEASE	ICD-10 CODE
BOTULISM	ICD-10 A05.1

1. Clinical features—Botulism is a severe neuroparalytic illness resulting from irreversible blockade of acetylcholine release from presynaptic nerve endings by botulinum toxin. Beyond infancy (i.e., > 1 year) it manifests as bilateral cranial nerve palsies followed by bilateral descending flaccid paralysis. Signs and symptoms typically include some or all of the following: ptosis, diplopia, blurred vision, dysphagia, dysarthria, and ophthalmoplegia. Autonomic symptoms such as constipation commonly occur. Patients maintain their baseline mental status. Gastrointestinal symptoms, including nausea, vomiting, and diarrhea, can occur in foodborne botulism. Illness may include respiratory failure and death if mechanical ventilation and supportive care are not provided. Most patients recover if diagnosed and treated promptly, but recovery may take months and some have residual weakness. Symptoms in infants younger than 1 year typically start with constipation and may include poor suck, altered cry, weakness, and loss of head control. Infant botulism ranges from a mild illness with gradual onset to severe paralysis and respiratory failure. Mortality from infant botulism is rare; the prevalence was about 0.1% during 2000–2009 in the USA, where 85% of all reported infant botulism cases occur.

2. Risk groups—Susceptibility to foodborne botulism is general. Persons who eat improperly home-preserved foods are at increased risk of foodborne botulism.

Almost all infants hospitalized with intestinal botulism are younger than 6 months. Infants younger than 1 year who are fed honey are at increased risk for infant botulism. Adult intestinal colonization is rare and poorly understood. Suspected risk factors include use of antimicrobial agents or presence of an anatomic or functional bowel abnormality. Persons who use injection drugs, particularly black tar heroin, are at increased risk of wound botulism. Persons who receive very high doses of botulinum toxin for therapeutic purposes may be at increased risk of iatrogenic botulism.

3. Causative agents—Botulinum toxin is a potent neurotoxin that is one of the most lethal substances known. Botulinum toxin is produced by *Clostridium botulinum*; it is also produced by some strains of *Clostridium butyricum*, *Clostridium baratii*, and *Clostridium argentinense*. These Gram-positive spore formers are present in the environment but only grow and produce toxin under specific conditions in food products (see Transmission in this chapter), in contaminated wounds, and in the intestinal tract of infants and adults with structurally or functionally compromised intestinal tracts (e.g., intestinal surgery, antibiotic use). Of the 7 recognized serotypes of botulinum toxin (types A–G), the most common serotypes associated with naturally occurring human illness are A, B, E, and F.

4. Diagnosis—Botulism is clinically diagnosed and confirmed by a laboratory. Other neurologic disorders resembling botulism in noninfants include myasthenia gravis, tick paralysis, and Guillain-Barré syndrome; those in infants include sepsis and electrolyte imbalances. Illnesses confused with botulism can be hard to differentiate in the early workup. Botulism should be considered and antitoxin administered early in the workup as more common diseases are evaluated. Routine hospital laboratory studies are not helpful in diagnosing botulism but may help rule out other illnesses. Electromyography can support the clinical diagnosis of botulism.

1) Foodborne: confirmed by detecting botulinum toxin in serum, stools, or gastric aspirate or through culture of botulinum toxin-producing clostridia from gastric aspirate or stools in a clinically compatible case. Laboratory confirmation of a foodborne case can also be achieved by detecting botulinum toxin in a food source known to have been consumed by the patient. Botulism is considered confirmed in persons with a consistent clinical syndrome who consumed a food item implicated in a laboratory-confirmed case.

2) Infant intestinal: confirmed by detecting botulinum toxin in clinical specimens (serum or stools) or by isolating botulinum toxin-producing clostridia from stool specimens from an infant younger than 1 year.

3) Wound: confirmed by culture of botulinum toxin-producing clostridia from a wound or detection of botulinum toxin in serum in a patient with a history of a contaminated wound or injection drug use within 2 weeks before onset of symptoms.

4) Other: a designation as other botulism occurs when a clinically compatible case is confirmed by a laboratory in a patient aged 1 year or older who has no history of ingestion of suspect food and has no wounds. Some of these cases are suspected to be adult intestinal colonization cases due to complicating medical factors and/or prolonged excretion of botulinum toxin-producing clostridia in stools.

5. Occurrence—Botulism is likely underrecognized and underreported. Although the worldwide incidence is unknown, cases have been reported in the Americas, Africa, Asia, Australia, Europe, and the Middle East. Outbreaks of foodborne botulism occur when food is prepared by methods that do not destroy spores and is preserved under conditions that permit toxin formation. The foods implicated reflect local eating habits and food-preservation procedures. Although primarily reported in the USA, infant and wound botulism have been reported in other countries.

6. Reservoirs—Botulinum toxin-producing clostridia are ubiquitous in soil. Spores are frequently recovered from agricultural products, including honey and vegetables, and are also found in dust, soil, lake and marine sediments, and the intestinal tracts of animals, including fish. Toxin is produced only under conditions that promote spore germination, growth, and toxin production.

7. Incubation period—Generally, the shorter the incubation period, the more severe the disease. Neurologic symptoms of foodborne botulism usually appear within 12 to 72 hours of toxin ingestion, but onset can range from 2 hours to 8 days. The incubation period of botulism due to intestinal colonization in infants is estimated to be up to 30 days but for adults is unknown (see Transmission in this chapter); the incubation period for iatrogenic botulism is unclear. For wound botulism, the incubation period is generally 4 to 14 days. The 3 known cases of inhalational botulism occurred among laboratory workers with a work-related exposure to botulinum neurotoxin; patients had neurologic symptoms similar to those in foodborne botulism and recovered within 2 weeks of the exposure.

8. Transmission—Person-to-person transmission does not occur. Mode of transmission varies by transmission category.

1) Foodborne: occurs by ingestion of preformed toxin in contaminated low-acid foods. Spores of botulinum toxin-producing clostridia present in food germinate and produce the toxin before the food is eaten; sufficient heating inactivates the toxin. Growth and toxin formation require an anaerobic environment, moisture, neutral-to-alkaline pH, and an energy source such as sugar or protein. These conditions are most often present in lightly preserved foods (such as fermented, lightly salted, or smoked fish and meat products) and in inadequately processed home-preserved foods (such as home-canned vegetables and garlic in oil) that are low in sugar, salt, and acid. Outbreaks have been linked to foods that have been inadequately stored, such as frozen chili product, chilled commercial soup, and flash pasteurized carrot juice. Occasionally, commercially prepared foods or restaurant-prepared foods are involved. However, foodborne botulism is more often due to home-canned vegetables such as green beans; home-canned tomatoes, formerly considered too acidic to support growth of *C. botulinum*, have been linked to botulism cases. Outbreaks have occurred following consumption of uneviscerated fish, baked potatoes, improperly handled commercially produced pot pies, pruno (an alcoholic beverage produced illicitly in prisons), sautéed onions, fermented bean curd, and minced garlic in oil.

   In Canada and the USA (specifically Alaska), outbreaks have been associated with seal meat, fermented whale blubber, salmon, salmon eggs, and other traditional foods that are processed and consumed without cooking. In Europe, most cases are associated with sausages and smoked or preserved meats; in Japan, with fermented fish. Foodborne transmission could hypothetically be used by bioterrorists for intentional exposure.

2) Intestinal (infant and adult): occurs after ingestion of botulinum spores rather than by ingestion of preformed toxin. Ingested spores germinate and produce botulinum toxin in the colon. Colonization is believed to occur in infants because normal bowel flora that compete with *C. botulinum* have not been fully established. Sources of spores for infant botulism include honey and dust, although the source is unknown in most cases. Adult intestinal botulism is poorly understood but typically occurs in adults who have altered intestinal flora because of antimicrobial use or because of anatomic or functional bowel abnormalities.

3) Wound: occurs when a wound is contaminated by *C. botulinum* spores that germinate and produce toxin inside the wound. Since the 1990s, wound botulism has emerged among chronic drug abusers in some parts of Europe and North America, primarily in

dermal abscesses from subcutaneous or intramuscular injection (skin or muscle popping) of black tar heroin. Wound botulism also results from contamination of wounds or open fractures with soil or gravel.

4) Inhalational: inhalation of aerosolized botulinum neurotoxin has been documented only once—among laboratory workers. This transmission mode could hypothetically be used by bioterrorists for intentional exposure.

5) Iatrogenic: commercial preparations of botulinum toxin are injected for cosmetic and other indications, including ophthalmologic disorders, movement disorders, neuromuscular disorders, and pain. Laboratory-confirmed iatrogenic botulism has occurred after injection of high doses of an unapproved botulinum toxin product.

9. Treatment—Supportive care, possibly including intensive care, and provision of botulinum antitoxin. Antitoxin is most effective when given early in the clinical course. Antibiotics do not have a role except in secondary infection.

10. Prevention—

1) Foodborne botulism can be prevented by sound food preparation practices, including proper canning of commercially canned foods.

   - Home-preserved foods should be prepared following directions such as those provided by the US Department of Agriculture (http://nchfp.uga.edu/publications/publications_usda.html) so that bacterial spores are inactivated and toxin is not produced.
   - Commercial heat pasteurization alone may not kill all spores, so a second barrier to organism growth and toxin production, such as acidification, should be considered for these products (e.g., vacuum-packed pasteurized and hot-smoked products).
   - Proper storage can prevent the growth of *C. botulinum* and toxin formation. Consumers should read and follow all manufacturers' recommendations for storage of food products, including temperature and shelf life.
   - Boiling of foods for 10 minutes may destroy the toxin; however, if food is suspected of containing botulinum toxin it should be discarded since there is a risk that uniform heating will not occur throughout the product.

2) Infants should not be fed honey. This may prevent some cases of infant botulism.

3) Adult intestinal colonization is poorly understood and prevention strategies are not known.

4) Wound botulism can be prevented by not using injection drugs (specifically black tar heroin) and by thorough cleaning of wounds contaminated by soil.

5) Iatrogenic botulism may be prevented by using commercially manufactured therapeutic botulinum toxin and by avoiding injections of doses higher than those recommended by the manufacturer and for conditions not approved by regulators.

11. Special considerations—

1) Reporting: reporting of suspected and confirmed cases is obligatory in most countries; an immediate phone report to public health authorities is indicated.

2) Outbreaks: a single case of suspected foodborne botulism should immediately raise suspicion of an outbreak. Home-preserved foods are the most common sources of foodborne botulism. However, in the rare situations when restaurant food or widely distributed commercially preserved food is contaminated, many people may be exposed, posing a major public health threat. Food implicated by epidemiologic or laboratory findings requires immediate recall. An immediate search for persons sharing the suspect food and for any remaining food from the same source should be performed. Suspected foods along with clinical specimens should be submitted for laboratory examination. International common source outbreaks have occurred from widely distributed commercial products; international efforts may be required to recover and test implicated foods.

3) Deliberate use: attempts to develop and use botulinum toxin as a bioweapon have been made. Although these attempts have been unsuccessful so far, foodborne, waterborne, and aerosolized toxin exposures could all hypothetically be caused intentionally. Outbreaks associated with commercial food products should be investigated with the possibility of intentional contamination in mind. The occurrence of several seemingly unrelated cases in the same time frame should raise the question of a contaminated commercially distributed food source or deliberate use of botulinum toxin. Suspicion of inhalational botulism, outside of a laboratory setting, would indicate intentional use.

[J. Hughes]

❖

BRUCELLOSIS
(undulant fever, Malta fever, Mediterranean fever)

DISEASE	ICD-10 CODE
BRUCELLOSIS	ICD-10 A23.9

1. Clinical features—Brucellosis is a systemic bacterial disease caused by small, Gram-negative, intracellular coccobacilli; it is associated with high morbidity in humans and animals. The disease is contracted as a result of contact between humans and infected animal fluids or tissue products and is a major cause of zoonoses worldwide. Brucellosis is characterized by both acute and chronic illness with a wide array of clinical symptoms but almost always includes fever with evidence of localized infection. Common features include headache, weakness, profuse sweating that can be malodorous, arthralgias, myalgias, fatigue, anorexia, back pain, weight loss, and depression. The fever may be undulant or variable if left untreated. Physical examination is non-specific, though generalized lymphadenopathy, hepatomegaly, or spleno-megaly is often present. A mild transaminitis is common and granulomas may be present on liver biopsy specimens. Hematologic abnormalities, such as cytopenias (typically leukopenia with relative lymphocytosis, anemia, throm-bocytopenia, or pancytopenia), may be seen but are usually mild when present. Osteoarticular complications occur in 20% to 60% of cases with sacroi-liitis being the most frequent joint manifestation. Genitourinary involvement is seen in 2% to 20% of cases, with orchitis and epididymitis as common mani-festations. Neurobrucellosis is a less common but more severe manifestation that occurs in approximately 10% of cases. Cerebrospinal fluid (CSF) typically includes a pleocytosis of 10 to 200 white blood cells (predominantly mono-nuclear cells), elevated protein levels, and hypoglycorrhachia. Similar to tuberculous meningitis, the CSF adenosine deaminase can be elevated.

Clinical symptoms occur 2 to 4 weeks after exposure and may last for days, months, or occasionally a year or longer if not adequately treated. Treatment with appropriate antibiotics leads to recovery but long-term dis-ability is often pronounced. Relapses have been reported in up to 15% of patients and usually occur within the first 6 months after appropriate treat-ment. Relapse is associated with objective clinical symptoms, such as fever and persistent localized foci of infection in addition to abnormal laboratory markers indicating sustained infection. Overall, mortality in appropriately treated cases is less than 1%, mostly attributed to endocarditis.

2. Risk groups—Brucellosis is predominantly an occupational disease of those working with infected animals, especially farm workers, veterinarians, and slaughterhouse workers, who are at increased risk for contracting the disease as a result of handling infected animal tissues or being exposed to their secretions. Medical personnel in endemic regions may be at risk when participating in activities characterized by gross exposure to contaminated fomites or tissues or as a result of massive bleeding, such as certain obstetric procedures. Brucellosis is among the most common laboratory-acquired bacterial infections and its high communicability warrants biosafety level 3 precautions. Persons consuming undercooked meat and unpasteurized dairy products are at increased risk.

3. Causative agents—Multiple species have been isolated with 4 main species found to be pathogenic in humans: *Brucella abortus, Brucella melitensis, Brucella suis*, and *Brucella canis*.

4. Diagnosis—*Brucella* can be isolated on culture, with the highest yield from bone marrow or blood specimens. Laboratory personnel should be notified in advance given the high risk of occupational exposure via aerosols or direct contact. Although most *Brucella* spp. reproduce in aerobic conditions, *B. abortus* and *B. suis* are microaerophilic and require 5% to 10% CO_2. Several polymerase chain reaction assays are currently available for isolates to identify *Brucella* at the species level. A 4-fold rise in *Brucella*-specific immunoglobulin class G antibody titers on a serum agglutination assay is the serologic method of choice in diagnosing acute, noncomplicated cases of brucellosis caused by *B. abortus, B. melitensis*, or *B. suis* and usually declines with treatment. For chronic, complicated, or neurobrucellosis cases, serologic assays other than agglutination, such as enzyme-linked immunosorbent assay, are recommended. Serologic tests to detect *B. canis* antibodies are not performed routinely by diagnostic laboratories.

5. Occurrence—Worldwide, especially in Mediterranean countries, the Middle East, Africa, Central Asia, India, Central and South America, and Mexico. Sources of infection and responsible organism vary according to geographic area. Cases are increasingly documented in nonendemic regions after international travel to endemic areas, import of infected livestock, as well as consumption of unpasteurized dairy products.

6. Reservoirs—Cattle, swine, goats, and sheep are most common. Infection can occur in camels, bison, elk, equids, caribou, and some species of deer. *B. canis* is an occasional challenge in laboratory dog colonies and kennels; a small percentage of pet dogs and a higher proportion of stray dogs have positive *B. canis* antibody titers. Marine mammals can be infected with *Brucella ceti* (whales, porpoises, dolphins) and *Brucella pinnipedialis* (seals, sea lions, walruses).

7. Incubation period—Variable and difficult to ascertain; 1 to 2 months is commonplace, with a range of 5 days to 5 months.

8. Transmission—Contact through mucous membranes and breaks in the skin with animal tissues, blood, urine, vaginal discharges, aborted fetuses, and especially placentas as well as ingestion of undercooked meat, raw milk, and dairy products (unpasteurized cheese) from infected animals. Airborne infection has been reported in laboratory and slaughterhouse workers. Isolated cases of infection with *B. canis* occur in animal handlers from contact with dogs and with *B. suis* in hunters from contact with feral swine and other game animals. Rare cases of infection with newly described marine-associated *Brucella* spp. have been reported. A small number of cases have resulted from accidental self-inoculation with *B. abortus* strain 19 animal vaccine or with the attenuated *B. abortus* RB51 cattle vaccine; the same risk is present when *B. melitensis* Rev-1 vaccine is handled. Person-to-person transmission is rare and is possibly related to sexual transmission. Breastfeeding women may transmit infections to their infants.

9. Treatment—

Drug	For uncomplicated brucellosis (no endocarditis, spondylitis, neurobrucellosis, or localized suppurative lesions): • Doxycycline 100 mg PO BID for 6 weeks AND • Streptomycin 1 g IM once daily for the first 14–21 days
Alternative drug	Gentamycin (5 mg/kg IM for the first 5–14 days) or rifampin (15 mg/kg, 600 mg, or 900 mg PO once daily for 6 weeks)[a] may be substituted for streptomycin. Alternatively, ciprofloxacin (500 mg PO BID for 6 weeks) may be substituted for doxycycline or rifampin but is not considered first-line treatment.
Special considerations and comments	• Monotherapy is usually not recommended and is associated with frequent therapeutic failures or relapses. • Spondylitis: treatment should consist of 2 antibiotic agents (preferably doxycycline and streptomycin) for at least 12 weeks. • Neurobrucellosis: treatment should consist of 2 or 3 antibiotics that cross the blood-brain barrier. Regimens include doxycycline, rifampin, and either ceftriaxone (dosed as 2 g IV every 12 hours) or TMP/SMX (1 double-strength tablet BID) for at least 12 weeks. • Endocarditis: treatment should include 2 or 3 drugs (inclusion of an aminoglycoside is favored) for at least 6 weeks to 6 months. Surgical intervention is almost always needed in addition to antibiotics. • Pregnancy: treatment should include rifampin (900 mg PO once daily) with either TMP/SMX (1 double-strength tablet BID) or ceftriaxone (2 g IV every 12 hours) for 6 weeks. • Children < 8 years with uncomplicated disease: TMP/SMX (TMP 10 mg/kg/day, ≤ 320 mg/day; SMX 50 mg/kg/day, ≤ 1.6 g/day) divided in 2 doses for 6 weeks PLUS rifampin (15–20 mg/kg/day, ≤ 900 mg/day) PO once daily for 6 weeks. • Children ≥ 8 years with uncomplicated disease: doxycycline (> 45 kg: 100 mg IV BID, THEN 100 mg PO BID; < 45 kg: 2.2 mg/kg IV BID, THEN 2.2 mg/kg PO) and rifampin (10–15 mg/kg/day IV as a single dose, THEN 10–15 mg/kg/day PO as a single dose) for 6 weeks. • Surgery may be warranted for localized abscess or neurologic deficit.

Note: BID = twice daily; IM = intramuscular(ly); IV = intravenous(ly); PO = oral(ly); TMP/SMX = trimethoprim-sulfamethoxazole.
[a]Rifampin dose based on clinical judgment.

10. Prevention—Prevention of human brucellosis rests on the elimination of the infection among domestic animals.

1) Educate the public (especially tourists) regarding the risks associated with consuming undercooked meat or unpasteurized dairy products.

2) Educate farmers and workers in slaughterhouses, meat-processing plants, and butcher shops about the nature of the disease and the risk in handling carcasses and products from potentially infected animals, particularly products of parturition, to reduce exposure.

3) Educate hunters to use protective outfits (gloves, clothing) when handling feral swine or other potentially infected wildlife (elk, bison, moose, and caribou/reindeer), to practice good hand hygiene techniques, to avoid eating meat from animals that appear sick, and to bury animal remains.

4) Search for infection among livestock by serologic testing or testing of cow's milk (ring test) and eliminate infected animals through segregation and/or slaughtering. Infection among swine usually requires slaughter of the herd. In high-prevalence areas, it is important to immunize young goats and sheep with *B. melitensis* Rev-1 vaccine as well as calves and (sometimes) adult animals with *B. abortus* strain 19. Since 1996, RB51 has largely replaced strain 19 for immunization of cattle against *B. abortus* in the USA. Currently, there is no vaccine for swine against *B. suis*.

5) Pasteurize milk and dairy products from cows, sheep, and goats. Boiling milk is effective when pasteurization is impossible.

6) Give emphasis to the importance of appropriate use of personal protective equipment and laboratory ventilation procedures for health care workers handling potentially infected specimens. Postexposure prophylaxis and periodic serologic testing should be considered in high-risk laboratory exposures.

7) Give care in handling and disposal of placentas, uterine discharges, and fetuses, and disinfect contaminated areas.

11. Special considerations—

1) Reporting: report cases to local health authorities, which is obligatory in most countries.

2) Epidemic measures: search for a common vehicle of infection, usually raw milk or milk products (especially cheese) from an infected herd. Recall incriminated products and stop production and distribution unless pasteurization is instituted.

3) The potential to infect humans and animals through aerosol exposure, combined with a low infectious dose of 10 to 100 organisms, has led

to *Brucella* spp. being considered as potential biologic weapons. CDC has classified brucellosis as a category B biologic weapon owing to the ease of facilitated transmission.

Bibliography

CDC. *Brucellosis Reference Guide: Exposures, Testing, and Prevention.* February 2017. Available at: https://www.cdc.gov/brucellosis/pdf/brucellosi-reference-guide.pdf. Accessed December 3, 2019.

[L. J. Gilbert, R. A. Ressner]

BURULI ULCER

DISEASE	ICD-10 CODE
BURULI ULCER	ICD-10 A31.1

1. Clinical features—Classically presents as a chronic painless skin ulcer with undermined edges and a necrotic white or yellow base (cotton wool appearance). Secondary bacterial infection may occur, causing the ulcer to become painful and giving the lesions a foul smell. Most lesions are located on the extremities and tend to be seen more frequently on lower rather than upper extremities. It often starts as a painless nodule or a papule, which eventually ulcerates; this progression usually takes between 3 weeks and 1 year. Other presentations may be seen, such as indurated plaques or edematous lesions; the latter represent a rapidly disseminating form that does not pass through a nodular stage. Ulcers may remain small and persist for years or may grow and extend widely. Bones and joints may be affected by direct spread from an overlying cutaneous lesion or through the bloodstream. Long-neglected or poorly managed patients usually present with scars that are sometimes hypertrophic or keloid with partially healed areas or disabling contractures, especially for lesions that cross joints. Marjolin ulcers (squamous cell carcinoma) may develop in unstable or chronic nonpigmented scars.

The differential diagnosis includes the following, by dermatologic manifestation:

1) Minor infections: insect bites and a variety of dermatologic conditions.
2) Nodules: cysts, lipomas, boils, onchocercomas, lymphadenitis, mycoses.
3) Plaques: leprosy, cellulitis, mycoses, psoriasis.

4) Edematous forms: cellulitis, elephantiasis, actinomycosis.
5) Ulcers: tropical phagedenic ulcer, diabetic ulcer, leishmaniasis, neurogenic ulcer, yaws, squamous cell carcinoma, pyoderma gangrenosum, noma.

2. Risk groups—Persons who reside in or travel to wetlands in endemic areas. Populations in rural wetlands can be at risk during manual farming activities. Human immunodeficiency virus infection is not a risk factor for *Mycobacterium ulcerans* infection but may exacerbate the clinical course of the disease.

3. Causative agents—*M. ulcerans*, an acid-fast bacillus, is a slow-growing environmental mycobacterium. *M. ulcerans* secretes mycolactone, a virulence factor that destroys tissues and locally suppresses immune activity. Three variants of cytopathic mycolactones may be produced by *M. ulcerans*, the type and amount varying by strain. African strains, which produce the greatest number and amount (and most potent variants) of mycolactone, are associated with the more severe forms of disease.

4. Diagnosis—An experienced clinician in endemic areas can usually diagnose on clinical grounds. Swabs, fine-needle aspirates, and biopsy specimens can be sent to the laboratory for confirmation by the Ziehl-Neelsen stain for acid-fast bacilli, culture, polymerase chain reaction (PCR), and histopathology. PCR is the most sensitive and specific method of diagnosis. Histopathologically, active lesions have contiguous coagulation necrosis of subcutaneous fat and acid-fast bacilli present.

5. Occurrence—*M. ulcerans* infection has been reported in more than 30 countries, mostly tropical, and tends to be seen most frequently in children younger than 15 years in rural areas. The global burden of the disease is yet to be determined. Based on the available data, Africa is the continent most affected, although disease also occurs in Australia, Japan, and South America. Numbers of reported cases have been increasing over the last 25 years, most strikingly in western Africa, where *M. ulcerans* disease is second only to tuberculosis in terms of mycobacterial disease prevalence following the elimination of leprosy as a public health problem in these countries. Australia has also been seeing increasing numbers of cases since 2013. In some endemic districts and communities, it is the most prevalent mycobacterial disease.

6. Reservoirs—Evidence points to the fauna, flora, and other ecologic aspects of tropical or subtropical wetlands. The bacterium has been identified as a commensal organism in insects, snails, and fish; further studies are needed to clarify their roles as natural hosts for *M. ulcerans*. In Australia, it has been described not only in humans but also in native animals including the koala (*Phascolarctos cinereus*), the brushtail and ringtail possums (family Phalangeridae), and the long-footed potoroo (*Potorous longipes*); infection has also been reported in a domesticated alpaca (*Lama pacos*). All of these infections, except for those in the potoroo, occurred in focal areas where human cases were known to have occurred.

7. Incubation period—Average of 2 to 3 months; however, anecdotal observations have suggested that *M. ulcerans* infections could exhibit longer periods of latency and some infections may progress over a matter of weeks. Similarly to tuberculosis, it is believed that only a small proportion of infected people develop clinically apparent disease.

8. Transmission—The mode of transmission is mostly speculative but regular contact with a contaminated aquatic environment and local trauma to the skin have been shown to be risk factors. In most studies, a significant number of patients had antecedent trauma at the site of the ulcer. Environmental changes that promote flooding, such as deforestation, dam construction, and irrigation systems, are often associated with outbreaks of Buruli ulcer. Lack of protected water supplies contributes to dependence on pond water for domestic use and potential exposure; aerosols arising from stagnant waters may disseminate *M. ulcerans*. Studies have shown a significant association between *M. ulcerans* in the environment and Buruli ulcer cases in neighboring villages; evidence suggests aquatic biting insects may also play a role in transmitting infection to humans. There is also some recent evidence suggesting that mosquitoes may be involved in transmission; however, this has not been definitively demonstrated. Only 1 case of possible direct human-to-human transmission of Buruli ulcer has been described. Factors that probably determine the type of disease are dose of agent, depth of inoculation, and host immunologic response. Bacillus Calmette-Guérin (BCG) neonatal vaccination appears to protect against *M. ulcerans* osteomyelitis in patients with skin lesions.

9. Treatment—

Drug	• Rifampicin • Clarithromycin • Streptomycin
Dose	• Rifampicin 10 mg/kg PO once daily PLUS • Clarithromycin 7.5 mg/kg PO BID OR • Rifampicin 10 mg/kg PO once daily PLUS • Streptomycin 15 mg/kg IM once daily
Route	• Rifampicin/clarithromycin PO • Rifampicin/streptomycin PO/IM

(Continued)

(Continued)

Alternative drug	• Moxifloxacin 400 mg PO once daily PLUS rifampicin 10 mg/kg PO once daily
Duration	• Rifampicin/clarithromycin 8 weeks • Rifampicin/streptomycin 8 weeks
Special considerations and comments	• Antibiotic treatment alone is highly effective for lesions < 10 cm diameter. • Wound care and physiotherapy should be included as a part of patient care to promote healing and prevent disability. • Adjunctive surgery (debridement, skin grafting) may be indicated after 4 weeks of antibiotic therapy for larger lesions. • Rifampicin PO plus amikacin IV may be useful in patients with severe extensive disease or in those with disease that involves tendons, muscles, nerves, joints, bones, or areas such as the face to minimize surgery.

Note: BID = twice daily; IM = intramuscular(ly); IV = intravenous(ly); PO = oral(ly).

10. Prevention—

1) Health education on the disease for populations at risk.
2) Wearing protective clothing and shoes covering the extremities.
3) Provision of a protected water supply.
4) Avoidance of insect bites, use of insect repellents.
5) BCG neonatal vaccination may provide short-term prophylaxis.
6) Prompt cleansing of abrasions or wounds antiseptically.

11. Special considerations—

1) Although neither notifiable nor contagious from person to person, it is recommended that cases be reported to local health authorities so that the geographic distribution can be clearly defined.
2) International measures: endemic countries should coordinate efforts across borders. Further information can be found at: http://www.who.int/buruli/en. It can also be found from WHO Collaborating Centres, which provide support as required, at: http://apps.who.int/whocc/Detail.aspx?cc_ref=BEL-40&cc_code=bel&cc_city=antwerp& and http://apps.who.int/whocc/Detail.aspx?cc_ref=AUS-95&cc_ref=aus-95&.

[D. Blaney]

CAMPYLOBACTER ENTERITIS

DISEASE	ICD-10 CODE
CAMPYLOBACTER ENTERITIS	ICD-10 A04.5

1. Clinical features—Prodromal fever and malaise often occur before diarrhea. Enteritis typically manifests as the abrupt onset of abdominal pain that can become continuous and is quickly accompanied by profuse watery stools. Stools often contain mucus and blood. Abdominal pain and fever are less common and nausea is more common among children than adults. Bacteremia occurs in approximately 1% of cases and can lead to localized intestinal complications and, occasionally, to seeding of extraintestinal foci. Endovascular infection, myopericarditis, and meningoencephalitis have been reported. Overall case fatality is approximately 0.1% in well-resourced settings. After acute illness, some patients (< 5%) develop reactive arthritis or, rarely (~ 0.1%), Guillain-Barré syndrome, typically within a few weeks of illness onset. *Campylobacter* infection has also been linked to development of irritable bowel syndrome. Infection with *Campylobacter fetus* is associated with persistent bacteremia and increased risk of extraintestinal infection.

2. Risk groups—Travelers to regions with higher incidence of campylobacteriosis than at home are at increased risk of infection. By contrast, persons who grow up in resource-poor settings may be protected from progression to clinical enteritis by immunity that develops from frequent childhood infections. People with decreased stomach acid levels, such as those taking proton pump inhibitors, are at increased risk of infection. People older than 80 years, those who are immunocompromised, or those with other serious comorbidities are at elevated risk of bacteremia. However, bacteremia can occur even among previously healthy people.

3. Causative agents—*Campylobacter jejuni* and, less commonly, *Campylobacter coli* are the usual causes of *Campylobacter* diarrhea. Several subtyping methods are available that may be helpful for epidemiologic purposes, especially in outbreak settings. Other *Campylobacter* spp., including *Campylobacter lari*, *C. fetus*, and *Campylobacter upsaliensis*, have been associated with illness among both normal and immunocompromised hosts.

4. Diagnosis—Definitive diagnosis is based on isolation of the organism from a clinical specimen. Selective media, microaerobic growth conditions, and incubation at 42°C (107.6°F) are recommended. Standard culture methods may not detect all species, particularly *C. fetus* and *C. upsaliensis*. Visualization of motile and curved, spiral, or S-shaped rods similar to those of *Vibrio cholerae* by stool phase contrast or dark-field microscopy can provide rapid presumptive evidence for *Campylobacter* infection. Culture-independent diagnostic tests (CIDTs), including nucleic acid and antigen-based methods, can detect *Campylobacter* (including *C. jejuni*, *C. coli*, and *C. upsaliensis*) in stool specimens. Diagnostic laboratories have been markedly increasing the use of CIDTs. However, a bacterial isolate is required for antibiotic susceptibility testing. Likewise, an isolate is required for whole-genome sequencing, which can be used for strain characterization and to predict likely resistance; whole-genome sequencing has also been used to help detect and identify the sources of outbreaks.

5. Occurrence—*Campylobacter* is an important cause of diarrheal illness worldwide. In industrialized countries, males and children younger than 5 years have the highest incidence of illness. In developing countries, illness is confined largely to children younger than 2 years. *Campylobacter* is a major cause of travelers' diarrhea. Common-source outbreaks are rarely detected. Those that are detected are most often associated with unpasteurized dairy products, undercooked poultry, and untreated water. In temperate areas, most infections occur in the warmer months, when there is a significant rise in *Campylobacter* prevalence among live chickens.

6. Reservoirs—Common hosts for *Campylobacter* spp. include animals (most frequently poultry and cattle, but also puppies, kittens, other pets, swine, sheep, rodents, and birds), and these animals may be sources of human infection. In many countries, raw poultry meat is commonly contaminated with *C. jejuni*. For example, in the USA, 24% of chicken tested from a sample of grocery stores yielded *Campylobacter* in 2015.

7. Incubation period—Usually 2 to 4 days, with a range of 1 to 10 days, depending on dose ingested and host.

8. Transmission—Through ingestion of the organisms in undercooked meat (particularly poultry), unpasteurized dairy products, or other contaminated food; untreated water; or from direct or indirect contact with infected animals, especially puppies, kittens, and farm animals. The infectious dose can be as little as 500 organisms. Infected persons not treated with antibiotics may excrete organisms for 2 to 7 weeks; however, person-to-person transmission is uncommon.

9. Treatment—The use of oral rehydration solution or intravenous fluids as needed is the mainstay of treatment. Antimotility agents should be avoided in children and in patients with bloody stools or fever.

Although antibiotics reduce duration of diarrhea by approximately 1.5 days and reduce bacterial shedding, the illness usually resolves on its own. Treatment is recommended if patients have severe disease or risk factors for severe disease, such as older age or an immunocompromising condition. Antibiotic choice should be guided by antimicrobial susceptibility: quinolone resistance is high in many regions and macrolide resistance has been increasing. Whenever possible, antibiotic susceptibility should be confirmed. Antibiotics should be continued for at least 3 days or until the resolution of symptoms (although in adults a single 1-g dose of azithromycin can be considered as an alternative); longer duration of therapy may be required for those with complications or underlying immunosuppression.

Patients with bacteremia should be investigated for a possible focal infection. The recommended empiric therapy for bacteremia varies by species; most species are resistant to ampicillin and cephalosporins, whereas *C. fetus* is usually susceptible.

Diagnosis	First Line	Second Line	Comment
Child: enteritis (high fever, blood in stools, or risk factors for severe disease[a])	• Azithromycin PO (10 mg/kg/day for ≥ 3 days) OR • Erythromycin PO (40 mg/kg/day QID for ≥ 5 days)	Consider ciprofloxacin[b,c] PO (10–20 mg/kg ≤ 750 mg/dose BID for ≥ 3 days).	Obtain stool culture before treatment to check antibiotic susceptibility (perform blood culture if risk of severe disease).
Adult: enteritis (high fever, blood in stools, or risk factors for severe disease[a])	• Azithromycin[d] PO (500 mg daily for ≥ 3 days) OR • Erythromycin PO (500 mg BID for ≥ 5 days)[b]	Consider ciprofloxacin[b] PO (500 mg BID for ≥ 3 days).	Obtain stool culture before treatment to check antibiotic susceptibility (perform blood culture if risk of severe disease).

Note: BID = twice daily; QID = 4 times daily.
[a]Risk factors for severe infection include being older than 80 years or being immunocompromised.
[b]In the USA, ~ 70% of isolates from travelers and 16% of isolates from other persons are resistant to ciprofloxacin; 7% of isolates from travelers and < 2% of isolates from others are resistant to azithromycin.
[c]In children, ciprofloxacin can sometimes be a reasonable first-line choice after assessment of risks and benefits of other choices.
[d]In adults, a single dose of azithromycin (1 g) is an alternative.

10. Prevention—

1) Control and prevention measures at all stages of the food chain, from agricultural production to processing, manufacturing, and preparation of foods in both commercial establishments and private homes.

2) Pasteurize all milk and chlorinate or boil water supplies. Thoroughly cook all foods of animal origin, especially poultry, which should reach a minimum internal temperature of 73.9°C (165°F). Avoid cross-contamination—for example, do not use the same cutting board for raw and cooked products and do not allow drippings from raw poultry to contaminate foods that are cooked or that will be eaten raw.

3) Reduce prevalence of *Campylobacter* in meat through specific interventions. Comprehensive control programs and hygienic measures (e.g., attention to biosecurity, changes of boots and clothes, full rather than partial depopulation of poultry houses followed by thorough cleaning and disinfection) can help prevent spread of organisms in poultry and animal farms. Vaccines and competitive exclusion are being investigated as control measures. The use of fly screens in chicken houses seems to reduce prevalence of *Campylobacter*-positive flocks significantly. Good slaughtering, handling, and processing practices, which can include testing of carcasses, can reduce contamination of carcasses and meat products. Further reduction of contamination can be achieved through freezing, chemical carcass decontamination, or irradiation.

4) Recognize, prevent, and control *Campylobacter* infections among domestic animals and pets. Puppies and kittens with or without diarrhea can transmit infection. Keep pets away from food preparation surfaces such as cutting boards and counter tops. Stress handwashing after animal contact.

5) Minimize contact with poultry and their feces. Do not let children younger than 5 years handle or touch chicks, ducklings, or other live poultry without adult supervision. Stress handwashing after contact with poultry and their environment when contact cannot be avoided. Keep backyard poultry out of the kitchen. Promote and use WHO's *Five Keys to Safer Food Manual* to achieve good preparation practices in commercial and domestic kitchens (https://www.who.int/foodsafety/publications/consumer/manual_keys.pdf).

11. Special considerations—Reporting: clinicians should report cases of campylobacteriosis to public health officials as required in each jurisdiction. Campylobacteriosis is nationally notifiable in the USA.

Bibliography

CDC. Campylobacter (campylobacteriosis). 2019. Available at: https://www.cdc.gov/campylobacter/index.html. Accessed May 17, 2018.

National Antimicrobial Resistance Monitoring System. *NARMS Integrated Report, 2015*. Laurel, MD: US Department of Health and Human Services, FDA; 2017.

WHO. 2019. Campylobacter. Available at: http://www.who.int/foodsafety/areas_work/foodborne-diseases/campylobacter/en. Accessed May 17, 2018.

[M. E. Laughlin, I. D. Plumb, K. Chatham-Stephens]

CANDIDIASIS
(moniliasis, thrush, candidosis)

DISEASE	ICD-10 CODE
CANDIDIASIS	ICD-10 B37

1. Clinical features—A mycosis that can cause mucocutaneous or invasive infections. Mucocutaneous infections involve the superficial layers of skin or mucous membranes, presenting clinically as oral thrush, intertrigo, vulvovaginitis, paronychia, or onychomycosis. Ulcers or pseudomembranes may form in the esophagus, stomach, or intestine. Repeated clinical skin or mucosal eruptions are common. Invasive candidiasis, including candidemia and intra-abdominal candidiasis, usually occurs in patients with specific risk factors for infection, such as premature birth, central venous catheters, immunosuppression, antibiotic therapy, abdominal surgery, or critical illness. Injection drug use is also becoming an increasingly commonly risk factor for candidemia. Candidemia may be uncomplicated or may disseminate and cause deep-seated infection in many organs, including the eyes, kidneys, liver, spleen, heart, and central nervous system.

2. Risk groups—Oral thrush is a common, usually benign condition during the first few weeks of life. Clinical disease occurs when host defenses are low. People with diabetes, those with human immunodeficiency virus (HIV) infection, and those treated with broad-spectrum antibiotics or corticosteroids are predisposed to superficial candidiasis. Women in the third trimester of pregnancy are prone to vulvovaginal candidiasis. Factors predisposing to invasive candidiasis include immunosuppression, indwelling intravenous catheters, neutropenia, hematologic malignancies, burns, postoperative complications, injection drug use, and very low birth weight in neonates. Urinary tract candidiasis usually arises as a complication of prolonged catheterization of the bladder or renal pelvis.

The frequent isolation of *Candida* spp. from sputum, throat, feces, and urine in the absence of clinical evidence of infection suggests a low level of pathogenicity or some level of immunity. Local factors contributing to superficial candidiasis include interdigital intertrigo and paronychia on hands with excessive water exposure (e.g., cannery and laundry workers or dishwashers) and intertrigo in moist skinfolds of obese individuals.

3. Causative agents—*Candida albicans*, *Candida* (formerly *Torulopsis*) *glabrata*, *Candida parapsilosis*, *Candida tropicalis*, and *Candida krusei* are most common. Numerous less common species, such as *Candida dubliniensis*, *Candida lusitaniae*, and the newly emerging multidrug-resistant species *Candida auris*, have also been reported to cause disease.

4. Diagnosis—Requires both laboratory and clinical evidence of candidiasis. The single most valuable laboratory test is microscopic demonstration of pseudohyphae or yeast cells in infected tissue or normally sterile body fluids. Culture confirmation is important, but isolation from sputum, bronchial washings, stools, urine, mucosal surfaces, skin, or wounds is not proof of a causal relation to the disease as the organism may be part of the transient flora. Severe or recurrent oropharyngeal infection in an adult with no obvious underlying cause should suggest the possibility of HIV infection. Polymerase chain reaction and other culture-independent diagnostic tests may play a role in early detection of candidemia. Specific biomarkers (i.e., β-D-glucan) could be useful for starting empirical therapy in some classes of high-risk critically ill patients. Culture independent diagnostic tests to detect invasive candidiasis are becoming increasingly common.

5. Occurrence—Worldwide. Many *Candida* spp. are part of the normal human flora.

6. Reservoirs—Humans and environment, depending on species.

7. Incubation period—Variable; 2 to 5 days for thrush in infants.

8. Transmission—Most *Candida* infections are thought to occur from overgrowth of endogenous flora; however, passage from mother to neonate during childbirth has been noted and hands of health care workers have been implicated in transmission of *C. parapsilosis*. The health care environment is thought to play a greater role in transmission of *C. auris*, resulting in outbreaks. The role of spread by the sexual route for vulvovaginal candidiasis is limited, although some studies have demonstrated significant asymptomatic male genital colonization with species of *Candida*, more commonly in male sexual partners of infected women.

9. Treatment—Improve conditions or reduce risk factors for candidiasis; for example, removal of indwelling central catheters in patients with candidemia may facilitate cure.

For complete treatment recommendations, refer to Infectious Diseases Society of America guidelines.[1] Therapy may be guided based on culture and susceptibility data. Growth of *Candida* from respiratory secretions usually indicates colonization and rarely requires antifungal treatment.

Vulvovaginal Candidiasis

Preferred therapy	Uncomplicated disease: • Topical antifungal agent (e.g., miconazole cream or intravaginal suppository); dose and duration depend on agent used[a]
	Severe disease: • Fluconazole 150 mg PO given every 72 hours for a total of 2 or 3 doses
Alternative therapy options	Uncomplicated disease: • Fluconazole 150 mg PO once

(Continued)

Vulvovaginal Candidiasis (Continued)

Special considerations and comments	For *Candida glabrata* not responsive to oral azoles, recommended treatment is • Topical intravaginal boric acid administered as a gelatin capsule 600 mg daily for 14 days OR • Nystatin intravaginal suppositories 100,000 units daily for 14 days OR • Topical 17% flucytosine cream alone or in combination with 3% AMB cream daily for 14 days
	For recurring vulvovaginal candidiasis[a]: • 10–14 days of induction therapy with a topical agent OR • Fluconazole PO THEN • Fluconazole 150 mg weekly for 6 months recommended

Note: AMB = amphotericin B; PO = oral(ly).
[a] For complete treatment recommendations, refer to CDC guidelines.[2]

Urinary Tract Infection: Asymptomatic Candiduria[a]

Preferred therapy	• Treatment of asymptomatic candiduria NOT recommended unless neutropenic host, very low birth weight infant (< 1,500 g), or patients who will undergo urologic manipulation. • Neutropenic patients and very low birth weight infants should be treated as invasive candidiasis/candidemia.
	Several days before or after the procedure, patients undergoing urologic procedures should be treated with • Fluconazole 400 mg (6 mg/kg) PO daily OR • AMB deoxycholate 0.3–0.6 mg/kg IV daily
Alternative therapy options	Not applicable
Special considerations and comments	• Azole antifungal agents have been associated with significant drug-drug interactions. Assess accordingly. • AMB has been associated with significant electrolyte abnormalities. Monitor serum creatinine, potassium, and magnesium closely. Supplemental electrolyte therapy may be warranted. To minimize infusion-related reaction, consider premedication with nonsteroidal anti-inflammatory agent OR acetaminophen with or without diphenhydramine 30–60 minutes prior to infusion. Rigors can be treated with meperidine. Premedicating with 0.9% normal saline 500 mL over 1 hour prior to infusion may also minimize renal toxicity.

Note: AMB = amphotericin B; IV = intravenous(ly); PO = oral(ly).
[a] For complete treatment recommendations, refer to Infectious Diseases Society of America guidelines[1] for symptomatic *Candida* cystitis, pyelonephritis, and urinary tract infections associated with fungal balls.

Oropharyngeal Candidiasis

Preferred therapy	Mild disease: • Clotrimazole troches 10 mg PO 5 times daily for 7–14 days; allow troche to dissolve slowly
	Moderate to severe disease: • Fluconazole 100–200 mg PO daily for 7–14 days
	Fluconazole-refractory disease: • Itraconazole solution 200 mg PO once daily for ≤ 28 days OR • Posaconazole suspension 400 mg PO BID for 3 days THEN • 400 mg PO daily for ≤ 28 days
Alternative therapy options	Mild disease: • Nystatin suspension 100,000 U/mL 4–6 mL swish and swallow QID for 7–14 days
	Fluconazole-refractory disease: • Voriconazole 200 mg PO BID for ≤ 28 days OR • AMB deoxycholate oral suspension 100 mg/mL PO QID for ≤ 28 days OR • Echinocandin IV (e.g., caspofungin 70 mg loading dose, THEN 50 mg daily; OR micafungin 100 mg daily; OR anidulafungin 200 mg loading dose, THEN 100 mg daily) for ≤ 28 days OR • AMB deoxycholate 0.3 mg/kg IV daily for ≤ 28 days
Special considerations and comments	• Chronic suppressive therapy is usually unnecessary. If considered for patients with recurrent infection, fluconazole 100 mg PO 3 times weekly is recommended. • HIV-infected patients should start antiretroviral therapy to reduce the incidence of recurrent infection. • For denture-related candidiasis, disinfection of denture in addition to antifungal therapy is recommended. • Azole antifungal agents have been associated with significant drug-drug interactions. Assess accordingly. • Posaconazole suspension should be taken with high-fat meal.

Note: AMB = amphotericin B; BID = twice daily; IV = intravenous(ly); HIV = human immunodeficiency virus; PO = oral(ly); QID = 4 times daily.

Esophageal Candidiasis

Preferred therapy	Fluconazole 200–400 mg (3–6 mg/kg) PO daily for 14–21 days
	For fluconazole-refractory disease: • Itraconazole solution 200 mg PO daily for 14–21 days OR • Voriconazole 200 mg (3 mg/kg) PO/IV BID for 14–21 days OR • Posaconazole suspension 400 mg PO BID for 14–21 days OR • Posaconazole extended release 300 mg PO daily for 14–21 days
Alternative therapy options	For patients who cannot tolerate oral therapy: • Fluconazole 400 mg (6 mg/kg) IV daily for 14–21 days OR • Echinocandin IV (e.g., caspofungin 70 mg loading dose, THEN 50 mg daily; OR micafungin 100 mg daily; OR anidulafungin 200 mg loading dose, THEN 100 mg daily) for 14–21 days OR • AMB deoxycholate 0.3–0.7 mg/kg IV daily for 14–21 days; consider de-escalating to PO therapy once the patient is able to tolerate it
	Alternatives for fluconazole-refractory disease: • Echinocandin IV (e.g., caspofungin 70 mg loading dose, THEN 50 mg daily; OR micafungin 100 mg daily; OR anidulafungin 200 mg loading dose, THEN 100 mg daily) for 14–21 days OR • AMB deoxycholate 0.3–0.7 mg/kg IV daily for 21 days
Special considerations and comments	• Recurrent esophagitis: chronic suppressive therapy with fluconazole 100–200 mg 3 times weekly is recommended. • HIV-infected patients should start antiretroviral therapy to reduce the incidence of recurrent infection. • Azole antifungal agents have been associated with significant drug-drug interactions. Assess accordingly. • AMB has been associated with significant electrolyte abnormalities. Monitor serum creatinine, potassium, and magnesium closely. Supplemental electrolyte therapy may be warranted. To minimize infusion-related reaction, consider premedication with nonsteroidal anti-inflammatory agent OR acetaminophen with or without diphenhydramine 30–60 minutes prior to infusion. Rigors can be treated with meperidine. Premedicating with 0.9% normal saline 500 mL over 1 hour prior to infusion may also minimize renal toxicity.

Note: AMB = amphotericin B; BID = twice daily; IV = intravenous(ly); HIV = human immunodeficiency virus; PO = oral(ly).

Invasive Candidiasis

Preferred therapy	Echinocandin IV (e.g., caspofungin 70 mg loading dose, THEN 50 mg daily; OR micafungin 100 mg daily; OR anidulafungin 200 mg loading dose, THEN 100 mg daily) for 2 weeks if no evidence of metastatic disease.
Alternative therapy options	For patients who are not critically ill and who are considered low risk for fluconazole-resistant *Candida* spp.: • Fluconazole 800 mg (12 mg/kg) IV/PO loading dose THEN • Fluconazole 400 mg (6 mg/kg) IV/PO daily for 2 weeks if no evidence of metastatic disease
Special considerations and comments	• Testing azole susceptibility is recommended for all bloodstream and other clinically relevant *Candida* isolates. • Transition to fluconazole (usually within 5–7 days) is recommended for patients who are clinically stable and have isolates susceptible to fluconazole with negative repeat blood cultures. • All patients with candidemia should have a dilated ophthalmologic examination, preferably performed by ophthalmologist within first week of diagnosis. For neutropenic patients, this should be performed within 1 week of recovery from neutropenia as ophthalmologic findings of chordial and vitreal infections are minimal until recovery from neutropenia. • Follow-up blood cultures should be performed every day or every other day to establish the time point at which candidemia has been cleared. Duration of therapy without obvious metastatic complication is for 2 weeks after documented clearance of blood cultures and resolution of symptoms. Presence of metastatic disease requires longer duration of treatment.[a] • Azole antifungal agents have been associated with significant drug-drug interactions. Assess accordingly. • AMB has been associated with significant electrolyte abnormalities. Monitor serum creatinine, potassium, and magnesium closely. Supplemental electrolyte therapy may be warranted. To minimize infusion-related reaction, consider premedication with nonsteroidal anti-inflammatory agent OR acetaminophen with or without diphenhydramine 30–60 minutes prior to infusion. Rigors can be treated with meperidine. Premedicating with 0.9% normal saline 500 mL over 1 hour prior to infusion may also minimize renal toxicity. *Candida glabrata:* • High-dose fluconazole 800 mg (12 mg/kg) IV/PO daily for 2 weeks (if no evidence of metastatic disease) may be considered if fluconazole susceptible dose dependent

(Continued)

Invasive Candidiasis (Continued)

Special considerations and comments	*Candida krusei*: • Echinocandin (e.g., caspofungin 70 mg loading dose, THEN 50 mg daily; OR micafungin 100 mg daily; OR anidulafungin 200 mg loading dose, THEN 100 mg daily) OR • Lipid formulation AMB 3–5 mg/kg IV once daily OR • Voriconazole 400 mg (6 mg/kg) IV/PO BID for 2 doses, THEN 200–300 mg (3–4 mg/kg) IV/PO BID
	For intolerance, limited availability, or resistance to other antifungal agents: • Lipid formulation AMB 3–5 mg/kg IV daily is a reasonable alternative
	Step-down PO therapy for select cases of candidemia due to *C. krusei* when susceptible: • Voriconazole 400 mg (6 mg/kg) PO BID for 2 doses THEN • 200 mg (3 mg/kg) BID is recommended

Note: AMB = amphotericin B; BID = twice daily; IV = intravenous(ly); PO = oral(ly).
[a]For complete treatment recommendations, refer to Infectious Diseases Society of America guidelines.

10. Prevention—

1) To prevent systemic spread, early detection and local treatment of any infection in the mouth, esophagus, or urinary bladder of those with predisposing systemic factors as described (see Risk Groups in this chapter). Maintenance and disinfection of central venous catheters can help prevent health care–associated candidemia. Fluconazole chemoprophylaxis decreases the incidence of invasive candidiasis following hematopoietic stem cell transplantation in some studies of high-risk critically ill patients and liver transplant recipients and in very low birth weight neonates. Antifungal prophylaxis may also be effective in preventing invasive candidiasis in hematopoietic stem cell transplant recipients with graft-versus-host disease and in patients with prolonged chemotherapy-induced neutropenia.

2) Management of contacts and the immediate environment: investigation of contacts and source of infection is not beneficial in most sporadic cases of candidiasis. However, identification of a case of *C. auris* requires a thorough epidemiologic investigation of health care contacts.

11. Special considerations—Outbreaks of candidiasis have occurred as a result of contaminated intravenous solutions and thrush in nurseries for newborns. Outbreaks of *C. parapsilosis* fungemia in neonatal intensive care units have been linked to transmission from health care workers. Concurrent disinfection and terminal cleaning, comparable to that used for epidemic diarrhea in hospital nurseries, is recommended (see "*E. coli* Diarrheal Diseases"). For *C. auris*, disinfection with an agent active against *C. auris* is recommended. Further information can be found at: https://www.cdc. gov/fungal/candida-auris/c-auris-infection-control.html.

C. auris is an emerging multidrug-resistant yeast that can cause invasive infections associated with high mortality and can be transmitted in health care settings. *C. auris* can be misidentified as other yeasts by many biochemical methods used for yeast identification. Detection of *C. auris* requires notifying public health agencies and prompt action with infection control measures to control transmission.

References

1. Pappas PG, Kauffman CA, Andes DR, et al. Clinical practice guideline for the management of candidiasis: 2016 update by the Infectious Diseases Society of America. *Clin Infect Dis*. 2016;62(4):e1–e50.
2. CDC. 2015. Sexually transmitted diseases treatment guidelines: vulvovaginal candidiasis. Available at: https://www.cdc.gov/std/tg2015/candidiasis.htm. Accessed January 3, 2020.

[S. Vallabhaneni]

CAPILLARIASIS

DISEASE	ICD-10 CODE
INTESTINAL CAPILLARIASIS	ICD-10 B81.1
HEPATIC CAPILLARIASIS	ICD-10 B83.8
PULMONARY CAPILLARIASIS	ICD-10 B83.8

1. Clinical features—Capillariasis is a zoonotic parasitic disease caused by infection with 3 different *Capillaria* spp. Clinical features depend on the location in the human body where the worm resides—intestines, liver, or respiratory tract.

1) Intestinal capillariasis is an enteropathy with fever, eosinophilia, massive protein loss due to predominantly chronic watery diarrhea, and a malabsorption syndrome, leading to progressive weight loss and emaciation. Fatal cases are characterized by the presence

of great numbers of parasites in the small intestine together with ascites and pleural transudate from hypoalbuminemia, abnormalities in electrolytes (in particular, hypokalemia), and cardiomyopathy. Case-fatality rates of 10% have been reported. Subclinical cases also occur but usually become symptomatic over time.

2) Hepatic capillariasis is an uncommon and occasionally fatal infection of the liver. The picture is that of an acute, or subacute, hepatitis, with fever, hepatomegaly, and marked eosinophilia resembling that of visceral larva migrans. Portions of the liver parenchyma may form necrotizing granulomas as a reaction to the eggs, leading to fibrosis. The organism can also disseminate to the lungs and other viscera.

3) Pulmonary capillariasis is associated with fever, cough, shortness of breath, and other symptoms of lower respiratory tract infection. Eggs may appear in the sputum in 4 weeks; symptoms may appear earlier or later. Pneumonitis may be severe; heavy infections may be fatal.

2. Risk groups—Men aged 20 to 45 years appear to be particularly at risk of intestinal capillariasis, especially those who consume raw fish. Hepatic capillariasis appears to affect malnourished children more often than any other group (especially ≤ 3 years and associated with pica) and children appear to be the main risk group for pulmonary capillariasis. Unsanitary environments, poor hygiene, and rodent infestation increase the risk of infections.

3. Causative agents—Intestinal capillariasis is caused by infection with *Capillaria philippinensis*; hepatic capillariasis by *Capillaria hepatica* (*Hepaticola hepatica*); and pulmonary capillariasis by *Capillaria aerophila* (*Thominx aerophila*).

4. Diagnosis—Diagnosis of intestinal capillariasis is based on clinical findings plus the identification of eggs, larvae, or adult parasites in the stool. The eggs measure 45 μm by 20 μm with plugs at each end and resemble those of *Trichuris trichiura*. Anthelmintic drugs stimulate their excretion and confirmation of diagnosis may sometimes only come after initiation of treatment. Serology using immunochromatographic tests (for cross-reactive antibodies against *Trichinella spiralis* larval antigen) may serve as a supportive diagnostic tool. Typically, bowel barium and computed tomography (CT) studies show continuous long segments of fold thickening and fold effacement. These radiologic studies also help in planning of endoscopic routes; jejunal and ileal biopsy may show worms in the mucosa.

Hepatic capillariasis is diagnosed by demonstrating eggs or the parasite in a liver biopsy or at necropsy (embryonated eggs are not passed in stools). These eggs also resemble *T. trichiura*. A hallmark of the parasite is the presence of a stichosome. Radiologic tests including ultrasonography and CT may help identify suspicious hepatic nodules. Serologic testing by indirect immunofluorescence assays may help.

Pulmonary capillariasis is diagnosed by demonstrating eggs in the sputum or bronchial biopsy specimen.

5. Occurrence—Intestinal capillariasis is endemic in the Philippines and Thailand; cases have been reported in Egypt, Japan, South Korea, and Taiwan (China). Isolated cases have also been reported in Colombia, India, Indonesia, and Iran. The disease was first described in the early 1960s in Luzon, the Philippines, where more than 1,800 cases have been seen since 1967.

Since hepatic capillariasis was identified as a human disease in 1924, about 30 cases have been reported in Africa, North and South America, Asia, Europe, and the Pacific area. This form appears to be more common in children younger than 3 years.

About 11 human cases of pulmonary capillariasis have been documented in Iran, Morocco, and Russia; animal infection has been reported in North and South America, Europe, Asia, and Australia.

6. Reservoirs—

1) Intestinal: unknown; possibly aquatic birds, where adult worms have also been found to reside. Fish are considered intermediate hosts.
2) Hepatic: primarily rats and other rodents but also a large variety of domestic and wild mammals. The adult worms live and produce eggs in the liver.
3) Pulmonary: cats, dogs, and other carnivorous mammals.

7. Incubation period—For intestinal capillariasis, the incubation period in humans is unknown. For hepatic capillariasis, the incubation period is 3 to 4 weeks. For pulmonary disease, the incubation period is also unknown; however it is currently thought to be 25 to 40 days.

8. Transmission—

1) Intestinal: *C. philippinensis* is transmitted to humans through ingestion of raw or inadequately cooked small fish, eaten whole. The life cycle of the parasite begins with fish-eating birds or humans passing unembryonated eggs in their stools into the environment. The eggs then become embryonated, develop infective larvae, and are eaten by freshwater fish. In the fish, these eggs hatch in the intestine; the larvae then penetrate the intestine to migrate to the tissues, which when eaten uncooked by humans (or by birds, monkeys, Mongolian gerbils) completes the infection cycle. Once ingested by humans, the adult nematodes reside in the small intestine and deposit unembryonated eggs. In rare instances, these become embryonated and can result in auto- and hyperinfection. *C. philippinensis* is not transmitted directly from person to person.

2) Hepatic: *C. hepatica* is transmitted to humans primarily through the ingestion of embryonated eggs in fecally contaminated (from rodents, or possibly pigs, carnivores, nonhuman and human primates) food, water, or soil. The adult worms produce fertilized eggs that remain in the liver of the host animal (e.g., rodents) until its death and decomposition or until it is eaten by a predator. When an infected liver is eaten, the eggs are freed by digestion, reach the soil in the feces, and develop to the infective stage in 2 to 4 weeks. When ingested by a suitable host, including humans, embryonated eggs hatch in the intestine; larvae migrate through the wall of the gut and are transported via the portal system to the liver, where they mature and produce eggs. Spurious findings of unembryonated eggs in human stools after consumption of infected liver—raw or cooked—occurs; however, since these eggs are not embryonated, infection cannot be established. The infection is not transmitted from person to person.

3) Pulmonary: humans become infected with *C. aerophila* through the ingestion of infective eggs in soil or in soil-contaminated food or water. The larvae migrate from the intestine (humans, cats, dogs, and other carnivorous mammals) to the lungs and live in tunnels in the epithelial lining of the trachea, bronchi, and bronchioles where they develop into the adult stage. Adults lay fertilized eggs, which are sloughed into the air passages, coughed up, swallowed, and discharged in the feces. In the soil, larvae develop in the eggs and remain infective for a year or longer.

9. Treatment—

Drug	• Albendazole • Mebendazole
Dose	• Albendazole 400 mg once daily • Mebendazole 200 mg BID
Route	PO
Alternative drug	Thiabendazole 25 mg/kg ($\leq$ 3 g) once daily
Duration	• Albendazole 10 days[a] • Mebendazole 20–30 days • Thiabendazole 30 days
Special considerations and comments	• Supportive fluids and nutritional supplements may be required. • Corticosteroids may help in the treatment of hepatic capillariasis by reducing associated inflammatory response. • There are no randomized controlled trials evaluating the approach to therapy or optimal duration.

Note: BID = twice daily; PO = oral(ly).
[a]Different strategies of extended or repeated treatment with albendazole have been used for hepatic capillariasis.

10. Prevention—

1) Avoid eating uncooked fish or other aquatic animal life in known endemic areas.
2) Avoid ingestion of dirt, whether directly (pica), in contaminated food or water, or on hands.
3) Protect water supplies and food from soil contamination.
4) Provide adequate facilities for the disposal of feces.

11. Special considerations—None.

Bibliography

Dubey A, Bagchi A, Sharma D, Dey A, Nandy K, Sharma R. Hepatic capillariasis—drug targets. *Infect Disord Drug Targets*. 2018;18(1):3–10.

Sadaow L, Sanpool O, Intapan PM, Sukeepaisarnjaroen W, Prasongdee TK, Maleewong W. A hospital-based study of intestinal capillariasis in Thailand: clinical features, potential clues for diagnosis, and epidemiological characteristics of 85 patients. *Am J Trop Med Hyg*. 2018;98(1):27–31.

Wang L, Zhang Y, Deng Y, et al. Clinical and laboratory characterizations of hepatic capillariasis. *Acta Trop*. 2019;193:206–210.

[V. Lee, Z. J. M. Ho]

CAT SCRATCH DISEASE
(cat scratch fever, benign lymphoreticulosis)

DISEASE	ICD-10 CODE
CAT SCRATCH DISEASE	ICD-10 A28.1

1. Clinical features—A subacute usually self-limited bacterial disease characterized by malaise, granulomatous lymphadenitis, and variable patterns of fever. Often preceded by a cat scratch, lick, or bite that produces a red papular lesion with involvement of a regional lymph node. The papule at the inoculation site can be found in 50% to 90% of cases. Lymphadenopathy occurs usually within 2 weeks, is usually painful, and may progress to suppuration. Axillary, epitrochlear, and cervical lymph nodes are most frequently involved. Parinaud oculoglandular syndrome (granulomatous conjunctivitis with pre-tragal adenopathy) can occur after conjunctival inoculation; approximately 10% of cases may be complicated by systemic disease including prolonged high fever, malaise, fatigue, myalgia, arthralgia, weight loss, or hepatosplenomegaly. Rarely neurologic complications such as encephalopathy and optic neuritis can also occur. Bacteremia, hepatic vascular proliferation resulting in blood-filled spaces in the liver (peliosis hepatis), and bacillary angiomatosis due to this infection may occur among young children and among immunocompromised persons, particularly those with advanced human immunodeficiency virus infection. Cat scratch disease (CSD) can be clinically confused with other diseases that cause regional lymphadenopathies (e.g., bacterial [staphylococcal and streptococcal] adenitis, tularemia, brucellosis, tuberculosis, atypical mycobacterial infections, plague, pasteurellosis, and lymphoma).

2. Risk groups—Children and young adults appear to be at greatest risk of infection.

3. Causative agents—*Bartonella* (formerly *Rochalimaea*) *henselae* has been implicated epidemiologically, bacteriologically, and serologically as the causal agent of most cases of CSD.

4. Diagnosis—A clinically compatible illness combined with serologic evidence of antibody to *B. henselae* by indirect immunofluorescence assay or enzyme immunoassay can establish the diagnosis. Antibodies usually become detectable within 1 to 2 weeks of symptom onset. Therefore, retrospective confirmation of the diagnosis via convalescent serology may be necessary. Cross-reactivity occurs with other species, in particular *Bartonella quintana*. Histopathologic examination of affected lymph nodes may show consistent characteristics but is not diagnostic. Although not specific for *Bartonella* spp. Warthin-Starry staining may aid in the visualization of the bacterium within tissues. Immunodetection and polymerase chain reaction are highly efficient in detecting *Bartonella* in biopsies or aspirates of lymph nodes. Although *Bartonella* can be isolated from blood or lymph node aspirates using blood agar in 5% CO_2, yield is low in patients with CSD and a prolonged incubation of up to 45 days may be required. Cell-based culture systems may be more sensitive but require special laboratory capabilities and are not widely available.

5. Occurrence—The disease has a worldwide distribution. It is more common in children and young adults. Familial clustering rarely occurs.

6. Reservoirs—Domestic cats are the main vectors and reservoirs for *B. henselae*; no evidence of clinical illness in cats even when chronic bacteremia has been demonstrated. Cat fleas (*Ctenocephalides felis*) and ticks may be infected, but their role in transmission to humans is not well defined.

7. Incubation period—Variable; usually 3 to 14 days from inoculation to primary lesion and 5 to 50 days from inoculation to lymphadenopathy.

8. Transmission—More than 90% of patients give a history of scratch, bite, lick, or other exposure to a healthy, usually young, cat or kitten. Dog scratch or bite, monkey bite, and contact with rabbits, chickens, or horses have also been reported prior to the syndrome, but cat involvement was not excluded in all cases. Cat fleas transmit *B. henselae* among cats but play no clear role in direct transmission to humans. The bacterium is not transmitted from person to person.

9. Treatment—

Drug	Azithromycin
Dose	500 mg on day 1 followed by 250 mg once daily on subsequent days
Route	PO
Alternative drug	• Clarithromycin 500 mg PO BID • Rifampin 300 mg PO BID • Trimethoprim-sulfamethoxazole 160–800 mg PO BID • Ciprofloxacin 500 mg PO BID
Duration	• Azithromycin 5 days • Alternative drugs 7–10 days • See next row for complicated disease
Special considerations and comments	• Aspiration of suppurative lymph nodes to relieve pain or corticosteroids in severe cases have been used. • Hepatosplenic disease: azithromycin PLUS rifampin for 14 days. • Neuroretinitis: doxycycline 100 mg PO BID PLUS rifampin for 4–6 weeks. • Endocarditis: doxycycline 100 mg PO BID for 6 weeks PLUS gentamycin 1 mg/kg IV every 8 hours for the first 2 weeks. • Bacillary angiomatosis or peliosis hepatis in those with AIDS: doxycycline 100 mg PO BID for 3–4 months.

Note: AIDS = acquired immunodeficiency syndrome; BID = twice daily; IV = intravenous(ly); PO = oral(ly).

10. Prevention—Avoidance of situations that may lead to cat scratches is advised. Thorough cleaning of cat scratches and bites may help. Flea control is very important to prevent continuing infection of cats and perhaps the spread to humans.

11. Special considerations—None.

[L. Blanton, D. Walker]

CHANCROID
(ulcus molle, soft chance)

DISEASE	ICD-10 CODE
CHANCROID	ICD-10 A57

1. Clinical features—An acute sexually transmitted bacterial infection usually localized in the genital area and characterized by a single or multiple painful necrotic ulcers that bleed on contact. Chancroid ulcers are more frequently found in uncircumcised men, on the foreskin, or in the coronal sulcus and may cause phimosis. These lesions are frequently accompanied by painful swollen suppurating regional lymph nodes. In women, minimally symptomatic or painless lesions may occur on the vaginal wall or cervix. Extragenital lesions have been reported. Chancroid ulcers, like other genital ulcers, are associated with an increased risk of acquiring human immunodeficiency virus (HIV).

2. Risk groups—It is more often diagnosed in uncircumcised men, sex workers, and clients of sex workers. In industrialized countries, cases are frequently linked to sex work, travel, or exposure to persons from endemic regions.

3. Causative agents—*Haemophilus ducreyi*, a Gram-negative coccobacillus.

4. Diagnosis—Genital ulcers may be difficult to distinguish clinically from syphilis and genital herpes.

Culture and polymerase chain reaction (PCR) tests are the preferred tests for definitive diagnosis, although PCR is not commonly available. Culture diagnosis is by isolation of the organism from lesion exudates on a selective medium incorporating vancomycin into chocolate horse blood agar enriched with fetal calf serum, IsoVitaleX, and activated charcoal. *H. ducreyi* grows best at 33°C (91.4°F).

5. Occurrence—Most prevalent in tropical and subtropical regions, including Africa and Southeast Asia. The disease is much less common in temperate zones, where it may occur in small outbreaks. In industrialized countries, outbreaks and some endemic transmission have occurred, but principally among high-risk groups. Prevalence appears to have declined substantially in many previously endemic areas, although the global prevalence is unknown.

6. Reservoirs—Humans.

7. Incubation period—From 3 to 5 days, up to 14 days.

8. Transmission—Through direct sexual contact with open lesions and pus from buboes. Autoinoculation to extragenital sites may occur in infected persons. The disease is communicable until the lesions are healed and the organism is cleared from discharging regional lymph nodes. Nonsexual transmission may occur from contact with open lesions. Beyond the neonatal period, sexual abuse must be considered when chancroid ulcers are found in children and young adults, especially in the genital and perineal region. However, *H. ducreyi* is recognized as a major cause of nonsexually transmitted cutaneous ulcers in children in tropical regions and, specifically, yaws-endemic countries. The acquisition of a lower extremity ulcer attributable to *H. ducreyi* in a child or young adult without genital ulcers and reported travel to a yaws-endemic region should not be considered evidence of sexual abuse.

9. Treatment—

Preferred therapy	• Azithromycin 1 g PO as a single dose OR • Ceftriaxone 250 mg IM as a single dose OR • Ciprofloxacin 500 mg PO BID for 3 days OR • Erythromycin 500 mg PO TID for 7 days
Special considerations and comments	• Data are limited regarding the current prevalence of antimicrobial resistance. However, intermediate resistance to either ciprofloxacin or erythromycin has been reported. Time of complete healing depends on the size of the ulcer but they usually improve within 7 days. • Uncircumcised men and persons with HIV infection may not respond as well to treatment. Persons with HIV infection might require repeated or longer courses of therapy. • Surgical drainage of buboes may be necessary.

Note: BID = twice daily; HIV = human immunodeficiency virus; IM = intramuscular(ly); PO = oral(ly); TID = thrice daily.

10. Prevention—

1) Perform testing for other sexually transmitted infections, including HIV infection.
2) Examine and treat sexual contacts of patients who have chancroid if they had sexual contact with the patient during the 10 days preceding the patient's onset of symptoms. Women without external signs of infection may have small inapparent intravaginal lesions. Sexual contacts even without obvious signs of disease should receive prophylactic treatment.

11. Special considerations—

1) Reporting: case reporting is obligatory in many countries.
2) Epidemic measures: empiric treatment of high-risk groups including sex workers, clients of sex workers, and patients with genital ulcers may be required to control outbreaks. Periodic presumptive treatment of sex workers and their clients has resulted in reduced incidence in some settings.
3) More information can be found at:

- http://www.cdc.gov/std/treatment
- http://www.who.int/topics/sexually_transmitted_infec-tions/en

[A. Ridpath]

CHLAMYDIAL INFECTIONS

DISEASE	ICD-10 CODE
CHLAMYDIAL DISEASE, SEXUALLY TRANSMITTED	ICD-10 A56
NONSPECIFIC URETHRITIS	ICD-10 N34.1
Chlamydial pelvic inflammatory disease	ICD-10 A56.11
Conjunctivitis (see "Conjunctivitis/Keratitis")	
Lymphogranuloma venereum (see "Lymphogranuloma Venereum")	
Pneumonia due to Chlamydia pneumoniae (see "Pneumonia")	
Pneumonia due to Chlamydia trachomatis (see "Pneumonia")	
Psittacosis (see "Psittacosis")	

1. Clinical features—Most chlamydial infections are asymptomatic. Symptomatic infections are difficult to distinguish clinically from gonorrhea and manifest in males primarily as urethritis (moderate or scanty mucopurulent discharge, dysuria, urethral itching) and in females as cervicitis (mucopurulent endocervical discharge, cervical friability). Rectal infection (asymptomatic or with proctitis) can be acquired through receptive anal intercourse or possibly via contiguous spread from the vagina. Less common manifestations of chlamydial infection include epididymitis in males; urethral syndrome (dysuria and pyuria), perihepatitis (Fitz-Hugh–Curtis syndrome), and bartholinitis in females; and conjunctivitis (acquired through contact with infected genital secretions) in either sex.

In females, untreated infection can ascend from the cervix to the uterus, fallopian tubes, and ovaries, causing pelvic inflammatory disease (PID); this may be asymptomatic (i.e., subclinical) or acute, with abdominal or pelvic pain and adnexal, uterine, or cervical motion tenderness. Both subclinical and acute PID can lead to long-term sequelae of chronic pelvic pain, ectopic pregnancy, and tubal factor infertility. Infection during pregnancy has been associated with preterm delivery and can result in conjunctival and pneumonic infection of the newborn.

Infants and young children may develop genitourinary infection because of perinatal infection; however, genitourinary infection in an older child or preadolescent should raise suspicion for sexual assault.

Chlamydial infection has been associated with an increased risk of acquiring human immunodeficiency virus. Reactive arthritis occurs as a sequela in a minority of chlamydial infections.

2. Risk groups—Sexually active persons, especially adolescents and young adults, and those with concurrent or multiple recent sex partners. Geographic and racial/ethnic disparities in chlamydia prevalence have been observed in some countries. Reinfection (with the same or different strains of chlamydia) is common and associated with increased risk of PID and long-term sequelae, including ectopic pregnancy and infertility in females. Infants born to mothers with untreated chlamydia infection are at risk for conjunctivitis and pneumonia.

3. Causative agents—*Chlamydia trachomatis* serovars B and D–K are responsible for sexually acquired genital infections in adolescents and adults and perinatally transmitted infections of the neonate and infant.

While *C. trachomatis* is the most frequently isolated causal agent of nongonococcal urethritis in males (isolated in 15%–40% of cases), other agents have been implicated (*Mycoplasma genitalium, Trichomonas vaginalis*, herpes simplex virus, Epstein-Barr virus, and adenovirus).

4. Diagnosis—Nucleic acid amplification tests offer excellent sensitivity and high specificity for diagnosing chlamydia. Nucleic acid amplification tests can be used with noninvasive and minimally invasive specimens, including vaginal swabs (patient or provider collected) and urine specimens. Culture is technically difficult and not as sensitive as molecular assays. Antigen detection using enzyme immunoassay has been shown not to be as sensitive as the molecular assays.

5. Occurrence—Chlamydia is the most common notifiable disease in the USA with nearly 1.8 million infections reported in 2018. Infections are common worldwide. Since infection is often asymptomatic, identification of infections is linked to availability of screening programs. Extension of screening has likely contributed to recently observed increases in case reports in many countries.

6. Reservoirs—Humans.

7. Incubation period—Poorly defined and variable, probably 7 to 14 days or longer.

8. Transmission—Sexual contact with the penis, vagina, mouth, or anus of an infected partner. Neonatal infection results from exposure to the mother's infected cervix. Infected individuals are presumed to be infectious. Without treatment, infection can persist for months.

9. Treatment—

	Adults and Adolescents	Pregnant Women	Infants and Children <8 Years[a] (Children ≥8 Years May Get the Adult and Adolescent Preferred Therapy)
Preferred therapy	• Azithromycin 1 g PO once OR • Doxycycline 100 mg PO BID for 7 days	• Azithromycin 1 g PO once	• <45 kg: erythromycin base or ethylsuccinate 12.5 mg/kg PO QID for 14 days • >45 kg: azithromycin 1 g PO once
Alternative therapy options	• Erythromycin base 500 mg PO QID for 7 days OR • Erythromycin ethylsuccinate 800 mg PO QID for 7 days OR • Levofloxacin 500 mg PO daily for 7 days OR • Ofloxacin 300 mg PO BID for 7 days	• Amoxicillin 500 mg PO TID for 7 days OR • Erythromycin base 500 mg PO QID for 7 days OR • Erythromycin base 250 mg PO QID for 14 days OR • Erythromycin ethylsuccinate 800 mg PO QID for 7 days OR • Erythromycin ethylsuccinate 400 mg PO QID for 14 days	• <45 kg: azithromycin 20 mg/kg PO daily for 3 days • Infant pneumonia: azithromycin 20 mg/kg PO daily for 3 days

(Continued)

(Continued)

	Adults and Adolescents	Pregnant Women	Infants and Children <8 Years[a] (Children ≥8 Years May Get the Adult and Adolescent Preferred Therapy)
Special considerations and comments		A test-of-cure culture to document chlamydial eradication (preferably by NAAT) 3–4 weeks after completion of therapy is recommended because severe sequelae can occur in mothers and neonates if the infection persists.	• Infants <6 weeks should be followed for infantile hypertrophic pyloric stenosis. • Topical antibiotic therapy alone is inadequate for treatment for ophthalmia neonatorum due to chlamydia and is unnecessary when systemic treatment is administered. • A test-of-cure culture to detect therapeutic failure ensures treatment effectiveness for infection of the nasopharynx, urogenital tract, and rectum. Therefore, this culture should be obtained at a follow-up visit approximately 2 weeks after treatment is completed.

Note: BID = twice daily; NAAT = nucleic acid amplification test; PO = oral(ly); TID = thrice daily; QID = 4 times daily.
[a]Data are limited on use of azithromycin in children <45 kg.

10. Prevention—

1) Health and sex education, same as for syphilis (see "Syphilis"), with emphasis on use of condoms.

2) Screening of women for *C. trachomatis* has been shown to reduce the risk of PID. Routine periodic screening for chlamydia is recommended for defined groups in some countries. In the USA, chlamydia screening is recommended yearly for all sexually active females younger than 25 years, older women with risk factors (e.g., new or multiple sex partners), and males who

have receptive anal sex; it is also recommended at the first prenatal care visit for all pregnant females. More frequent screening may be performed based on patient risk factors. Current tests for *C. trachomatis* infection enable use of noninvasive or minimally invasive specimens, including vaginal swabs (patient or clinician collected) and urine. All partners of persons with chlamydia should be evaluated, tested, and offered presumptive treatment if they have had sexual contact during the preceding 60 days. The most recent sex partner should be evaluated and treated even if the last sexual contact occurred more than 60 days prior.

11. Special considerations—

1) Because repeat infections are common, all patients diagnosed with chlamydia should be rescreened approximately 3 months after treatment.

2) Reporting: case reporting is required in the USA and some other countries.

3) More information can be found at:

- http://www.cdc.gov/std/treatment
- http://www.who.int/topics/sexually_transmitted_infections/en

[G. Anyalechi]

CHOLERA AND OTHER VIBRIOSES

DISEASE	CAUSATIVE AGENT	ICD-10 CODE
CHOLERA	Toxigenic *Vibrio cholerae* serogroups O1 and O139	ICD-10 A00
VIBRIO PARAHAEMOLYTICUS INFECTION	*Vibrio parahaemolyticus*	ICD-10 A05.3
VIBRIO VULNIFICUS INFECTION	*Vibrio vulnificus*	ICD-10 A05.5
OTHER *VIBRIO* INFECTIONS	Other non-O1 and -O139 serogroups of *V. cholerae*, *Vibrio mimicus*, *Vibrio alginolyticus*, and others	ICD-10 A05.8

I. CHOLERA

1. Clinical features—Following an incubation period of 1 to 2 days, patients develop profuse watery diarrhea, which is classically described as having a rice water consistency. Patients may have abdominal cramping but do not generally have any abdominal pain. Vomiting with watery emesis can also occur. Severity of the illness is determined by the rate of fluid and electrolyte losses, which can be as high as 1 liter per hour in the most severe cases owing to the secretory nature of the diarrhea, resulting in rapid dehydration with high mortality.

As a result of this rapid volume loss, patients may be noted to have sunken eyes, dry mouth, and cold skin with decreased turgor; patients may also be lethargic with apathy. Rapid pulse and hypotension may be found on examination; patients may have other manifestations of electrolyte disturbances, such as muscle weakness and cramping related to losses of calcium and potassium.

Laboratory testing may reveal hyponatremia or hypernatremia, hypokalemia, hypocalcemia, and a metabolic acidosis due to gastrointestinal losses of sodium bicarbonate. Renal failure due to prerenal azotemia or acute tubular necrosis may also be noted. Hypoglycemia, especially in children, can also be seen owing to depletion of glycogen stores.

2. Risk groups—Cholera continues to cause pandemics in all age groups in the modern era, notably following natural disasters; it is also endemic to resource-limited countries throughout Africa and Asia. Prior large epidemics include a 1992 outbreak in India and Bangladesh and a 2010 outbreak in Haiti; in the latter, the bacterium was introduced by a humanitarian worker following an earthquake. In 2016, WHO identified an ongoing outbreak in Yemen, which is the largest outbreak of cholera in recorded history. Climate change and severe weather events are also likely to increase vulnerability to outbreaks; this has been demonstrated following flooding from Cyclone Idai and Cyclone Kenneth in Mozambique in 2019.

3. Causative agents—Cholera is caused by infection with toxin-producing strains of the Gram-negative bacterium *Vibrio cholerae*, specifically strains that produce toxins O1 and O139. This bacterium is ubiquitous in aquatic environments. O1 and O139 are the strains that have been recognized to cause large epidemics; however, among the more than 200 identified serogroups, others have also been found to cause sporadic diarrheal illnesses.

4. Diagnosis—Cholera should be presumptively diagnosed in patients who present with acute watery diarrhea, especially in the context of a known outbreak or in a region where it is endemic. In nonendemic settings, cholera should be considered in travelers returning from endemic areas.

The differential diagnosis for cholera includes other pathogens known to cause acute watery diarrhea, which can be due to viruses and other bacteria, depending on local epidemiology.

For microbiologic diagnosis, stool culture using selective media such as thiosulfate-citrate-bile salts-sucrose agar or taurocholate-tellurite-gelatin agar can be used. Biochemical testing can be done on cultured isolates, including specific antibody tests to detect serogroup O1 and O139 to confirm cholera toxin–producing strains. Dark-field microscopy of fresh stools can show the shooting star–like motion of *Vibrio* spp., which is then inhibited by adding specific antibodies. Most relevant at point of care, rapid lateral flow assays can identify O1 and O139 antigens directly from stool samples.

5. Occurrence—Cholera is a diarrheal disease that has caused catastrophic epidemics throughout human history, including pandemics in the 19th and 20th centuries. Prior to identification of the causative organism, in 1849 John Snow famously demonstrated that an epidemic in London could be stopped by blocking access to contaminated water. Shortly thereafter, the curved bacillus *V. cholerae* was identified in the stools of affected patients by several investigators, including Pacini and Koch.

6. Reservoirs—Humans and the environment (such as copepods and other zooplankton).

7. Incubation period—From a few hours to 5 days.

8. Transmission—Cholera is spread by the fecal-oral route. Production of the cholera toxin by the bacterium results in severe secretory diarrhea through its actions on the intestinal epithelial cells. An infective dose of the bacterium is ingested through consumption of water or food contaminated by the fecal matter of infected individuals. Drinking water can be contaminated at its source, during transportation, or during home storage. Food can be contaminated by soiled hands, either during preparation or while eating. In funeral ceremonies of persons who have died of cholera, transmission may occur through consumption of food and beverages prepared by family members after they have handled the corpse.

An infected person can transmit cholera as long as they shed the bacteria in their stools, usually for 2 to 3 days after resolution of symptoms. Chronic fecal bacterial shedding for months to years is uncommon but has been documented.

9. Treatment—The primary and immediate goal of treatment is fluid resuscitation to replace fluid losses within 3 to 4 hours of presentation, followed by maintenance fluid administration. Assessment of the severity of the dehydration determines whether resuscitation can be oral or should be intravenous.

For mild to moderately ill patients, WHO currently recommends reduced osmolarity oral rehydration solutions (ORSs), with dosing of approximately

100 mL/kg initially. Continued close monitoring of the patient's volume status is crucial while fluids are being replaced to ensure adequate rehydration.

For severely ill patients (e.g., presenting in shock) or those who cannot tolerate oral intake, intravenous fluids should be urgently administered over the first 3 hours, approximately 100 mL/kg, with 30 mL/kg given over the first half-hour. Intravenous Ringer's lactate is the best solution to use in this setting, given its potassium and bicarbonate content because these are lost in the stools. Normal saline is not recommended as it will not correct metabolic acidosis. Alternative locally produced fluids, such as the Dhaka solution, are also acceptable for use.

Antibiotics are considered adjunctive therapy for cholera. Antibiotics can shorten the duration of diarrhea and stool volume and should be considered in patients with moderate-to-severe disease. They are also useful to reduce the duration of fecal shedding and thus may have a role in reducing transmission during outbreaks. Tetracyclines have the most evidence for efficacy, with a single high dose of doxycycline 300 mg orally being similarly effective to a 2-day course of tetracycline. However, resistance to these agents is common, thus fluoroquinolones (e.g., ciprofloxacin 1 g orally once) and macrolides (e.g., azithromycin 1 g orally once) should be considered if tetracycline-resistant strains are endemic. Weight-based doses of macrolides such as azithromycin and erythromycin can be used in children.

Restoring nutritional intake and enteral feeding is an important aspect in management of cholera. Once the initial volume deficit has been corrected, the patient should be encouraged to resume eating. Infants with cholera should be encouraged to breastfeed, along with rehydration.

10. Prevention—Prevention of cholera and management of epidemics is primarily focused on interrupting the fecal-oral transmission of the organism by ensuring access to safe, potable drinking water; proper sanitation and waste disposal; and appropriate hygiene including handwashing. Persons should avoid raw fruits and vegetables and food from street vendors as well as raw or undercooked seafood.

Vaccination is a critical component of outbreak control and disease prevention. Three oral vaccines are licensed internationally for this purpose. The bivalent killed whole-cell vaccine (Shanchol; Shantha Biotechnics; Hyderabad, India) contains whole cells of both *V. cholerae* serotype O1 and *V. cholerae* serotype O139 and has been found to have efficacy of 53% to 67% in clinical trials, with protection lasting 5 years and declining over this period. Two doses are recommended for most patients. Another whole-cell vaccine protective against serotype O1 only (Dukoral; SBL Vaccines; Stockholm, Sweden) is also used as a 2-dose series, with studies showing 78% protection in outbreak settings. Additionally, a similar vaccine with protection against both serotypes O1 and O139 (Euvichol; Eubiologics; Seoul, South Korea) is available. Herd immunity due to these vaccines also occurs once high levels of vaccine coverage are attained. These 3 vaccines have been prequalified by WHO for use in outbreak control, with Shanchol and Euvichol included in the global oral cholera vaccine stockpile.

Another oral vaccine (Vaxchora; PaxVax; Redwood City, CA), which is also effective against serotype O1, is the only cholera vaccine approved by FDA and is indicated as a single dose for travelers to endemic regions, including aid and health care workers. This vaccine has been found to have a greater than 90% efficacy 10 days after administration and 80% at 3 months.

A summary of cholera vaccines is given in Table 1.

Table 1. Cholera Vaccines

Trade Name	Shanchol	Dukoral	Euvichol	Vaxchora
Constituent	Killed whole cell	Killed whole cell	Killed whole cell	Live attenuated
Route	PO	PO	PO	PO
Dose	2	2	2	1
Toxin	O1, O139	O1	O1, O139	O1

Note: PO = oral(ly).

11. Special considerations—

1) Reporting: under the International Health Regulations (IHR), governments are required to report cholera cases and outbreaks or epidemics of acute watery diarrhea to WHO when they are unusual or unexpected or when they present significant risk of international spread or of international travel or trade restrictions. The reporting as cholera caused by non-O1 or non-O139 serogroups of *V. cholerae* is not correct (even if these strains possess the cholera toxin gene) and therefore leads to confusion. In addition, nontoxigenic *V. cholerae* O1 should not be reported as cholera.

2) Epidemic measures:

- Educate the population at risk concerning the need to seek appropriate treatment for dehydration without delay.
- Provide effective treatment facilities.
- Adopt emergency measures to ensure a safe water supply.
- Chlorinate public water supplies, even if the source water appears uncontaminated. Chlorinate or boil water used for drinking, cooking, and washing dishes and food containers, unless the water supply is already adequately chlorinated. Households that store drinking water should ensure that protective storage containers are used to prevent recontamination of treated water by hands or objects during storage.

- Ensure careful preparation and supervision of food and drinks. After cooking food or boiling water, protect against contamination by flies and unsanitary handling; leftover foods should be thoroughly reheated (70°C [158°F] for at least 15 minutes) before ingestion. Persons with diarrhea should not prepare food or haul water for others.
- Food served at funerals of cholera victims may be particularly hazardous if the body has been prepared for burial by persons in contact with the diseased person without stringent precautions; this practice should be discouraged during epidemics and handwashing promoted.
- Initiate a thorough investigation designed to find the predominant vehicle(s) of infection and circumstances (time, place, and person) of transmission; plan control measures accordingly.
- Provide appropriate safe facilities for sewage disposal. Oral cholera vaccines may be used as an additional public health tool in outbreak control but should not replace other recommended control measures or detract from clinical management of cases. Priority measures during cholera outbreaks should focus on access to life-saving treatment (ORSs in particular) and provision of safe drinking water.

3) Disaster implications: outbreak risks are high in endemic areas if large groups of people are crowded together without sufficient quantities of safe water, adequate food handling facilities, or sanitary facilities.

4) Measures applicable to ships, aircraft, and land transport arriving from cholera areas are to be applied within the framework of the IHR.

5) International travelers: no country is authorized under the IHR to require proof of cholera vaccination as a condition of entry and the International Certificate of Vaccination no longer provides a specific space for recording cholera vaccination. Immunization with either of the oral vaccines can be recommended for individuals traveling to areas of endemic or epidemic cholera but should not replace the need to be sure that drinking water is safe. Further information can be found at: http://www.who.int/csr/disease/cholera.

II. *VIBRIO PARAHAEMOLYTICUS* INFECTION

1. Clinical features—*Vibrio parahaemolyticus* is a Gram-negative bacterium that causes diarrheal illness associated with seafood consumption as well as wound infections and septicemia. This bacterium causes an intestinal disorder characterized by watery diarrhea and abdominal cramps in most cases, often with nausea, vomiting, and headache. About one-fourth of patients experience a dysentery-like illness with bloody or mucoid stools. Wound infections can also occur. Typically, it is a disease of moderate severity lasting 1 to 7 days; systemic infection and death rarely occur.

The most common clinical presentation of infection with this organism is gastroenteritis, predominantly diarrhea. Patients also present with abdominal cramping, nausea, vomiting, and fevers. The median incubation period is 17 hours with a mean duration of illness of 2.4 days. Less commonly, wound infections occur when a wound is exposed to contaminated water; these infections can be particularly severe in patients with underlying conditions such as liver disease, diabetes mellitus, and alcoholism as they are at higher risk of severe infection, with death in up to 3% of cases. In immunocompromised patients, bacteremia can also occur, with much higher case fatality.

2. Risk groups—Those with decreased gastric acidity, liver disease, or immunosuppression.

3. Causative agents—Isolates may be subtyped into O and K serotypes. More than 30 different O:K serotypes are found in the USA, but O3:K6, O4:K12, and O6:K18 have been identified from recent outbreaks. Clinical isolates from humans are generally (but not always) capable of producing a characteristic hemolytic reaction (the Kanagawa phenomenon) and carriage of 2 hemolysin genes correlates with diarrheal disease. More than 90% of isolates from ill persons carry 1 or both of these genes compared with less than 1% of isolates from food or environmental sources.

4. Diagnosis—By isolation of *V. parahaemolyticus* from stools, blood, or another clinical specimen. No serodiagnostic or rapid tests have been developed.

5. Occurrence—Sporadic cases and common-source outbreaks are reported in many parts of the world, particularly Japan, southeastern Asia, and the USA. Cases occur primarily in warm months. In 1998, 2 large outbreaks caused by serotype O3:K6, a common strain in Asia, occurred in the USA linked to consumption of raw oysters. This strain eventually emerged in South America and Africa, causing additional large outbreaks. Other genotypically similar serotypes, such as O4:K68 and O1:K untypable, have also spread worldwide and together are referred to as the *V. parahaemolyticus* pandemic clone. In the USA, the incidence of reported cases of *V. parahaemolyticus* has been increasing, reaching 0.7 cases per 100,000 population in 2017.

6. Reservoirs—Marine coastal environments are the natural habitat of these bacteria. During the cold season, organisms are found in marine silt; during the warm season, they are found free in coastal waters and in fish and shellfish. Increased overall colony counts are found in warmer water, suggesting that climate change may increase its future prevalence.

7. Incubation period—Usually about 24 hours but can range from 4 to 96 hours.

8. Transmission—By ingestion of raw or inadequately cooked seafood, especially oysters or other shellfish. Not normally communicable from person to person.

9. Treatment—Treatment consists of rehydration as appropriate, similar to the management of cholera infection. For septicemia or wound infection, effective antimicrobials (aminoglycosides, third-generation cephalosporins, fluoroquinolones, tetracycline) are recommended, in addition to supportive care.

10. Prevention—Key aspects of prevention of *V. parahaemolyticus* infection consist of educating consumers about the risks associated with eating raw or undercooked seafood, especially oysters and other shellfish. Consumers in high-risk groups should not eat raw or undercooked seafood. In addition, seafood handlers and processors should be informed of the importance of ensuring that seafood reaches temperatures adequate to kill the organism by thoroughly cooking it. Cooked seafood should also be handled carefully to avoid contamination from raw seafood or contaminated seawater, with appropriate refrigeration used as well. For oyster harvesting, several methods such as using high hydrostatic pressure, heat-cool pasteurization, and individual quick-freezing can reduce—but may not eliminate—*Vibrio* contamination.

Wounds exposed to sea or brackish waters should be cleaned thoroughly with soap and water.

11. Special considerations—Reporting of cases to a local health authority is recommended and is obligatory in some countries. Recognition and reporting of cases associated with recent shellfish consumption is especially important for follow-up investigation.

III. *VIBRIO VULNIFICUS* INFECTION

1. Clinical features—*Vibrio vulnificus* is a Gram-negative bacterium that can cause severe wound infections with septicemia, as well as diarrhea, especially in patients with chronic underlying illness, such as liver disease, alcohol abuse, diabetes mellitus, and hereditary hemochromatosis. Like *V. parahaemolyticus*, this is a free-living bacterium of saltwater marshes and river estuaries. Oysters in such waters may have high concentrations of this bacterium.

Wound infections occur as a result of exposure of the wound to salt water containing the organism. Several infections were noted in August and September 2005 following Hurricane Katrina in Louisiana, mostly in patients with underlying chronic diseases. The bacterium has especially been noted to grow in iron-rich environments and cause more severe disease in those patients with higher iron concentrations, such as hemochromatosis. The bacterium produces several toxins that are thought to mediate clinical disease. Wound infections are sometimes complicated by severe myositis and necrotizing fasciitis. Septicemia with shock is also a common presentation, with high associated mortality, especially in those with underlying chronic liver disease, chronic alcoholism, hemochromatosis, or immunocompromising conditions. Intestinal infection rarely occurs. Fever, chills, and hypotension are common, as are distinctive bullous skin lesions that progress to necrotic ulcers. About 50% of patients with septicemia die. *V. vulnificus* can also cause wound infection when preexisting or new skin lesions are exposed to seawater or brackish water or to sea life; these infections range from mild, self-limited lesions to rapidly progressive cellulitis, myositis, and septicemia. Others can be infected and can develop gastroenteritis but do not usually present with septicemia.

2. Risk groups—Persons with cirrhosis, hemochromatosis and other chronic liver diseases, or immunocompromising conditions are at increased risk for the infection and for the septicemic form of disease.

3. Causative agents—These bacteria are halophilic and are commonly found in marine environments. Three biogroups have been identified. Biogroup 1 is an opportunistic human pathogen usually associated with the consumption of raw oysters, although wound infections can occur after trauma and exposure to a contaminated marine environment. Biogroup 2 strains are rarely found outside of Europe; they are isolated predominantly from diseased eels but are occasionally isolated from human septicemia and wound infections acquired from handling eels. Biogroup 3 has been isolated only from Israeli patients with wound infections and bacteremia. These cases are associated with exposure to live fish (tilapia and carp) grown in aquaculture environments.

4. Diagnosis—*V. vulnificus* infection is usually diagnosed by isolation of the organism from blood or a wound, usually on blood agar. No serodiagnostic or rapid tests have been developed.

The bacterium will grow on standard nonselective media, but thiosulfate-citrate-bile salts-sucrose medium can also be used. However, the diagnosis and empiric treatment should be considered in any patient with a typical presentation of shock with characteristic skin lesions, given the high mortality of this disease.

5. Occurrence—It is the most common agent of serious infections caused by *Vibrio* spp. in North America and has been reported in many areas of the world (e.g., Israel, Japan, South Korea, Spain, Taiwan, and Turkey).

6. Reservoirs—*V. vulnificus* is a free-living autochthonous element of flora of estuarine environments. It is recovered from estuarine waters and from shellfish, particularly oysters. During summer, it can often be isolated routinely from oysters.

7. Incubation period—Usually 12 to 72 hours after eating raw or undercooked seafood.

8. Transmission—This organism is transmitted through ingestion of raw or undercooked seafood, after exposure of wounds to marine or estuarine water (e.g., in boating accidents), or from occupational wounds (in oyster shuckers, fishermen). Not transmitted directly from person to person.

9. Treatment—Similar principles as for *V. parahaemolyticus* infection. Antibiotic therapy is a combination of a tetracycline (e.g., doxycycline or minocycline) with a third-generation cephalosporin (e.g., cefotaxime or ceftriaxone) as a first-line regimen. Fluoroquinolones (e.g., levofloxacin) can also be used as monotherapy. Aggressive surgical debridement is generally needed for severe wound infections.

10. Prevention—Similar measures to those for *V. parahaemolyticus* infection. Two key features: (a) avoidance of exposing open wounds to seawater and (b) careful washing of wounds that have been exposed to sea or brackish waters with soap and clean water. Prevention of disease also involves avoiding consumption of raw or undercooked shellfish, especially in persons with chronic high-risk diseases.

11. Special considerations—

1) Reporting of cases to local health authorities is recommended and is obligatory in some countries. Recognition and reporting of cases associated with recent shellfish consumption is especially important for further investigation.
2) Disaster implications: a potential hazard in environmental disaster situations, such as hurricanes, in which wounds and exposure to seawater are widespread among those at risk. Healthy persons with a wound can develop infection but their risk is much lower than that for people in risk groups.

IV. OTHER *VIBRIO* INFECTIONS

1. Clinical features—There are more than 100 species of *Vibrio* that have been identified. Species associated with the most severe diseases have been discussed in the previous sections. Other *Vibrio* spp. cause a range of clinical syndromes. Many of these can cause gastroenteritis that ranges from mild to severe but they have not caused large epidemics. Certain species in particular, such as *Vibrio alginolyticus*, cause otitis externa, otitis media, and cellulitis. Other less commonly identified *Vibrio* spp. cause wound and septicemic illnesses.

2. Risk groups—Immunosuppressed; alcohol abuse. Septicemia develops most commonly in persons with immunocompromising conditions, chronic liver disease, or severe malnutrition.

3. Causative agents—Multiple *Vibrio* spp., as detailed earlier, including non–O1- and non–O139-producing strains of *V. cholerae, Vibrio mimicus, Vibrio fluvialis, Vibrio furnissii,* and *V. alginolyticus.* Additional species have also been identified from human specimens but it is not yet clear if they cause human disease.

Isolates of *V. cholerae* O1 and O139 that do not produce cholera toxin are known to occur but, as is the case with nontoxigenic non-O1/non-O139 strains, these strains do not cause large cholera epidemics but are usually associated with sporadic diarrheal disease. Isolates of non-O1/non-O139 *V. cholerae* can cause illness because they can possess a variety of virulence factors, sometimes including production of cholera toxin. However, cholera toxin–producing strains of non-O1 *V. cholerae* are rarely encountered. In the USA, toxigenic strains of *V. cholerae* serogroups O75 and O141 are associated with sporadic cholera-like illness that is usually attributed to consumption of undercooked seafood; on average fewer than 10 cases a year are detected. Some *V. cholerae* strains that do not agglutinate in O1 or O139 antiserum and produce a heat-stable enterotoxin (ST) are referred to as nonagglutinable-ST strains. Certain other species in the family Vibrionaceae can cause human illness, including diarrhea, septicemia, and other extraintestinal infections. These include *V. mimicus, Grimontia hollisae* (formerly *Vibrio hollisae*), *V. furnissii, V. fluvialis, V. alginolyticus,* and *Photobacterium damselae* (formerly *Vibrio damsela*). Some strains of *V. mimicus* produce cholera toxin and have been associated with outbreaks of severe watery diarrhea. Most septicemic infections occur in immunocompromised individuals or persons with underlying liver disease.

4. Diagnosis—Diagnosis is by isolation of the organism from clinical specimens. No serodiagnostic or rapid tests have been developed.

5. Occurrence—These other *Vibrio* spp. are uncommon causes of diarrheal, wound, and septicemic illness, mainly in tropical and coastal areas. Most are of little public health importance, though small outbreaks have been reported.

6. Reservoirs—*Vibrio* spp. are found in aquatic environments worldwide, particularly in brackish waters and salt waters. *Vibrio* counts vary seasonally, peaking in warm seasons. In brackish waters, they are often found adherent to chitinous zooplankton and shellfish. Isolates can survive and multiply in a variety of foods.

7. Incubation period—This generally ranges from 12 to 24 hours depending on the particular species.

8. Transmission—Cases of gastroenteritis are usually linked to consumption of raw or undercooked seafood, particularly shellfish. In tropical endemic areas, some infections may be due to ingestion of surface waters. Wound infections arise from environmental exposure, usually to brackish waters or salt water or to sea life. In high-risk hosts, septicemia may result from a wound infection or from ingestion of contaminated seafood.

9. Treatment—Similar to treatment of other *Vibrio* infections as detailed previously.

10. Prevention—Same as for other *Vibrio* spp. as detailed previously.

11. Special considerations—Reporting to national health authorities is recommended and may be mandatory in some areas. Clinicians who report non-O1/non-O139 *V. cholerae* infections or nontoxigenic *V. cholerae* O1 infection should clearly distinguish these infections from those due to cholera toxin–producing strains.

[E. Talbot, M. Abel]

CHROMOMYCOSIS
(chromoblastomycosis, dermatitis verrucosa)

DISEASE	ICD-10 CODE
CHROMOMYCOSIS	ICD-10 B43

1. Clinical features—Considered by WHO to be a neglected tropical disease, chromomycosis occurs as a chronic spreading mycosis of the skin and subcutaneous tissues, usually of the lower extremities although other areas can be involved. The initial lesion appears as a papule or a nodule. Progression to contiguous tissues is slow, over a period of years, with eventual large, nodular, verrucous, or even cauliflower-like masses. Invasion to muscle or bone can occur, although disseminated disease is rare. Rarely is a cause of death.

2. Risk groups—Primarily a disease of barefoot rural agricultural workers in tropical regions, probably due to frequent traumatic inoculation. The disease is most common among men aged 30 to 50 years.

3. Causative agents—Dematiaceous fungi, including *Fonsecaea (Phialophora) pedrosoi*, *Phialophora verrucosa*, *Cladosporium carrionii*, *Rhinocladiella aquaspersa*, *Botryomyces caespitatus*, *Exophiala spinifera*, and *Exophiala jeanselmei*.

4. Diagnosis—The most useful technique is direct microscopic examination of scrapings or biopsies of lesions with 10% potassium hydroxide. Characteristic muriform cells (or Medlar bodies) are large, brown, thick-walled, rounded cells that divide by fission in 2 planes. Cells are pathognomonic for chromomycosis; however, this does not distinguish between organisms. Confirmation of diagnosis should be made by biopsy and attempted cultures of the fungus. Molecular taxonomy, using sequencing of specific genes, has been shown to be useful for the correct identification of isolates at the species level.

5. Occurrence—Worldwide; predominantly in tropical and subtropical regions, particularly Latin America, the Caribbean, Asia, and Africa. Causative organism differs by region; for example, *C. carrionii* is more common in dry climates. Occurs more commonly in men and in those with professions working outdoors (e.g., farming, agriculture).

6. Reservoirs—Wood, soil, and decaying vegetation.

7. Incubation period—Unknown; likely months to years.

8. Transmission—Inoculation via superficial, minor, penetrating trauma/injuries (e.g., usually a sliver of contaminated wood or other material). Not transmitted from person to person.

9. Treatment—

Preferred therapy	Small and few lesions:
	• Surgical excision or cryosurgery with liquid nitrogen
	Chronic, extensive, or burrowing lesions:
	• Itraconazole 200–400 mg PO every 24 hours OR 400 mg pulse therapy once daily for 1 week monthly for 6–12 months (or until response)

(Continued)

(Continued)

Alternative therapy options	• Terbinafine 500–1,000 mg once daily for 6–12 months (or until response). • For refractory cases, consider itraconazole PLUS terbinafine combination OR other expanded spectrum triazoles (i.e. posaconazole). • Physical therapeutic methods are typically used as adjuvant therapy to systemic antifungals and include surgical resection, cryotherapy, heat therapy, laser therapy, and/or photodynamic therapy. • Experts have also cited sources that have had success in using topical imiquimod in conjunction with systemic antifungal therapy. • Topical ajoene (a garlic extract) and 5-fluorouracil have been reported to be effective against disease secondary to *Cladosporium carrionii*.
Special considerations and comments	• Chromomycosis is difficult to cure and relapse is an issue. Treatment typically involves many months of therapy, including both physical therapeutic methods and systemic antifungal therapy. • Terbinafine should be avoided in patients with chronic or acute liver disease.

Note: PO = oral(ly).

10. Prevention—Education of those at risk, especially in agricultural professions in tropical and subtropical regions. Protect against small puncture wounds by wearing gloves, shoes, or protective clothing.

11. Special considerations—None.

[D. Caceres, S. Tsay]

COCCIDIOIDOMYCOSIS
(valley fever, San Joaquin fever, desert fever, desert rheumatism, coccidioidal granuloma)

DISEASE	ICD-10 CODE
COCCIDIOIDOMYCOSIS	ICD-10 B38

1. Clinical features—The primary infection may be entirely asymptomatic or may present as a respiratory illness with fever, chills, fatigue, cough, dyspnea, headache, night sweats, myalgias, arthralgias, and weight loss.

About one-fourth of recognized cases involve erythema nodosum. Primary infection may resolve without detectable sequelae. However, about 5% to 10% of symptomatic patients may develop long-term complications, such as fibrosis, a pulmonary nodule with or without calcified areas, a persistent thin-walled cavity, or disseminated disease.

Fewer than 1% of symptomatic coccidioidomycosis cases involve dissemination beyond the lungs. Disseminated coccidioidomycosis is a progressive, severe granulomatous disease characterized by lesions in nearly any part of the body, especially in subcutaneous tissues, skin, bone, and meninges. Coccidioidal meningitis can resemble tuberculous meningitis but runs a more chronic course, often requiring lifelong therapy. Disseminated infection is fatal without treatment.

2. Risk groups—Coccidioidomycosis is a common cause of pneumonia and influenza-like illness among persons visiting or living in endemic areas. Occupations and activities with high dust exposure (such as construction, agriculture, field archaeology, and military exercises) have caused coccidioidomycosis outbreaks. The disease affects all races and age groups, with the incidence of symptomatic disease being highest in the elderly. Risk factors for severe or disseminated infection include acquired immunodeficiency syndrome (AIDS), immunosuppressive medications, organ transplant, diabetes mellitus, pregnancy (especially during third trimester), and African or Filipino race/ethnicity. Latent infection can occur, with reactivation in people who become immunocompromised.

3. Causative agents—*Coccidioides immitis* and *Coccidioides posadasii*, dimorphic fungi. The 2 species cannot be distinguished morphologically. *Coccidioides* spp. grow in soil and culture media as saprophytic molds that reproduce by arthroconidia; in tissues and under special conditions, the parasitic form grows as spherical cells (spherules) that reproduce by formation of endospores.

4. Diagnosis—Serologic antibody tests are most commonly used. Enzyme immunoassay (EIA) is a sensitive and commonly used method that can detect immunoglobulin class M (IgM) and immunoglobulin class G (IgG) antibodies. IgM antibodies appear approximately 1 to 2 weeks after symptom onset and typically persist for several months. False-positive EIA IgM results have been reported. IgG antibodies can be associated with recent infection and persist for approximately 6 to 8 months, though with considerable variation. Samples positive by EIA are commonly sent for reference laboratory testing by immunodiffusion, which detects presence of IgM, IgG, and complement fixation (CF), which detects presence of IgG. CF testing can yield quantitative results helpful in monitoring response to therapy. Serologic tests may be negative in the immunocompromised (e.g., those with AIDS). Antigen testing is not widely used but may be useful in making the diagnosis in immunocompromised patients with severe disease; however, cross-reactivity with histoplasmosis and blastomycosis antigen occurs.

Microscopic examination or culture of tissues or respiratory specimens can be used to detect *Coccidioides*. Although these methods are highly specific, they have low sensitivity. Handling cultures of the agent is extremely hazardous and must be carried out in a class II biologic safety cabinet under biosafety level (BSL) 3 containment. Clinical specimens should be handled under BSL-2 containment.

5. Occurrence—Primary infections are common in arid and semiarid endemic areas of the western hemisphere: in the USA, *Coccidioides* is known to be endemic in Arizona, California, Nevada, New Mexico, Texas, Utah, and as far north as south-central Washington. The disease also occurs in Mexico, Central America, and parts of South America (Argentina, Columbia, Venezuela, and northeastern Brazil). Disease has occurred in people who have merely traveled through endemic areas.

Infections occur year round. In the USA, incidence increases in the late summer and fall. Infects humans, cattle, cats, dogs, horses, and many other animals.

6. Reservoirs—Soil in endemic areas.

7. Incubation period—In primary infection, 1 to 3 weeks. Dissemination may develop insidiously years after the primary infection, sometimes without recognized symptoms of primary pulmonary infection.

8. Transmission—Typically through inhalation of infective arthroconidia from soil. Infection can occur from improper handling of cultures producing arthroconidia. Rare transmissions have been reported via solid organ transplantation, pregnancy, and exposure to fomites containing dust from endemic areas. *Coccidioides* is highly infectious; disease may occur after inhalation of only a few arthroconidia. While the parasitic form is not normally infective, accidental inoculation of infected pus or culture suspension into the skin or bone can result in granuloma formation. No direct person-to-person or animal-to-human transmission. *Coccidioides* spp. from skin abscesses may rarely change from the parasitic to the infective saprophytic form.

9. Treatment—Consult Infectious Diseases Society of America (IDSA) guidelines (https://www.idsociety.org/practice-guideline/coccidioidomy-cosis). Some infections can be followed until resolution without antifungal treatment. Antifungal treatment and sometimes surgery are indicated for patients with severe disease and those at elevated risk for complications. Patients with disseminated disease may need lifelong antifungal therapy to prevent relapses.

In case treatment is warranted (i.e., severe disease), fluconazole 400 mg orally once daily for 3 to 6 months is an option. For severe disease in immunocompromised individuals, the addition of liposomal amphotericin B is suggested, dosed at 4 to 6 mg/kg per day, plus fluconazole 400 mg orally daily until clinical improvement.

IDSA guidelines referenced earlier address several specific scenarios that may vary from those described here.

10. Prevention—It is difficult to avoid breathing in *Coccidioides* arthroconidia where they are common in the environment. People who live in or visit these areas can try to avoid spending time in dusty places or inhaling dust as much as possible. Examples of activities and events involving increased dust exposure include gardening, construction, excavation, wildland firefighting, and dust storms.

11. Special considerations—

1) Reporting: reporting cases to local health authority may be required.
2) Outbreaks occur when groups of susceptible persons are infected by airborne arthroconidia.

[O. Z. McCotter, B. Jackson]

COMMON COLD AND OTHER ACUTE VIRAL RESPIRATORY DISEASES

DISEASE	ICD-10 CODE
COMMON COLD	ICD-10 J00
OTHER ACUTE FEBRILE RESPIRATORY ILLNESSES	ICD-10 J01–J06; J12
Influenza (see "Influenza")	
Severe acute respiratory syndrome (see "SARS, MERS, and Other Coronavirus Infections")	
Streptococcal pharyngitis (see "Streptococcal Diseases")	

Numerous acute respiratory illnesses of known and presumed viral etiology are grouped here. Clinically, infections of the upper respiratory tract (above the epiglottis) can be designated as acute viral rhinitis or acute viral pharyngitis (common cold); infections involving the lower respiratory tract (below the epiglottis) can be designated as croup (laryngotracheitis and sometimes laryngotracheobronchitis), acute viral tracheobronchitis, bronchitis, bronchiolitis, or acute viral pneumonia. These respiratory syndromes are associated with a large number of viruses that can produce a wide spectrum of acute respiratory illnesses and differ in etiology between children and adults.

The illnesses, caused by known agents, have important common epidemiologic attributes, such as reservoir and mode of transmission. Many of the viruses invade any part of the respiratory tract; others show a predilection for certain anatomic sites. Some predispose to bacterial complications. Morbidity and mortality from acute respiratory diseases are especially significant in children. In adults, relatively high incidence and resulting disability, with consequent economic loss, make acute respiratory diseases a major health problem worldwide. As a group, acute respiratory diseases constitute one of the leading causes of death from any infectious disease.

Several other infections of the respiratory tract are presented as separate chapters because they are sufficiently distinctive in their manifestations and occur in regular association with a single infectious agent: examples include influenza, psittacosis, hantavirus pulmonary syndrome, chlamydial pneumonia, vesicular pharyngitis (herpangina), epidemic myalgia (pleurodynia), and severe acute respiratory syndrome and other coronavirus infections. Symptoms of upper respiratory tract infection, mainly pharyngotonsillitis, can be produced by bacterial agents, among which group A *Streptococcus* is the most common, although recent etiologic studies involving respiratory pathogens do not support this. Viral infections should be differentiated from bacterial or other infections for which specific antimicrobial measures are available.

I. COMMON COLD (acute viral rhinitis, rhinitis, coryza [acute])

1. Clinical features—An acute catarrhal infection of the upper respiratory tract characterized by coryza, sneezing, lacrimation, irritation of the nasopharynx, chills, and malaise lasting 2 to 7 days. Fever is uncommon in children older than 3 years and rare in adults. White blood cell counts are usually normal. Illness may be accompanied by laryngitis, tracheitis, or bronchitis and may predispose individuals to more serious complications, such as sinusitis and otitis media. Fatalities are not associated with common colds, although severe illness may progress through a catarrhal phase, such as in debilitated persons or in those with secondary infections. Disability due to common colds is important because it affects work performance and industrial and school absenteeism.

2. Risk groups—Susceptibility is universal.

3. Causative agents—Rhinoviruses, of which there are more than 100 recognized serotypes, are the major known causal agents of the common cold in adults; they account for about 30% to 50% of infections, especially in the fall. Coronaviruses are responsible for about 10% to 15% of common colds in adults. Other known respiratory viruses account for a small proportion of common colds in adults. In infants and children, parainfluenza viruses, respiratory syncytial virus (RSV), adenoviruses, certain enteroviruses, and coronaviruses may cause illnesses similar to the common cold (see Other Acute Febrile Respiratory Illnesses in this chapter). The cause of about half of common colds has not been identified.

4. Diagnosis—Primary diagnosis should be based on clinical parameters as patients with common cold essentially present without any clinical features of pneumonia, such as absence of increased work of breathing, especially in children. Adult patients with common cold may present without a fever but with a productive purulent cough and chest pain. Specific clinical, epidemiologic, and other manifestations aid differentiation from similar diseases due to toxic, allergic, physical, or psychologic stimuli. Cell or organ culture studies of nasal secretions may be done to identify known viruses. Polymerase chain reaction (PCR) methods can also be used to detect respiratory viruses.

5. Occurrence—Worldwide, both endemic and epidemic. In temperate zones, incidence rises in fall, winter, and spring; in tropical settings, incidence is highest in the rainy season. Many people have 1 to 6 colds yearly. Incidence is highest in children younger than 5 years and gradually declines with increasing age.

6. Reservoirs—Humans.

7. Incubation period—Between 12 hours and 5 days, usually 48 hours, varying with the agent.

8. Transmission—Presumably through direct contact or exposure of mucous membranes to respiratory droplets and indirect transmission through hands and articles freshly soiled by nose and throat discharges of an infected person. Contaminated hands carry rhinovirus, RSV, and probably other similar viruses to the mucous membranes of the eye or nose. Nasal washes carried out 24 hours before onset and for 5 days after onset have produced symptoms in experimentally infected volunteers. Inapparent infections occur; some viruses, notably rhinoviruses and adenoviruses, have been detected in asymptomatic persons.

9. Treatment—

Drug	• Mainly symptomatic treatment. • Nasal clearance is the mainstay of treatment. It can be done using a nasal decongestant such as saline in the case of nasal congestion. • Use antipyretic in case of fever/malaise if needed.

(Continued)

(Continued)

Dose	Nasal drops:
	• Adults: xylometazoline 2 or 3 drops adult formula (0.1%) 2 or 3 times daily
	• Children < 12 years: xylometazoline 1 or 2 drops children's formula (0.05%) in each nostril 1 or 2 times daily (not to be used in infants < 3 months)
	• Younger infants < 3 months: normal saline 1 or 2 drops in each nostril 3–4 hourly recommended
	Antipyretics:
	• Adults: acetaminophen 500 mg tablet 6–8 hourly (≤ 8 tablets/day)
	• Children: 15–20 mg/kg/dose 6–8 hourly
Route	Nasal drops:
	• In nostrils
	Antipyretics
	• PO
Alternative drug	Adequate fluid intake, adequate rest, avoid crowds, hand-washing after cleaning nose and eyes.
Duration	Treatment should be continued until symptoms subside, usually 3–5 days.
Special considerations and comments	• Adequate rest and avoid crowding.
	• Adequate fluid intake.
	• Maintain personal hygiene and handwashing after cleaning nose, eyes, etc.
	• Appropriate disposal of nasal secretions.

Note: PO = oral(ly).

10. Prevention—

1) Practice good personal hygiene, such as covering the mouth when coughing and sneezing, sanitary disposal of oral and nasal discharges, and hand hygiene.

2) When possible, avoid crowding in living and sleeping quarters, especially in institutions, in barracks, and aboard ships. Provide adequate ventilation.

3) Oral live adenovirus vaccines are administered to US military recruits to prevent adenovirus type 4 and type 7 infections but are not indicated in civilian populations because of the low incidence of specific disease.

4) Avoid smoking and passive smoke exposure. The risk of pneumonia increases among infected children exposed to passive smoke.

11. Special considerations—None.

II. OTHER ACUTE FEBRILE RESPIRATORY ILLNESSES

1. Clinical features—Viral diseases of the respiratory tract may be characterized by fever, cough, increased respiratory rate, chills, headache, general aches, malaise, anorexia, and, occasionally, gastrointestinal symptoms. Localizing signs also occur at various sites in the respiratory tract, either alone or in combination, such as rhinitis, pharyngitis or tonsillitis, laryngitis, laryngotracheitis, and pneumonia in both adults and children. However, bronchitis and pneumonitis may occur in adults and bronchiolitis in young children (2 weeks to 18 months). There may be associated conjunctivitis. Upper respiratory tract infection symptoms and signs usually subside in 2 to 5 days without complications. Lower respiratory tract infections may be severe or complicated by bacterial infections.

2. Risk groups—Susceptibility is universal. Illness is more frequent and more severe in infants, children, and older adults. Infection induces specific antibodies that are usually short-lived. Reinfection with RSV and parainfluenza viruses is common but illness is generally milder. Individuals with compromised cardiac, pulmonary, or immune systems are at increased risk of severe illness. Those at high risk of RSV-related complications include infants and children younger than 2 years who have congenital heart disease or required medical treatment for chronic lung disease within 6 months of the RSV season and premature infants of less than 35 weeks' gestation at birth. Children infected with human immunodeficiency virus have a greater risk of hospitalization for RSV-associated lower respiratory illness and a higher case-fatality rate, which may be related to heightened susceptibility to coinfection with other pathogens, including bacteria and *Pneumocystis jiroveci.*

3. Causative agents—Viruses considered etiologic agents of acute febrile respiratory illnesses are RSV; parainfluenza virus types 1, 2, 3, 4; human metapneumovirus; adenoviruses; rhinoviruses; certain coronaviruses; and certain enteroviruses, including some types of coxsackievirus groups A and B, and echoviruses. Influenza virus (see "Influenza") can produce a similar clinical picture. Some of these agents tend to cause more severe illnesses; others are more commonly detected in certain age groups and populations. RSV, the major viral respiratory tract pathogen of early childhood irrespective of geography, produces illness with greatest frequency during the first 2 years of life; it is the major known causal agent of bronchiolitis and one of the main causes of viral pneumonia and croup in children, and bronchitis, otitis media, and febrile upper respiratory tract illness mostly in adults. The parainfluenza viruses are the major known causal agents of croup; they also cause pneumonia, bronchiolitis, and febrile upper respiratory tract illness, particularly in children. Human metapneumovirus causes upper and lower respiratory tract illness in children. RSV, parainfluenza viruses, and human metapneumovirus may cause symptomatic disease in adults, particularly older adults and persons with chronic cardiopulmonary conditions or immunosuppression. Adenoviruses are associated with several forms of respiratory disease; types 4 and 7 are common causes of acute respiratory disease in nonimmunized military recruits.

4. Diagnosis—Should be primarily diagnosed on the basis of clinical features. Usually is associated with increased work of breathing. However, isolation of the causal agent from respiratory secretions in appropriate cell or organ cultures and identification of viral antigen in nasopharyngeal cells by fluorescent antibody, enzyme-linked immunosorbent assay, and radio-immunoassay tests and/or antibody studies of paired sera may help with the diagnosis. PCR methods can also be used to detect respiratory viruses in respiratory specimens, such as nasopharyngeal or oropharyngeal swab specimens.

5. Occurrence—Worldwide. Seasonal in temperate zones, with greatest incidence during fall and winter and occasionally spring. In tropical zones, respiratory infections tend to be more frequent in wet and in colder weather. In large communities, some viral illnesses are constantly present, usually with little seasonal pattern; others tend to occur in seasonal outbreaks (e.g., RSV).

Annual incidence is high, particularly in infants and children, with 2 to 6 episodes per child per year, and depends on the number of susceptibles and the virulence of the virus.

6. Reservoirs—Humans. Some viruses produce inapparent infections; some cause similar infections in many animal species but are thought to be of minor importance as sources of human infections.

7. Incubation period—From 1 to 10 days, depending on the viral pathogen.

8. Transmission—Directly through oral contact or droplet spread; indirectly from hands, handkerchiefs/tissues, eating utensils, or other articles freshly soiled with respiratory discharges of an infected person. Enteroviruses and adenoviruses may be transmitted by the fecal-oral route. Outbreaks of illness due to adenovirus have been related to swimming pools. Infections are communicable shortly prior to, and for the duration of, active disease; limited information is available about subclinical or asymptomatic infections.

9. Treatment—

Drug	Antipyretic (acetaminophen) for fever (if needed)
	Antibiotic for LRTI (if needed):
	• Amoxicillin is the drug of choice; for those who require hospitalization, consider amoxicillin with clavulanic acid PLUS macrolide antibiotic (such as clarithromycin or azithromycin)

(Continued)

(Continued)

Dose	Acetaminophen:
	• Adults: 500 mg tablet 6–8 hourly ($\leq$ 8 tablets/day) • Children: 15–20 mg/kg/dose syrup 6–8 hourly
	• Amoxicillin or amoxicillin with clavulanic acid: ○ Adults: 500 mg capsule 8 hourly for 5–7 days ○ Children: 40–50 mg/kg/dose syrup 12 hourly PLUS • Clarithromycin: ○ Adults: 500 mg tablet 12 hourly for 7 days ○ Children: 7.5 mg/kg/dose syrup 12 hourly
	• Bronchodilator in case of wheezing (all ages): 3–4 mg/kg/dose PO • Nebulization with albuterol solution: 0.03 mL/kg/dose with 2.5–3 mL normal saline 8 hourly if needed • Note that bronchodilator does not have any role in children with bronchiolitis and only works in children with asthma or postinfective wheeze and in adults with asthma or chronic bronchitis
Route	Antipyretic:
	• PO
	Antibiotic:
	• PO or IV
	Bronchodilator:
	• PO or through nebulization/inhaler
Alternative drug	Alternative antibiotic for nonhospitalized cases:
	• Adults: azithromycin (500 mg tablet PO once daily for 3–5 days) or levofloxacin (500–750 mg PO once daily for 7–10 days) • Children: azithromycin (10 mg/kg PO once daily for 3–5 days) or cefixime (8–10 mg/kg/day PO as a single dose or every 12 hours for 5–7 days)
Duration	Acetaminophen:
	• Need to continue until fever subsides
	Antibiotic:
	• Need to continue for 5–7 days
	Bronchodilator:
	• Need to continue until wheezing subsides only in asthma/postinfective wheeze/chronic bronchitis. • Avoid the use of bronchodilator in other respiratory illnesses, especially in children, because it provokes heart failure.

(Continued)

(Continued)

Special considerations and comments	• Adequate rest • Adequate fluid intake • Maintain personal hygiene • Avoid crowding • If needed, oxygen inhalation

Note: IV = intravenous(ly); LRTI = lower respiratory tract infection; PO = oral(ly).

10. Prevention—

1) As for common cold. See Prevention under Common Cold in this chapter.

2) Infants at high risk of RSV-related complications (see Risk Groups under Other Acute Febrile Respiratory Illnesses in this chapter) may benefit from palivizumab prophylaxis. Palivizumab is a monoclonal antibody preparation against RSV that is given monthly (intramuscularly) in some countries during the course of the RSV season. Palivizumab has reduced RSV-related hospitalization by about half in such infants.

11. Special considerations—None.

[K. Zaman]

CONJUNCTIVITIS AND KERATITIS

DISEASE	ICD-10 CODE
CONJUNCTIVITIS, BACTERIAL	ICD-10 A48.4
KERATOCONJUNCTIVITIS, ADENOVIRAL	ICD-10 B30.0
KERATOCONJUNCTIVITIS, MICROSPORIDIAL	ICD-10 B60.13
HEMORRHAGIC CONJUNCTIVITIS, ADENOVIRAL AND ENTEROVIRAL	ICD-10 B30.1 (adenoviral) ICD-10 B30.3 (enteroviral)
CHLAMYDIAL CONJUNCTIVITIS	ICD-10 A74.0
Gonococcal conjunctivitis (see "Gonococcal Infections")	
Trachoma (see "Trachoma")	

I. CONJUNCTIVITIS, BACTERIAL (pinkeye, sticky eye, Brazilian purpuric fever)

1. Clinical features—A clinical syndrome beginning with lacrimation, irritation, and hyperemia of the palpebral and bulbar conjunctivae of 1 or both eyes, followed by edema of eyelids and mucopurulent discharge. In severe cases, ecchymoses of the bulbar conjunctiva and marginal infiltration of the cornea with mild photophobia may occur. Nonfatal (except as noted later), the disease may last between 2 days and 2 to 3 weeks; many patients have no more than hyperemia of the conjunctivae and slight exudate for a few days. If the eyes are glued shut, there is a 15:1 chance that the infection is bacterial and not viral.

2. Risk groups—Children younger than 5 years are most often affected; incidence decreases with age. The very young, the debilitated, and the aged are particularly susceptible to staphylococcal infections. Immunity after attack is low grade and varies with the infectious agent.

3. Causative agents—*Haemophilus influenzae* biogroup *aegyptius* (Koch-Weeks bacillus) and *Streptococcus pneumoniae* appear to be the most important; *H. influenzae* type b, *Branhamella* spp., *Neisseria meningitidis*, and *Corynebacterium diphtheriae* may also produce the disease. *H. influenzae* biogroup *aegyptius*, gonococci (see "Gonococcal Infections"), *S. pneumoniae*, *Streptococcus viridans*, various Gram-negative enteric bacilli, and, rarely, *Pseudomonas aeruginosa* may produce the disease in newborn infants. *Staphylococcus aureus* is the most common cause in adults, especially in contact lens wearers.

4. Diagnosis—Diagnosis through microscopic examination of a stained smear. Culture to exclude other causative agent. Broad-spectrum antimicrobial therapy should initially be instituted while awaiting specific diagnosis.

5. Occurrence—Widespread and common worldwide, particularly in warmer climates; frequently epidemic. Infection due to other organisms occurs throughout the world, often associated with acute viral respiratory disease during cold seasons. Occasional cases of systemic disease have occurred among children in several communities in Brazil 1 to 3 weeks after conjunctivitis due to a unique invasive clone of *H. influenzae* biogroup *aegyptius*. This severe Brazilian purpuric fever had a 70% case-fatality rate among more than 100 cases recognized over a wide area of Brazil covering 4 states. The causal agent has been isolated from conjunctival, pharyngeal, and blood cultures.

6. Reservoirs—Humans. Carriers of *H. influenzae* biogroup *aegyptius* and *S. pneumoniae* are common in many areas during interepidemic periods.

7. Incubation period—Usually 24 to 72 hours.

8. Transmission—Contact with discharges from conjunctivae or upper respiratory tracts of infected people; contaminated fingers, clothing, and other articles, including shared eye-makeup applicators, multiple-dose eye medications, and inadequately sterilized instruments such as tonometers. Eye gnats or flies may transmit the organisms mechanically in some areas but their importance as vectors is undetermined and probably differs from area to area.

9. Treatment—

Preferred therapy	<ul><li>Ofloxacin 0.3% solution: 1 or 2 drops in affected eye every 2–4 hours for 2 days then QID for 5 days</li><li>Trimethoprim/polymyxin B solution: 1 drop in affected eye QID for 5–7 days</li><li>Erythromycin 0.5% ointment: instill 1 cm ribbon to affected eye ≤ 6 times daily</li></ul>
Alternative therapy options	<ul><li>Besifloxacin 0.6% suspension: 1 drop in affected eye TID for 7 days</li><li>Tobramycin 0.3% solution: 1 or 2 drops in affected eye every 4 hours for mild to moderate infection. For severe infections, could instill 2 drops in affected eye every hour until improvement</li><li>Bacitracin/neomycin/polymyxin ointment: apply every 3–4 hours for 7–10 days</li></ul>
Special considerations and comments	Reevaluate in 24–36 hours.

Note: QID = 4 times daily; TID = thrice daily.

Given the small benefit that has been observed with topical antibiotic therapy, treatment may be deferred when the etiology of conjunctivitis is unclear (e.g., viral vs. bacterial). Corneal involvement must be ruled out to be eligible for the wait-and-watch approach. Topical corticosteroids are not recommended in bacterial conjunctivitis.

10. Prevention—Personal hygiene, hygienic care, and treatment of affected eyes.

11. Special considerations—

1) Reporting: report to local health authority obligatory for epidemics in some countries; no case report for classic disease.
2) Epidemic measures:

- Prompt and adequate treatment of patients and their close contacts.

- In areas where insects are suspected of mechanically transmitting infection, measures to prevent access of eye gnats or flies to the eyes of sick and well people.
- Insect control, based on the suspected vector.

II. KERATOCONJUNCTIVITIS, ADENOVIRAL (epidemic keratoconjunctivitis, shipyard conjunctivitis, shipyard eye)

1. Clinical features—An acute viral disease of the eye, with unilateral or bilateral inflammation of conjunctivae and edema of the lids and periorbital tissue. Onset is sudden with pain, photophobia, and blurred vision; occasionally low-grade fever, headache, malaise, and tender preauricular lymphadenopathy. Approximately 7 days after onset in about half the cases, the cornea exhibits several small, round subepithelial infiltrates; these may eventually form punctate erosions that stain with fluorescein. Duration of acute conjunctivitis is about 2 weeks; it may continue to evolve, leaving discrete subepithelial opacities that may interfere with vision for a few weeks. In severe cases, permanent scarring may result.

2. Risk groups—Trauma, even minor, and eye manipulation increase the risk of infection. There is usually complete type-specific immunity after adenoviral infections. People who are eye-rubbers.

3. Causative agents—Typically, adenovirus types 8, 19, and 37 are responsible, though other adenovirus types have been involved. Most severe disease has been found in infections caused by types 5, 8, and 19.

4. Diagnosis—The clinical appearance, history, and preauricular lymph node is 90% positive. Confirmed by recovery of virus from appropriate cell cultures inoculated with eye swabs or conjunctival scrapings; virus may be visualized through fluorescent antibody staining of scrapings or through immune electron microscopy; viral antigen may be detected by enzyme-linked immunosorbent assay (ELISA) testing. Serum neutralization or hemagglutination inhibition tests may identify type-specific titer rises. A rapid, FDA-approved, point-of-care antigen-based immunoassay is available to detect adenoviral conjunctivitis (sensitivity 40%–85%; specificity 96%–98%).

5. Occurrence—Presumably worldwide. Both sporadic cases and large outbreaks have been reported in Asia, Europe, the Pacific Islands, and North America.

6. Reservoirs—Humans.

7. Incubation period—Between 5 and 12 days, but in many instances longer.

8. Transmission—Direct contact with eye secretions of an infected person and, indirectly, through contaminated surfaces, instruments, or solutions. The infection is communicable from late in the incubation period to 14 days after onset. Prolonged viral shedding has been reported.

9. Treatment—

Preferred therapy	• Artificial tears (hydroxypropyl methylcellulose): 1 or 2 drops into eyes as required to relieve symptoms • Possibly cycloplegic drugs • If associated with pain, photophobia, visual alteration, a course of mild topical corticosteroids in addition to cycloplegics may be beneficial
Alternative therapy options	• 10% povidone-iodine swabbing OR • 2% povidone-iodine drops QID
Special considerations and comments	• Cold compresses • Handwashing • Workplace hygiene • Disposal of contaminated contact lenses and solutions

Note: QID = 4 times daily.

10. Prevention—

1) Ensure personal hygiene and avoid sharing towels, eyedroppers, eye makeup, and toilet articles. Educate patients to minimize hand-to-eye contact.
2) Wash hands properly before doing any ophthalmologic procedures, such as examining the patient, and properly sterilize instruments after use. Use clean gloves to examine eyes. Any ophthalmic medicines or droppers that have come into contact with eyelids or conjunctivae must be discarded. Medical personnel with overt conjunctivitis should not have physical contact with patients.
3) With persistent outbreaks, patients with epidemic keratoconjunctivitis should be seen in physically separate facilities. Ophthalmic equipment must be sterilized between patients.
4) Use safety measures such as goggles in high-risk areas.

11. Special considerations—

1) Reporting: obligatory report to local health authority of epidemics in some countries; no individual case report.
2) Epidemic measures: strictly apply prevention recommendations discussed earlier and organize convenient facilities for prompt diagnosis, with no or only minimal contact between infected and uninfected individuals.

III. KERATOCONJUNCTIVITIS, MICROSPORIDIAL

1. Clinical features—Clinical symptoms include foreign body sensations, moderate-to-intense pain, redness, light sensitivity, excessive tearing, swelling of eyelid, itchiness, and impaired eyesight. Ocular manifestations include superficial punctate keratoconjunctivitis and corneal stromal keratitis. Duration of symptoms lasts between 4 days and 18 months. Disease commonly causes symptoms in immunocompromised patients but also has been documented in immunocompetent persons.

2. Risk groups—Those in contact with unclean contaminated river water, contaminated rain, soil, and mud. Patients with human immunodeficiency virus/acquired immunodeficiency syndrome and contact lens wearers who frequent hot tubs.

3. Causative agents—Microsporidia—obligate, intracellular, spore-forming protozoa belonging to the phylum Microspora. Keratoconjunctivitis is caused by *Encephalitozoon* spp. and stromal keratitis is caused by *Nosema* spp. and *Microsporidium* spp. *Vittaforma corneae* (syn. *Nosema corneum*) causes keratoconjunctivitis and urinary tract infections in humans.

4. Diagnosis—By corneal scraping/conjunctival smear for microsporidia. Culture to exclude other causative agents. Laboratory methods to assist diagnosis include light microscopy using various stains, such as Gram stains (microsporidia spores are Gram-positive, stain dark violet, and become readily visible under the microscope), modified trichrome stains (e.g., trichrome blue), Warthin-Starry silver stains, Giemsa, and chemofluorescent agents such as Calcofluor. *V. corneae* and *Nosema* spp. measure 1.5 to 4 mm under the microscope. IF assays and molecular techniques are emerging methods for diagnosis. Transmission electron microscopy is the gold standard for identifying specific species.

5. Occurrence—Cases of microsporidial keratoconjunctivitis are reported worldwide among immunocompromised humans but cases in immunocompetent persons are seen in India and Singapore.

6. Reservoirs—Contaminated river water; contaminated rain, soil, and mud.

7. Incubation period—Usually from 2 to 30 days.

8. Transmission—Generally through contact with mud, soil, river water, and rain water contaminated with spores of *V. corneae* and *Nosema* spp. Predisposing factors include exposure to contaminated river water, rain, soil, and mud during swimming and outdoors activities such as cricket, rugby, soccer, and golf. It can occur in both immunocompromised and immunocompetent individuals. Person-to-person transmission has not been reported.

9. Treatment—

Preferred therapy	<ul><li>Fumagillin solution (3 mg/mL in saline): 2 drops[a] every 2 hours for 4 days THEN 2 drops[a] QID. Eye drops[a] should be continued indefinitely, relapse is common.</li><li>Albendazole 400 mg PO BID if systemic infection is present.</li></ul>
Alternative therapy options	No well-recognized options
Special considerations and comments	<ul><li>Long-term therapy is necessary.</li><li>Consider cornea transplantation.</li></ul>

Note: BID = twice daily; PO = oral(ly); QID = 4 times a day.
[a]An eye can only hold 1/5 of a drop.

10. Prevention—Avoid playing on very muddy, waterlogged pitches, in unclean rivers, and in contaminated rain; avoid contact with soil and mud. If these cannot be avoided, regular, thorough washing of face and eyes immediately after contact with mud, soil, and unclean water sources is advised.

11. Special considerations—None.

IV. HEMORRHAGIC CONJUNCTIVITIS, ADENOVIRAL (pharyngoconjunctival fever) AND ENTEROVIRAL (Apollo 11 disease, acute hemorrhagic conjunctivitis)

1. Clinical features—In adenoviral hemorrhagic conjunctivitis, lymphoid follicles usually develop, the conjunctivitis lasts 7 to 15 days, and there are frequently small subconjunctival hemorrhages. In 1 adenoviral syndrome, pharyngoconjunctival fever (PCF), there is upper respiratory disease and fever with minor corneal epithelial inflammation (epithelial keratitis). In enteroviral acute hemorrhagic conjunctivitis (AHC), onset is sudden, with redness, swelling, and pain often in both eyes; the course of the inflammatory disease is 4 to 6 days, during which subconjunctival hemorrhages appear on the bulbar conjunctiva as petechiae that enlarge to form confluent subconjunctival hemorrhages. Large hemorrhages gradually resolve over 7 to 12 days. In major outbreaks of enteroviral origin, there has been a low incidence of a polio-like paralysis, including cranial nerve palsies, lumbosacral radiculomyelitis, and lower motor neuron paralysis. Neurologic complications start a few days to a month after conjunctivitis and often leave residual weakness.

2. Risk groups—Institutional populations associated with overcrowding.

3. Causative agents—Adenoviruses and picornaviruses. Most adenoviruses can cause PCF, but types 3, 4, and 7 are the most common causes.

The most prevalent picornavirus type is enterovirus 70; this and a variant of coxsackievirus A24 have caused large outbreaks of AHC.

4. Diagnosis—Laboratory confirmation of adenovirus infections is through isolation of the virus from conjunctival swabs in cell culture, rising antibody titers, detection of viral antigens through immunofluorescence (IF), or identification of viral nucleic acid with a deoxyribonucleic acid (DNA) probe. Enterovirus infection is diagnosed by isolation of the agent, IF, demonstration of a rising antibody titer, or polymerase chain reaction.

5. Occurrence—Widespread and common worldwide, especially in warmer climates. PCF occurs during outbreaks of adenovirus-associated respiratory disease or as summer epidemics in temperate climates associated with swimming pools. Smaller outbreaks have occurred in Europe, usually associated with eye clinics.

6. Reservoirs—Humans.

7. Incubation period—For adenovirus infection, 4 to 12 days, with an average of 8 days. For enteroviral infection, 12 hours to 3 days.

8. Transmission—Direct or indirect contact with discharge from infected eyes. Person-to-person transmission is most noticeable in families, where high attack rates often occur. Adenovirus can be transmitted in poorly chlorinated swimming pools and also transmitted through respiratory droplets. Large AHC epidemics are often associated with overcrowding and low hygiene standards, especially among school children, which can result in rapid dissemination of AHC throughout communities. Adenovirus infections may be communicable up to 14 days after onset; picornavirus at least 4 days after onset.

9. Treatment—

Preferred therapy	• Artificial tears (hydroxypropyl methylcellulose): 1 or 2 drops into eyes as needed to relieve symptoms • Possibly cycloplegic drugs • If associated with pain, photophobia, visual alteration, a course of mild topical corticosteroids in addition to cycloplegics may be beneficial
Alternative therapy options	• 10% povidone-iodine swabbing OR • 2% povidone-iodine drops QID
Special considerations and comments	• Cold compresses • Handwashing • Workplace hygiene • Disposal of contaminated contact lenses and solutions

10. **Prevention**—No effective treatment; prevention is critical.

   1) Personal hygiene should be emphasized, including use of non-shared towels and avoidance of overcrowding.
   2) Maintain strict asepsis in eye clinics; proper handwashing before examining patients and carrying out procedures. Eye clinics must ensure high-level disinfection of potentially contaminated equipment.
   3) Adequate chlorination of swimming pools. Closing schools may be necessary in an outbreak.

11. **Special considerations**—

   1) Reporting: obligatory report of epidemics to local health authority in some countries.
   2) Epidemic measures: organize adequate facilities for the diagnosis and symptomatic treatment of cases; improve standards of hygiene and limit overcrowding wherever possible.

V. CHLAMYDIAL CONJUNCTIVITIS (inclusion conjunctivitis, paratrachoma, neonatal inclusion blennorrhea, sticky eye)

1. Clinical features—In the newborn, an acute conjunctivitis with purulent discharge, usually recognized within 5 to 12 days after birth. The acute stage usually subsides spontaneously in a few weeks; inflammation of the eye may persist for more than a year if untreated, with mild scarring of the conjunctivae and infiltration of the cornea (micropannus). Chlamydial pneumonia (see "Pneumonia" and "Chlamydial Infections") occurs in some infants with concurrent nasopharyngeal infection. Gonococcal infection must be ruled out. In children and adults, an acute follicular conjunctivitis is seen typically with preauricular lymphadenopathy on the involved side, hyperemia, infiltration, and a slight mucopurulent discharge, often with superficial corneal involvement. In adults, there may be a chronic phase with scant discharge and symptoms that sometimes persist for more than a year if untreated. The agent may cause symptomatic infection of the urethral epithelium and the cervix, with or without associated conjunctivitis.

2. Risk groups—Diabetics and infants of infected mothers.

3. Causative agents—*Chlamydia trachomatis* serovars D-K. Feline strains of *Chlamydia psittaci* have also caused acute follicular keratoconjunctivitis in humans.

4. Diagnosis—Laboratory methods to assist diagnosis include isolation in cell culture, antigen detection using IF staining of direct smears, ELISA, and DNA probe.

5. Occurrence—Sporadic cases of conjunctivitis are reported worldwide among sexually active adults. Neonatal conjunctivitis due to *C. trachomatis* is common and occurs in 15% to 35% of newborns exposed to maternal infection. Among adults with genital chlamydial infection, 1 in 300 develops chlamydial eye disease.

6. Reservoirs—Humans for *C. trachomatis*; cats for *C. psittaci*.

7. Incubation period—In newborns, 5 to 12 days, ranging from 3 days to 6 weeks; in adults, 6 to 19 days.

8. Transmission—Generally transmitted in adults during sexual intercourse; the genital discharges of infected people are infectious. In the newborn, conjunctivitis is usually acquired by direct contact with infectious secretions during transit through the birth canal. In utero infection may also occur. The eyes of adults become infected by the transmission of genital secretions to the eye, usually by the fingers. Children may acquire conjunctivitis from infected newborns or other household members; cases in children should be assessed for sexual abuse as appropriate. Outbreaks reported among swimmers in nonchlorinated pools have not been confirmed by culture and may be due to adenoviruses or other known causes of swimming pool conjunctivitis.

The disease is communicable while genital or ocular infection persists; carriage on mucous membranes has been observed for as long as 2 years after birth.

9. Treatment—

Preferred therapy	• Azithromycin 1 g PO once OR • Doxycycline 100 mg PO BID for 21 days
Alternative therapy options	• Tetracycline 250 mg PO QID for 14 days OR • Azithromycin 1% drops: instill 1 drop[a] into affected eye(s) QID for 7 days OR • Erythromycin ointment 0.5%: instill approximately 1 cm ribbon into affected eye(s) BID to QID for 3–4 weeks OR • Sulfacetamide ointment 10%: instill approximately 1 cm ribbon BID to QID for 3–4 weeks
Special considerations and comments	Identify contacts.

Note: BID = twice daily; PO = oral(ly); QID = 4 times daily.
[a]An eye can only hold 1/5 of a drop.

10. Prevention—

1) Correct and consistent use of condoms to prevent sexual transmission; prompt treatment of persons with chlamydial urethritis and cervicitis, including pregnant women.

2) General preventive measures as for other sexually transmitted infections; see "Syphilis."

3) Sanitary control of swimming pools; ordinary chlorination suffices.

4) Identification of infection in high-risk pregnant women by culture or antigen detection. Treatment of cervical infection in pregnant women will prevent subsequent transmission to the infant. Erythromycin base is usually effective, but frequent gastrointestinal side effects interfere with compliance and treatment must be observed to ensure completion. If compliance is a problem, consideration may be given to the use of other macrolides.

5) Routine prophylaxis for gonococcal ophthalmia neonatorum is effective against chlamydial infection and should be practiced. The method of choice is a single application into the eyes of the newborn within 1 hour after delivery of 1 of the following: povidone-iodine (2.5% solution); tetracycline 1% eye ointment; erythromycin 0.5% eye ointment; or silver nitrate eye drops (1%). Ocular prophylaxis does not prevent nasopharyngeal colonization and risk of subsequent chlamydial pneumonia. Penicillin is ineffective against chlamydiae.

11. Special considerations—Reporting: case report of neonatal cases obligatory in many countries.

[R. Abel Jr]

CRYPTOCOCCOSIS
(torula)

DISEASE	ICD-10 CODE
CRYPTOCOCCOSIS	ICD-10 B45

1. Clinical features—Primary pulmonary infection in immunocompetent persons is commonly asymptomatic but may present with fever and dry cough. Meningoencephalitis: in immunocompromised persons, signs and symptoms often develop after hematogenous spread to the meninges, with subacute or chronic encephalomeningitis; symptoms include headache, fever, visual disturbance, and confusion. Other sites of disseminated infection include the kidneys, prostate, bone, and skin (pustules, papules, plaques, ulcers, or subcutaneous masses). Untreated meningitis leads to death within weeks to months.

2. Risk groups—Acquired immunodeficiency syndrome (AIDS) has been a major risk factor, with hundreds of thousands of illnesses annually worldwide in this group. Other patients with impaired T-cell immunity (e.g., from glucocorticoids, malignancy) are also at risk.

3. Causative agents—*Cryptococcus neoformans* var. *neoformans, Cryptococcus neoformans* var. *grubii*, and *Cryptococcus gattii*. However, the taxonomy of these organisms is under debate and division into 7 instead of 2 species has been proposed.

4. Diagnosis—Lumbar puncture for cerebrospinal fluid analysis (CSF) is used to evaluate for cryptococcal meningoencephalitis in patients with consistent signs and symptoms, particularly in immunocompromised patients and in those with positive serum cryptococcal antigen (CrAg) testing. CSF cell count, protein, and glucose may be abnormal, but these values are normal in some patients with culture-confirmed cryptococcal meningoencephalitis. Microscopic examination of CSF with India ink staining can identify the characteristic capsular halo or budding forms, allowing rapid identification and treatment; however, this test requires an experienced microbiologist and sensitivity is 80% or less. CSF CrAg testing is highly sensitive and specific: a positive test makes cryptococcal meningoencephalitis highly likely, although false-positive results can rarely occur. Polymerase chain reaction testing is increasingly available and further evaluation of testing characteristics is needed. Diagnosis is confirmed through histopathology or culture.

5. Occurrence—Cases of *C. neoformans* infection occur worldwide and tend to follow the AIDS epidemic in a given country or region. However, cases also occur in immunocompromised patients with conditions other than AIDS (e.g., organ transplant, hematologic malignancy, glucocorticoid therapy) and rarely in immunocompetent individuals with environmental exposures. Infection is more frequent in adults than in children and in males slightly more frequently than in females. *C. gattii* is more frequent in tropical or subtropical regions, such as Australia, Africa, tropical South America, and the southern Pacific coast of the USA. *C. gattii* cases regularly occur along the west coast of North America and sporadically elsewhere in the USA.

6. Reservoirs—Saprophytic growth in the environment. *C. neoformans* can be isolated consistently from old pigeon nests and pigeon droppings and from soil in many parts of the world. *Cryptococcus* spp. have been isolated from leaves and bark of many tree species. Infection also occurs in cats, dogs, horses, camelids, and other animals.

7. Incubation period—Unknown for *C. neoformans*. Limited data suggest a median incubation period of approximately 6 months for *C. gattii*, ranging from several weeks to more than 1 year. Pulmonary disease may precede brain infection by months or years.

8. Transmission—Presumably by inhalation of the fungal spores. No person-to-person or animal-to-person transmission.

9. Treatment—Consult the Infectious Diseases Society of America (IDSA) guidelines[1] for further information. WHO guidelines[2] include a focus on resource-limited settings. Note that for patients with HIV, WHO guidelines recommend a higher dose of flucytosine during induction phase compared with IDSA guidelines. WHO also recommends 1 week of AMB PLUS flucytosine for induction phase (vs. 2 weeks per IDSA guidelines).

Preferred therapy	Mild-to-moderate pulmonary disease:
	• Fluconazole 400 mg PO/IV daily for 6–12 months
	Severe pulmonary disease or meningoencephalitis:

	• Induction phase: treat for ≥ 2 weeks for transplant patients and those with HIV and ≥ 4 weeks in nonimmunocompromised patients
	  ○ AMB deoxycholate 0.7–1.0 mg/kg IV daily PLUS flucytosine 100 mg/kg PO daily in 4 divided doses (IV formulations, where available, okay in severe cases) for ≥ 2 weeks
	  OR
	  ○ AMB lipid formulations, including liposomal AMB, 3–4 mg/kg IV daily OR AMB lipid complex 5 mg/kg IV daily ≥ 2 weeks as possible substitutes among patients with or predisposed to renal dysfunction
	• Consolidation phase:
	  ○ Fluconazole 400–800 mg PO daily for 8 weeks
	• Maintenance phase:
	  ○ Fluconazole 200 mg PO daily for 6–12 months (in patients with HIV, continue until CD4+ count is > 200 for 6 months)

(Continued)

(Continued)

Alternative therapy options	Mild-to-moderate pulmonary disease: • Itraconazole 200 mg PO BID for 6–12 months • Voriconazole 200 mg PO BID for 6–12 months • Posaconazole delayed-release tablets 300 mg PO BID for 2 doses, THEN 300 mg PO daily OR posaconazole suspension 200 mg PO QID, THEN 400 mg PO BID after stabilization of disease for 6–12 months

	Severe pulmonary diseases or meningoencephalitis:
	
	• Induction phase:
	  ○ Liposomal AMB 3–4 mg/kg IV every 24 hours OR AMB lipid complex 5 mg/kg IV every 24 hours PLUS fluconazole 800–1,200 mg IV/PO daily for 2 weeks
	  ○ Liposomal AMB 3–4 mg/kg IV every 24 hours OR AMB lipid complex 5 mg/kg IV every 24 hours OR AMB deoxycholate 0.7–1 mg/kg IV every 24 hours for 4–6 weeks
	  ○ Fluconazole 800–1,200 mg IV/PO daily PLUS flucytosine 25 mg/kg PO every 6 hours for 4–6 weeks
	  ○ Fluconazole 1,200–2,000 mg PO daily for 10–12 weeks

Special considerations and comments	• Management of elevated intracranial pressure in patients with meningeal involvement, through manometry and periodic therapeutic lumbar punctures, is essential. • In patients with HIV, initiation of ART is usually delayed for ≥ 2 weeks following initiation of therapy for cryptococcal meningoencephalitis to reduce risk of IRIS; WHO recommends delaying ART initiation for 4–6 weeks following start of antifungal therapy. • To minimize the risks of toxicity with AMB, it is recommended to administer normal saline, acetaminophen, and diphenhydramine prior to administration of the IV amphotericin product. It is also recommended to closely monitor electrolytes (potassium and magnesium) and provide supplementation if/when needed. • Avoid use of liposomal AMB doses higher than 3–4 mg/kg/day given no improved efficacy data and increased risks for toxicity. • It is recommended to monitor flucytosine levels when possible, given that higher levels are associated with increased risks of bone marrow toxicity.

Note: AMB = amphotericin B; ART = antiretroviral therapy; BID = twice daily; CD4+ = cluster of differentiation 4; HIV = human immunodeficiency virus; IRIS = immune reconstitution inflammatory syndrome; IV = intravenous(ly); PO = oral(ly); QID = 4 times daily.

10. Prevention—No specific measures to prevent exposure. In patients with advanced human immunodeficiency virus disease, a detectable serum CrAg may prompt the use of oral fluconazole, which may prevent development of meningoencephalitis.

11. Special considerations—Reporting: report to local health authority is required in some areas as a possible manifestation of AIDS. Within the USA, *C. gattii* is a notifiable disease in Oregon and Washington states.

References

1. Perfect JR, Dismukes WE, Dromer F, et al. Clinical practice guidelines for the management of cryptococcal disease: 2010 update by the Infectious Diseases Society of America. *Clin Infect Dis.* 2010;50(3):291-322.
2. WHO. *Guidelines for the Diagnosis, Prevention and Management of Cryptococcal Disease in HIV-Infected Adults, Adolescents and Children.* March 2018. Available at: https://www.who.int/hiv/pub/guidelines/cryptococcaldisease/en. Accessed November 20, 2019.

[B. Jackson]

CRYPTOSPORIDIOSIS

DISEASE	ICD-10 CODE
CRYPTOSPORIDIOSIS	ICD-10 A07.2

1. Clinical features—*Cryptosporidium* is an intracellular protozoan parasite that was first recognized as a causative agent of diarrhea in 1976. This parasitic infection affects epithelial cells of the gastrointestinal, biliary, and respiratory tracts. The major symptom is diarrhea, which may be profuse and watery and is associated with cramping abdominal pain. The diarrhea is preceded by anorexia and vomiting in children but general malaise, fever, anorexia, nausea, and vomiting occur less often in adults. Symptoms often wax and wane but remit in less than 15 days in most immunologically healthy people. Overall, however, no specific signs or symptoms implicate *Cryptosporidium* over other organisms that cause diarrhea such as rotavirus, enterotoxigenic *Escherichia coli*, adenovirus, or even *Shigella* or *Campylobacter*, which are also important causes of watery diarrhea in children. Severity is correlated with parasite burden, at least in patients with acquired immunodeficiency syndrome (AIDS), in whom histopathologic diseases correlate with parasite load. Immunocompetent people may have asymptomatic or self-limited symptomatic infections; it is not clear whether reinfection and latent infection with reactivation can occur. Immunodeficient individuals generally clear their infections when factors contributing to immunosuppression (including malnutrition or intercurrent viral infections such as measles) are ameliorated or controlled. In those with human immunodeficiency virus (HIV) infection, the clinical course may vary and asymptomatic periods may occur but the infection usually persists throughout the illness unless highly active antiretroviral therapy is successful. Symptoms of cholecystitis may occur in biliary tract infections; the relationship between respiratory tract infections and clinical symptoms is unclear.

In addition to diarrhea, asymptomatic intestinal infection with *Cryptosporidium* has been associated with poor child growth.

2. Risk groups—Children younger than 2 years, animal handlers, travelers, men who have sex with men, and close personal contacts of infected individuals (families, health care and day care workers) are particularly prone to infection. Hospital experience indicates that 10% to 20% of patients with AIDS develop the infection at some time during their illness. In immunodeficient persons, especially those infected with HIV, who may be unable to clear the parasite, the disease has a prolonged and fulminant clinical course contributing to death.

3. Causative agents—*Cryptosporidium hominis* and *Cryptosporidium parvum*, coccidian protozoa, are the 2 species most often associated with human infection. Several other species of *Cryptosporidium* have also been identified in humans, such as *Cryptosporidium meleagridis* and many others. However, it is now generally accepted that *C. hominis* is the main cause globally in childhood diarrhea.

4. Diagnosis—Generally through identification of oocysts in fecal smears or of life cycle stages of the parasites in intestinal biopsy sections. Oocysts are small (2–4 μm) and may be confused with yeast unless appropriately stained. Most commonly used stains include auramine-rhodamine, a modified acid-fast stain, and safranin-methylene blue. Several FDA-approved enzyme-linked immunosorbent assays (ELISAs), rapid tests, and immunofluorescent antibody tests are also commercially available from different sources, including TechLab (Blacksburg, VA). A fluorescein-tagged monoclonal antibody is useful for detecting oocysts in stools and in environmental samples. Infection with this organism is not easily detected unless looked for specifically. Serologic assays may help in epidemiologic studies. Molecular tests, such as polymerase chain reaction, are increasingly being used; for example, the FilmArray Gastrointestinal Pathogen Panel (Biofire Diagnostics, Salt Lake City, UT) and the xTAG Gastrointestinal Pathogen Panel (Luminex, Austin, TX). These diagnostics detect more than a dozen enteropathogens, including *Cryptosporidium*, and are highly sensitive compared with microscopy or ELISA; however they are costly.

5. Occurrence—Worldwide. *Cryptosporidium* oocysts have been identified in human fecal specimens from both developed and developing countries. In industrialized countries, prevalence of infection is fewer than 1% to 4.5% of individuals surveyed by stool examination. In developing regions, prevalence ranges from 3% to 20%. The Global Enteric Multicenter

Study identified *Cryptosporidium* as 1 of the 4 major contributors to moderate-to-severe diarrheal diseases during the first 2 years of life at all sites and showed *Cryptosporidium* as a key pathogen in diarrheal disease, even among otherwise healthy children.

6. Reservoirs—Humans and various animals. The parasite infects more than 45 vertebrate species, including birds, fish, reptiles, and mammals.

7. Incubation period—Variable; 1 to 12 days is the likely range, with an average of about 7 days.

8. Transmission—Fecal-oral, which includes person-to-person, animal-to-person, waterborne, and foodborne transmission. Outbreaks have been reported in day care centers around the world and have also been associated with drinking water (at least 3 major outbreaks involved public water supplies); recreational use of water including waterslides, swimming pools, and lakes; and consumption of contaminated beverages.

The parasite infects intestinal epithelial cells and multiplies initially by merogony (schizogony), followed by a sexual cycle resulting in fecal oocysts. Oocysts, the infectious stage, appear in the stools at the onset of symptoms and are infectious immediately upon excretion. Excretion continues in stools for several weeks after symptoms resolve; outside the body, oocysts may remain infective for 2 to 6 months or longer in a moist environment. Oocysts are highly resistant to chemical disinfectants used to purify drinking water. One or more autoinfectious cycles may occur in humans.

9. Treatment—

Preferred therapy	Nitazoxanide 500 mg PO BID for 3 days
	Pediatric recommendations:
	<ul><li>1–3 years: nitazoxanide 100 mg PO BID for 3 days</li><li>4–11 years: nitazoxanide 200 mg PO BID for 3 days</li></ul>
Alternative therapy options	Paromomycin for adults only in patients with AIDS.
Special considerations and comments	<ul><li>Typical therapy for childhood diarrhea, including that caused by *Cryptosporidium*, is supportive care with rehydration. Only in severe and laboratory-confirmed cases is drug therapy pursued.</li><li>Nitazoxanide is the only drug that is approved by FDA for the treatment of cryptosporidiosis.</li><li>Nitazoxanide is not useful in patients with AIDS; optimizing antiretroviral therapy is the preferred treatment.</li><li>Encourage adequate hydration.</li><li>May consider use of antidiarrhea agents, if needed (i.e. loperamide or diphenoxylate/atropine).</li></ul>

Note: AIDS = acquired immunodeficiency syndrome; BID = twice daily; PO = oral(ly).

10. Prevention—Given the difficulty in treating cryptosporidiosis, prevention is important. The infectious dose is low and the parasite is relatively resistant to chlorination. The following measures should be taken to prevent *Cryptosporidium* infection:

1) Educate the public about personal hygiene, especially the need for handwashing before handling food, before eating, and after toilet use.
2) Dispose of feces in a sanitary manner; use care in handling animal or human excreta.
3) Have those in contact with calves and other animals with diarrhea (scours) wash their hands carefully.
4) Boil drinking water supplies for 1 minute; chemical disinfectants are not effective against oocysts in drinking water. Filters capable of removing particles 0.1 to 1.0 mm in diameter should be considered.

11. Special considerations—

1) Reporting: report to local health authority; case report to local health authorities required in some countries.
2) Epidemic measures: epidemiologic investigation of clustered cases in an area or institution to determine source of infection and mode of transmission; search for common vehicle, such as recreational water, drinking water, raw milk, or other potentially contaminated food or drink; and institution of applicable prevention or control measures. Control of person-to-person or animal-to-person transmission requires emphasis on personal cleanliness and safe disposal of feces.

Bibliography

Checkley W, White AC, Jagnath D, et al. A review of global burden, novel diagnostics, therapeutics, and vaccine targets for cryptosporidium. *Lancet Infect Dis*. 2015;15 (1):85–94.

Korpe PS, Haque R, Gilchrist C, et al. Natural history of cryptosporidiosis in a longitudinal study of slum-dwelling Bangladeshi children: association with severe malnutrition. *PLoS Negl Trop Dis*. 2016;10(5):e0004564.

Liu J, Platts-Mills JA, Juma J, et al. Use of quantitative molecular diagnostic methods to identify causes of diarrhoea in children: a reanalysis of the GEMS case-control study. *Lancet*. 2016;388(10051):1291–1301.

[R. Haque]

CYCLOSPORIASIS

DISEASE	ICD-10 CODE
CYCLOSPORIASIS	ICD-10 A07.8

1. Clinical features—An infection of the upper small bowel with a clinical syndrome that consists of watery diarrhea, nausea, anorexia, abdominal cramps/bloating, fatigue, myalgia, and weight loss. Vomiting, fever, and influenza-like symptoms are less common. Persistence of symptoms, with remitting and relapsing episodes, is typical. If untreated, diarrhea in the immunocompetent usually lasts for 10 to 24 days but is self-limited; in the immunocompromised, who appear more susceptible to infection, diarrhea can last for months in some patients. Some infected persons are asymptomatic, particularly in settings where cyclosporiasis is endemic. Although not life threatening, *Cyclospora* infection occurring in individuals who are not treated or not treated promptly has been associated with complications including malabsorption, cholecystitis, Guillain-Barré syndrome, and reactive arthritis. Health care providers should consider the diagnosis of *Cyclospora* infection in persons with prolonged diarrheal illness, particularly in travelers to tropical and subtropical regions, and should request stool specimens so that specific tests for this parasite can be made.

2. Risk groups—Persons of all ages are at risk for infection. Persons living or traveling in the tropics and subtropics may be at increased risk because cyclosporiasis is endemic in some countries. Those with human immunodeficiency virus (HIV) and HIV/tuberculosis coinfection are particularly susceptible to infection.

3. Causative agents—*Cyclospora cayetanensis*, a single-celled sporulating coccidian protozoan.

4. Diagnosis—Historically via identification in the stools of the 8 to 10 μm size oocysts, about twice the size of *Cryptosporidium parvum* (*Cyclospora* is sometimes refer to as giant crypto) in wet mount under phase contrast microscopy. A modified acid-fast stain or modified safranin technique can be used. Organisms autofluoresce under ultraviolet illumination. Diagnosis can be difficult in part because even patients who are symptomatic might not shed enough oocysts in their stools to be readily detectable by laboratory examinations. Commercially available gastrointestinal molecular diagnostic testing (polymerase chain reaction) panels are more sensitive than traditional microscopic examinations of stools.

5. Occurrence—*Cyclospora* infection is transmitted by ingesting infective *Cyclospora* oocysts (e.g., in contaminated food or water).

Foodborne outbreaks of cyclosporiasis in the USA have been linked to various types of imported fresh produce. *Cyclospora* is endemic in many developing countries. The disease is most common in tropical and subtropical countries, where asymptomatic infections are not infrequent. It has also been associated with diarrhea in travelers to Asia, the Caribbean, and Latin America. In the USA, most reported cases have occurred during the months of May through August, peaking in June and July.

6. Reservoirs—Humans. Several *Cyclospora* spp. are known to infect primates; whether this is the case for *C. cayetanensis* is still unclear.

7. Incubation period—Approximately 1 week.

8. Transmission—Occurs either through drinking (or swimming in) contaminated water or through consumption of contaminated fresh fruits and vegetables. *C. cayetanensis* has been responsible for multiple food-borne outbreaks in North America. In the USA, foodborne outbreaks of cyclosporiasis have been linked to various types of imported fresh produce from developing countries, such as raspberries, basil, snow peas, mesclun lettuce, and cilantro; no commercially frozen or canned produce has been implicated to date. *Cyclospora* oocysts in freshly excreted stools are not infectious; they require days to weeks outside the host to sporulate and become infectious, making person-to-person transmission unlikely. The mechanism of contamination of water and food has not been fully elucidated. Mean duration of organism shedding was 23 days in Peruvian children.

9. Treatment—

Drug	TMP-SMX
Dose	1 double-strength tablet (TMP 160 mg/SMX 800 mg) BID
Route	PO
Alternative drug	• No highly effective alternatives have been identified for persons who are allergic to (or are intolerant of) TMP-SMX. • May consider ciprofloxacin 500 mg PO BID in HIV-infected patients.
Duration	7–10 days
Special considerations and comments	• Immunocompromised patients may require longer treatment durations. • Suppressive treatment (1 double-strength tablet 3 times/week) may be required to prevent recurrence in immunocompromised patients.

Note: BID = twice daily; HIV = human immunodeficiency virus; PO = oral(ly); SMX = sulfamethoxazole; TMP = trimethoprim.

10. Prevention—Produce should be washed thoroughly before it is eaten, although this practice does not eliminate the risk of cyclosporiasis. *Cyclospora* is unlikely to be killed by routine chemical disinfection or sanitizing methods and is resistant to chlorination. Avoiding food or water that might have been contaminated with stools is the best way to prevent infection. Symptomatic reinfection can occur.

11. Special considerations—Reporting: in jurisdictions where formal reporting mechanisms are not yet established, clinicians and laboratory workers who identify cases of cyclosporiasis are encouraged to inform the appropriate health departments.

[P. Robben, C. F. Decker]

CYTOMEGALOVIRUS DISEASE

DISEASE	ICD-10 CODE
CYTOMEGALOVIRUS DISEASE	ICD-10 B25
CONGENITAL CYTOMEGALOVIRUS INFECTION	ICD-10 P35.1

1. Clinical features—While infection with cytomegalovirus (CMV) is common, it often passes undiagnosed as a febrile illness without specific characteristics. Serious manifestations of infection vary depending on the age and immunocompetence of the individual.

The most severe form of the disease develops in approximately 10% of infants infected in utero, who show signs and symptoms of severe generalized infection, especially involving the central nervous system and liver. Lethargy, convulsions, jaundice, petechiae, purpura, hepatosplenomegaly, chorioretinitis, intracerebral calcifications, intrauterine growth restriction, and pulmonary infiltrates may occur. Survivors may show developmental delays, microcephaly, motor disabilities, hearing loss, and/or evidence of chronic liver disease. Death may occur in utero; the neonatal case-fatality rate is high for severely affected infants.

Primary infection in an immunocompetent person acquired later in life is usually asymptomatic but may cause a syndrome clinically and hematologically similar to Epstein-Barr virus mononucleosis and hepatitis, distinguishable by virologic or serologic tests and the absence of heterophile antibodies. Disseminated infection, with pneumonitis, retinitis, gastrointestinal tract disorders (gastritis, enteritis, colitis), and hepatitis, occurs in immunodeficient and immunosuppressed patients, including those with acquired immunodeficiency syndrome.

CMV is a common cause of posttransplant infection, for both solid organ and bone marrow transplants; symptomatic infection occurs in about 10% to 40% of transplant recipients.

2. Risk groups—Fetuses, infants born prematurely or with a very low birth weight, patients with immunosuppressive conditions, including persons with human immunodeficiency virus infection, those on immunosuppressive drugs, and especially organ allograft recipients (kidney, heart, bone marrow), are more susceptible to overt and severe disease.

3. Causative agents—Human (beta) herpesvirus 5 (human CMV), a member of the subfamily Betaherpesvirinae of the family Herpesviridae; includes 4 major genotypes and many strains, although there often is cross-antigenicity among genotypes and strains.

4. Diagnosis—Optimal diagnosis in the newborn is through virus isolation or polymerase chain reaction (PCR), usually from urine or saliva, in the first 2 to 3 weeks of life. A strongly positive CMV-specific immunoglobulin class M (IgM) antibody test at birth can also be helpful, but commercial assays vary in sensitivity and specificity. Diagnosis of CMV disease in adults is made difficult by the high frequency of asymptomatic and recurrent infections. Multiple diagnostic modalities should be used if possible. Virus isolation, CMV antigen detection (which can be done within 24 hours), and CMV deoxyribonucleic acid detection by PCR or in situ hybridization can be used to demonstrate virus in organs, blood, respiratory secretions, or urine. Serologic studies can be done to demonstrate the presence of CMV-specific IgM antibody, seroconversion (4-fold rise in immunoglobulin class G [IgG] antibody titer), or IgG antibody avidity. Interpretation of the results requires knowledge of the patient's clinical and epidemiologic background.

5. Occurrence—Worldwide, the birth prevalence of congenital CMV infection is approximately 0.6% and tends to be higher in countries with high CMV seroprevalence. The reported birth prevalence of congenital CMV infection in developing countries ranges from 0.6% to 6.1%, higher than in developed countries (0.2%-2.0%). Seroprevalence among young adults varies from 30% in highly industrialized countries to almost 100% in some developing countries; it is higher among women than among men and is related to socioeconomic status or ethnic group in some countries.

6. Reservoirs—Humans are the only known reservoir of human CMV; strains found in many animal species are not infectious for humans.

7. Incubation period—The incubation period for horizontally transmitted infections is not known. Illness following a transplant of an infected allograft, or transfusion with infected blood, begins within 3 to 8 weeks. Perinatal or early postnatal infection from breast milk is usually demonstrable 3 to 12 weeks after birth.

8. Transmission—Intimate exposure through mucosal contact with infectious tissues, secretions, and excretions, including saliva, breast milk, cervical secretions, and semen. Transmission through sexual intercourse is common and is reflected by the almost universal infection of men who have many male sexual partners. Viremia may be present in asymptomatic people, so the virus may be transmitted by blood transfusion, probably associated with leukocytes.

The fetus may be infected in utero from either a primary maternal infection, maternal reinfection with a new CMV strain, or reactivation of latent maternal infection. Most intrauterine infections are due to maternal reactivation or reinfection. Fetal infection with manifest disease at birth occurs most commonly following maternal primary infection but has also been reported in populations with high seroprevalence, in whom recurrent infections are more likely. Perinatal transmission through exposure to infected cervical secretions at delivery or early postnatal transmission via breast milk may occur among infants born to CMV-seropositive mothers.

Virus is excreted in urine and saliva for many months and may persist or be episodic for several years following primary infection. Many children in day care centers excrete CMV; this may represent a community reservoir. Children with congenital CMV infection may excrete virus for as long as 5 to 6 years. Adults appear to excrete virus for shorter periods. CMV persists as a latent infection. Excretion recurs with immunodeficiency and immunosuppression.

9. Treatment—

Drug	Congenital CMV:
	• Valganciclovir
	CMV retinitis in immunocompromised adults:
	• Valganciclovir
	CMV prophylaxis in posttransplant patients:
	• Valganciclovir
Dose	Congenital CMV:
	• 16 mg/kg/dose BID
	CMV retinitis in immunocompromised adults:
	• Induction: 900 mg BID • Maintenance: 900 mg daily
	CMV prophylaxis in posttransplant patients:
	• $[7 \times BSA \times CrCl]$ (< 900 mg daily)
Route	• Ganciclovir IV • Valganciclovir PO
Alternative drug	Congenital CMV:
	• Ganciclovir 6 mg/kg/dose BID (switch to valganciclovir when able to tolerate)
	CMV retinitis in immunocompromised adults:
	• Ganciclovir: induction 5 mg/kg/dose BID, THEN maintenance 5 mg/kg/dose daily
	CMV prophylaxis in posttransplant patients:
	• Ganciclovir 5 mg/kg/dose BID for 7–14 days, THEN 5 mg/kg/dose daily

(Continued)

(Continued)

Duration	Congenital CMV:
	• 6 months
	CMV retinitis in immunocompromised adults:
	• Induction: 14–21 days • Maintenance: ongoing
	CMV prophylaxis in posttransplant patients:
	• Depends on type of transplant: 100–200 days
Special considerations and comments	• Valganciclovir should be given with food. • Both ganciclovir and valganciclovir require renal dosing for renal impairment.

Note: BID = twice daily; BSA = body surface area; CMV = cytomegalovirus; CrCl = creatinine clearance; IV = intravenous(ly); PO = oral(ly).

10. Prevention—

1) Take care in handling diapers/nappies; wash hands after diaper changes and toilet care of newborns and infants.

2) Health care personnel should follow standard precautions. Workers in day care centers and preschools should observe strict standards of hygiene, including handwashing after contact with urine or saliva.

3) CMV transmission through transfusion of blood products to newborns or immunocompromised persons can be prevented by freezing red blood cells in glycerol before administration, by removal of the buffy coat, by filtration to remove white blood cells, or by use of CMV antibody-negative donors. However, screening of blood products for CMV may not be routinely performed in all countries or may not be a feasible strategy in countries with high CMV seroprevalence.

4) Avoid transplanting organs from CMV-seropositive donors to seronegative recipients. If unavoidable, hyperimmune immunoglobulin or prophylactic or preemptive administration of antivirals may be helpful. Antivirals are also helpful in seropositive bone marrow transplant recipients who carry latent CMV.

11. Special considerations—None.

[M. L. Donahue]

DENGUE

(dengue fever, dengue hemorrhagic fever/dengue shock syndrome, severe dengue)

DISEASE	ICD-10 CODE
DENGUE FEVER	ICD-10 A90
DENGUE HEMORRHAGIC FEVER	ICD-10 A91

1. Clinical features—Dengue is a mild to moderately severe acute febrile illness that usually follows 3 phases: febrile, critical, and convalescent. Patients with dengue often have sudden onset of fever, which lasts for 2 to 7 days and may be biphasic. Other signs and symptoms include intense headache, myalgia, arthralgia, bone pain, retro-orbital pain, anorexia, vomiting, macular or maculopapular rash, and minor hemorrhagic manifestations, including petechiae, ecchymosis, purpura, epistaxis, bleeding gums, hematuria, or a positive tourniquet test. Some patients have injected oropharynx and facial erythema in the first 24 to 48 hours after onset. Warning signs of progression to severe dengue occur in the late febrile phase, around the time of defervescence, and include persistent vomiting, severe abdominal pain, mucosal bleeding, fluid accumulation and difficulty breathing, signs of hypovolemic shock, lethargy, hepatomegaly, and rapid decline in platelet count with an increase in hematocrit (hemoconcentration).

The critical phase of dengue begins at defervescence and typically lasts 24 to 48 hours. Most patients improve clinically during this phase but those with significant plasma leakage develop severe dengue as a result of a marked increase in vascular permeability. Initially, physiologic compensatory mechanisms maintain adequate circulation, which narrows pulse pressure as diastolic blood pressure increases. Patients may appear to be well despite early signs of shock. However, once hypotension develops, systolic blood pressure rapidly declines and irreversible shock and death may ensue despite resuscitation. Patients with severe plasma leakage have pleural effusions or ascites, hypoproteinemia, and hemoconcentration. Patients can also develop hemorrhagic manifestations, including severe frank hemorrhage, hematemesis, hematochezia, melena, or menorrhagia, especially if they have prolonged shock. Patients with severe dengue may also present clinically with hepatitis, myocarditis, pancreatitis, and encephalitis.

The convalescent phase begins when plasma leakage subsides and extravasated fluids (intravenous, pleural, abdominal) reabsorb, hemodynamic status stabilizes, and diuresis ensues. The hematocrit stabilizes or may fall because of the dilutional effect of the reabsorbed fluid; the white cell count usually starts to rise, followed by a slow recovery of platelet count. Patients may develop a generalized erythematous rash with circular areas of nonerythematous skin. This convalescent-phase rash may desquamate and be pruritic.

Laboratory findings commonly include leukopenia, thrombocytopenia, hyponatremia, elevated aspartate aminotransferase and alanine aminotransferase, and a normal erythrocyte sedimentation rate in most patients. Some patients may have an elevated partial thromboplastin time and a decreased fibrinogen level (with a normal prothrombin time).

Differential diagnosis includes chikungunya and other epidemiologically relevant diseases listed under Arboviral Fevers in "Arboviral Diseases"; influenza; measles; rubella; malaria; leptospirosis; melioidosis; typhoid; scrub typhus; and other systemic febrile illnesses, especially those accompanied by rash.

The revised 2009 WHO case classification guidelines require dividing the illness into dengue with and without warning signs and severe dengue. Dengue hemorrhagic fever (DHF) and dengue shock syndrome (DSS) are further classified as subsets of severe dengue. Timely identification of patients with dengue with warning signs is critical to ensure proper anticipatory guidance and initiation of supportive treatment to reduce mortality. Severe dengue can occur in both children and adults and is more likely to occur with the individual's second infection, probably because of immune enhancement (see later).

2. Risk groups—People of all ages living in dengue-endemic areas should be considered at risk for infection. In most areas, disease incidence is highest in children, although increasing numbers of adult cases are being reported from both rural and urban areas. Perinatal dengue virus (DENV) transmission can occur, with most reported cases being febrile, but temperature instability can also occur similar to other perinatal infections. Other findings have included hemorrhagic manifestations, hepatomegaly, and hypotension. In addition, infants infected with DENV at 6 to 12 months and born to mothers previously infected with DENV are at increased risk for severe dengue. This is thought to occur because of waning levels of transplacentally transferred maternal immunoglobulin class G (IgG) anti-DENV and immune-enhanced DENV infection.

Persons from dengue-nonendemic areas traveling to dengue-endemic areas for recreation, for work, or to live are at risk for DENV infection and dengue. Dengue is the leading cause of febrile illness among travelers to the Caribbean, South America, and South Central/Southeast Asia.

3. Causative agents—DENVs are flaviviruses and include 4 types (serotypes DENV-1, -2, -3, -4). All 4 DENV serotypes can cause dengue and have been associated with severe dengue, including DHF/DSS with increased mortality. The majority (75%) of DENV infections are asymptomatic in both children and adults. Long-term serotype-specific protective immunity is produced by infection with each serotype but there is no long-term cross-protective immunity following infection. An increased risk of severe dengue is associated with the presence of heterotypic antibody and with viral strains that have greater virulence and/or epidemic potential. DENV serotypes can be further defined into genotypes based on differences in the envelope gene sequence; molecular epidemiologic studies may assist in tracking disease transmission patterns.

4. Diagnosis—Laboratory confirmation of the clinical diagnosis of dengue can be made using a single serum specimen obtained during the febrile phase of the illness (days 0-7 after onset of fever) to detect DENV and immunoglobulin class M (IgM) anti-DENV. DENV viremia occurs for 5 to 6 days before and after fever onset. Molecular diagnostics by nucleic acid amplification, such as by reverse transcriptase polymerase chain reaction (RT-PCR), can detect DENV ribonucleic acid with a higher sensitivity than virus isolation by cell culture, and multiplex RT-PCR provides serotype-specific results. Molecular diagnostics are now available in many dengue-endemic areas. DENV can also be detected by an immunoassay for the nonstructural protein 1 (NS1) antigen, a soluble antigen present during the viremic period. Although somewhat less sensitive than DENV detection by RT-PCR, NS1 antigen detection tests have become commercially available in many dengue-endemic areas. Detection of IgM anti-DENV in the febrile phase may indicate a current or recent DENV infection or, in some settings, infection with another flavivirus because of antibody cross-reactivity. IgM anti-DENV becomes detectable in about 30% of patients with dengue on the third day after fever onset and in almost all patients 6 to 7 days after fever onset. IgM capture anti-DENV enzyme-linked immunosorbent assay testing is widely available; evaluation studies have identified commercially available microplate tests with high sensitivity and specificity and low cross-reactivity with other flaviviruses. Testing for IgG anti-DENV is not useful for dengue diagnosis since a high proportion of persons in endemic areas have pre-existing cross-reactive IgG antibody from previous DENV infections (secondary DENV infection). In summary, molecular diagnostics (and testing of nonstructural proteins when appropriate) will help avoid the diagnostic pitfalls of cross-reactivity among the arboviruses that occur with the use of immunologic techniques.

5. Occurrence—Dengue virus transmission has now become endemic in most countries located in the tropics and subtropics. In dengue-endemic areas, transmission occurs year-round with peak disease incidence usually occurring during the rainy season and in areas of high *Aedes aegypti* prevalence. Most dengue-endemic areas experience epidemic cycles at 2- to 5-year intervals, with disease incidence exceeding the expected annual increase in incidence. In most endemic areas, more than 1 DENV serotype will circulate over time and usually 2 or more serotypes circulate simultaneously. In some island nations, DENV is reintroduced periodically and produces large epidemics, with little or no transmission between introductions. In addition, places such as Taiwan and Queensland, Australia, have annual DENV introductions with transmission and disease occurring only during a single dengue season. All tropical and subtropical regions of Asia, the Americas, the Caribbean, Oceania, and Africa should be considered at risk for dengue. Areas that border dengue-endemic regions (e.g., northern Argentina and Brazil, USA-Mexico border) have experienced DENV introductions and epidemics. Epidemics may occur wherever vectors are present and DENV is introduced, whether in urban or rural areas. Good risk maps for dengue are available as well as mapping programs with real-time reporting of reported dengue activity.

6. **Reservoirs**—Where endemic, DENV is maintained in a human/*A. aegypti* mosquito cycle, in which human infections are either with or without symptoms. There is a sylvatic monkey/mosquito cycle, which may spill over into human populations of southeastern Asia and western Africa.

7. **Incubation period**—From 3 to 14 days, commonly 4 to 7 days.

8. **Transmission**—Bite of infective mosquitoes, principally *A. aegypti*. This is a day-biting species, with increased biting activity for 2 hours after sunrise and several hours before dusk. Dengue outbreaks have been attributed to *A. aegypti* and, to a lesser extent, *Aedes albopictus*. The latter is a periurban species abundant in Asia that has now spread to the USA, the Caribbean, Central and South America, the Pacific, parts of southern Europe, and Africa. *A. albopictus* is less anthropophilic than *A. aegypti* and hence a less efficient epidemic vector. Other *Aedes* spp. mosquitoes associated with DENV transmission include *Aedes polynesiensis* and several species of the *Aedes scutellaris* complex. Each of these species has a particular ecology, behavior, and geographic distribution. Patients are infective for mosquitoes during their period of viremia, from shortly before until the end of the febrile period. The mosquito becomes infective 8 to 12 days after the viremic blood meal and remains so for life. During the 7-day viremia in infected persons, bloodborne transmission is possible through exposure to infected blood, organs, or other tissues. In addition, perinatal DENV transmission occurs with the highest risk among infants born to mothers acutely ill around the time of delivery.

9. **Treatment**—Supportive measures. Early detection of warning signs may be life-saving.

10. **Prevention**—

1) Presently no chemoprophylaxis or antiviral agent is available to prevent or treat dengue; prevention of bites from the vector mosquito is the only means of prevention. Vector control includes public education and community programs to eliminate mosquito vector larval habitats, which for *A. aegypti* include water-holding containers close to or inside human habitation (e.g., old tires, flowerpots, trash, food, or water storage containers). Community surveys to determine the density of vector mosquitoes and identify

productive larval habitats should complement plans for the elimination, management, or treatment of mosquito production sites with appropriate larvicides. Communities should be educated about personal protection against day-biting mosquitoes by using repellents, screening, and protective clothing (see "Malaria"). Prevention measures are required year-round; once increased dengue activity is identified it is usually too late for reactive vector control activities to be effective.

2) Because vector control and personal protection have generally been ineffective in preventing seasonal and epidemic increases in dengue or mitigating an epidemic once it has begun, timely identification of cases and good clinical management of patients with dengue to prevent mortality and morbidity are essential. These should include ongoing education of the public about dengue and warning signs, ongoing education of health care professionals in best clinical practices, evaluation of health care practices related to clinical outcomes, and planning by health care facilities to meet demands placed upon them by the annual seasonal increase in cases or by periodic epidemics.

3) Currently, a tetravalent combination of 4 monovalent chimeric live attenuated viruses has been licensed in 19 countries for use in persons 9 years or older. Because of increased hospitalization as a result of severe DENV in 2- to 5-year-old children who were DENV naive prior to vaccination, in April 2018 the WHO Scientific Advisory Group of Experts recommended conducting serologic testing of DENV immune status before vaccine administration and avoiding vaccinating DENV-naive persons.

11. Special considerations—

1) Reporting: obligatory reporting of dengue cases according to national health authority regulations. Dengue is a reportable condition in the USA and in most dengue-endemic countries. Dengue is a reportable condition under the International Health Regulations.

2) "Dengue has a wide spectrum of clinical presentations, often with unpredictable clinical evolution and outcome."[1] Criteria for the diagnosis of presumptive dengue are living in/traveling to dengue-endemic area plus fever and 2 of the following:

- Nausea, vomiting
- Rash
- Aches and pains
- Tourniquet test positive
- Leukopenia

- Warning signs (which include abdominal pain or tenderness, persistent vomiting, clinical fluid accumulation, mucosal bleeding, lethargy/restlessness, liver enlargement greater than 2 cm, increase in hematocrit test concurrent with rapid decrease in platelet count)

3) Epidemic measures: epidemics can be extensive and affect a high percentage of the population. Response should include establishing enhanced surveillance for acute febrile illness or conducting seroincidence surveys to determine the extent of the epidemic; ensuring availability of dengue diagnostic testing; ensuring appropriate medical care for patients and surge capacity in medical facilities to handle the increase in cases; coordinating community messages to ensure persons with symptoms seek medical attention; conducting vector surveys and source reduction activities; providing education in use of mosquito repellents for people exposed to vector mosquitoes; and, where appropriate, applying indoor residual spraying to reduce adult mosquito populations guided by information from the vector surveys.

4) Improve international surveillance and exchange of data between countries. Further information can be found at:

- http://www.cdc.gov/dengue
- http://www.who.int/tdr/publications/training-guideline-publications/dengue-diagnosis-treatment/en
- http://www.healthmap.org/dengue/index.php

References

1. WHO. *Dengue: Guidelines for Diagnosis, Treatment, Prevention and Control.* 2009. Available at: https://apps.who.int/iris/handle/10665/44188. Accessed January 14, 2020.

[J. Andrus]

DIPHTHERIA

DISEASE	ICD-10 CODE
DIPHTHERIA	ICD-10 A36

1. Clinical features—An acute bacterial disease primarily involving the mucous membrane of the upper respiratory tract (nose, tonsils, pharynx, larynx), skin, or rarely other mucous membranes (e.g., conjunctivae, vagina, or ear). Inapparent infections (colonization) outnumber clinical cases. The characteristic lesion, caused by reaction to a potent exotoxin, is an asymmetrical adherent grayish white membrane with surrounding inflammation. In moderate-to-severe cases of respiratory diphtheria, the throat may be moderately to severely sore with enlarged and tender cervical lymph nodes and, together with marked swelling of the neck, can give rise to a bull neck appearance. Pharyngeal membranes may extend into the trachea or progress to cause airway obstruction. Nasal diphtheria can be mild and chronic with one-sided serosanguineous nasal discharge and excoriations. The lesions of cutaneous diphtheria are variable and may be indistinguishable from impetigo. Absorption of diphtheria toxin can lead to myocarditis, with heart block and progressive congestive failure beginning about 1 week after onset. Neurologic complications may occur about 2 weeks after onset of illness and include polyneuropathies that can mimic Guillain-Barré syndrome. The case-fatality rate is 5% to 10% for respiratory diphtheria even with treatment and has changed little in the past 50 years.

Respiratory diphtheria should be suspected in the differential diagnosis of membranous pharyngitis, which includes streptococcal pharyngitis, Vincent angina, infectious mononucleosis, oral syphilis, oral candidiasis, and adenoviruses.

2. Risk groups—Occurs primarily in nonimmunized or underimmunized children younger than 15 years but may be found among adult population groups with low vaccination coverage. Infants born to immune mothers have passive protection, which is usually lost before the sixth month. Disease or inapparent infection may induce long-lasting or lifelong immunity but do not always do so.

Immunization with diphtheria toxoid produces prolonged but not lifelong immunity. Immunity wanes with increasing age. Serosurveys in developed countries indicate that more than 40% of adults lack protective levels of circulating antibodies. Older adults may have immunologic memory and may be protected against disease after exposure. Immunity induced by diphtheria toxoid protects against toxin-mediated systemic disease but not against colonization in the nasopharynx.

3. Causative agents—Toxin-producing strains of *Corynebacterium diphtheriae*. There are 4 biotypes: gravis, mitis, intermedius, and belfanti. Toxin production results when bacteria are infected by corynebacteriophage containing the diphtheria toxin gene *tox*. Nontoxigenic strains may cause a sore throat but rarely produce membranous lesions; however, they are increasingly associated with infective endocarditis.

4. Diagnosis—Presumptive diagnosis is based on observation of an asymmetrical, adherent grayish membrane associated with tonsillitis, pharyngitis, or a serosanguineous nasal discharge. The diagnosis is confirmed by bacteriologic examination of lesions. If respiratory diphtheria is strongly suspected, specific treatment with antitoxin and antibiotics should be initiated without awaiting laboratory confirmation by culture and continued even if the laboratory report is negative. Delay in starting treatment is associated with increased risk for complications and death.

5. Occurrence—A disease of colder months in temperate zones. In the tropics, seasonal trends are less distinct; inapparent, cutaneous, and wound diphtheria are much more common. Diphtheria epidemics can occur in susceptible populations. In 1990, for example, a massive outbreak began in Russia after diphtheria immunization was stopped; diphtheria spread to all countries of the former Soviet Union and Mongolia, where immunizations had also been stopped. The outbreak was responsible for more than 150,000 reported cases and 5,000 deaths between 1990 and 1997.

In Ecuador, an outbreak of about 200 cases occurred in 1993–1994; about 50% of cases occurred in persons aged 15 years or older. In both epidemics, control was achieved through mass immunization campaigns. More recently, outbreaks have occurred in Haiti, Sudan, Indonesia, Thailand, and Laos.

6. Reservoirs—Humans.

7. Incubation period—Usually 2 to 5 days, occasionally longer.

8. Transmission—Contact with a patient or carrier; more rarely, contact with articles soiled with discharges from lesions of infected people including raw milk that has served as a vehicle. Period of communicability is variable until virulent bacilli have disappeared from discharges and lesions: usually 2 weeks or less, seldom more than 4 weeks for respiratory diphtheria. The rare chronic carrier may shed organisms for 6 months or more. Effective antibiotic therapy promptly terminates shedding.

9. Treatment—

1) Use diphtheria antitoxin to stop toxin produced by the bacteria.
2) Give oral penicillin V 250 mg 4 times instead of injections to persons who can swallow.

Drug	Erythromycin
Dose	40 mg/kg/day (≤ 2 g/day)
Route	PO or IM
Alternative drug	Penicillin G IM daily (300,000 units every 12 hours for ≤ 10 kg and 600,000 units every 12 hours for > 10 kg) for 14 days.

(Continued)

(Continued)

Duration	14 days
Special considerations and comments	Not applicable

Note: IM = intramuscular(ly); PO = oral(ly).

10. Prevention—

1) Educational measures are important: inform the public, particularly parents of young children, of the hazards of diphtheria and the need for active immunization.

2) The only effective control is widespread active immunization with diphtheria toxoid. Immunization should be initiated in infancy with a formulation containing diphtheria toxoid, tetanus toxoid, and either diphtheria/tetanus and acellular pertussis vaccine (DTaP) or diphtheria/tetanus and whole-cell pertussis vaccine (DTwP). Some currently available formulations combine DTwP or DTaP with 1 or more of the following: *Haemophilus influenzae* type b vaccine (Hib), inactivated poliomyelitis vaccine, or hepatitis B vaccine.

3) The schedule recommended in developing countries is at least 3 primary intramuscular doses at 6, 10, and 14 weeks old; and a DTwP booster at 1 to 6 years old. The following schedules are recommended for use in industrialized countries (some countries may recommend different ages or dosages):

- Recommended immunization schedule for persons 0 to 18 years old: vaccination is recommended with a primary series of diphtheria toxoid combined with other antigens, such as DTaP, DTaP-Hib, or DTaP-Hib–inactivated polio vaccine. The first 3 doses are given at 4- to 8-week intervals beginning when the infant is 6 to 8 weeks old; a fourth dose is given 6 to 12 months after the third dose. This schedule should not entail restarting immunizations because of delays in administering scheduled doses. A fifth dose is given at 4 to 6 years old, prior to school entry; this dose is not necessary if the fourth dose was given after the fourth birthday. If the pertussis component of the vaccine is contraindicated, diphtheria/tetanus vaccine for children should be substituted. A booster dose with an adult formulation—tetanus, diphtheria, and acellular pertussis (Tdap; or tetanus and diphtheria [Td] if Tdap is unavailable)—is recommended at 11 to 18 years old.

- Previously unvaccinated persons older than 7 years: because adverse reactions may increase with age, a preparation with a reduced concentration of diphtheria toxoid (adult Td) is usually given after the seventh birthday for booster doses. For a previously unimmunized person, a primary 3-dose series of adsorbed Td toxoids is advised. Two doses are given at a 4- to 8-week interval; the third dose is given 6 months to 1 year after the second dose. If the person is 10 years or older, a dose of Tdap may be substituted for a single Td dose in the series. Limited data from Sweden suggest that the 3-dose Td regimen may not induce protective diphtheria antibody levels in most adults and additional doses may be needed.
- Active protection should be maintained by administering a dose of Td every 10 years thereafter. A onetime dose of Tdap may be substituted for the next Td dose in persons aged 19 to 64 years for added protection against pertussis.

4) Special efforts should be made to ensure that those who are at higher risk of patient exposure, such as health workers, are fully immunized and receive a booster dose of Td every 10 years.
5) For those who are severely immunocompromised or infected with human immunodeficiency virus, diphtheria immunization is indicated with the same schedule and dose as for immunocompetent persons even though immune response may be suboptimal.

11. Special considerations—

1) Reporting: case report to local health authority is obligatory in most countries.
2) Outbreaks can occur when social or natural conditions lead to crowding of susceptible groups, especially infants and children. This frequently occurs when there are large-scale movements of susceptible populations.
3) Epidemic measures:

- Immunize the largest possible proportion of the population group involved, especially infants and preschool children. In an epidemic involving adults, immunize groups that are most affected or at high risk. Repeat immunization procedures 1 month later to provide at least 2 doses to recipients.
- Identify close contacts and define population groups at special risk. In areas with appropriate facilities, carry out a prompt field investigation of reported cases to verify the diagnosis and to determine the biotype and toxigenicity of *C. diphtheriae*.

4) People traveling to or through countries where either respiratory or cutaneous diphtheria is common should receive primary immunization if necessary or a booster dose of Td for those previously immunized.

5) Further information can be found at:

- https://www.cdc.gov/diphtheria/clinicians.html
- https://www.cdc.gov/diphtheria/dat.html

[O. A. Khan, E. Healy]

DRACUNCULIASIS

(Guinea worm disease, dracunculiasis)

DISEASE	ICD-10 CODE
DRACUNCULIASIS	ICD-10 B72

1. Clinical features—An infection of the subcutaneous and deeper tissues by a large nematode. A blister appears, often on a lower extremity (especially the foot), when the gravid adult (60–100 cm long) female worm is ready to discharge its larvae. Burning and itching of the skin in the area of the lesion and frequently fever, nausea, vomiting, diarrhea, dizziness, generalized urticaria, and eosinophilia may accompany or precede blister formation. After the blister ruptures, the worm discharges larvae whenever the affected part is immersed in fresh water. The prognosis is good unless bacterial infection of the lesion occurs; such secondary infections may produce arthritis, synovitis, ankylosis, and contractures of the involved limb. Tetanus infections may occur via the site of the lesion. Secondary infection may be life-threatening.

2. Risk groups—Susceptibility is universal. Multiple and repeated infections may occur in the same person or animal (most often domestic dogs).

3. Causative agents—*Dracunculus medinensis*, a nematode (roundworm).

4. Diagnosis—By visual recognition of the adult worm protruding from a skin lesion. For programmatic purposes (not clinical use), *Dracunculus* can also be identified by microscopic identification of larvae within a worm specimen and the species determined by polymerase chain reaction.

5. Occurrence—Nearing eradication. Transmission of the parasite is limited to Africa, remaining in 5 countries in 2019: Angola, Chad, Ethiopia, Mali, and South Sudan. As of 2019, dracunculiasis has been eliminated from 17 formerly endemic countries. WHO has certified 199 countries, territories, and areas as being free of dracunculiasis transmission as of April 2019.

6. Reservoirs—Humans, domestic dogs and cats, olive baboons, and paratenic hosts in areas where transmission remains endemic. (A paratenic host [also known as a transfer or transport host] is an intermediate host in which no development of the parasite occurs but that can maintain the parasite until it enters the definitive host, where the parasite reaches maturity.)

7. Incubation period—Approximately 10 to 14 months.

8. Transmission—Larvae discharged by the female worm into stagnant fresh water are ingested by minute crustacean copepods (*Cyclops* spp.), which are the obligatory intermediate hosts of the parasite. In about 2 weeks, the larvae develop into the infective stage. People unwittingly ingest the infected copepods in drinking water from infested wells, ponds, and other stagnant surface water or possibly from poorly cooked or cured aquatic animals harboring infective larvae in their guts or somatic tissues (paratenic hosts). The larvae are then liberated in the person's stomach, cross the duodenal wall, migrate through the connective tissue, mate, and become adults. The worms mate 60 to 90 days postinfection. Only a gravid female worm causes a patent infection. Once gravid she continues to grow and develop to full maturity while migrating to the subcutaneous tissues (most frequently a lower limb), where a painful burning blister is created on the skin. The period of communicability lasts for as long as the infected person with an emerging worm seeks relief by immersing the affected limb in stagnant sources of drinking water. In water, the larvae are infective for the copepods for about 3 to 5 days. After ingestion by the copepods, the larvae become infective for people after 12 to 14 days at temperatures above 25°C (77°F). There is no direct person-to-person transmission. *D. medinensis* from both human and animal infections are genetically indistinguishable.

9. Treatment—Drugs, including thiabendazole, albendazole, ivermectin, and metronidazole, have no therapeutic value.

Roll the emerging worm around a piece of gauze and assist the patient to slowly pull the worm out, a few centimeters per day. Use antiseptics to clean the wound and provide local treatment with antibiotic ointment and occlusive bandaging. Give tetanus toxoid, as required. Aseptic surgical extraction just prior to worm emergence is possible for some individuals but not applicable as a public health measure of eradication.

10. Prevention—Prevention of people or animals with emerging worms from contaminating water supplies; provision of copepod-free water from protected water sources and flowing surface water; filtration of drinking water; treatment of stagnant water with the insecticide temephos; and health education of the populations at risk, including dissemination of information about the disease and about cash rewards for information leading to confirmation of human cases or animal infections.

1) Provide behavior change education programs in endemic communities to convey 4 messages:

- Guinea worm infection comes from drinking unsafe water and possibly from consuming insufficiently cooked or cured aquatic animals.
- In endemic areas, people and animals with blisters or ulcers should not enter any source of water.
- Drinking water from stagnant sources should be filtered through fine mesh cloth (e.g., nylon gauze with a mesh size of 100 μm) or through pipe filters (with the same mesh size) to remove copepods.
- Aquatic animals should be thoroughly cooked or cured and their entrails buried or burned to prevent ingestion by domestic animals.

2) Provide safe drinking water. Construct and maintain protected drinking water sources, such as boreholes, protected wells, protected springs, and rainwater catchments, which provide water uncontaminated by copepods.

3) Train and empower at-risk resident populations without access to safe drinking water to properly use filter cloths and pipe filters provided by the Dracunculiasis Eradication Program.

4) Apply temephos, where feasible, every 28 days to suppress copepod populations in unsafe sources of drinking water (e.g., ponds, tanks, reservoirs, and unprotected wells). Prompt treatment of contaminated water sources with temephos within 14 days of suspected contamination by infected humans or animals can prevent transmission.

11. Special considerations—

1) Reporting: human case or animal infection report to local health authority required wherever the disease occurs as part of the national eradication program.

2) Epidemic measures: wherever human cases or animal infections are identified, conduct community surveys to determine prevalence, obtain information as to sources of drinking water and food consumption patterns during probable time of infection

(10-14 months earlier), and guide control/eradication measures as described under Prevention in this chapter.

3) Further information can be found at: https://www.cdc.gov/parasites/guineaworm.

[S. Roy, E. Ruiz-Tiben]

EBOLA-MARBURG VIRAL DISEASES

(African hemorrhagic fever, Ebola virus disease, Marburg virus hemorrhagic fever)

DISEASE	ICD-10 CODE
EBOLA VIRUS DISEASE	ICD-10 A98.4
MARBURG VIRUS DISEASE	ICD-10 A98.3

1. Clinical features—Infection with Ebola, previously known as Ebola hemorrhagic fever, is now known as Ebola virus disease (EVD). Infection consists of a wide range of clinical manifestations from asymptomatic infection to severe disease. There is significant variability in morbidity and case fatality, ranging from 24% to 81%. Prior to the West African Ebola epidemic in 2013-2016, descriptions of the clinical manifestations of Ebola infection were based on clinical observations of patients involved in smaller outbreaks. This more recent experience suggests that hemorrhage and bleeding complications are less common than previously described and that hypovolemia due to severe vomiting and diarrhea is a more prominent clinical feature than previously understood. As of 2014, the name of the disease was changed from Ebola hemorrhagic fever to EVD in scientific and public health literature.

Asymptomatic (3%-27.1%) and minimally symptomatic (8.3%) infections have been described in household transmission studies and in large serosurveys of populations exposed to Ebola virus in West Africa and among populations with no history of Ebola outbreaks in Central Africa.

Approximately 6 to 12 days (range, 2-21 days) after exposure, symptomatic infection presents with the abrupt onset of symptoms of an initial influenza-like illness. Symptoms of the initial syndrome can be nonspecific and consist of malaise, myalgia, anorexia, headache, high fever, and chills, followed by gastrointestinal symptoms such as nausea, vomiting, and diarrhea. Fever is the most commonly observed symptom but may not be present in all patients; some may develop a nonspecific maculopapular rash, commonly presenting on the upper arms, flexor forearms, and upper legs. Rare symptoms include conjunctival injection, localized pain in the chest, abdomen, muscles, or joints, and hiccups.

Fluid losses from profuse watery diarrhea and vomiting can be severe and lead to significant electrolyte disturbances, including hypomagnesemia and hypoalbuminemia and moderate hypo- and hypernatremia, hypokalemia, and hypocalcemia. Without supportive care, reduced vasculature volume and electrolyte deficiencies can progress to multisystem organ hypoperfusion, shock, and death. EVD resembles bacterial septic shock in systemic inflammation, cytokine dysregulation, and multiorgan failure without intense supportive care. Severe hypovolemia can contribute to renal failure that may require renal replacement therapy.

Many patients develop hemorrhagic complications. The most common observation is oozing from intravenous sites and bleeding gums; less frequent observations include ecchymoses, mucosal hemorrhage, hematemesis, melena, and severe hemorrhage. However, although hemorrhage was once considered a hallmark of EVD, it was a relatively uncommon symptom during the 2013–2016 West African outbreak.

Other manifestations of EVD during the acute phase include pericarditis, myocarditis, tachypnea, and shortness of breath with hypoxia or hypoventilation that can progress to respiratory failure. Neurologic symptoms, including meningoencephalitis seizures and coma, and ocular symptoms, such as conjunctival injection and/or signs and symptoms of uveitis including blurred vision, photophobia, and vision loss, can also be present. During EVD convalescence, uveitis is the most common observation and may lead to severe vision impairment or blindness in up to 40% of affected individuals.

Pregnant women may present with nonspecific illness and some of the more atypical manifestations of EVD, including abdominal pain, and/or pregnancy complications, such as preterm labor, vaginal bleeding, or premature rupture of membranes. Pregnant women with EVD face high mortality as well as a high risk of miscarriage and stillbirth.

Fatal disease has been characterized by more severe clinical signs and symptoms early during infection, with progression to multiorgan failure and death typically occurring in the second week. Early supportive care, prior to development of more severe hemodynamic and metabolic abnormalities, is associated with improved survival. Other favorable prognostic factors include younger age, the absence of diarrhea, and a lower Ebola viral load.

Patients who survive typically begin to recover during the second week of illness. EVD survivors often have a variety of disabling symptoms during the convalescent period. Survivors may experience musculoskeletal symptoms, including weakness, fatigue, and muscle and joint pain; insomnia; headache; hearing loss; retro-orbital pain; uveitis; and memory loss and other neuropsychiatric conditions such as depression and anxiety. Disabling conditions can persist for extended periods.

Infection with Marburg virus causes a severe hemorrhagic fever known as Marburg hemorrhagic fever (MHF). Acute illness caused by Marburg virus is abrupt and typically begins with high fever, severe malaise, headache, and muscle aches and pains. The third day of illness gives way to gastrointestinal symptoms, such as cramping, nausea, vomiting, and severe watery diarrhea that can persist for up to a week. During the severe phase of illness, neurologic symptoms like confusion, irritability, and aggression have been observed. Orchitis (inflammation of 1 or both testicles) has also been observed in a rare number of cases during the late phase of disease. MHF is characterized by volume and hemodynamic abnormalities that can lead to multiorgan failure and shock, coagulation abnormalities and bleeding, sustained high fevers, and a high case-fatality rate, with most deaths occurring between 8 and 9 days after symptom onset. The total number of known MHF cases is approximately 450. The range of clinical symptoms and disease severity as well as the onset and disease course of MHF are similar to EVD, but there are currently insufficient clinical data available to precisely define the disease processes and clinical manifestations of Marburg infection.

2. Risk groups—All ages are susceptible. Ebola and Marburg infect indiscriminately and transmission is driven by direct contact with infected blood or bodily fluids. The main human groups at risk are patients who are injected with contaminated needles and syringes that are not properly sterilized; caregivers in affected communities and health care workers in contact with infected patients and their bodily fluids; laboratory workers processing clinical specimens or working in research laboratories; people working with wildlife, in particular nonhuman primates (NHPs) in Central Africa or bats; and people working in bat-inhabited locations, such as mines.

The environmental source of Ebola and Marburg virus is still not well defined, but activities (e.g., hunting, cleaning, and preparing bushmeat) placing humans in close proximity to suspected animal reservoirs (bats, NHPs) and animal products in defined endemic regions increases risk of infection. Family and/or household members living alongside a patient with · EVD and other community contacts are at high risk of exposure to bodily fluids carrying virus. Funeral attendees that directly touch the body of a deceased EVD patient, a common cultural practice in many places where EVD occurs, are at high risk for exposure. Prior to recognition of an outbreak and widespread uptake and utilization of personal protective equipment (PPE), health care workers are at high risk. In this situation, health care workers and patients in the health care system are at high risk for nosocomial transmission. Persons responsible for biologic waste management may be exposed to infectious fluids. Sexual partners of survivors are also at risk for infection as Ebola virus persists in semen and genital secretions beyond recovery from acute infection.

3. Causative agents—Ebola and Marburg viruses are negative-sense, single-stranded ribonucleic acid filoviruses in the family Filoviridae that can cause severe hemorrhagic fever in humans and NHPs. The genus *Ebolavirus* comprises 5 species: *Bundibugyo ebolavirus* (BEBOV/BDBV), *Reston ebolavirus* (REBOV/RESTV), *Sudan ebolavirus* (SEBOV/SUDV), *Taï Forest ebolavirus* (formerly *Côte d'Ivoire ebolavirus*, CIEBOV/TAFV), and *Zaire ebolavirus* (ZEBOV/EBOV). Four species of *Ebolavirus* identified to date are known to cause human disease and have caused major outbreaks in Africa: *Zaire, Sudan, Bundibugyo,* and *Taï Forest. Bundibugyo* and *Sudan* have caused outbreaks primarily in South Sudan and Uganda, while *Zaire* has caused major outbreaks in Gabon, Guinea, and the Democratic Republic of the Congo (DRC). The *Zaire* strain was responsible for both the 2013–2016 West African outbreak and the ongoing outbreak in DRC. A single Marburg virus species, *Marburg marburgvirus,* has been identified and is known to cause disease in humans; it has most recently caused small outbreaks in Uganda.

4. Diagnosis—Ebola or Marburg infection can be confirmed by direct detection of virus in blood or tissue samples by virus isolation, conventional or real-time polymerase chain reaction (PCR), antigen-detection enzyme-linked immunosorbent assay, immunohistochemistry on formalin-fixed tissues, or detection of virus-specific immunoglobulin class M antibodies or rising immunoglobulin class G antibody titers.

Because the early presentation of EVD and MHF is similar to other more common infections, diagnostic evaluation is largely influenced by clinical suspicion and the epidemiologic context (e.g., presence of a current outbreak, known exposure to Ebola). Evaluation of all patients with suspected EVD and MHF should be done in consultation with local and state health departments; any presumptive positive Ebola test should be confirmed at CDC.

Experience from the 2013–2016 West Africa outbreak has informed new guidance from CDC about the evaluation and management of patients with suspected EVD. A biosafety level 4 laboratory is required for evaluation of clinical samples and CDC provides guidance on the safe collection and handling of specimens from patients with suspected EVD.

Currently there is no FDA-approved diagnostic for detection of any *Ebolavirus* spp. All diagnostics available have an emergency use authorization (EUA) from FDA that strictly defines use of each diagnostic. Therefore, health care providers should consult the FDA factsheet included with each authorization when using any diagnostic assay for Ebola or Marburg virus.

For all persons whose clinical symptoms and risk factors are consistent with infection by *Ebolavirus* or Marburg virus, the local health department should be notified for further coordination with CDC and other health agents. These departments can assist in preparing a sample for submission through the Laboratory Response Network (LRN), which has the capability to definitively test a presumptive sample.

Ebola virus is generally detectable in blood samples by real-time reverse transcription polymerase chain reaction (RT-PCR) within 3 days after the onset of symptoms; a negative RT-PCR test that is collected 72 hours or longer after the onset of symptoms excludes EVD according to current CDC guidelines. Nucleic acid testing (RT-PCR) is the most sensitive test available. FDA issued an EUA for presumptive detection of ZEBOV using the FilmArray NGDS BT-E Assay (BioFire, Salt Lake City, UT) in patient serum, plasma, and whole blood and the Xpert Ebola Assay (Cepheid, Sunnyvale, CA) in venous whole-blood samples.

Point-of-care commercial kits are available through EUA waivers; rapid lateral-flow chromatographic immunoassays include: (a) ReEBOV Antigen Rapid Test for detection of viral protein in whole blood (fingerstick or venipuncture), serum, and plasma (Zalgen Labs Germantown, MD); (b) OraQuick Ebola Rapid Antigen Test for testing whole blood (fingerstick or venipuncture) and cadaveric oral fluid (OraSure Technologies Bethlehem, PA). Both tests have limited sensitivity and can generate false-negative test results; rapid diagnostic tests are also prone to high false-positive rates and should only be used to presumptively identify a case of EVD.

Other tests have been approved under an FDA EUA and can be found on the FDA website. Regardless of access to in-house EVD testing, all samples should be submitted to the LRN for confirmatory testing.

5. Occurrence—Ebola disease was first recognized in 1976 when 2 outbreaks of hemorrhagic fever, caused by 2 different species of *Ebolavirus*, occurred in northern Zaire (now DRC) and South Sudan. Since then outbreaks of EVD have occurred in several countries in sub-Saharan Africa (see Table 1 in this chapter). The largest outbreak to date was centered in the West African countries of Guinea, Liberia, and Sierra Leone between 2013 and 2016. Additional cases associated with this outbreak among travelers and health care workers were identified in other countries in the region: Nigeria, Senegal, and Mali. Additional cases also occurred among travelers and health care workers in Europe and the USA. This outbreak overwhelmed the limited public health surveillance, infection control, treatment, and response resources available. WHO declared the outbreak a public health emergency of international concern (PHEIC) in August 2014. This declaration led to a broad and intensive international response that contributed to ending the outbreak in July 2016. At the conclusion of the outbreak, there were more than 28,000 cases and 11,325 deaths.

Table 1. Ebola Virus Outbreaks Since 1976

Year	Location	Cases	*Ebolavirus* Strain
1976	DRC	318 cases; 280 deaths	*Zaire*
1976	Sudan	284 cases; 151 deaths	*Sudan*
1977	DRC	1 fatal case	*Zaire*
1979	Sudan	34 cases; 22 deaths	*Sudan*
1994	Côte d'Ivoire	1 mild case	*Taï Forest*
1994–1996	Gabon, Republic of South Africa	3 outbreaks (149 cases; 97 deaths); a fatal secondary infection occurred in a nurse in South Africa	*Zaire*
1995	DRC	315 cases; 250 deaths	*Zaire*
2000–2001	Uganda	425 cases; 224 deaths	*Sudan*
2001–2003	Gabon, DRC	Several outbreaks (300 cases; 254 deaths); high numbers of deaths were simultaneously reported among wild animals in the region, particularly nonhuman primates	*Zaire*
2004	Sudan	17 cases; 7 deaths	*Sudan*
2007	DRC	264 cases; 187 deaths	*Zaire*
2007–2008	Uganda	131 cases; 42 deaths	*Bundibugyo*
2008–2009	DRC	32 cases; 15 deaths	*Sudan*
2011	Uganda	1 fatal case	*Sudan*
2012	Uganda	2 outbreaks (31 cases; 21 deaths)	*Sudan*
2012	DRC	53 cases; 29 deaths	*Bundibugyo*
2013–2016	Guinea, Liberia, Sierra Leone, Nigeria, Senegal	3,707 confirmed, probable, and suspected cases; 1,848 deaths	*Zaire*
2018	DRC (Équateur province)	54 confirmed, probable, and suspected cases; 33 deaths	*Zaire*
2018–ongoing	DRC (North Kivu province), Uganda (Kasese district)	3,298 confirmed, probable, and suspected cases; 2,196 deaths	*Zaire*

Note: DRC = Democratic Republic of the Congo.

The next largest outbreak began in 2018 in the Équateur province of DRC. The outbreak spanned from early May to late July; there were 38 confirmed and 16 probable cases and 33 deaths. A subsequent outbreak began in August 2018 in the North Kivu province of DRC bordering Uganda and Rwanda, a region marred by ongoing refugee and security crises. As of November 2019, the outbreak has resulted in more than 3,298 cases and more than 2,196 deaths. In June 2019, the outbreak spread to neighboring Uganda, where to date there have been 3 confirmed cases and 1 death. National and international response efforts have been hampered by insecurity, ongoing conflict including violence directed at health care workers, and significant community mistrust. As of July 17, 2019, WHO declared the ongoing outbreak in DRC a PHEIC.

Marburg disease was first recognized in 1967 during an outbreak of hemorrhagic fever among laboratory workers exposed to African green monkeys imported from Uganda. Since then, there have been 2 large outbreaks in sub-Saharan Africa and, between 2012 and 2017, small sporadic outbreaks in Uganda (see Table 2 in this chapter).

Table 2. Marburg Virus Outbreaks Since 1967

Year	Location	Cases
1967	Germany, Yugoslavia	31 cases; 7 deaths
1975	South Africa	3 cases; 1 death
1980	Kenya	2 cases; 1 death
1987	Kenya	1 fatal case
1998–2000	DRC	154 cases; 128 deaths
2005	Angola	252 cases; 227 deaths
2007	Uganda	4 cases; 2 deaths
2008	Netherlands, USA	2 cases among tourists from the Netherlands (fatal) and USA after a trip to Uganda
2012	Uganda	23 cases; 15 deaths
2014	Uganda	1 fatal case
2017	Uganda	3 fatal cases

Note: DRC = Democratic Republic of the Congo.

6. Reservoirs—Ebola virus is an animal-borne (zoonotic) pathogen; forest-dwelling fruit bats (of the Pteropodidae family) are the most likely natural reservoir. However, the exact reservoir species is not definitively known.

The reservoir host of Marburg virus is the African fruit bat. Fruit bats infected with Marburg virus do not show obvious signs of illness. Further study is needed to determine if other species serve as reservoirs.

Ebola and Marburg viruses have also been identified in multiple species of NHPs in which highly lethal outbreaks have occurred, although these are likely incidental hosts and not reservoirs of these viruses.

7. Incubation period—The incubation period is 2 to 21 days for both EVD and Marburg virus disease.

8. Transmission—Marburg infection of index cases has occurred among individuals with exposure to bat-inhabited confined spaces (e.g., caves, mines) and among those with close contact with bats.

Ebola infection of index cases in Central Africa has occurred among individuals exposed to infected wild mammals while hunting for bushmeat or while handling animals found dead in the forest. As fruit bats are thought to be the virus's natural reservoir, humans are likely infected by direct or indirect contact with infected bats as well.

Person-to-person transmission of Ebola and Marburg diseases occurs through direct contact with the blood and bodily fluids of infected living or deceased individuals. Risk during the asymptomatic incubation period appears to be negligible and communicability increases with stage of illness. Risk is highest during the late stages of illness and during funerals involving unprotected exposure during body preparation. Under natural conditions, airborne transmission among humans has not been documented. Nosocomial infections have been frequent. The virus can persist in a variety of bodily fluids (e.g., urine, semen); transmission through semen appears to be rare but has occurred up to 7 weeks after clinical recovery.

9. Treatment—There is currently no licensed therapeutic agent against Ebola or Marburg disease. After the 2013–2016 Ebola epidemic in West Africa, a multidisciplinary panel of experts convened to develop evidence-based guidelines on the delivery of supportive care in Ebola treatment units in resource-limited settings. According to the expert panel, treatment of affected hospitalized patients should consist of early and aggressive supportive care, including oral or intravenous rehydration and electrolyte replacement; systematic monitoring and charting of vital signs and volume status; analgesic therapy (including the prescription of opioids) for patients experiencing pain; and ventilatory support if necessary. Broad-spectrum antibiotics and antimalarials are recommended for patients at high risk of concomitant infections. Experience from the West African outbreak also underscored the provision of critical care as required and when possible, given the similarities between severe EVD and septic and hypovolemic shock.

During the West African outbreak and subsequent outbreaks, several investigational therapies that aim to inhibit viral replication, including antiviral medications, convalescent plasma/whole blood, combination and single monoclonal antibodies, and antimalarials, were administered under compassionate use and/or under research protocol. However, none is currently a licensed product.

During the ongoing EVD outbreak in the North Kivu province of DRC, 4 investigational therapeutics have been approved for compassionate use under an expanded access protocol; all 4 are currently being assessed in a randomized controlled trial.

- ZMapp is a combination of 3 humanized recombination monoclonal antibodies (a cocktail), which showed antiviral activity in NHP studies. A randomized controlled trial assessing its efficacy against EVD in humans was performed during the West African epidemic; however, sample size limitations as the epidemic waned meant that a statistically significant difference in mortality could not be observed in the study. Administering ZMapp during the outbreak proved to be logistically challenging as well because the product needed to be stored and transported on cold chain.

- REGN3470-3471-3479 is a coformulation of 3 monoclonal antibodies that target 3 nonoverlapping epitopes of the Ebola virus glycoprotein, which may result in potent neutralizing activity from a single dose or infusion of the agent. Also referred to as REGN-EB3, this therapeutic agent was efficacious in NHP studies and was safe and tolerable when administered as a single dose in a phase I study.

- mAb114 is a single monoclonal antibody that was isolated from a survivor of EVD and has shown strong neutralizing activity and protection against lethal infection in NHP challenge studies. Compared with monoclonal antibody cocktails, single monoclonal antibodies are easier and less expensive to manufacture.

- Remdesivir is a nucleoside analog that has been shown to be highly efficacious against EVD in NHPs when administered intravenously and had a good safety profile when evaluated in phase I studies.

10. Prevention—

1) Vaccination: there are currently no licensed preventive or therapeutic vaccines for Marburg or Ebola virus infection, though clinical development of multiple vaccine candidates was accelerated during the 2013–2016 West African outbreak and these candidates are currently being assessed in clinical trials.

Based on prior research and experiences from the ring vaccination strategy of vaccinating contacts and contacts of contacts during the West African outbreak, the investigational vaccine rVSV-ZEBOV (VSV) is recommended by the WHO Strategic

Advisory Group of Experts on Immunization for use during outbreaks of the *Zaire* strain. This vaccine has been used under expanded access/compassionate use in an outbreak setting and has been the most widely used vaccine against Ebola. The VSV vaccine has been shown to be safe and to rapidly induce immunity; it may also be effective for postexposure prophylaxis. However, questions remain about the vaccine's efficacy and further evaluations in clinical trials are required before licensure. Furthermore, there are logistical challenges in supplying and distributing vaccines in the field as they are required to be frozen at −80°C (−176°F) and are often transported to remote locations.

Immunization response efforts using the VSV vaccine were initiated shortly after the 2018 DRC outbreak started. Despite immense security challenges and an environment of community mistrust and misinformation about EVD, field laboratories and Ebola treatment centers were rapidly established and a ring vaccination campaign was implemented under WHO's expanded access framework. Compared with the ring vaccination efforts of the 2013–2016 West African outbreak, a notable facet of the 2018 DRC ring vaccination campaign was that, in addition to vaccination of sick contacts and first-line health care workers, other individuals who are likely to come into contact with sick people in the local context (i.e., taxi drivers and motorcyclists transporting sick patients, traditional healers, religious leaders) were also vaccinated.

2) Outbreak response and infection control: several concurrent strategies should be employed to prevent the spread of Ebola virus. A maximally effective public health response should include active engagement of government authorities, the health care community, local leaders, and both affected and at-risk populations.

Strict infection control measures are necessary to prevent transmission to health care workers and to prevent nosocomial transmission to patients being evaluated for possible EVD. These measures include isolation of hospitalized patients with known or suspected EVD; standard, contact, and droplet precautions; the avoidance of aerosol-generating procedures, if possible; and the correct use of appropriate PPE. Detailed guidelines are available from CDC and WHO. Environmental infection control measures are also essential and include frequent cleaning, environmental decontamination, and medical waste management.

Persons who have had a possible exposure to Ebola virus should be monitored for signs and symptoms of disease.

Monitoring should continue for 21 days after the last known exposure. In addition, precautions should be taken to reduce the risk of transmission during convalescence because patients who have recovered from EVD and are no longer viremic continue to shed infectious virus in several bodily fluids, including urine, breast milk, and semen, long after recovery. For example, several cases of EVD have been attributed to sexual transmission. Current CDC and WHO recommendations are for abstinence or condoms if abstinence is not possible. However, it is not known when unprotected sexual activity can be safely resumed; thus, current recommendations are to perform serial testing of semen beginning 3 months after the onset of infection and repeated testing until negative prior to resuming unprotected sexual activity. If semen testing is unavailable, men who have recovered from EVD should use condoms for at least 12 months after the initial onset of illness.

Ebola virus has been isolated from breast milk and can be transmitted through breastfeeding and close contact. Current CDC recommendations are to (a) avoid breastfeeding in mothers being evaluated for EVD, in those with confirmed infection, or in those who have recently recovered until serial laboratory test results of breast milk are negative or (b) weigh the risks and benefits of cessation of breastfeeding in settings where this is not easily implemented.

11. Special considerations—

1) Reporting of suspected/confirmed cases: in many countries, Ebola and Marburg virus infections are reportable as viral hemorrhagic fever. Suspected cases should be reported to the national health authorities and to a WHO Collaborating Centre (Hamburg, Germany; Salisbury, UK; Atlanta, GA, USA; Winnipeg, Canada; Johannesburg, South Africa) for diagnostic support. In the USA, persons under investigation for suspected EVD infection and laboratory-confirmed cases are to be reported to CDC and the National Notifiable Disease Surveillance System. Occurrence of Ebola or Marburg infections likely constitutes an International Health Regulations notifiable event to WHO. Additionally, isolation of Ebola or Marburg viruses must be reported to the national biosecurity agencies in several countries.

2) PPE: infection control recommendations for patients who present with acute *Ebolavirus* infection include the correct use of appropriate PPE. Depending on the patient's clinical presentation, the type of PPE in use and careful donning and doffing of the

equipment are essential for preventing nosocomial transmission.

CDC and WHO have developed guidelines on the use of PPE for patients with suspected or confirmed EVD. These recommendations include full coverage of PPE on all clothing and skin while in contact with a patient, frequent disinfection of gloved hands and contaminated PPE, repeated training of health care workers in correct donning and doffing of PPE, and provision of trained monitors to actively observe and coach health care workers when donning and doffing PPE. More detailed recommendations on the use of PPE during a filovirus disease outbreak have been produced by CDC (https://www.cdc.gov/vhf/ebola/healthcare-us/ppe/guidance.html) and WHO (https://www.who.int/csr/resources/publications/ebola/personal-protective-equipment/en).

3) Travel restrictions and considerations: currently, there is no ban on international travel for travelers to and from areas where EVD occurs. Ebola transmission requires contact with blood and other bodily fluids; there have not been any documented cases of airborne transmission of EVD. Despite the low risk of transmission during air travel, travelers should exercise correct hand hygiene. Current guidance from CDC on handwashing and EVD prevention (https://www.cdc.gov/vhf/ebola/prevention/handwashing.html) is:

- Use alcohol-based hand sanitizer when hands are not visibly dirty. These products usually contain 60% to 95% ethanol or isopropanol. Alcohol-based hand sanitizer should not be used when hands are visibly soiled with dirt, blood, or other bodily fluids.
- Use soap and water when hands are visibly soiled with dirt, blood, or other bodily fluids and as an alternative to alcohol-based hand sanitizer. Antimicrobial soaps are not proven to offer benefits over washing hands with plain soap (not containing antimicrobial compounds) and water.
- Use mild (0.05%) chlorine solution in settings where hand sanitizer and soap are not available. Repeated use of 0.05% chlorine solution may cause skin irritation.

The 2013–2016 West African outbreak was one of few outbreaks in history that constituted a PHEIC, during which there were considerable restrictions on travel and trade to control transmission. In 2014, WHO advised those with recent travel to Ebola-affected countries to take the following precautions for 21 days after returning from a trip:

- Stay within reach of a good quality health care facility.
- Be aware of the symptoms of infection (sudden fever, intense weakness, muscle pain, headache, vomiting, diarrhea, rash, and sometimes bleeding).
- Immediately report a fever of 38°C (100.4°F) or higher to the local medical emergency service (ideally by phone) and mention the travel history.

Lessons and guidelines that emerged from the 2013-2014 outbreak continue to be applicable in current outbreak settings.

[P. Scott, A. Parikh, S. Mate, M. Amare, J. Jones, K. Modjarrad]

ECHINOCOCCOSIS

DISEASE	ICD-10 CODE
CYSTIC ECHINOCOCCOSIS	ICD-10 B67.0–B67.4
ALVEOLAR ECHINOCOCCOSIS	ICD-10 B67.5–B67.7
POLYCYSTIC ECHINOCOCCOSIS	ICD-10 B67.9

1. Clinical features—The larval (hydatid cyst or solid and multi-vesiculated lesions) stages of *Echinococcus* spp. tapeworm produce disease in humans and animals; disease characteristics depend upon the infecting species. Cysts and lesions usually develop in the liver or the lungs but also develop in other viscera, nervous tissue, or bone. They can be cystic, alveolar, and/or polycystic.

1) Cystic: larval stages of the tapeworm *Echinococcus granulosus*, the most common *Echinococcus* spp., cause cystic echinococcosis or hydatid disease. Hydatid cysts enlarge slowly and require several years to develop. Developed cysts range from 1 to 15 cm in diameter but may be larger. Infections may be asymptomatic until cysts cause noticeable mass effect; signs and symptoms vary according to location, cyst size, cyst type, and numbers. Ruptured or leaking cysts can cause severe anaphylactoid reactions and may release protoscolices that can produce secondary echinococcosis. One or several cysts—typically spherical, thick-walled, and consisting of a single cavity (unilocular)—are most frequently found in the liver and lungs, although they may occur in other organs.

Differential diagnoses include benign tumor, malignancies, amebic abscesses, and congenital cysts.

2) Alveolar: a highly invasive, destructive disease. Lesions are usually found in the liver; because a thick laminated cyst wall does not restrict their growth, they expand at the periphery to produce solid, tumor-like masses. Metastases can result in secondary cysts and larval growth in other organs. Clinical manifestations depend on the size and location of cysts but are often confused with hepatic carcinoma and cirrhosis.

3) Polycystic: this disease occurs in the liver, lungs, and other viscera. Symptoms vary depending on cyst size and location. The polycystic lesion is unique in that the germinal membrane proliferates externally to form new cysts and internally to form septae that divide the cavity into numerous microcysts. Brood capsules containing many protoscolices develop in the microcysts.

2. Risk groups—Children, who are more likely to have close contact with infected dogs and less likely to have adequate hygienic habits, are at greater risk of cystic echinococcosis, especially in rural areas. Alveolar echinococcosis usually affects adults.

3. Causative agents—

1) Cystic: *E. granulosus*
2) Alveolar: *Echinococcus multilocularis*
3) Polycystic: *Echinococcus vogeli* and *Echinococcus oligarthrus*

4. Diagnosis—

1) Cystic: based on signs and symptoms compatible with a slowly growing tumor, a history of residence in an endemic area, and an association with canines. Ultrasonography, computerized axial tomography, and serologic testing are useful for supporting diagnosis, with ultrasonography the method of first choice. WHO has developed a classification of ultrasound images of liver cystic echinococcosis for diagnostic and prognostic purposes and determination of the type of intervention required (see Treatment in this chapter). Definitive diagnosis in seronegative patients, however, requires microscopic identification from specimens obtained at surgery or by percutaneous aspiration; the potential risks of this (anaphylaxis, spillage) can be avoided by ultrasound guidance and anthelmintic coverage. Species identification is based on finding thick laminated cyst walls and protoscolices as well as on the structure and measurements of protoscolex hooks.

Molecular techniques are now available to identify the species from biopsies.

2) Alveolar: diagnosis is often based on histopathology (i.e., evidence of the thin host layer and multiple microvesicles formed by external proliferation). Humans are an abnormal host and the lesions rarely produce brood capsules, protoscolices, or calcareous bodies. Serodiagnosis using purified or recombinant *E. multilocularis* antigen is highly sensitive and specific. A staging and classification system proposed by WHO, named PNM, is based on hepatic localization of the parasite (P), extrahepatic involvement of neighboring organs (N), and metastases (M).

3) Polycystic: immunodiagnosis using a purified antigen of *E. vogeli* does not always allow differentiation from alveolar echinococcosis, which does not co-occur in South America. The causative agents are distinguished by the form and size of their rostellar hooks from protoscolices.

5. Occurrence—

1) Cystic: all continents except Antarctica; depends on close association of humans and infected dogs. Especially common in grazing countries where dogs eat viscera containing cysts. Transmission has been eliminated in Iceland and greatly reduced in Tasmania (Australia), Cyprus, and New Zealand. Control programs exist in Argentina, Brazil, China, Kenya (Turkana district), Spain, Uruguay, and other countries, including those of the Mediterranean basin.

2) Alveolar: distribution is limited to areas of the northern hemisphere (China, Russia, northern Japan, Turkey, central Europe, Alaska, Canada, and, rarely, north-central USA). The disease is usually diagnosed in adults.

3) Polycystic: Central and South America.

6. Reservoirs—

1) Cystic: the domestic dog and other canids, definitive hosts for *E. granulosus*, may harbor thousands of adult tapeworms in their intestines without signs of infection. Intermediate hosts include herbivores—primarily sheep, cattle, goats, pigs, horses, camels—and other animals.

2) Alveolar: adult tapeworms are largely restricted to wild animals such as foxes, raccoons, dogs, and coyotes; the associated disease is commonly maintained in nature in fox-rodent cycles. Dogs and cats can be sources of human infection if hunting wild (and rarely

domestic) intermediate hosts such as rodents, including voles, lemmings, and mice.

3) Polycystic: natural definitive hosts are bush dogs (for *E. vogeli*) and wild felids (for *E. oligarthrus*), while intermediate hosts are rodents. Domestic dogs can act as occasional definitive hosts for *E. vogeli*.

7. Incubation period—12 months to years, depending on number and location of cysts and how rapidly they grow.

8. Transmission—

1) Cystic: human infection often takes place directly via hand-to-mouth transfer of eggs after association with infected dogs or indirectly via contaminated food, water, soil, or fomites. In some instances, flies have dispersed eggs after feeding on infected feces. Adult worms in the small intestines of canines produce eggs containing infective embryos (oncospheres); these are passed in feces and may survive for several months in pastures or gardens. When ingested by susceptible intermediate hosts, including humans, eggs hatch, releasing oncospheres that migrate through the mucosa and are carried in the blood to organs, primarily the liver (first filter) and then the lungs (second filter), where they form cysts. Strains of *E. granulosus* vary in their ability to adapt to infect various hosts as well as in their infectivity to humans. Not directly transmitted from person to person or from one intermediate host to another. Dogs become infected by eating animal viscera containing hydatid cysts and begin to pass eggs 5 to 7 weeks later. Most canine infections resolve spontaneously by 6 months; however, some adult worms may survive for up to 2 to 3 years. Dogs may become infected repeatedly. Sheep and other intermediate hosts are infected while grazing in areas contaminated with dog feces containing parasite eggs.

2) Alveolar: ingestion of eggs passed in the feces of dogs and cats that have fed on infected rodents. Fecally soiled dog hair, harnesses, and environmental fomites also serve as vehicles of infection.

3) Polycystic: ingestion of eggs passed in the feces of definitive hosts that have hunted or fed on infected rodents.

9. Treatment—Percutaneous drainage or surgical removal of cysts. Medical treatment, cyst puncture, or PAIR (percutaneous aspiration, injection of chemicals, and respiration) are alternatives to surgery.

Treatment with albendazole has been successful. Albendazole dosing is 10 to 15 mg/kg body weight per day (≤ 800 mg orally in 2 doses). Mebendazole is a second choice but is not as readily available in the USA.

In the case of a ruptured primary cyst, treatment with a proctoscolicidal agent such as praziquantel may reduce the probability of secondary cysts.

10. Prevention—

1) Avoid ingestion of raw vegetables and water that may have been contaminated with the feces of infected dogs. Emphasize basic hygiene practices such as handwashing and washing of fruits and vegetables. Educate those at risk on avoidance of exposure to dog feces.

2) Interrupt transmission from intermediate to definitive hosts by preventing access of dogs to potentially contaminated (uncooked) viscera, by inspecting livestock carcasses and organs after slaughter, and by condemning and safely disposing of infected viscera. Disposal should be by incineration or deep burial.

3) Periodically treat high-risk dogs, and all dogs in high-risk areas, with praziquantel; encourage responsible dog ownership and implement programs aimed at reducing dog populations in compliance with principles of animal welfare.

4) Field and laboratory personnel must observe strict safety precautions to avoid ingestion of tapeworm eggs.

11. Special considerations—Control the movement of dogs from known enzootic areas.

[O. A. Khan]

E. COLI DIARRHEAL DISEASES

DISEASE	ICD-10 CODE
SHIGA TOXIN–PRODUCING *E. COLI*	ICD-10 A04.3
ENTEROTOXIGENIC *E. COLI*	ICD-10 A04.1
ENTEROPATHOGENIC *E. COLI*	ICD-10 A04.0
ENTEROINVASIVE *E. COLI*	ICD-10 A04.2
INTESTINAL *E. COLI* INFECTION, OTHER	ICD-10 A04.4

I. SHIGA TOXIN–PRODUCING *E. COLI* (STEC) (verotoxin-producing *E. coli*, enterohemorrhagic *E. coli*, formerly called Shiga-like toxin-producing *E. coli*)

1. Clinical features—Shiga toxin–producing *Escherichia coli* (STEC) O157 diarrhea can range from mild and nonbloody to stools that are virtually all blood. It typically progresses from watery to bloody stools in 2 to 3 days. Abdominal cramps are often severe and tenderness can result in mistaken diagnoses of appendicitis or intussusception. Illness lasts an average of 6 to 8 days but can range from 1 to 10 days. STEC non-O157 diarrhea and clinical symptoms are similar to those of STEC O157. However, bloody diarrhea, abdominal cramping, and vomiting occur less often.

The most severe manifestation of STEC infection is hemolytic uremic syndrome (HUS), a thrombotic microangiopathy that is typically diagnosed a week after onset of illness, often after diarrhea has resolved. HUS is characterized by hemolytic anemia, thrombocytopenia, and acute renal dysfunction; some patients have neurologic abnormalities. STEC are the primary cause of HUS. A white blood cell count higher than 10,500/μL is associated with increased risk for diarrhea-associated HUS (D+HUS) among children. Some adults with D+HUS are misdiagnosed as having thrombotic thrombocytopenic purpura (TTP), a different thrombotic microangiopathy unrelated to STEC infection. STEC O157 causes the vast majority of D+HUS cases worldwide. Approximately 15% of young children and 6% of people overall with laboratory-confirmed STEC O157 diarrhea develop HUS. Although only 1% of non-O157 STEC infections result in HUS, some strains have higher risk. In an outbreak setting, a higher than expected proportion of patients with STEC infection resulting in HUS suggests either incomplete diarrheal case ascertainment or a strain with unusual virulence properties. An example of the latter scenario is an outbreak in Germany caused by a STEC O104:H4 strain that also had features of enteroaggregative *E. coli*. About 55% of patients with D+HUS required dialysis and 3% to 5% died. Long-term sequelae for D+HUS include hypertension, long-term renal insufficiency, and, rarely, chronic neurologic deficits, diabetes mellitus, pancreatic insufficiency, and other gastrointestinal complications.

2. Risk groups—Infection and HUS occur in persons of all ages. Children aged 1 to 4 years have the highest rate of infection and are at greatest risk of developing HUS. Older adults are at highest risk of death from STEC infection, with or without HUS.

3. Causative agents—STEC are a heterogeneous group of bacteria that express potent cytotoxins called Shiga toxins 1 and 2 (Stx1 and Stx2; also called verotoxins). Stx1 is essentially identical to the toxin produced by *Shigella dysenteriae* 1; D+HUS is also a complication of *S. dysenteriae* 1 infection. In STEC, the toxins are carried on bacterial phages. These toxins can cross the intestinal mucosal border into the bloodstream and then bind to renal endothelium, activate platelets, and stimulate release of proteases, tissue factor, and complement, causing HUS. HUS is more commonly associated with STEC strains that produce only Stx2 than with those that produce both toxins or only Stx1. Certain Stx subtypes, especially Stx2a, have been more strongly linked to HUS than other subtypes in some analyses. In the USA, approximately 65% of D+HUS cases reported in children have laboratory evidence of STEC infection; approximately 90% of these are STEC O157 and virtually all produce Stx2. However, STEC is likely responsible for a higher proportion of D+HUS cases, as stool samples are often collected when diarrhea is resolving and the pathogen may no longer be present. After O157, the most common serogroups isolated from persons with diarrheal illness in the USA are O26, O103, O111, O121, O45, and O145; about 95% of O121 and 50% of O145 isolates produce only Stx2; the percentages are lower for the other major serogroups. In the EU, the most common non-O157 serogroups are O26, O103, O146, O91, O145, and O128. STEC strains vary considerably in virulence and some appear to only cause disease in animals. In addition to the Shiga toxins, STEC bacteria must also express intestinal adherence factors to cause disease; most produce the adherence factor intimin, encoded by *eae* genes (see Enteropathogenic *E. coli* in this chapter).

4. Diagnosis—Specimens should be collected as close to the onset of symptoms as possible because the phages that carry the Stx genes are sometimes lost during illness. Clinical laboratories commonly screen for STEC using a polymerase chain reaction (PCR) for Stx1 and Stx2 genes. A positive test should be followed by culture of the same specimen to isolate STEC and to quickly determine whether illness is caused by STEC O157. All clinical laboratories, but especially those that do not screen stools for Stx genes, should test specimens for STEC O157, which is easily identified on sorbitol-MacConkey medium. STEC that do not agglutinate in O157 antisera should be serotyped, usually in a reference laboratory. All STEC (or, if STEC not isolated, Stx-positive broths) should be sent to a public health laboratory for isolation and characterization, including pulsed-field gel electrophoresis or whole-genome sequencing, which is critical for outbreak detection.

5. Occurrence—STEC is estimated to cause over 2 million illnesses and 269 deaths globally each year—an important problem in Canada, the USA, Europe, Japan, Australia, and the southern cone of South America. The incidence of STEC O157 infection is higher in Canada and northern US states than in southern US states and Mexico, higher in northern than southern Europe, and higher in Argentina than in the northern part of South America. About 15% of non–O157 STEC infections, but only 3% of STEC O157 infections, in the USA occur among persons with recent international travel.

6. Reservoirs—Cattle shed STEC in their feces and are the most important reservoir of STEC O157; cattle also harbor many non-O157 STEC. Other ruminants, including sheep, goats, and deer, can shed STEC in their feces.

7. Incubation period—For *E. coli* O157 the median is 3 to 4 days but can range from 1 to 10 days; not well described for other STEC. In 2011, the median incubation period was 8 days for the *E. coli* O104:H4 outbreak in Germany.

8. Transmission—Mainly through ingestion of food contaminated with ruminant feces and direct contact with animals or their environment. Outbreaks have primarily occurred from beef (usually as inadequately cooked hamburgers) and leafy green vegetables. Outbreaks have also been linked to other produce (e.g., sprouts, melons), unpasteurized products (e.g., apple cider, milk), and other vehicles (e.g., flour, soynut butter). Outbreaks among children have occurred after visits to petting zoos where children touched animals' environments. Direct person-to-person transmission (fecal-oral) occurs most commonly in families, child care centers, and custodial institutions. Waterborne transmission occurs from both contaminated drinking water and recreational waters. The infectious dose is very low. The median duration of excretion is 39 days among children but is much shorter among adults. Prolonged carriage is uncommon.

9. Treatment—Primary treatment should focus on ensuring appropriate hydration. Early use of intravenous fluids may decrease the risk of oligoanuric renal failure. Antibiotics are not recommended because administration may increase the risk of HUS; when used, no definitive improvement has been demonstrated. Antimotility agents should be avoided because they may increase the risk of toxic megacolon and HUS.

Administration of antibiotics may increase the risk of HUS; when used, no definitive improvement has been demonstrated. Antimotility agents should be avoided because they may increase the risk of toxic megacolon and HUS.

10. Prevention—

1) Wash hands thoroughly with soap and water for 20 seconds after using the toilet or after contact with animals or their environments (e.g., in petting zoos; before, during, and after preparing food; and before eating). If soap and water are not available, hand sanitizer that contains 60% or more alcohol can be used.

2) Take food safety universal/standard precautions, including the following:

   - Clean: wash utensils, cutting boards, and countertops with hot, soapy water. Wash fruits and vegetables, particularly if eaten raw.

   - Separate: use separate cutting boards, plates, and knives for produce and raw meat, poultry, and seafood, and wash thoroughly with hot, soapy water after use. Keep raw meat, poultry, and seafood separate from other foods in the refrigerator and in the grocery cart.

- Cook: use a food thermometer and cook food to at least the minimum recommended temperature. More information can be found at: https://www.foodsafety.gov/keep/charts/mintemp.html.
- Chill: never leave perishable food out at room temperature for more than 2 hours. Maintain a refrigerator temperature of less than 40°F (4.5°C). Thaw frozen food in the refrigerator, in cold water, or in the microwave—never on the countertop—because parts can get warm, which allows pathogens to proliferate.

3) Access to safe water is important for preventing illness. General measures include the following:

- Where the safety of the water is uncertain, drink only unopened, factory-sealed bottled or canned beverages and beverages made with boiled water (e.g., tea, coffee); avoid ice and raw produce including salads.
- Drinking water may be disinfected by boiling or by adding one-eighth of a teaspoon (or 8 drops) of regular, unscented, liquid household bleach for each gallon of water at least 30 minutes before drinking.
- The safest way to feed an infant younger than 6 months is to breastfeed exclusively. If the infant is fed formula prepared from commercial powder, the powder should be reconstituted with water within 30 minutes after boiling the water. Cool formula to a safe temperature before feeding and use within 2 hours of preparation.
- Chlorinate swimming pools to at least 1 ppm and hot tubs and spas to 3 ppm, with a pH of 7.2 to 7.8.

4) Some foods pose higher risks for contamination with STEC than others. Therefore, the following are recommended:

- Ensure beef, especially ground beef, is cooked to an internal temperature of 70°C (160°F).
- Ensure milk is pasteurized, juices and ciders are heat-treated (pasteurized), and dairy products are made with pasteurized milk.
- Do not serve raw sprouts to persons most susceptible to complications of foodborne infections, such as young children, the elderly, pregnant women, and persons with compromised immune systems.

11. Special considerations—Reporting: reporting of STEC infections to the local health authority is obligatory in all US states and many countries. The potential severity of some types of STEC infections calls for early involvement of local health authorities to identify the source and apply preventive measures. Report at once to the local health authority any group of persons with acute bloody diarrhea, D+HUS, or TTP (TTP clusters may represent misdiagnosed HUS cases), even if no causal agent has been identified.

II. ENTEROTOXIGENIC *E. COLI* (ETEC)

1. Clinical features—Diarrhea is watery without blood or mucus and ranges from mild to severe. Fever is uncommon. Abdominal cramping, vomiting, and dehydration can occur with severe disease. Symptoms usually last less than 5 days but may last longer in infants and children.

2. Risk groups—Children younger than 5 years in developing countries and travelers visiting developing countries have the highest rates of infection. Multiple infections with different serotypes are required to develop broad-spectrum immunity. Preexisting malnutrition, including micronutrient deficiency, can lead to more severe infection.

3. Causative agents—Enterotoxigenic *E. coli* (ETEC) are a heterogeneous group of noninvasive *E. coli* that colonize the small intestine and produce a heat-labile enterotoxin (LT), a heat-stable enterotoxin (ST), or both (LT/ST). The enterotoxin genes are carried on plasmids. These toxins deregulate ion absorption and secretion, resulting in free water in the intestinal lumen. Strains that produce ST (with or without LT) have been associated with more severe disease than those that produce only LT. Strains that produce only ST or both ST and LT have caused the most ETEC outbreaks in the USA. Serotypes O6:H16 and O169:H41 have been implicated in most outbreaks in the USA. More than 20 O antigens and more than 30 H antigens have been identified among ETEC strains.

4. Diagnosis—Some culture-independent diagnostic PCR tests available in clinical laboratories identify ETEC by detecting the genes that encode ST and LT toxins. Otherwise, testing is only available through reference or public health laboratories. Studies are needed to guide the interpretation of results when multiple pathogens are detected or when ETEC are identified, as little is known about the epidemiology of ETEC within the USA.

5. Occurrence—ETEC are estimated to cause more than 240 million illnesses and nearly 74,000 deaths globally each year. Their role as a cause of sporadic diarrhea in developed countries is largely unknown. During the first 3 years of life, children in developing countries experience multiple ETEC infections that lead to the acquisition of immunity. The frequency of infections increases again after age 15 years, suggesting waning immunity. ETEC is the most frequently identified cause of traveler's diarrhea in European and North American travelers to developing countries.

6. Reservoirs—Although ETEC infections occur in animals, people constitute the main reservoir for strains causing diarrhea in humans.

7. Incubation period—24 to 48 hours in adult volunteer studies. Incubations as short as 10 to 12 hours have been observed in outbreaks and in volunteer studies with certain LT-only and ST-only strains.

8. Transmission—Fecal-oral, through contaminated food and water. Transmission via contaminated weaning foods may be particularly important in infants. Direct contact transmission through feces-contaminated hands is believed to be rare.

9. Treatment—Primary treatment should focus on ensuring appropriate hydration. Empirical antibiotic treatment before ruling out STEC might increase the risk of HUS. Antibiotics should be avoided for mild illness, can be considered for moderate diarrhea, and should be used for severe diarrhea. Loperamide can be used for patients aged 2 years or older: 4-mg first dose and 2 mg after each loose stool, not to exceed 16 mg in a 24-hour period.

Drug	Azithromycin (moderate-to-severe disease)
Dose	1,000 mg (adults); 10 mg/kg (children)
Route	PO
Duration	• Adults and children: single dose unless not resolved in 24 hours, THEN daily for ≤ 3 days OR • Adults only (additional option): 500 mg daily for 3 days
Alternative drug	• Levofloxacin 500 mg PO as a single dose or 3-day course OR • Ciprofloxacin 750 mg PO as a single dose or 500 mg PO for 3 days OR • Ofloxacin 400 mg PO as a single dose or 3-day course OR • Rifaximin 200 mg PO TID for 3 days

(Continued)

(Continued)

Special considerations and comments	• Use of an antibiotic should be weighed against illness severity, likelihood of pathogen resistance, and the risk of adverse effects.
	• Administration of antibiotics before ruling out STEC may increase the risk of HUS.
	• Do not use rifaximin if *Campylobacter, Salmonella,* or *Shigella,* or other causes of invasive diarrhea, are suspected.
	• Fluoroquinolones are not approved for this indication in patients < 18 years.

Note: HUS = hemolytic uremic syndrome; PO = oral(ly); STEC = Shiga toxin–producing *Escherichia coli*; TID = thrice daily.

10. Prevention—

1) Fecal-oral spread of infection is prevented through proper hygiene, sanitation, access to safe water, and food safety practices (see Shiga Toxin-Producing *E. coli* in this chapter for general handwashing, food safety, and safe water recommendations).

2) Some foods pose a higher risk when traveling. Therefore, the following preventive measures are recommended:

   • Fruits without peels should be avoided and fruits with peels should be peeled by the person who will consume them.
   • If feeding an infant with formula, consider bringing enough for the entire trip as manufacturing standards vary widely.

3) The use of prophylactic bismuth subsalicylate may be considered for adults traveling for short periods to high-risk areas where it is not easy to obtain safe food or water.

4) Travelers should consider bringing packets of oral rehydration salts, which can be added to boiled or bottled water and ingested soon after symptom onset to ensure fluid and electrolyte balance is maintained.

5) Prophylactic antibiotics should be considered only for travelers going to a resource-poor area and who also have an illness that predisposes them to complications. Rifaximin is the best drug for prophylaxis.

11. Special considerations—

1) Reporting: varies by state, but is not a nationally notifiable infection in the USA.

2) Epidemic measures: during an outbreak, an epidemiologic investigation is indicated to determine how transmission is occurring. Targeted testing should be considered for patients with

compatible symptoms who recently traveled to a less industrialized country and whose stool specimens tested negative for routine enteric pathogens.

III. ENTEROPATHOGENIC *E. COLI* (EPEC)

1. Clinical features—Diarrhea is watery and ranges from mild to severe and acute to persistent; fever and vomiting may also be present. High case-fatality rates have been seen in newborn nurseries.

2. Risk groups—Children younger than 2 years are most susceptible. Infection is less common in breastfed infants.

3. Causative agents—Enteropathogenic *E. coli* (EPEC) are a heterogeneous group of *E. coli* that produce an attaching and effacing (A/E) lesion on intestinal epithelial cells and do not produce Shiga toxin. The pathogenesis involves virulence factors that induce diarrhea through several mechanisms, including malabsorption secondary to decreased enterocyte surface area and increased secretions due to deregulation of ion channels. Local inflammation with altered intestinal permeability may be a contributory factor. The bacteria produce the protein Tir and insert it into the enterocyte, where it acts as a receptor for intimin, a protein encoded by the *eae* gene, which facilitates adherence of EPEC to the enterocyte. This process leads to a compromise of the enterocyte structure, resulting in the A/E lesion. EPEC are further classified by the presence or absence of the EPEC adherence factor plasmid, for which the bundle-forming pilus gene (*bfpA*) serves as the marker. Typical EPEC (tEPEC) are *E. coli* with both *eae* and *bfpA*. Atypical EPEC (aEPEC) possess *eae* but not *bfpA*; virulence features that differentiate those that are pathogenic for humans have not yet been determined. Traditional EPEC strains that have caused outbreaks fall into serogroups O55, O111, O114, O119, O125, O127, O128, O142, and O157 (non-Shiga toxin–producing O157:H45). Many STEC and *Escherichia albertii* also have the *eae* gene.

4. Diagnosis—Most culture-independent PCR tests currently available in clinical laboratories rely on only the *eae* gene for detecting EPEC (and report the test as positive if the specimen does not also test positive for STEC, which usually also has the *eae* gene). This method cannot discriminate between tEPEC and aEPEC. Some PCR tests identify EPEC by targeting the *bfpA* as well as the *eae* genes; these provide more reliable identification. Testing is also available through public health laboratories. Interpretation of PCR test results that rely on only the *eae* gene can be difficult because asymptomatic persons, and those whose illness is caused by another pathogen, can carry organisms with the *eae* gene. Most tEPEC strains are multidrug-resistant; antimicrobial susceptibility testing can help inform treatment.

5. Occurrence—Frequent EPEC outbreaks among hospitalized infants were reported in the first half of the 20th century, with mortality rates of up to 50%. Since the late 1960s, tEPEC has largely disappeared as an important cause of outbreaks of infant diarrhea in North America and Europe. However, tEPEC remains a major agent of infant diarrhea in less developed areas. Atypical EPEC are common in stool specimens in both developed and developing countries, but not all cause diarrhea.

6. Reservoirs—Humans are the reservoir for tEPEC. Atypical EPEC have been isolated from humans and many animal species.

7. Incubation period—7 to 16 hours in adult volunteer studies. The incubation period for infants is 2 to 12 days.

8. Transmission—Fecal-oral, primarily through contaminated surfaces, weaning fluids, and human carriers. Outbreaks from contaminated food and water have occurred.

9. Treatment—For treatment recommendations, see Enterotoxigenic *E. coli* in this chapter.

10. Prevention—

1) In this chapter, see Shiga Toxin–Producing *E. coli* for general handwashing, food safety, and safe water recommendations and Enterotoxigenic *E. coli* for recommendations for travelers.
2) Ensure health professionals are trained to support and instruct mothers on breastfeeding and safe preparation of powdered formula.
3) Maintain high sanitary standards in facilities for infants. Provide individual equipment for each infant, including thermometers and stethoscopes, whenever possible. Clean and disinfect equipment that is to be shared, e.g., scales, between each use.
4) Practice rooming-in for mothers and infants in maternity facilities, unless there is a firm medical indication for separation. If mother or infant has a gastrointestinal or respiratory infection, keep the pair together but isolate them from healthy persons. In special care facilities, separate infected infants from those who are premature or ill.

11. Special considerations—Reporting: reporting to local health authorities is required in a small number of US states. In some countries, reporting of epidemics to local health authorities is obligatory. Two or more concurrent cases of diarrhea requiring treatment for these symptoms in a nursery or among those recently discharged should be interpreted as a possible outbreak requiring investigation.

IV. ENTEROINVASIVE *E. COLI* (EIEC)

1. Clinical features—Symptoms and course can closely resemble *Shigella*. Diarrhea is often watery and some patients have fever. Illness may be accompanied by tenesmus, abdominal cramps, or malaise. Illness usually lasts 4 to 7 days.

2. Risk groups—Children in and travelers visiting developing countries have the highest rates of infection.

3. Causative agents—Enteroinvasive *E. coli* (EIEC) are a heterogeneous group of invasive *E. coli*. An invasion plasmid contains the *ipaH* and *ipaC* genes and other factors that allow EIEC to multiply within mucosal cells of the colon and extend into adjacent cells, causing inflammation. Characteristic serogroups include O124, O143, and O164. By phylogenetic analysis, EIEC is highly related to *Shigella*. The 2 groups share many characteristics, including virulence factors.

4. Diagnosis—Culture-independent PCR tests available in clinical laboratories detect the *ipaH* or *ipaC* genes common to EIEC and *Shigella*. Otherwise, testing is available through reference or public health laboratories.

5. Occurrence—EIEC infections are endemic in developing countries. However, the burden of illness is not clearly understood. Its similarity to *Shigella* poses diagnostic challenges and most large-scale surveys do not distinguish between the 2 infections. A community-based study has estimated an attributable fraction for EIEC of 0.8% when comparing children aged 12 to 24 months with and without diarrhea. Rarely, infections and outbreaks of EIEC diarrhea have been reported in industrialized countries.

6. Reservoirs—Humans are currently the only known reservoir.

7. Incubation period—Average incubation periods of 10 hours and 18 hours have been reported in volunteer studies and outbreaks, respectively.

8. Transmission—Fecal-oral, based on scant available evidence, through contaminated food and water.

9. Treatment—For treatment recommendations, see Enterotoxigenic *E. coli* in this chapter.

10. Prevention—Prevention is the same as for ETEC (in this chapter, see Shiga Toxin–Producing *E. coli* for general handwashing, food safety, and safe water recommendations and Enterotoxigenic *E. coli* for recommendations specific for travelers).

11. Special considerations—None.

V. INTESTINAL E. COLI INFECTION, OTHER (enteroaggregative E. coli [EAEC], diffuse-adherent E. coli [DAEC])

1. Clinical features—Diarrhea due to both enteroaggregative *E. coli* (EAEC) and diffuse-adherent *E. coli* (DAEC) is typically watery and non-bloody. EAEC diarrhea has been further described as often containing mucus and having an acute onset; fever, vomiting, and bloody stools can also occur. EAEC has also been associated with persistent (> 14 days) diarrhea in children. The roles of EAEC and DAEC as enteric pathogens are not fully understood.

2. Risk groups—For EAEC, those at risk are infants and young children, particularly malnourished children living in developing countries, human immunodeficiency virus (HIV)–infected persons, and international travelers to developing countries. Little is known about host risk factors. For DAEC, based on a few epidemiologic studies, children aged 1 to 5 years appear to be at increased risk (though not infants, possibly owing to lack of the cellular receptor for DAEC adherence among infants).

3. Causative agents—EAEC are a heterogeneous group of *E. coli* that exhibit adherence to Hep-2 cells in a pattern resembling stacked bricks. Adherence to small intestinal epithelium results in increased secretion of mucus, which forms a biofilm that entraps the bacteria onto the epithelium. Strains vary considerably in virulence; pathogenic strains have been identified in outbreak investigations. Most strains carry the aggregative adherence plasmid, which contains the *aggR* regulatory gene and *aatA* outer protein gene. The adhesins for many EAEC have not been identified.

DAEC are a heterogeneous group of *E. coli* that exhibit a diffuse pattern of adherence to Hep-2 cells in culture. This pattern is due to the action of fimbrial (Dr) or afimbrial (Afa) adhesins. Binding of bacterial adhesins to the decay-accelerating factor receptor on epithelial cells induces a cytopathic effect, accompanied by activation of signal transduction cascades including the ability to cause epithelial cells to secrete a high amount of interleukin-8, which might be linked to pathogenesis. A role has been proposed for DAEC in inflammatory bowel disease by promoting pro-inflammatory responses through the interaction of adhesins with host membrane–bound receptors.

4. Diagnosis—Some culture-independent diagnostic PCR tests available in clinical laboratories identify EAEC by targeting the *aggR* and *aatA* genes. Otherwise, testing is available through reference or public health laboratories.

No commercial kits or reagents are available for diagnosing DAEC. Some research laboratories have PCR assays to detect the *daaC* gene and the Afa and Dr adhesins.

5. Occurrence—EAEC are associated with acute and persistent diarrhea among children and adults in developing and developed countries. Reports associating EAEC with infant diarrhea, including persistent diarrhea, have come from Latin America, Asia, and sub-Saharan Africa. In case-control studies in Europe and the USA, approximately 5% of cases (people presenting with diarrhea, vomiting, or both) and 2% of controls tested positive for EAEC. EAEC have also been associated with diarrhea among HIV-infected adults and international travelers returning from developing countries. A small number of outbreaks have been reported.

Unlike EAEC, preliminary evidence suggests DAEC are more pathogenic among children aged 3 to 5 years than among infants and toddlers. However, 2 DAEC strains failed to cause diarrhea when fed to volunteers, and no outbreaks have been recognized. Additionally, a case-control study conducted in Europe found that approximately equal proportions (~4%) of cases and controls tested positive for DAEC.

6. Reservoirs—Humans are the likely reservoir for both EAEC and DAEC, but animals are possible.

7. Incubation period—Estimated 20 to 48 hours for EAEC; periods as short as 8 hours have been observed. Unknown for DAEC.

8. Transmission—Fecal-oral, likely through food or water for EAEC. Unknown for DAEC.

9. Treatment—For treatment recommendations, see Enterotoxigenic *E. coli* in this chapter.

10. Prevention—Prevention is the same as for ETEC. In this chapter, see Shiga Toxin–Producing *E. coli* for general handwashing, food safety, and safe water recommendations and Enterotoxigenic *E. coli* for recommendations specific for travelers.

11. Special considerations—Optimal diagnostic testing methods are lacking, and a way to determine which strains are pathogens has not been identified.

[D. M. Tack, A. Winstead, N. A. Strockbine, P. M. Griffin]

EHRLICHIOSIS AND ANAPLASMOSIS

DISEASE	ICD-10 CODE
EHRLICHIOSIS	ICD-10 A77.4
EHRLICHIOSIS, UNSPECIFIED	ICD-10 A77.40
EHRLICHIA CHAFFEENSIS	ICD-10 A77.41
OTHER EHRLICHIOSES (may be used for anaplasmosis)	ICD-10 A77.49

DISEASE IN HUMANS	CAUSATIVE AGENTS	VERTEBRATE RESERVOIRS	GEOGRAPHIC DISTRIBUTION OF HUMAN ILLNESS
EHRLICHIOSIS	Ehrlichia chaffeensis	White-tailed deer, dogs, goats	North America (especially southeastern and south-central USA)
	Ehrlichia ewingii	Dogs, white-tailed deer	North and South America (especially southeastern and south-central USA), Africa
	Ehrlichia muris eauclairensis	Small rodents	USA (Minnesota and Wisconsin)
ANAPLASMOSIS	Anaplasma phagocytophilum	Ruminants, deer, field rodents, dogs	North America, Asia, Europe

I. EHRLICHIOSIS (ehrlichiosis caused by *Ehrlichia chaffeensis, Ehrlichia ewingii,* and *Ehrlichia muris eauclairensis*)

1. Clinical features—Ehrlichiosis is an acute febrile illness caused by a group of small pleomorphic obligate intracellular bacteria that survive and reproduce in the phagosomes of mononuclear or polymorphonuclear leukocytes of the infected host. The organisms are sometimes observed within these cells in the peripheral blood. Ehrlichiosis caused by *Ehrlichia chaffeensis* primarily affects monocytes and tissue macrophages, while ehrlichiosis caused by *Ehrlichia ewingii* affects neutrophils. Ehrlichiosis caused by *Ehrlichia muris eauclairensis* has recently been described and the target cell type is unknown. Ehrlichiosis is most commonly caused by *E. chaffeensis* and generally presents as a moderate-to-severe illness, which can be fatal in some cases. Ehrlichiosis caused by *E. ewingii* and *E. muris eauclairensis* usually presents as a milder disease than that caused by *E. chaffeensis*; no fatalities have been reported.

Ehrlichiosis caused by *E. chaffeensis* presents with nonspecific symptoms, including fever, headache, malaise, and myalgia. Gastrointestinal manifestations, including nausea, vomiting, and diarrhea, have also been reported and are more common among children. Ehrlichiosis can be confused clinically with Rocky Mountain spotted fever (RMSF), although skin rash is less commonly reported with *E. chaffeensis* and direct vasculitis and endothelial injury are rare in ehrlichiosis. Up to one-third of patients can develop a skin rash, which typically occurs a median of 5 days after illness onset. Many of the clinical manifestations are a reflection of the host systemic inflammatory response rather than direct effects of the pathogen. Laboratory findings include leukopenia, thrombocytopenia, hyponatremia, and elevated hepatic transaminases. Anemia can also occur later in the clinical course. Neurologic manifestations, such as meningitis and meningoencephalitis, are reported in approximately 20% of patients. Other severe manifestations include acute respiratory distress syndrome (ARDS), toxic shock-like or septic shock-like syndromes, renal failure, hepatic failure, coagulopathies, and, occasionally, hemorrhagic manifestations. Infection with *E. chaffeensis* can cause severe illness or death; reported case-fatality rates range from 1% to 3%. There is no current evidence of persistent infection in humans.

Symptoms of *E. ewingii* and *E. muris eauclairensis* infections are usually milder and nonspecific and can include fever, headache, malaise, and myalgia. Laboratory findings are also similar. To date, these infections have not been reported to be associated with fatalities.

Differential diagnosis for ehrlichiosis includes various viral syndromes (including Heartland and Bourbon viruses), RMSF, sepsis, toxic shock syndrome, gastroenteritis, meningoencephalitis, tularemia, Colorado tick fever, tickborne encephalitis, babesiosis, Lyme borreliosis, leptospirosis, hepatitis, typhoid fever, murine typhus, and blood malignancies.

2. Risk groups—Severity of ehrlichiosis depends, in part, on host factors such as age and immune status. Persons with compromised immunity caused by immunosuppressive therapies (e.g., corticosteroids, cancer chemotherapy, or long-term immunosuppressive therapy following organ transplant), human immunodeficiency virus infection, or splenectomy appear to develop more severe disease and can have higher case-fatality rates. Reinfection with *E. chaffeensis* has been described in an immunosuppressed patient; however, the frequency of reinfection in immunocompetent persons is unknown. Travel history to endemic areas should raise suspicion for ehrlichiosis.

3. Causative agents—See the earlier table. These bacterial organisms are members of the family Anaplasmataceae, order Rickettsiales.

4. Diagnosis—Diagnosis is based on clinical signs and symptoms and later confirmed by laboratory findings and molecular or immunologic test results. Treatment should never be delayed pending the receipt of laboratory test results or be withheld based on an initial negative laboratory result.

During the acute phase of illness, a sample of ethylenediamine-tetraacetic acid (EDTA)–anticoagulated whole blood can be tested by polymerase chain reaction (PCR) assay. This method is most sensitive in the first week of illness and quickly decreases in sensitivity following the administration of doxycycline (within 24–48 hours). Because organisms for *E. ewingii* have not been cultured, antigen for serologic testing is not available, and *E. muris eauclairensis* antigen is not yet available commercially. However, both infections can generate cross-reactive antibodies with *E. chaffeensis* antigen. Thus, *E. ewingii* and *E. muris eauclairensis* infections are specifically diagnosed by molecular detection methods: *E. ewingii* and *E. muris eauclairensis* deoxyribonucleic acid (DNA) is detected in a clinical specimen via amplification of a specific gene target.

The gold standard test for serologic diagnosis of ehrlichiosis is the indirect immunofluorescence assay (IFA) using *E. chaffeensis* antigen, performed on paired serum samples. To demonstrate a significant (4-fold) rise in antibody titers, the first sample should be taken during the acute phase of illness (within 1–2 weeks of illness onset) and before treatment; the second sample should be taken 2 to 4 weeks later. In most cases of ehrlichiosis, the first immunoglobulin class G (IgG) IFA titer is typically low or seronegative and the second typically shows at least a 4-fold increase in IgG antibody levels. Immunoglobulin class M (IgM) antibodies are less specific and can produce false-positive results, so it is not recommended to use IgM test results alone as diagnostic support criteria. IgG antibodies to *E. chaffeensis* can remain elevated for months, or longer, after the disease has resolved or can be detected in persons who were previously exposed to antigenically related organisms. Up to 12% of currently healthy people in some areas may have elevated antibody titers due to past exposure to *Ehrlichia* spp. or related organisms. Therefore, a diagnosis of ehrlichiosis cannot be confirmed on the basis of only 1 serologic result.

Serologic tests based on enzyme immunoassay (EIA) technology are available from some commercial laboratories. However, currently available EIA tests are qualitative rather than quantitative, meaning they only provide a positive/negative result and are not designed to measure changes in antibody titers between paired specimens. Furthermore, some EIAs rely on the evaluation of IgM antibody alone, which can have a higher frequency of false-positive results and persist for periods long beyond the acute infection.

Blood smear examination is not generally recommended as the most sensitive method of detection but, in some cases, stained blood smears or buffy coat smears may show characteristic inclusions (morulas) during the acute stage of illness. *E. chaffeensis* most commonly infects monocytes, whereas *E. ewingii* more commonly infects granulocytes. The observance of morulas in a particular cell type cannot conclusively identify the infecting species. Culture isolation of *Ehrlichia* is only available at specialized laboratories; routine hospital blood cultures cannot detect *Ehrlichia*. Culture and immunohistochemistry of bone marrow or necropsy tissues can be used for diagnosis in fatal cases.

5. Occurrence—See the earlier table for the geographic distribution of human illness. The distribution of the organisms in their animal and vector reservoirs can extend beyond the areas where human cases occur. Travel-associated infections have been reported both domestically and internationally.

6. Reservoirs—See the earlier table. A number of vertebrate reservoirs have been identified for each pathogen and the ecology can be complex.

7. Incubation period—5 to 14 days for *E. chaffeensis*; the incubation periods for *E. ewingii* and *E. muris eauclairensis* have not been established but are likely similar.

8. Transmission—*E. chaffeensis* and *E. ewingii* are transmitted through the bite of a lone star tick, *Amblyomma americanum*, in North America. *E. muris eauclairensis* has been reported from *Ixodes scapularis* in the upper Midwestern USA; similar organisms have been identified in *Ixodes persulcatus* and *Haemaphysalis flava* ticks in certain parts of the world. Transmission of both *E. chaffeensis* and *E. ewingii* via transfusion of infected blood products has been reported infrequently. Cases of solid tissue organ transplant–acquired ehrlichiosis have been reported. No evidence of other person-to-person transmission has been demonstrated.

9. Treatment—

Drug	Doxycycline
Dose	<ul><li>Adults: 100 mg BID</li><li>Children < 45 kg: 2.2 mg/kg BID; short courses of doxycycline (≤ 10 days), such as that recommended for ehrlichiosis, have not been shown to cause tooth staining in children < 8 years</li><li>≤ 100 mg/dose</li></ul>
Route	PO or IV

(Continued)

(Continued)

Alternative drug	In cases of life-threatening allergies to doxycycline and in some pregnant patients for whom the clinical course of ehrlichiosis appears mild, physicians may need to consider alternate antibiotics. Rifampin appears effective against *Ehrlichia* in laboratory settings. However, rifampin is not effective in treating RMSF, a disease that may be confused with ehrlichiosis. Health care providers should be cautious when exploring treatments other than doxycycline, which is highly effective in treating both diseases.
Duration	≥ 3 days after fever subsides and until evidence of clinical improvement is noted; minimum treatment course of 5–7 days.
Special considerations and comments	• Doxycycline is the first-line treatment for adults and children of all ages and should be initiated immediately whenever ehrlichiosis is suspected. • Receiving a sulfonamide antimicrobial agent may worsen the course of illness. • There is no evidence supporting prophylactic treatment of rickettsial diseases.

Note: BID = twice daily; IV = intravenous(ly); PO = oral(ly); RMSF = Rocky Mountain spotted fever.

10. Prevention—Measures to avoid tick bites (see Lyme Disease and Tickborne Spotted Fevers in "Rickettsioses") should be employed to prevent ehrlichiosis.

11. Special considerations—Reporting: case reporting to the local health authority is required in most counties and states. These data are compiled for national surveillance and provide important clues to changing trends in tickborne rickettsial diseases.

II. ANAPLASMOSIS (*Anaplasma phagocytophilum*)

1. Clinical features—Anaplasmosis is caused by *Anaplasma phagocytophilum*, an obligate intracellular bacterium that is found predominantly within granulocytes of the infected host. The organisms are sometimes observed within these cells in stained peripheral blood smears or buffy coat preparations.

Anaplasmosis, known as human granulocytic anaplasmosis (formerly human granulocytic ehrlichiosis), ranges from a mild to a moderate illness and is characterized clinically by acute and usually self-limited fever, headache, malaise, myalgia, and chills. Gastrointestinal symptoms occur in about 20% of cases. Skin rash is uncommon, occurring in fewer than 10% of patients. Nervous system involvement is rare. Patients with anaplasmosis typically seek medical care later in the course of illness (4–8 days after onset) than patients with other tickborne rickettsial diseases (2–4 days after onset). Common laboratory findings may include thrombocytopenia, leukopenia, mild-to-moderate elevations in hepatic transaminases, increased numbers of immature neutrophils, and mild anemia. Abnormal laboratory findings can be present in the first week of illness; however, normal laboratory findings do not rule out possible infection. Severe or life-threatening manifestations are less frequent with anaplasmosis than with RMSF or ehrlichiosis. However, ARDS, peripheral neuropathies, disseminated intravascular coagulation–like coagulopathies, hemorrhagic manifestations, rhabdomyolysis, pancreatitis, and acute renal failure have been reported. Case-fatality rate is less than 1%. There is no current evidence of persistent infection in humans. Coinfections with *Borrelia burgdorferi*, *Babesia* spp., and tickborne encephalitis viruses may occur; if a patient is not responding to appropriate treatment, consideration and treatment of these coinfections should be considered.

Differential diagnosis can be broad and includes various viral syndromes, RMSF, sepsis, toxic shock syndrome, gastroenteritis, meningoencephalitis, tularemia, Colorado tick fever, tickborne encephalitis, babesiosis, Lyme borreliosis, leptospirosis, hepatitis, typhoid fever, murine typhus, and blood malignancies among others.

2. Risk groups—Predictors of a more severe course of anaplasmosis include advanced age; immunosuppression; comorbid medical conditions, such as diabetes; and delay in diagnosis and treatment. Reinfection is rare. Travel history to an endemic area (domestic or international) should increase suspicion for anaplasmosis.

3. Causative agents—See the earlier table. These organisms are members of the family Anaplasmataceae, order Rickettsiales.

4. Diagnosis—Diagnosis is based on clinical signs and symptoms and later confirmed by laboratory findings.

PCR amplification is performed on DNA extracted from EDTA-anticoagulated whole-blood specimens. This method is most sensitive in the first week of illness and decreases in sensitivity following the administration of appropriate antibiotics (within 24–48 hours). Although a positive PCR result is confirmatory, a negative result does not rule out the diagnosis and treatment should not be withheld owing to a negative result. PCR might also be used to amplify DNA in solid tissue and bone marrow specimens.

The standard serologic test for diagnosis of anaplasmosis is the IFA assay for IgG using *A. phagocytophilum* antigen. IgG IFA assays should be performed on paired acute and convalescent serum samples collected 2 to 4 weeks apart to demonstrate evidence of a 4-fold seroconversion. Antibody titers are frequently negative in the first week of illness. Anaplasmosis cannot be confirmed using single acute antibody results and results are greatly strengthened by paired testing. While IgM IFA assays may also be offered by reference laboratories, IgM antibodies are long-lasting and thus not necessarily indicators of acute infection. It is not recommended to use IgM test results alone as diagnostic support criteria and physicians requesting IgM serologic titers should also request a concurrent IgG titer.

Serologic tests based on EIA technology are available from some commercial laboratories. However, currently available EIA tests are qualitative rather than quantitative, meaning they only provide a positive/negative result and are not designed to measure changes in antibody titer between paired specimens. Furthermore, some EIAs rely on the evaluation of IgM antibody alone, which may not be diagnostically reliable.

IgG antibodies to *A. phagocytophilum* can remain elevated for many months after the disease has resolved. In certain persons, high titers of antibodies against *A. phagocytophilum* have been observed for more than 4 years after the acute illness. Between 5% and 10% of healthy people in some areas can have elevated antibody titers due to past exposure to *A. phagocytophilum* or similar organisms. Comparison of paired, and appropriately timed, serologic assays provides the best evidence of recent infection. Single, or inappropriately timed, serologic tests, in relation to clinical illness, can lead to misinterpretation of results.

During the first week of illness, a microscopic examination of a stained peripheral blood smear can reveal morulas (microcolonies of anaplasmas) in the cytoplasm of granulocytes; these are highly suggestive of anaplasmosis. However, blood smear examination is relatively insensitive and should not be relied upon solely to diagnose anaplasmosis. Moreover, the observance of morulas in a particular cell type cannot conclusively differentiate between *Anaplasma* and *Ehrlichia* spp.

Culture isolation and immunohistochemical (IHC) assays of *A. phagocytophilum* are only available at specialized laboratories; routine hospital blood cultures cannot detect the organism. PCR, culture, and IHC assays can also be applied to autopsy tissue specimens. If a bone marrow biopsy is performed as part of the investigation of cytopenia, immunostaining of the bone marrow biopsy specimen can confirm *A. phagocytophilum* infection.

5. Occurrence—See the earlier table for the geographic distribution of human illness. The distribution of the organisms in their reservoirs can extend beyond the areas where human cases occur. Travel-associated infections have been reported.

6. Reservoirs—See the earlier table. A number of vertebrate reservoirs have been identified for the pathogen and the ecology can be complex; the earlier table provides the animals most prominent in transmission.

7. Incubation period—5 to 14 days for *A. phagocytophilum*.

8. Transmission—*Ixodes* spp., including *I. scapularis*, *Ixodes ricinus*, *Ixodes pacificus*, *Ixodes trianguliceps*, *Ixodes spinipalpis*, and *I. persulcatus* ticks.

There is a risk of transmission of *A. phagocytophilum* through blood transfusions. *A. phagocytophilum* has been shown to survive for more than a week in refrigerated blood. Several cases of transfusion-transmitted anaplasmosis have been reported, including in cases of asymptomatic donors. Use of leukoreduced blood products might reduce the risk of *Anaplasma* transmission but does not eliminate it. Among tickborne rickettsial diseases, anaplasmosis is the most frequently associated with transfusion-acquired infection.

9. Treatment—

Drug	Doxycycline
Dose	<ul><li>Adults: 100 mg BID</li><li>Children < 45 kg: 2.2 mg/kg BID; short courses of doxycycline (≤ 10 days) have not been shown to cause tooth staining in children < 8 years</li><li>≤ 100 mg/dose</li></ul>
Route	PO or IV
Alternative drug	In cases of life-threatening allergies to doxycycline and in some pregnant patients for whom the clinical course of anaplasmosis appears mild, physicians may need to consider alternate antibiotics. Rifampin appears effective against *Anaplasma phagocytophilum* in laboratory settings. However, rifampin is not effective in treating RMSF, a disease that might be confused with anaplasmosis, nor is it an effective treatment for potential coinfection with Lyme disease. Health care providers should be cautious when exploring treatments other than doxycycline, which is highly effective in treating both. Although recommended as a second-line therapeutic alternative to treat RMSF, chloramphenicol is not recommended for the treatment of anaplasmosis as studies have shown a lack of efficacy.
Duration	Patients with suspected anaplasmosis should be treated with doxycycline for 10–14 days to provide appropriate length of therapy for possible concurrent Lyme disease infection.
Special considerations and comments	<ul><li>Doxycycline is the first-line treatment for adults and children of all ages and should be initiated immediately whenever anaplasmosis is suspected.</li><li>Sulfonamide antimicrobials are associated with increased severity of tickborne rickettsial diseases.</li><li>There is no evidence supporting prophylactic treatment of rickettsial diseases.</li></ul>

Note: BID = twice daily; IV = intravenous(ly); PO = oral(ly); RMSF = Rocky Mountain spotted fever.

10. Prevention—Measures to avoid tick bites (see Lyme Disease and Tickborne Spotted Fevers in "Rickettsioses") should be employed to prevent anaplasmosis.

11. Special considerations—Reporting: case reporting to the local health authority is required in most counties and states. These data are compiled for national surveillance and provide important clues to changing trends in tickborne rickettsial diseases.

[K. Nichols Heitman, D. Cherry-Brown, W. L. Nicholson]

ENTEROBIASIS
(pinworm infection, oxyuriasis)

DISEASE	ICD-10 CODE
ENTEROBIASIS	ICD-10 B80

1. Clinical features—A common intestinal helminthic infection that may range from asymptomatic to recurrently symptomatic. The most common clinical feature is perianal itching, especially at night, which may lead to disturbed sleep, irritability, and secondary bacterial infection of scratched skin. Other clinical manifestations include vulvovaginitis, salpingitis, and pelvic and liver granulomata. Appendicitis, eosinophilic enterocolitis without systemic eosinophilia, and enuresis have also been reported as possible associated conditions.

2. Risk groups—Differences in frequency and intensity of infection are due primarily to differences in exposure. Infection often occurs in more than 1 family member. Prevalence can be high in domiciliary institutions. Those most likely to be infected with pinworm are children younger than 18 years, people who take care of infected children, and people who are institutionalized. In these groups, the prevalence can reach up to 50%.

3. Causative agents—*Enterobius vermicularis*, a small intestinal nematode helminth, also called pinworm, that can be seen with the naked eye as a tiny white thread. The male worm measures 2 to 4 mm in length, while the female measures 8 to 12 mm. The worm is oviparous, and the adults are found in the lumen of the cecum, appendix, and occasionally the ascending colon and ileum. Eggs measure 50×25 μm and are flattened on one side, resulting in a bean-shaped appearance. A second species, *Enterobius gregorii*, has been reported in Europe, Asia, and Africa and has similar appearance and clinical manifestations to *E. vermicularis*.

4. Diagnosis—The diagnosis can be made by demonstrating the presence of worms or their eggs. Female adult worms can be seen in the perianal region 2 to 3 hours after the infected person goes to sleep. Eggs can be demonstrated by applying transparent adhesive tape (tape swab or pinworm paddle) to the perianal region and examining the tape or paddle microscopically for eggs; material for examination is best obtained at night or first thing in the morning before bathing or passage of stools. Examination should be repeated over 3 or more consecutive days before accepting a negative result. Eggs are sometimes found on microscopic stool and urine examination, nail washings, and bed linen. Female worms may be found in feces and in the perianal region during rectal or vaginal examinations. However, since eggs and worms are usually sparse in stools, routine stool examination for diagnosis is not recommended. There is no serologic test available for diagnosis.

5. Occurrence—Worldwide, affecting all socioeconomic classes, with high rates in some areas. It is the most common worm infection in countries with a temperate climate, including the USA. Prevalence is highest in school-aged children (in some groups, near 50%), followed by preschoolers, and is lowest in adults except for caregivers of infected children.

6. Reservoirs—Humans. Pinworms of other animals are not transmissible to humans.

7. Incubation period—The incubation period ranges between 1 month and 2 months. Symptomatic disease with high worm burdens results from successive reinfections occurring within months of initial exposure.

8. Transmission—By direct transfer of infective eggs by hand from anus to mouth of the same or another person, or indirectly through clothing, bedding, food, or other articles contaminated with parasite eggs. Dust-borne infection is possible in heavily contaminated households and institutions. Eggs become infective within a few hours after being deposited on perianal skin by migrating gravid females; eggs survive less than 2 weeks outside the host. Larvae from ingested eggs hatch in the small intestine; young worms mature in the cecum and upper portions of the colon. Gravid worms usually migrate actively from the rectum and may enter adjacent orifices. People who are infected with pinworm can transfer the parasite to others as long as there is a female pinworm depositing eggs on the perianal skin. A person can also self-reinfect or be reinfected by eggs from another person.

9. Treatment—

Drug	Pyrantel pamoate
Dose	11 mg/kg/day ($\leq$ 1 g)
Route	PO

(Continued)

(Continued)

Alternative drug	• Albendazole 400 mg/day PO OR • Mebendazole 100 mg/day PO
Duration	2 doses taken 2 weeks apart
Special considerations and comments	• Children < 2 years: there are limited studies of the recommended medications in children < 2 years; consideration of risks and benefits to treatment should be considered. Albendazole dose for children aged 12–23 months is 100 mg/day, repeated once 2 weeks after initial dose. • Pregnant women: the above medications are pregnancy class C. If infection is compromising the pregnancy, treatment can be considered but should be delayed until the third trimester. • Lactation: all 3 medications may be used during breastfeeding.

Note: PO = oral(ly).

10. Prevention—

1) Educate the public in personal hygiene, particularly the need to wash hands with soap and water after defecation, after changing of diapers, and before eating or preparing food. Keep nails short; discourage nail biting and scratching of the anal area.

2) Daily morning bathing with showers (or stand-up baths) is preferred to bathing in tub baths.

3) Change to clean underclothing, nightclothes, and bedsheets frequently, preferably after bathing.

4) Reduce overcrowding in living accommodations.

5) Provide adequate toilets; maintain cleanliness in these facilities.

11. Special considerations—Multiple cases in schools and institutions can best be controlled through systematic treatment of all infected individuals and household contacts.

[M. L. Donahue]

ENTEROVIRUS DISEASES

DISEASE	CAUSATIVE AGENTS	ICD-10 CODE
ENTEROVIRAL VESICULAR PHARYNGITIS	*Enterovirus A* serotypes CV-A1 to 10, 16, 22, and EV-A71	ICD-10 B08.5
ENTEROVIRAL VESICULAR STOMATITIS WITH EXANTHEM	Predominantly CV-A16 and EV-A71, but includes other *Enterovirus A* serotypes. Less frequently associated with *Enterovirus B* serotypes CV-B2 and CV-B5	ICD-10 B08.4
ENTEROVIRAL LYMPHONODULAR PHARYNGITIS	*Enterovirus A* serotype CV-A10	ICD-10 B08.8
MYALGIA, EPIDEMIC	Predominantly associated with *Enterovirus B* serotypes CV-B1 to 3, 5, 6, and E-1, 6. Sporadically associated with other *Enterovirus A* and *B* serotypes	ICD-10 B33.0
VIRAL CARDITIS	Primarily *Enterovirus B* serotypes CV-B1 to 5, CV-A9, and CV-A23, but occasionally *Enterovirus A* serotypes CV-A4 and CV-A16, *Enterovirus C* serotype CV-A1, and other enteroviruses	ICD-10 B33.2
Enteroviral hemorrhagic conjunctivitis (see "Conjunctivitis and Keratitis")		
Meningitis (see "Meningitis")		

Enteroviruses are members of the Picornaviridae family along with parechoviruses and share a genus with rhinoviruses, coxsackieviruses, and polioviruses.

I. ENTEROVIRAL VESICULAR PHARYNGITIS (herpangina), ENTEROVIRAL VESICULAR STOMATITIS WITH EXANTHEM (hand, foot, and mouth disease)

1. Clinical features—Hand, foot, and mouth disease is a brief, usually mild, febrile illness with papulovesicular rashes over the palms and soles, with or without multiple painful mouth ulcers. Sometimes, the rash may be of maculopapular type without vesicles. It may also involve the buttocks, knees, or elbows, particularly in younger children and infants. In the 2012 CV-A6 outbreaks in North America and Europe, patients most typically had perioral and perirectal papules in addition to vesicles on the dorsum of their hands. The skin lesions, which heal spontaneously without scarring, may last for 3 to 5 days after the onset of illness. Secondary bacterial skin infection is very unusual.

Herpangina is characterized by a brief, generally mild, febrile illness with multiple painful mouth ulcers that predominantly affect the posterior oral cavity, including the anterior pharyngeal folds, uvula, tonsils, and soft palate. In some children, the ulcers may affect other parts of the mouth, including the buccal mucosa and tongue. The oral lesions may persist for 3 to 5 days after the onset of illness.

The most common clinical problems associated with these 2 closely related conditions are odynophagia and dehydration. The odynophagia may be severe in young children and result in inadequate fluid intake and dehydration. Recent epidemics of hand, foot, and mouth disease in Asia have shown that infection caused by EV-A71, in contrast to that caused by other enteroviruses, may be associated with central nervous system (CNS) complications, including aseptic meningitis, encephalitis, and acute flaccid paralysis. Children, particularly those aged 5 years or younger, are at risk of acute severe pulmonary edema or hemorrhage and cardiac dysfunction, which can rapidly progress to death/coma within 3 to 5 days of symptom onset. The warning signs of CNS involvement and systemic complications include persistent fever for more than 48 hours, body temperature higher than 39°C, recurrent vomiting, unexplained irritability, lethargy, myoclonus, focal limb weakness, truncal/eye ataxia, nystagmus, signs of respiratory distress, and skin mottling.

Important differential diagnoses for hand, foot, and mouth disease and herpangina include aphthous stomatitis, herpetic gingivostomatitis, and scabies. Aphthous stomatitis is characterized by larger ulcerative lesions of the lips, tongue, and buccal mucosa that are painful but lack constitutional symptoms. It is benign and noncontagious, and commonly affects older children and adults. Recurrence is common. Patients with herpetic gingivostomatitis are usually febrile and toxic. The gingiva is typically inflamed and may be bleeding. There may be circumoral ulcers or vesicles and associated cervical lymphadenopathy without extremity involvement. Scabies infestation may sometimes be confused with hand, foot, and mouth disease because it also causes pustules, vesicles, or nodular lesions over the hands and feet. Intense itch and interdigital space involvement are useful clinical clues to the parasitic infestation.

2. Risk groups—Children younger than 10 years have the highest incidence of *Enterovirus* infections. These diseases frequently occur in outbreaks among groups of children (e.g., in nursery schools, child care centers, and large households with many young children).

3. Causative agents—See earlier table. The enteroviruses often cocirculate, usually with one predominant serotype during outbreaks of hand, foot, and mouth disease and herpangina, and result in clinically indistinguishable skin and mucosal lesions.

4. Diagnosis—To date, more than 110 different enterovirus serotypes have been described. With such a large number of serotypes and overlapping clinical syndromes, cross-reactivity will confound the interpretation of any laboratory results, limiting the usefulness of serology for confirmatory diagnosis. Current diagnostic tools for identification of enteroviruses involve detection of viral ribonucleic acid by the reverse transcription polymerase chain reaction (RT-PCR). These methods (i.e., RT-PCR, multiplex or real-time RT-PCR) typically target the 5 untranslated region of the enterovirus genome to identify the genus and one or more of the structural genes (VP1 predominantly, VP2, and VP4) for serotyping. These methods are useful as they can be performed directly on primary clinical specimens and identify the probable causative agent. Confirmatory diagnosis can be achieved by virus isolation from cell culture, followed by molecular typing, preferably from the infected site. If not feasible, virus isolation and molecular identification from secondary sites (e.g., throat swabs, feces, blood) can provide information on the likely causative agent.

5. Occurrence—Worldwide, sporadic, and epidemic occurrence. In temperate regions the peak incidence is during summer and early fall, whereas in the tropics infections occur throughout the year. Since 1997, epidemics of hand, foot, and mouth disease have been reported in many parts of Asia; the occurrence is perennial or cyclical with an interval of 2 to 3 years. A large outbreak of EV-D68 occurred in the USA from mid-August, 2014, to January 15, 2015; public health laboratories confirmed 1,395 people in 49 states and the District of Columbia with respiratory illness.

6. Reservoirs—Human.

7. Incubation period—Usually 3 to 5 days.

8. Transmission—Direct contact with nasal and oral secretions, vesicular fluid, and stools of infected individuals, as well as contaminated articles such as toys and surfaces, is the most important route of transmission. Spread through aerosol droplets may occur. Asymptomatic individuals, including adults, are an important source of infection. There is no reliable evidence of spread through insects, water, food, or sewage. The disease is most contagious during the first week of illness. Viral shedding may occur for as long as 2 and 11 weeks in throat secretions and stools, respectively.

9. Treatment—There is no specific treatment for enterovirus infections.

10. Prevention—Limit person-to-person contact, where practicable, by measures such as crowd reduction and isolating infected children. Promote handwashing with soap and water and other hygienic measures.

11. Special considerations—

1) Reporting: obligatory report of epidemics in some countries.
2) Epidemic measures: give general notice to physicians/health care providers of increased incidence of the disease, together with a description of onset, clinical characteristics, and precautions. Isolate diagnosed cases and all children with fever, pending diagnosis, with special attention to proper handling of respiratory secretions and feces.

II. MYALGIA, EPIDEMIC (epidemic pleurodynia, Bornholm disease, devil's grippe)

1. Clinical features—Pleurodynia is an uncommon complication of *Enterovirus B* infection. It is characterized by paroxysmal spasmodic pain in the chest or abdomen, which may be intensified by movement, and is usually accompanied by fever and headache. The pain tends to be more abdominal than thoracic in infants and young children, while the reverse applies to older children and adults. Most patients recover within 1 week of onset, but relapses occur; no fatalities have been reported. It is important to differentiate from more serious medical or surgical conditions. Complications occur infrequently, including orchitis, pericarditis, pneumonia, and aseptic meningitis.

Localized epidemics are characteristic. During outbreaks of epidemic myalgia, cases of *Enterovirus B* (serotypes CV-B1 to 5) myocarditis of the newborn have been reported. While myocarditis in adults is a rare complication, the possibility should always be considered.

2. Risk groups—No specific risk group.

3. Causative agents—See the earlier table.

4. Diagnosis—See Enteroviral Vesicular Stomatitis with Exanthem in this chapter.

5. Occurrence—An uncommon disease, occurring in summer and early fall; usually occurs in youths aged 5 to 15 years, but all ages may be affected. Multiple cases in a household can occur frequently. Outbreaks have been reported in Europe, Australia, New Zealand, and North America.

6. Reservoirs—Humans.

7. Incubation period—Usually 3 to 5 days.

8. Transmission—Directly by fecal-oral or respiratory droplet contact with an infected person, or indirectly by contact with articles freshly soiled with feces or throat discharges of an infected person. *Enterovirus B* (serotypes CV-B1 to 5) has been found in sewage and flies, though the relationship to transmission of human infection is not clear. Stools may contain virus for several weeks.

9. Treatment—There is no specific treatment for enterovirus infections.

10. Prevention—Avoid fecal-oral contact and/or respiratory droplet contact with infected persons and/or associated materials.

11. Special considerations—

1) Reporting: obligatory report of epidemics to the local health authority.
2) Epidemic measures: general notice to physicians and health care providers of the presence of an epidemic and the necessity for differentiation of cases from more serious medical or surgical emergencies.

III. VIRAL CARDITIS (enteroviral carditis)

1. Clinical features—An acute or subacute viral myocarditis or pericarditis, occurring as a manifestation of infection with enteroviruses, especially *Enterovirus B*. The enteroviruses are commonly identified etiologies of myocarditis. The myocardium is affected, particularly in neonates, in whom fever and lethargy may be followed rapidly by heart failure with pallor, cyanosis, dyspnea, tachycardia, and enlargement of heart and liver. Heart failure may be progressive and fatal or recovery may take place over a few weeks; some cases run a relapsing course over months and may show residual heart damage (dilated cardiomyopathy). In young adults, pericarditis is the more common manifestation, with acute chest pain, disturbance of heart rate, and often dyspnea. It may mimic myocardial infarction but is frequently associated with pulmonary or pleural manifestations (pleurodynia). The disease may be associated with aseptic meningitis; hepatitis; orchitis; pancreatitis; pneumonia; hand, foot, and mouth disease; rash; or epidemic myalgia (see Myalgia, Epidemic in this chapter).

2. Risk groups—Neonates, young infants, and young adults are susceptible to *Enterovirus B*–associated myocarditis.

3. Causative agents—See earlier table.

4. Diagnosis—See Enteroviral Vesicular Stomatitis with Exanthem in this chapter.

5. Occurrence—The enteroviruses have long been known to be important causes of acute myocarditis. The true incidence of acute myocarditis is unknown, as is the true incidence of an enterovirus etiology. The etiology of most cases of myocarditis is probably not determined. However, it is estimated that enteroviruses may cause 25% to 35% of cases of myocarditis for which a cause is found. This estimate is based on serologic study, nucleic acid hybridization, and PCR-based studies of endomyocardial biopsy and autopsy specimens.

6. Reservoirs—Not applicable.

7. Incubation period—Not applicable.

8. Transmission—See Myalgia, Epidemic in this chapter.

9. Treatment—While there were some studies on pleconaril to treat severe infections in various age groups from neonates, to adolescents, to adults, the effect was inconclusive. No specific treatment for enterovirus infections.

10. Prevention—Avoid fecal-oral and respiratory droplet contact with infected persons and associated materials.

11. Special considerations—See Myalgia, Epidemic in this chapter.

[I. Chuang]

EPSTEIN-BARR VIRUS INFECTIONS

DISEASE	ICD-10 CODE
MONONUCLEOSIS, INFECTIOUS	ICD-10 B27
BURKITT'S LYMPHOMA	ICD-10 C83.7
NASOPHARYNGEAL CARCINOMA	ICD-10 C11
OTHER MALIGNANCIES POSSIBLY RELATED TO EPSTEIN-BARR VIRUS	
HODGKIN'S DISEASE	ICD-10 C81
NON-HODGKIN'S LYMPHOMAS	ICD-10 B21.2, C83.0, C83.8, C83.9, C85

I. MONONUCLEOSIS, INFECTIOUS (gammaherpesviral mononucleosis, mononucleosis due to Epstein-Barr virus [EBV], glandular fever, monocytic angina, kissing disease)

1. Clinical features—An acute viral syndrome characterized clinically by fever, sore throat (often with exudative pharyngotonsillitis), lymphadenopathy (especially posterior cervical), and splenomegaly; characterized hematologically by mononucleosis and lymphocytosis of 50% or greater, including 10% or more atypical cells; and characterized serologically by the presence of Epstein-Barr virus (EBV) antibodies. Recovery usually occurs in a few weeks, but a very small proportion of individuals can take months to regain their former level of energy. There is no evidence that this is due to abnormal persistence of the infection in a chronic form.

In young children the disease is generally mild and more difficult to recognize. Jaundice occurs in about 4% of infected young adults, although 95% have abnormal liver function tests; splenomegaly occurs in 50%. Duration is from 1 to several weeks; the disease is rarely fatal and is more severe in older adults.

The causal agent, EBV, is also closely associated with the pathogenesis of several lymphomas and nasopharyngeal cancer (see Nasopharyngeal Carcinoma in this chapter). Fatal immunoproliferative disorders involving a polyclonal expansion of EBV-infected B lymphocytes may occur in persons with an X-linked recessive immunoproliferative disorder; they can also occur in persons with acquired immune defects, including those with human immunodeficiency virus (HIV), transplant recipients, and persons with other conditions requiring long-term immunosuppressive therapy.

A syndrome resembling infectious mononucleosis is caused by cytomegalovirus and accounts for 5% to 7% of the *mono* syndrome (see "Cytomegalovirus Disease"); other rare causes are toxoplasmosis and herpesvirus type 6 (see "Exanthema Subitum") following rubella. A mononucleosis-like illness may occur early in HIV-infected patients; differentiation depends on laboratory results that include the EBV immunoglobulin class M (IgM) test.

2. Risk groups—Reactivation of latent EBV, or seroconversion in the setting of organ transplantation when donor-recipient status is discordant, may occur in immunodeficient individuals and may result in increased viral replication (manifested by increased EBV viral load); it may also precipitate the development of lymphoproliferative disorders.

3. Causative agents—EBV, also called human (gamma) herpesvirus 4. It is closely related to other herpesviruses morphologically, yet is distinct serologically; it infects and transforms B lymphocytes.

4. Diagnosis—Laboratory diagnosis may include the finding of a lymphocytosis exceeding 50% (including 10% abnormal forms) and abnormalities in liver function tests (aspartate aminotransferase). EBV antibody tests are not usually needed to diagnose infectious mononucleosis; however, antibody tests may be beneficial in identifying the cause of illness, particularly in those individuals who do not have a typical case of infectious mononucleosis. Heterophile antibody testing remains useful in patients with typical illness, particularly in older children and young adults. Incidence of positive test results increases in the second and third week of illness. The most beneficial EBV antibody tests include measuring antibodies to the viral capsid antigen (VCA) and the EBV nuclear antigen (EBNA). A positive anti-VCA IgM response or a strong anti-VCA immunoglobulin class G response coupled with a negative anti-EBNA response is indicative of a current or recent EBV infection. The presence of both anti-VCA and anti-EBNA antibodies during a period of 4 weeks after onset of clinical symptoms suggests evidence of a past EBV infection. In rare cases, individuals with active EBV infections may not have detectable EBV-specific antibodies. Since most adults have been infected with EBV, they will have elevated anti- VCA and anti-EBNA antibody titers for years.

5. Occurrence—Worldwide. Typical infectious mononucleosis occurs primarily in industrialized countries, where age of infection is delayed until older childhood and young adulthood, so that it is most commonly recognized in high school and college students. About 50% of those infected develop clinical infectious mononucleosis; the others are mostly asymptomatic. Infection is common and widespread in early childhood in developing countries and in socioeconomically depressed population groups in some industrialized countries, where it is usually mild or asymptomatic.

6. Reservoirs—Humans.

7. Incubation period—4 to 6 weeks.

8. Transmission—Person-to-person spread by the oropharyngeal route, via saliva. Young children may be infected by saliva on the hands of nurses and other attendants and on toys, or by pre-chewing of baby food by the mother—a practice in some countries. Kissing facilitates spread among young adults. Spread may also occur via blood transfusion to susceptible recipients, but ensuing clinical disease is uncommon. Reactivated EBV may play a role in the interstitial pneumonia of HIV-infected infants and in hairy leukoplakia and B-cell tumors in HIV-infected adults.

The period of communicability is prolonged; pharyngeal excretion may persist in cell-free form for a year or more after infection; 15% to 20% or more of EBV antibody-positive healthy adults are long-term oropharyngeal carriers.

9. Treatment—The treatment of EBV-mediated mononucleosis is supportive. Steroid use should be discouraged for common symptoms such as fatigue, yet can be lifesaving in cases of impending airway obstruction, severe inflammatory complications (e.g., liver failure), and immunologic complication (e.g., aplastic anemia).

Antiviral therapies such as aciclovir do not have a positive clinical benefit in any EBV-mediated syndrome. It is essential, therefore, when managing an EBV-mediated lymphoproliferative disorder, to reduce the degree of exogenous immune suppression to allow host innate immunity to recover and suppress viral activity.

10. Prevention—Use hygienic measures, including handwashing, to avoid salivary contamination from infected individuals through intimate or other contact; avoid drinking beverages from a common container in order to minimize contact with saliva.

11. Special considerations—None.

II. BURKITT'S LYMPHOMA (BL, African Burkitt's lymphoma, endemic Burkitt's lymphoma, Burkitt's tumor)

Burkitt's lymphoma (BL) is a tumor of B-cell origin characterized by activation of the *c-MYC* oncogene. Three distinct clinical types of BL have been described by WHO: endemic (African), sporadic (nonendemic), and immunodeficiency-associated. They all have similar histopathologic features, with germinal centroblasts and similar clinical behavior, but differ in epidemiology, clinical presentation, EBV association, and genetics. The translocation of most endemic cases involves the heavy-chain joining region, while in sporadic cases the heavy-chain switch region is most often involved. Translocations in BL are likely followed by several other additional genetic abnormalities, which are commonly found in all BL cases, in order for tumorigenesis to occur.

The endemic type occurs in regions where altitudes are typically lower than 1,000 m (3,000 ft) and rainfall is higher than 1,000 mL (40 inches) a year, such as in equatorial Africa and lowland Papua New Guinea. The incidence rate in these areas is around 50 per year per million children younger than 18 years, with peak incidence occurring in children aged around 6 years. BL accounts for more than 90% of childhood lymphomas and commonly presents with jaw and facial bone involvement.

Sporadic BL is much less common and is seen mostly in North America, Europe, and East Asia. Incidence rates vary but have been reported to be around 3 per million (children and adults combined) per year in North America and Western Europe; they account for around 30% of all childhood lymphomas and fewer than 1% of adult lymphomas. Incidence rates peak for children aged around 11 years and for adults aged around 30 years. Patients commonly present with abdominal disease.

The immunodeficiency-associated type is mostly seen in patients with HIV and less commonly in patients with organ transplant and hereditary immunodeficiency, such as familial X-linked immunodeficiency. Patients usually present with nodal and central nervous system (CNS) disease. In patients with BL and HIV, cluster of differentiation 4 glycoprotein (CD4+) counts are typically high and present during the early stages of HIV infection.

EBV plays an important pathogenic role in almost all cases of endemic BL, where EBV infection occurs in infancy, and where malaria, an apparent cofactor, is holoendemic. For sporadic BL, EBV association rates vary geographically and are not well characterized; rates range from less than 25% in North America to 85% in northern Brazil, and disease is not malaria-related. In HIV-associated BL, EBV positivity has been reported to be around 30% to 40%. In general, the estimated time range of tumor development is 2 to 12 years from primary EBV infection but is much shorter in patients with HIV.

BL is a highly aggressive tumor, yet can nevertheless be cured in 90% of cases with intensive multiple-agent chemotherapy. Prevention of EBV infection early in life and control of malaria (see "Malaria") might reduce tumor incidence in Africa and Papua New Guinea. Subunit vaccines against EBV are at the trial stage. Cases should be reported to a tumor registry.

III. NASOPHARYNGEAL CARCINOMA

Nasopharyngeal carcinoma is a malignant tumor of the epithelial cells of the nasopharynx that usually occurs in adults aged 20 to 40 years. Incidence is particularly high (10-fold when compared with the general population) among groups from China (Taiwan and southern China), even in those who have moved elsewhere. This risk decreases in subsequent generations after emigration from Asia.

Immunoglobulin class A (IgA) antibody to the EBV VCA in both serum and nasopharyngeal secretions is characteristic of the disease and has been used in China as a screening test for the tumor. Its appearance may precede the clinical appearance of nasopharyngeal carcinoma by several years and its reappearance after treatment heralds recurrence.

The serologic and virologic evidence relating EBV to nasopharyngeal carcinoma is similar to that for BL (high EBV antibody titers, genome in tumor cells); this genetic relationship has been found without respect to the geographic origin of the patient. The tumor occurs worldwide but is highest in southern China, southeastern Asia, northern and eastern Africa, and the Arctic. Male cases outnumber female cases by about a 2:1 ratio. Chinese individuals with human leukocyte antigen (HLA) class II and Singapore 2 (SIN 2) antigen profiles are at particularly high risk.

EBV infection occurs early in life in settings where nasopharyngeal carcinoma is most common, yet the tumor does not appear until age 20 to 40 years, which suggests the occurrence of some secondary reactivating factor, with epithelial invasion later in life. Repeated respiratory infections or chemical irritants, such as nitrosamines in dried foods, may play a role. The higher frequency of the tumor in persons of southern Chinese origin without respect to later residence, and the association with certain HLA haplotypes, suggests a genetic susceptibility. A lower incidence among those who have migrated to the USA and elsewhere suggests that one or more environmental factor(s)—suspected are the nitrosamines present in smoked fish and other foods—may be associated cofactors. Early detection in highly endemic areas (screening for EBV IgA antibodies to VCA) permits early treatment. A subunit vaccine against EBV infection is under study. Chemotherapy after early recognition is the only specific therapy for nasopharyngeal carcinoma. Cases should be reported to a tumor registry.

IV. OTHER MALIGNANCIES POSSIBLY RELATED TO EBV

Hodgkin's disease is a tumor of the lymphatic system occurring in 4 histologic subtypes: nodular sclerosis, lymphocyte predominance, mixed cellularity, and lymphocyte depletion. The histology shows the presence of a highly specific but nonpathognomonic cell, the Reed-Sternberg cell—also seen in cases of infectious mononucleosis. The cause of Hodgkin's disease is not certain, but laboratory and epidemiologic evidence associates EBV in at least half the cases. The disease is more common in industrialized countries, but age-adjusted incidence is relatively low. It is more common in higher socioeconomic settings, in smaller families, and in Caucasians than in Americans of African origin.

Hodgkin's disease may develop after infectious mononucleosis and occur some 10 years later; Hodgkin's disease in older adults, if EBV-associated, is thought to be the result of virus reactivation in the presence of a naturally deteriorating immune system. The high frequency of EBV found in cases of Hodgkin's disease diagnosed among HIV-infected patients and the relatively short incubation period appear related to the severe immunodeficiency of HIV infection; whether the presence of EBV in the tumor cell is cause or effect is not known. Among HIV-infected patients, particularly those infected through intravenous drug use, a higher proportion of Hodgkin's disease is EBV-associated. Cases should be reported to a tumor registry.

For non-Hodgkin's lymphomas (NHLs), the incidence of lymphomas in patients with acquired immunodeficiency syndrome (AIDS) is about 50 to 100 times that in the general population. While these lymphomas may be related to EBV, HIV is the virus most associated with NHL tumors such as high-grade and CNS lymphomas. Since 1980, NHL has shown a dramatic increase among young, single white men with AIDS in the USA. About 4% of AIDS patients present with lymphoma, and perhaps 30% will eventually develop lymphoma if untreated for their HIV infection and survival is sufficiently long. Whether EBV is a causal factor in EBV-associated lymphomas in HIV-infected patients, or simply enters the tumor cell after it has been formed, is not clear, but accumulating evidence points to the former possibility. A marked increase in NHL not explained by the increase in the number of patients with AIDS has been noted in recent years. The disease commonly occurs in the presence of other forms of immunodeficiency, such as in posttransplant patients, people given immunosuppressive drugs, and people with inherited forms of immuno-deficiency. There are few epidemiologic indications as to the risk factors responsible. Altered antibody patterns to EBV, characteristic of those seen in immunodeficiency states, occur in many cases of NHL; these changes have been shown to precede the development of NHL. Molecular techniques have demonstrated the EBV genome in 10% to 15% of tumor cells of the spontaneous form of NHL. Cases should be reported to a tumor registry.

[D. Cohen]

ERYTHEMA INFECTIOSUM
(fifth disease)

DISEASE	ICD-10 CODE
ERYTHEMA INFECTIOSUM	ICD-10 B08.3

1. Clinical features—A usually mild childhood viral exanthematous disease, with low-grade or no fever, occurring sporadically or in epidemics. Characteristic is a striking erythema of the cheeks (slapped cheek appearance), frequently associated with a lace-like rash on the trunk and extremities, which fades but may recur for 1 to 3 weeks or longer on exposure to sunlight or heat (e.g., when bathing). Itch may occur on the rash-affected skin and on the palm/sole. Mild constitutional symptoms may precede onset of rash. Immunocompetent children and young adults may have an atypical rash that can be rubelliform or petechial—papular-purpuric gloves-and-socks syndrome with painful and pruritic papules, petechiae, and purpura of the hands and feet. In adults, the rash is often atypical or absent, but polyarthropathy (arthralgia or arthritis) may occur. Arthropathy is uncommon in children but occurs in 50% of adults, more commonly in women; distribution is symmetric with involvement of small joints of hands and occasionally ankles, knees, and wrists. Arthropathy may last for days to months but then resolves. Twenty-five percent or more of infections may be asymptomatic.

Differentiation from rubella, scarlet fever, dengue fever, and chikungunya fever is necessary. Usually the rash of erythema infectiosum (commonly called fifth disease) does not have a raised maculopapular appearance, unlike in the aforementioned diseases. On dark skin, the rash is very often missed on examination.

Complications are unusual, but persons with hemolytic anemias (e.g., sickle cell disease) may develop transient aplastic crisis, often even in the absence of a preceding rash. Intrauterine infection in the first half of pregnancy results in hydrops fetalis and fetal death in fewer than 10% of infections; intrauterine infection also infrequently results in fetal anemia that persists in the infant after birth. Immunosuppressed people may develop severe, chronic anemia. Red cell aplasia has been reported. Several diseases (e.g., rheumatoid arthritis, systemic vasculitis, fulminant hepatitis, and myocarditis) have been reported in association with erythema infectiosum, but no causal link has been established.

2. Risk groups—Universal susceptibility in persons with blood group P antigen, the receptor for human parvovirus B19 (B19) in erythroid cells. Attack rates among susceptible individuals can be high: 50% in household contacts and 10% to 60% in the day care or school setting during a 2- to 6-month outbreak period. Those with hemolytic anemia or immunodeficiency and pregnant women not immune to B19 are most at risk of serious complications.

3. Causative agents—B19, a 20- to 25-nm deoxyribonucleic acid (DNA) virus belonging to the family Parvoviridae, genus *Erythroparvovirus*. The virus replicates primarily in erythroid precursor cells. B19 is resistant to inactivation by various methods, including heating to 80°C (176°F) for 72 hours.

4. Diagnosis—Usually on clinical and epidemiologic grounds. Can be confirmed by detection of B19-specific immunoglobulin class M (IgM) antibodies or by a rise in immunoglobulin class G antibody titers. IgM titers begin to decline 1 to 2 months after the onset of symptoms. Diagnosis of B19 infection is ideally made by detecting viral DNA by nucleic acid amplification by polymerase chain reaction (PCR), which is highly sensitive and specific and will often remain positive during the first month of acute infection and for prolonged periods in some people, showing that the infection is chronic in some.

5. Occurrence—Worldwide, common in children; both sporadic and epidemic. In temperate zones, epidemics tend to occur in winter and spring, with a periodicity of 3 to 7 years in a given community.

6. Reservoirs—Humans.

7. Incubation period—Variable; 4 to 20 days to development of rash or symptoms of aplastic crisis.

8. Transmission—Primarily through contact with respiratory secretions; also from mother to fetus and through transfusion of blood and blood products. The child with disease is infectious starting from a few days before onset of rash until the rash has faded—usually a span of 1 week to 10 days. Those who have an aplastic crisis may be infectious longer. Those with chronic infection may remain infectious for longer periods of time; immunosuppressed persons with chronic infection and severe anemia are infectious for months to years. Transmission as a result of transfusion is mostly from pooled blood components.

9. Treatment—There is no targeted antiviral therapy available. Supportive care is recommended. Intravenous immunoglobulin may be used for chronic infection in immunodeficient hosts.

Blood transfusion for aplastic crisis or hydrops fetalis may be considered.

10. Prevention—

1) As the disease is generally benign, prevention efforts should focus on preventing complications in those most likely to develop them, who should avoid exposure to potentially infectious people in hospital or outbreak settings.

2) Susceptible women who are pregnant or who might become pregnant, and have continued close contact with people with B19 infection (e.g., at school, home, or in health care facilities), should be advised of the potential for acquiring infection and of the potential risk of complications to the fetus. Pregnant women with sick children at home are advised to keep a reasonable physical distance, wash hands frequently, and avoid sharing eating utensils.

3) Health care workers should be advised of the importance of following good infection control measures. Rare nosocomial outbreaks have been reported. Strict handwashing is required after patient contact.

4) Plasma pools should be screened by PCR (nucleic acid amplification) and positive pools should be discarded.

11. Special considerations—

1) Reporting: any detected outbreak should be reported to the local health authority.

2) During outbreaks in school or day care settings, those with hemolytic anemia or immunodeficiency and pregnant women should be informed of the possible risk of acquiring and transmitting infection.

[M. L. Donahue]

❖

EXANTHEMA SUBITUM

DISEASE	ICD-10 CODE
EXANTHEMA SUBITUM	ICD-10 B08.2

1. Clinical features—Exanthema subitum results from primary infection with a human herpesvirus (HHV) type 6, particularly the 6B species (HHV-6B), in children younger than 2 years. It is unusual in children older than this and in adults, where primary infection causes a mild glandular fever-like illness in some individuals. Most infections with HHV are asymptomatic or cause a nonspecific fever. About 20% of HHV-6B infections result in exanthema subitum presenting as an acute febrile illness, up to 41°C (106°F), which subsides in 3 to 5 days, followed a few days later by a maculopapular rash on the trunk and later on the remainder of the body, which then fades rapidly. Symptoms are generally mild, but febrile seizures and more severe illness, such as meningoencephalitis or hepatitis, occur in a small proportion.

Occasionally, exanthema subitum is caused by other viruses, such as enteroviruses and adenoviruses. Also, it may clinically resemble other viral exanthems such as measles, rubella, and parvovirus B19 (erythema infectiosum) infection. However, the mild nature of the illness and the gap between resolution of the fever and onset of the rash are important diagnostic clues.

2. Risk groups—Infection rates in infants younger than 6 months are low, possibly owing to temporary protection from transplacentally acquired maternal antibodies, but increase rapidly thereafter. Most children are infected within the first 2 years of life so that disease is uncommon after that age. Immunosuppressed individuals, including those with organ transplants, are at increased risk of severe disease owing to both primary infection and reactivation.

3. Causative agents—HHV-6B (family Herpesviridae, subfamily Betaherpesvirinae, genus *Roseolovirus*) is the most common cause of exanthema subitum, with occasional cases due to HHV-7 and possibly HHV-6A. As with the other herpesviruses, primary infection is followed by lifelong latent infection, mainly in the salivary glands and monocytes/macrophages. Reactivations occur regularly and are usually asymptomatic. Immunosuppressed individuals may develop severe disease owing to both primary infection and reactivation, including fever, encephalitis, pneumonitis, hepatitis, and bone marrow suppression.

4. Diagnosis—Virus can be detected by polymerase chain reaction (PCR) in saliva, peripheral blood, urine, cervical secretions, and other sites during primary infection and reactivation, though titers are higher in primary infection. Peripheral blood PCR assays are usually reserved for immuno-suppressed patients. Serologically, primary infection is indicated by immunoglobulin class G (IgG) seroconversion or a rise in IgG over the course of 7 to 14 days, with detectable immunoglobulin class M (IgM) appearing 1 week after onset and disappearing after 3 to 4 weeks. Reactivations are usually marked by a rapid rise in IgG with or without the detection of IgM.

5. Occurrence—Worldwide, the incidence peaks at age 6 to 13 months, with 65% to 100% seroprevalence by age 2 years. Seroprevalence in women of childbearing age ranges from 80% to 100% in most parts of the world, although rates as low as 20% have been observed in Morocco and 49% in Malaysia. HHV-6 infections and exanthema subitum occur year-round, though a seasonal predilection (late winter, early spring) has been described in Japan.

6. Reservoirs—Latently infected humans are the only known reservoir of infection.

7. Incubation period—10 days, with a usual range of 5 to 15 days. For susceptible organ transplant recipients, onset of illness after primary infection is usually 2 to 4 weeks after transplantation.

8. Transmission—Infection is most likely acquired by direct or indirect contact with saliva from individuals with primary infection or reactivation, especially within household or day care settings. Transplacental transmission occurs but is uncommon and rarely causes adverse fetal outcomes, while the virus can also be transmitted by transfusion of blood or blood products. Organ transplant recipients may acquire infection from the transplant, though currently there is no standard recommendation for HHV-6 testing or matching of infected donors and recipients. Other potential modes of transmission, including breastfeeding and sexual contact, do not appear to be important.

9. Treatment—No specific therapy is currently recommended for exanthema subitum.

10. Prevention—No specific preventive measures are recommended. Screening of donors and recipients before organ transplants is not routinely performed.

11. Special considerations—None.

[D. Smith]

FASCIOLIASIS

DISEASE	ICD-10 CODE
FASCIOLIASIS	ICD-10 B66.3

Fasciola hepatica and *Fasciola gigantica* are the zoonotic foodborne trematodes that cause fascioliasis. *F. hepatica* is the only trematode with a worldwide distribution and adapted to very high altitudes. An estimated 2.4 to 17 million people worldwide are infected with *Fasciola*. In addition, *Fasciola* represents a significant burden to the global livestock industry.

1. Clinical features—Most persons infected with *Fasciola* in the community are asymptomatic. Patients seeking medical care can present with acute or chronic symptoms, reflecting the complex life cycle of the parasite. Shortly after ingesting metacercariae in aquatic plants or water, the juvenile parasites start their migration through the liver parenchyma, causing fever, right upper quadrant pain, and hypereosinophilia that can last 3 to 4 months (see Figure 1 in this chapter). Later, when the parasites have reached the biliary tree, patients present with chronic obstructive biliary symptoms that include intermittent right upper quadrant pain, jaundice, and dyspepsia. Mature parasites produce eggs that are passed in the stools. Untreated, chronic infection may last more than 10 years. Ectopic infection most often affects the subcutaneous tissues, causing migrating nodules associated with hypereosinophilia.

2. Risk groups—In endemic areas, persons ingesting aquatic plants or water contaminated with metacercariae are at risk of infection. Certain local beverages prepared with herbs (*emoliente*) have been associated with transmission. In developed countries (i.e., USA, France, Portugal) transmission has been associated with ingestion of wild watercress.

3. Causative agents—The trematodes *F. hepatica* and *F. gigantica*.

4. Diagnosis—During the acute infection, while juveniles migrate through the liver, the diagnosis relies on clinical findings and serology, which turns positive as early as 2 to 3 weeks after infection. Enzyme-linked immunosorbent assay tests using different *F. hepatica* antigens (i.e., crude excretory/secretory product, Fas2) are available and vary in sensitivity and specificity. An immunoblot assay using recombinant *Fasciola* antigens with over 90% sensitivity and specificity is available through CDC.

During chronic infection, *Fasciola* eggs can be detected by microscopy. The Kato-Katz test and flotation and sedimentation methods are used to detect the large parasite eggs in the stools. However, microscopy has low sensitivity and therefore it is necessary to use multiple tests and stool samples to make the diagnosis. Eggs may not be detected by routine ova and parasite testing.

5. Occurence—Human infection has been reported from 81 countries, on all continents except Antarctica. The highest prevalence occurs in sheep- and cattle-raising areas. *F. hepatica* is more widespread than *F. gigantica*, which is only found in Africa and some Asian countries. In endemic countries of South America, more than half the children may be infected in some communities. It has been estimated that half of the global burden relating to *Fasciola* affects poor persons in Bolivia, Ecuador, and Peru. In the USA and other developed countries, most cases of fascioliasis occur in travelers and migrants. However, sporadic autochthonous human transmission has been reported in the USA, Spain, Portugal, and France, among other countries.

6,7. Reservoirs and incubation period—Cattle, sheep, and other livestock are the most common definitive hosts for *Fasciola*. However, a wide variety of animals, including ungulates and rodents, can harbor the parasite in nature. Humans can be sporadic hosts or, in highly endemic areas, an important part of the transmission cycle. Eggs passed in stools of definitive hosts generate miracidia in fresh water. This free-swimming form infects lymnaeid snails (i.e., *Galba truncatula*), going through cycles of asexual division to generate hundreds of cercariae. Cercariae leave the snails and encyst, forming metacercariae in water or on the surface of leafy plants such as watercress. Upon ingestion by a suitable host, metacercariae excyst, releasing juvenile *Fasciola* in the small intestine, which then pass through the intestinal wall and migrate through the peritoneum and liver parenchyma until reaching the biliary tree. Once in the biliary tree, juveniles attach to the epithelium and mature to adult parasites that produce eggs that will be passed in the stools to complete the cycle.

8. Transmission—Metacercariae constitute the infecting stage. The infection is transmitted through ingestion of water or vegetables containing metacercariae. Infection is not transmitted from person to person or through ingestion of raw liver infected with *Fasciola*.

9. Treatment—

Drug	Triclabendazole
Dose	10 mg/kg every 12–24 hours for 2 doses
Route	PO
Alternative drug	Nitazoxanide 500 mg PO every 12 hours
Duration	7 days
Special considerations and comments	• Triclabendazole has not been studied in children younger than 6 years or pregnant women. Nonrandomized trials suggest that triclabendazole can safely be used in children aged ≥ 3 years. • Individuals with heavy infections (> 300 eggs/g of stool) should receive treatment under observation. • Right upper abdominal pain is not uncommon after treatment and responds well to antispasmodic medications.

Note: PO = oral(ly).

10. Prevention—

1) Educate the public in endemic areas with reference to avoiding eating uncooked watercress and other aquatic plants. In highly endemic areas, water should be boiled or filtered to eliminate metacercariae. Vegetables grown in fields that might have been irrigated with contaminated water should be thoroughly cooked.

2) Control the growth and sale of watercress and other edible water plants.

3) Mass treatment in communities with high prevalence has proven to be effective in reducing the prevalence and burden of infection. However, the emergence of resistance in livestock and humans in some areas may preclude the use of this approach in certain endemic areas. Given the zoonotic nature of the infection and wide range of possible domestic and sylvatic hosts, elimination of the infection is unlikely.

4) The use of chemical molluscicides to eliminate snails in endemic areas may be a temporary measure. This approach as a sole measure is likely to be ineffective, as the reintroduction of snails may occur rapidly.

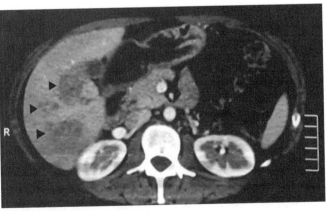

Photo Credit: Courtesy of M. M. Cabada.
Note: Arrowheads indicate hypodense lesions in the liver parenchyma caused by the parasite migration.

Figure 1. Abdominal Computed Tomography Scan With Contrast of a Patient With Acute *Fasciola* Infection.

11. Special considerations—None

Bibliography

Fürst T, Keiser J, Utzinger J. Global burden of human food-borne trematodiasis: a systematic review and meta-analysis. *Lancet Infect Dis.* 2012;12(3):210–221.

Mas-Coma MS, Esteban JG, Bargues MD. Epidemiology of human fascioliasis: a review and proposed new classification. *Bull World Health Organ.* 1999;77(4):340–346.

Torgerson PR, Devleesschauwer B, Praet N, et al. World Health Organization estimates of the global and regional disease burden of 11 foodborne parasitic diseases, 2010: a data synthesis. *PLoS Med.* 2015;12:e1001920.

Webb CM, Cabada MM. Recent developments in the epidemiology, diagnosis, and treatment of Fasciola infection. *Curr Opin Infect Dis.* 2018;31:409–414.

[M. M. Cabada, C. M. Webb, M. Tanabe]

FASCIOLOPSIASIS

DISEASE	ICD-10 CODE
FASCIOLOPSIASIS	ICD-10 B66.5

1. Clinical features—Caused by the intestinal fluke *Fasciolpsis buski.* It is a zoonotic trematode infection of the small intestine, particularly the duodenum. Many infections are probably asymptomatic. When they do occur, symptoms are nausea, vomiting, diarrhea, fever resulting from local inflammation, ulceration of the intestinal wall, and systemic toxic effects. Diarrhea usually alternates with constipation; vomiting and anorexia occur commonly. Large numbers of flukes may produce acute intestinal obstruction. Patients may show edema of the face, abdominal wall, and legs within 20 days after massive infection, and ascites is common. Eosinophilia is usual; secondary anemia may occur. Death is rare. As noted, some infections are asymptomatic.

2. Risk groups—Risk for infection occurs in those who eat uncooked aquatic plants (owing to the parasite encysting on these plants). In malnourished individuals, ill effects are pronounced; the number of worms influences the severity of the disease.

3. Causative agents—*F. buski*, a large trematode, 2 to 4 cm long, but reaching lengths up to 7 cm.

4. Diagnosis—Through detection of the large flukes or characteristic eggs in stools or vomitus.

5. Occurrence—Widely distributed in rural southeastern Asia, especially central and south China, parts of India, and Thailand. Prevalence is often high in pig-rearing areas.

6. Reservoirs—Swine and humans are definitive hosts and reservoirs of adult flukes; dogs less commonly.

7. Incubation period—Eggs appear in feces about 3 months after infection.

8. Transmission—Acquired by eating uncooked aquatic plants. Eggs passed in human and swine feces develop in water within 3 to 7 weeks under favorable conditions; miracidia hatch and penetrate planorbid snails as intermediate hosts; cercariae develop, are liberated, and encyst on aquatic plants to become infective metacercariae.

In China, chief sources of infection are the nuts of the red water caltrop (*Trapa bicornis, Trapa natans*), grown in enclosed ponds, and tubers of the so-called water chestnut (*Eleocharis tuberosa*) and water bamboo (*Zizania aquatica*). Infection can result when the hull or skin is peeled off with the teeth and lips; less often from metacercariae in pond water. The period of communicability lasts as long as viable eggs are discharged in feces—without treatment, probably for 1 year. No direct person-to-person transmission.

9. Treatment—Praziquantel is recommended for treatment of fasciolopsiasis. One-day dosing is adequate, 25 mg/kg 3 times over 1 day, or 15 mg/kg in a single dose (based on 1 clinical trial in schoolchildren). Caution is advised in pregnancy and breastfeeding and in children younger than 1 year.

10. Prevention—

1) Educate the population at risk in endemic areas on the mode of transmission and life cycle of the parasite.
2) Sanitary disposal of human waste. Prevent human and pig fecal contamination of water where aquatic plants are grown.
3) Prohibit swine from entering contaminating areas where water plants are growing; do not feed water plants to pigs.
4) Dry suspected plants, or if plants are to be eaten fresh dip them in boiling water for a few seconds; both methods kill metacercariae.

11. Special considerations—Reporting: some endemic areas may require a case report to be submitted to the local health authority.

Bibliography

Bunnag D, Radomyos P, Harinasuta T. Field trial on the treatment of fasciolopsiasis with praziquantel. *Southeast Asian J Trop Med Public Health*. 1983;14(2):216–219.

CDC. Fasciolopsiasis FAQs. 2014. Available at: https://www.cdc.gov/parasites/fasciolopsis/faqs.html. Accessed October 28, 2019.

Chai J-Y. Praziquantel treatment in trematode and cestode infections: an update. *Infect Chemother.* 2013;45(1):32–43.

[O. A. Khan]

FILARIASIS

DISEASE	ICD-10 CODE
BANCROFTIAN FILARIASIS	ICD-10 B74.0
MALAYAN FILARIASIS	ICD-10 B74.1
TIMOREAN FILARIASIS	ICD-10 B74.2
DIROFILARIASIS	ICD-10 B74.8
OTHER NEMATODES PRODUCING MICROFILARIAE IN HUMANS: MANSONELLOSIS	ICD-10 B74.4
Loiasis (see "Loiasis")	
Onchocerciasis (see "Onchocerciasis")	

The term "filariasis" denotes infection with any of several nematodes (roundworms) belonging to the superfamily Filarioidea. Eight filarial species are known to use humans as their definitive hosts: 3 closely related species causing lymphatic filariasis, 3 causing various subcutaneous infections (onchocerciasis, loiasis, and mansonellosis), and 2 causing serous cavity diseases.

I. BANCROFTIAN FILARIASIS, MALAYAN FILARIASIS (Brugian filariasis), TIMOREAN FILARIASIS

1. Clinical features—Chronic parasitic infection with any of the 3 filarial species (*Wuchereria bancrofti, Brugia malayi, Brugia timori*) that inhabit human lymphatic vessels and subcutaneous tissues. Depending upon species, chronicity, and intensity of exposure to infective insect bites, various clinical presentations may include a symptomatic, parasitologically negative form; asymptomatic microfilaremia; recurrent filarial fevers accompanied by lymphadenitis and retrograde lymphangitis and usually without microfilaremia; the chronic lymphedema that is pathognomonic; and a tropical pulmonary eosinophilic syndrome. In endemic areas, about two-thirds of filarial cases are clinically asymptomatic, and symptomatic cases can show considerable overlap in clinical complexes.

Earlier manifestations include filarial fever (self-limited episodes of high fever), acute adenolymphangitis (ADL), and acute dermatolymphangioadenitis (DLA). ADL is often the first manifestation of infection, believed to be due to the host immune response to dying adult worms. Characterized by sudden onset of high fever and painful lymphadenopathy, ADL often involves an unusual retrograde spread of inflammation extending distally from inflamed lymph nodes. DLA is manifested by systemic symptoms including high fever, myalgia, and headache along with edematous, clearly demarcated inflammatory plaques. Believed to be due to superficial bacterial infection, DLA often occurs on areas of the skin that have been previously traumatized (e.g., burn, insect bites, radiation). Chronic manifestations of filariasis typically occur after many years of lymphostasis and thus are rare in children; symptoms are often painful and profoundly disfiguring and debilitating. Lymphatic damage caused by adult parasites progresses to lymphedema (limb swelling due to chronic inflammation of the lymphatic vessels), often associated with secondary bacterial infections. Manifestations include hydrocele; lymphedema and elephantiasis of the limbs, breasts, and genitalia; and chyluria (milky urine due to impairment of the renal lymphatics). Bancroftian, Malayan, and Timorean filariasis have similar clinical findings, with some exceptions: the acute, recurrent attacks of adenitis and retrograde lymphangitis associated with fever are more severe in Brugian filariasis. Chyluria, elephantiasis, hydrocele, and breast lymphedema are much more common in Bancroftian filariasis. In Brugian filariasis, elephantiasis is usually confined to the distal extremities (frequently the legs below the knees) and hydrocele and breast lymphedema are rarely, if ever, seen.

Tropical pulmonary eosinophilia (TPE) is a distinct syndrome of Bancroftian or Malayan filariasis characterized by gradual onset of paroxysmal, nocturnal asthma and dry, hacking, nonproductive cough; recurrent low-grade fever; weight loss; and pronounced eosinophilia. Usually occurring in young adults, especially males, TPE is believed to be due to an immune hyperresponse to microfilariae trapped within the lung and reticuloendothelial organs. Left untreated, it may progress to chronic restrictive lung disease and interstitial fibrosis.

2. Risk groups—Adult worms do not replicate within the human host; thus, repeated exposure to infected mosquitoes over a prolonged stay in an endemic area is usually required for infection. In endemic areas, universal susceptibility to infection is probable, with infection typically acquired in childhood and prevalence increasing with advancing age, with most residents exposed by their third or fourth decade. Considerable geographic difference occurs in type and severity of disease related to filarial species, extent and duration of exposure (insect bites), individual host immune response, and fungal and/or bacterial coinfections.

3. Causative agents—*W. bancrofti*, *B. malayi*, and *B. timori*—microscopic, threadlike worms.

4. Diagnosis—Usually based on a combination of epidemiologic history, physical findings, and laboratory tests. In endemic areas, physical findings of lymphedema in the extremities or male genitalia without other obvious causes are likely due to filarial infection. Definitive diagnosis can be made microscopically or with antigen or deoxyribonucleic acid (DNA) testing, but diagnosis cannot be excluded in the absence of parasites or circulating filarial antigens because disease persists with low-level microfilaremia or amicrofilaremia.

Microscopic diagnosis is through detection of microfilariae in peripheral blood smears, best achieved on smears collected during hours of maximal microfilaremia (i.e., nocturnally for Brugian filariasis and some Bancroftian filariasis, with the greatest microfilariae concentrations found in blood smears collected between 10 PM and 2 AM; Bancroftian filariasis also has a form showing diurnal subperiodicity, in which microfilariae circulate continuously in the peripheral blood but occur in greater concentration in the daytime). Live microfilariae can be detected under low power in a drop of peripheral blood (finger prick) on a slide or in hemolyzed blood in a counting chamber. Giemsa or hematoxylin-and-eosin–stained blood smears (thick or thin) permit species identification and differentiation based on morphology. For increased sensitivity, concentration techniques may be used, including filtration of anticoagulated blood through a Nucleopore filter (2–5 μm pore size), in a Swinnex adapter, or by the Knott technique (centrifugal sedimentation of the blood sample lysed in 2% formalin). Circulating filarial antigen assays permit diagnosis of *W. bancrofti* infections with or without microfilaremia and can be collected regardless of time of day. Two highly specific (100%) and sensitive (96%-100%) tests for *W. bancrofti* are available—an Og4C3 monoclonal antibody–based enzyme-linked immunosorbent assay (ELISA) and a rapid immunochromatic test permitting point-of-care diagnosis; neither are as yet FDA approved. There are currently no similar tests for *Brugia* infections. Polymerase chain reaction assays for DNA of *W. bancrofti* and *B. malayi* are available; however, performance is not good compared with the ELISA. Antibody tests detecting elevated immunoglobulin class G (IgG) and IgG4 antibodies are available but many commercial assays lack specificity (cannot distinguish between various filarial infections and may cross-react with antigens from other helminths). A sensitive, rapid immunochromatographic test using Wb123monoplex-IgG4 antibodies for the detection of *W. bancrofti* is available internationally but is not licensed for use in the USA. For diagnosis of *Brugia* in international settings, the Brugia Rapid Test (Reszon Diagnostics, Malaysia) can be used (not FDA approved).

Lymphoscintigraphic imaging and ultrasonography can be used to detect lymphatic abnormalities and living adult worms in damaged lymphatic vessels (especially the scrotum) can demonstrate a distinctive pattern of movement (filarial dance sign). Dead, calcified worms can sometimes be detected on X-ray or in biopsy specimens of lymphatic tissue. Peripheral blood eosinophilia is common in lymphatic filariasis and may be profound (e.g., in TPE). In TPE, microfilariae typically are not detectable in peripheral blood—nor, often, is circulating filarial antigen detectable; however, marked elevations in filarial antibody titers support the diagnosis.

5. Occurrence—In tropical and subtropical climates, where conditions favor breeding of vector mosquitoes (see Transmission in this chapter), including rural, peri-urban, and (increasingly) urban areas. *W. bancrofti*— estimated to account for 90% of lymphatic filariasis globally—is the most widespread of the 3 parasites and occurs predominantly in sub-Saharan Africa and Southeast Asia. Scattered foci exist in Egypt, Sudan, Yemen, India, several western Pacific Islands, and parts of Latin America including Hispaniola (the Dominican Republic and Haiti) and coastal areas of South America (Guyana and a few areas of Brazil). In general, nocturnal subperiodicity in *Wuchereria*-infected areas of the Pacific is found west of 140°E longitude and diurnal subperiodicity east of 180°E longitude. *B. malayi* occurs in China, rural southwestern India, southeastern Asia, the Philippines, and several Pacific island groups (e.g., Indonesia and the Philippines). *B. timori* occurs in Timor-Leste and on the rural islands of Flores, Alor, and Roti in southeastern Indonesia.

6. Reservoirs—Humans with microfilariae in the blood are the only hosts for *W. bancrofti*, periodic *B. malayi*, and *B. timori*. In Malaysia, southern Thailand, the Philippines, Timor-Leste, and Indonesia, cats, civets (*Viverra tangalunga*), and nonhuman primates are reservoirs for subperiodic *B. malayi*, but zoonotic transmission is thought to be of limited significance.

7. Incubation period—Microfilariae may not appear in the blood until after 3 to 6 months in *B. malayi* and 6 to 12 months in *W. bancrofti* infections.

8. Transmission—Person-to-person through the bite of a mosquito harboring infective larvae. The mosquito vectors vary geographically: *W. bancrofti* is transmitted by several mosquito species, most commonly *Culex, Anopheles,* and *Aedes* spp. *B. malayi* is transmitted by various species of *Mansonia, Anopheles,* and *Aedes. B. timori* is transmitted by *Anopheles barbirostris*. The mosquito becomes infective 12 to 14 days after an infected blood meal. In the female mosquito, ingested microfilariae penetrate the stomach wall and develop in the thoracic muscles into elongated, infective filariform larvae that migrate to the proboscis. When the mosquito feeds, the larvae emerge and are deposited near the punctured skin; within a few minutes, they make their way through the skin to enter the local lymphatic vessels. A large number of infected mosquito bites are typically required to initiate infection in the human host. In the host, larval worms travel via the lymphatics, where they molt twice before becoming adults over approximately 6 to 9 months. Adult worms mate and release millions of microfilariae (microscopic worms) that circulate in the blood. Humans can infect mosquitoes when microfilariae are present in the peripheral blood; microfilaremia may persist for 5 to 10 years or longer after initial infection.

9. Treatment—Infection with all 3 species can be treated effectively with single-dose antibiotic therapy. The drug of choice is dependent upon age, pregnancy status, and whether onchocerciasis or loiasis are coendemic.

Drug	DEC
Dose	6 mg/kg
Route	PO
Alternative drug	Ivermectin 150 µg/kg
Duration	Single dose
Special considerations and comments	• DEC is not commercially available in the USA but can be obtained from CDC under an Investigational New Drug protocol. • DEC should be avoided in children < 18 months and during pregnancy. It is considered safe during lactation. • DEC is contraindicated in patients who may also have onchocerciasis owing to the possibility of severe exacerbations of skin and eye involvement (Mazzotti reaction). It should be used cautiously in patients with *Loa loa*, particularly infection with high circulating levels, owing to the possibility of serious side effects (e.g., encephalopathy, renal failure). • Doxycycline (200 mg/day for 4–6 weeks) has demonstrated efficacy against *W. bancrofti* and *B. malayi* infections, likely acting by treating *Wolbachia*, a symbiotic bacterial infection present in microfilariae. Doxycycline is contraindicated in pregnant women and young children.

Note: DEC = diethylcarbamazine; PO = oral(ly).

10. Prevention—In endemic areas:

1) Educate inhabitants on the mode of transmission and methods of preventing mosquito bites (e.g., long sleeves and trousers, using mosquito repellant on exposed skin, sleeping under nets or in an air-conditioned room).

2) Promote vector control: identify the vectors by detecting infective larvae in mosquitoes caught; identify times and places of mosquito biting; and locate breeding places. If indoor night-biters are

responsible, screen houses or use bed nets (preferably impregnated with synthetic pyrethroid) and insect repellents. Eliminate mosquito breeding places (e.g., standing water in open latrines, tires, coconut husks) and treat with polystyrene beads or larvicides. Where *Mansonia* spp. are vectors, clear ponds of vegetation (*Pistia*), which serves as a source of oxygen for the larvae. Long-term vector control may involve changes in housing construction to include screening and environmental control in order to eliminate mosquito breeding sites.

3) People with lymphedema and hydrocele can benefit from careful hygiene and management to prevent bacterial infections.

4) Where onchocerciasis is not endemic, WHO recommends mass treatment with single-dose diethylcarbamazine (DEC) and albendazole, annually for at least 5 years; addition of a single dose of ivermectin (i.e., triple drug therapy) may be beneficial in certain settings with high filariasis prevalence. In areas where onchocerciasis is coendemic, WHO recommends mass drug administration using single-dose ivermectin and albendazole, annually. In areas with concurrent loiasis, mass drug administration with either DEC or ivermectin is contraindicated at present owing to the risk of severe adverse reactions in patients with high-density *Loa loa* infections; WHO recommends use of albendazole during mass drug administration, twice annually, in these areas. DEC salt is no longer recommended by WHO as a primary strategy.

11. Special considerations—

1) Reporting: may be required in some endemic regions; reporting of cases with demonstrated microfilariae or circulating filarial antigen provides information on areas of transmission.

2) In 2000, WHO launched its Global Program to Eliminate Lymphatic Filariasis through an alliance of 72 endemic countries and partners from the public and private sectors. The strategy, promoting mass drug administration campaigns to stop the spread of infection and access to a basic package of care to manage chronic disease, has been adopted in 70 countries as of 2018, and 14 countries have already been validated by WHO as having met elimination goals. Cases of lymphatic filariasis are estimated to have declined from about 53 million in 2000 to 29 million in 2016. More information can be found at:

- http://www.filariasis.org
- http://www.cdc.gov/parasites/lymphaticfilariasis
- https://www.who.int/lymphatic_filariasis/en

II. DIROFILARIASIS (zoonotic filariasis)

Certain species of filariae commonly seen in wild or domestic animals occasionally infect humans, but microfilaremia occurs rarely. The genus *Dirofilaria* causes pulmonary and cutaneous disease in humans. Human infection with *Dirofilaria immitis*, the dog heartworm, has been reported from most parts of the world, including Australia, Europe, Canada, the USA, Japan, and other parts of Asia. Transmission to humans is by mosquito bite. The worm lodges in a pulmonary artery, where it may form the nidus of a thrombus; this can then lead to vascular occlusion, coagulation, necrosis, and fibrosis. Symptoms are chest pain, cough, and hemoptysis. Eosinophilia is infrequent. A fibrotic nodule, 1 to 3 cm in diameter, which is most commonly asymptomatic, is recognizable by X-ray as a coin lesion.

Various species cause subcutaneous lesions, including *Dirofilaria tenuis*, a parasite of the raccoon in the USA; *Dirofilaria ursi*, a parasite of bears in Canada; and *Dirofilaria repens*, a parasite of dogs and cats in Europe, Africa, and Asia. The worms develop in, or migrate to, the conjunctivae and the subcutaneous tissues of the scrotum, breasts, arms, and legs, but microfilaremia is rare. Animal species of *Brugia* cause zoonotic infections and localize in lymph nodes; they have been reported from North and South America and Africa. Similarly, animal species of *Onchocerca* have increasingly been reported to cause zoonotic infections, typically localized in demarcated nodules, and have been reported from North America, Europe, Eurasia, North Africa, Japan, and the Arabian Peninsula. Diagnosis is usually made by the finding of worms in tissue sections of surgically excised lesions.

III. OTHER NEMATODES PRODUCING MICROFILARIAE IN HUMANS

Several other nematodes may infect humans and produce microfilariae. These include *Onchocerca volvulus* and *Loa loa*, which cause onchocerciasis and loiasis, respectively (see "Onchocerciasis" and "Loiasis"). Other infections are forms of mansonellosis: *Mansonella perstans* is widely distributed in western Africa and northeastern South America; the adult is found in the body cavities and the unsheathed microfilariae circulate with no regular periodicity. Infection is usually asymptomatic, but eye infection from immature stages has been reported. In some countries of western and central Africa, infection with *Mansonella* is common and is suspected of causing cutaneous edema and thickening of the skin, hypopigmented macules, pruritus, and papules. Adult worms and unsheathed microfilariae occur in the skin as in onchocerciasis. *Mansonella ozzardi* occurs from the Yucatan Peninsula in Mexico to northern Argentina and in the West Indies; diagnosis is based on demonstration of the circulating unsheathed nonperiodic microfilariae. Infection is generally asymptomatic but may be associated with allergic manifestations such as arthralgia, pruritus, headaches, and lymphadenopathy. *Culicoides* midges are the main vectors for *Mansonella streptocerca*, *M. ozzardi*, and *M. perstans*; in the Caribbean area, blackflies also transmit *M. ozzardi*. *Mansonella rodhaini*, a parasite of chimpanzees, was found in 1.7% of skin snips taken from humans in Gabon. DEC is effective against *M. streptocerca* and occasionally against *M. perstans* and *M. ozzardi*. Combination regimens of DEC and mebendazole have been found effective against *M. perstans*, and ivermectin has been effective in treating *M. ozzardi* in small trials. The utility of doxycycline in *Mansonella* infections has not yet been evaluated.

[M. Kamb]

FOODBORNE INTOXICATIONS

DISEASE	ICD-10 CODE
FOODBORNE STAPHYLOCOCCAL INTOXICATION	ICD-10 A05.0
FOODBORNE *CLOSTRIDIUM PERFRINGENS* INTOXICATION	ICD-10 A05.2
FOODBORNE *BACILLUS CEREUS* INTOXICATION	ICD-10 A05.4
SEAFOOD POISONING	
SCOMBROID FISH POISONING	ICD-10 T61.1
PUFFER FISH POISONING (TETRODOTOXIN)	ICD-10 T61.2
CIGUATERA FISH POISONING	ICD-10 T61.0
PARALYTIC SHELLFISH POISONING	ICD-10 T61.2
NEUROTOXIC SHELLFISH POISONING	
DIARRHETIC SHELLFISH POISONING	ICD-10 T61.2
AMNESIC SHELLFISH POISONING	ICD-10 T61.2
AZASPIRACID POISONING	ICD-10 T61.2

Foodborne illness can occur when a person consumes a food or beverage contaminated with pathogenic bacteria, parasites, viruses, heavy metals, chemicals, or toxins. This chapter deals specifically with toxin-related foodborne illnesses, with the exception of botulism, which is addressed in the relevant chapter.

I. FOODBORNE STAPHYLOCOCCAL INTOXICATION

1. Clinical features—Characterized by abrupt and sometimes violent onset of nausea, cramps, and vomiting, often accompanied by diarrhea. Fever is uncommon. Illness commonly lasts no more than 24 hours. The intensity of symptoms occasionally requires hospitalization; deaths are rare.

2. Risk groups—Specific risk groups for intoxication have not been identified, but those more susceptible to dehydration, such as children and older adults, should be closely monitored.

3. Causative agents—Staphylococci are Gram-positive bacteria that can grow in temperatures ranging from 7°C to 48°C (44.6°F–118.4°F) and in sodium chloride concentrations up to 15%. Staphylococci produce toxins during growth; while heating contaminated foods will destroy these bacteria, the toxins are heat stable and can survive even the high temperatures associated with commercial canning. Foodborne staphylococcal intoxications are principally due to *Staphylococcus aureus*.

4. Diagnosis—For sporadic cases, diagnosis of possible toxin-mediated foodborne illness is presumptive. Outbreak-associated cases can be confirmed via isolation of the same organism from stools or vomitus from 2 or more ill persons, detection of enterotoxin in epidemiologically linked food, or isolation of 10^5 organisms per gram from implicated food.

5. Occurrence—Widespread and relatively frequent; one of the most common foodborne intoxications worldwide.

6. Reservoirs—Principally humans; also found in domesticated animals, such as cows, pigs, poultry, dogs, and cats.

7. Incubation period—Interval between eating the contaminated food and onset of symptoms ranges from 30 minutes to 8 hours, usually 2 to 4 hours.

8. Transmission—Through ingestion of food containing staphylococcal enterotoxin. When contaminated foods are not properly heated or cooled, the bacteria can multiply and produce heat-stable toxins at dangerous levels. Commonly implicated foods include pork products, such as ham, poultry, beef, sandwiches, milk, cheese, and cream-filled pastries, but can vary by country owing to different consumption patterns. Often, foods are contaminated by an infected food handler, but some foods, such as milk or cheese, are contaminated before or during production.

9. Treatment—Supportive treatment for approximately 24 hours.

10. Prevention—Food handlers should wash hands and under fingernails thoroughly with soap and water before handling and preparing food; ill persons should not prepare food. Wounds or sores on hands should be cleaned, properly dressed, and covered with gloves before food is handled. Hot food should be kept hot ($\geq 60°C$ [$140°F$]) and cold food should be cold ($\leq 4°C$ [$39.2°F$]). Unconsumed food should be stored in wide, shallow containers and refrigerated no later than 2 hours after preparation.

11. Special considerations—Swift, accurate outbreak investigations are needed to identify contaminated commercially produced foods quickly and to prevent additional cases.

II. FOODBORNE *CLOSTRIDIUM PERFRINGENS* INTOXICATION (including enteritis necroticans [pigbel])

1. Clinical features—An illness characterized by sudden onset of diarrhea and abdominal cramps; vomiting and fever are infrequently reported. Duration is usually approximately 24 hours. Hospitalizations and deaths are uncommon. While severe disease is rare, necrotizing enteritis was reported in Denmark and Germany after World War II and in Papua New Guinea, where the disease was termed "pigbel." It is characterized by vomiting, bloody diarrhea, and acute abdominal pain. Small intestine ulceration and perforation of the intestinal wall can occur, leading to peritonitis, shock, and death.

2. Risk groups—Most people are likely susceptible. Although very rare, necrotizing enteritis is a risk among the malnourished, those with drug-induced constipation, and persons with comorbidities, such as diabetes.

3. Causative agents—*Clostridium perfringens* is a Gram-positive anaerobic spore-forming bacterium. *C. perfringens* type A causes foodborne intoxication through production of heat-labile *C. perfringens* enterotoxin in the small intestine. *C. perfringens* type C causes necrotizing enteritis through production of β-toxin.

4. Diagnosis—Clinical suspicion can be confirmed via isolation of 10^6 organisms per gram from stools or detection of enterotoxin in the stools, but such tests are rarely performed because the illness is of brief duration. Outbreak etiology can be confirmed via stool isolation or enterotoxin detection in 2 or more ill persons or through isolation of 10^5 organisms per gram from epidemiologically implicated food.

5. Occurrence—Widespread and relatively frequent.

6. Reservoirs—Gastrointestinal tract of healthy people and animals (e.g., cattle, fish, pigs, and poultry) and soil.

7. Incubation period—From 6 to 24 hours, usually 9 to 12 hours.

8. Transmission—Through ingestion of food containing 10^5 organisms or more per gram. If *C. perfringens* spores survive the cooking process, they can germinate and multiply rapidly, particularly if food is stored at temperatures ranging from 20°C to 60°C (68°F–140°F) or if it is inadequately reheated. Commonly implicated foods include beef, poultry, pork, soups, stews, and bean dishes.

9. Treatment—Supportive treatment is only for self-limited foodborne *Clostridium perfringens* intoxications. Treatment for necrotizing enterocolitis varies by stage of the condition, from vigorous supportive care to surgery. Duration is approximately 24 hours.

10. Prevention—Food should be cooked to a safe internal temperature and then kept at 60°C (140°F) or higher or refrigerated at 4°C (39.2°F) or lower until served. Large amounts of food, such as soups, stews, and big cuts of meats (e.g., roasts), should be divided into small quantities for refrigeration and stored in wide, shallow containers. Leftovers should be reheated to 75°C (167°F) or higher before serving. Contaminated foods may not taste, smell, or look different.

11. Special considerations—See Foodborne Staphylococcal Intoxication in this chapter.

III. FOODBORNE *BACILLUS CEREUS* INTOXICATION

1. Clinical features—*Bacillus cereus* is the cause of 2 toxin-mediated illnesses—1 emetic and 1 diarrheal. The emetic illness is characterized principally by vomiting, nausea, and abdominal cramps. The diarrheal illness tends to be more severe and involves abdominal cramps and watery diarrhea. Duration of illness is approximately 24 hours. Hospitalizations and deaths are uncommon but fulminant liver failure has occurred following illness owing to the emetic toxin.

2. Risk groups—Most people are likely susceptible. Risk factors for *B. cereus*-induced fulminant liver failure have not been determined.

3. Causative agents—*B. cereus* strains are Gram-positive aerobic and facultatively anaerobic spore-forming bacteria. They produce 2 enterotoxins—1 heat-stable and 1 heat-liable. The former causes the emetic form of illness and the latter causes the diarrheal form.

4. Diagnosis—Diagnosis of single cases is usually presumptive, based on symptoms and food history. Laboratory confirmation during outbreaks occurs via isolation of the organism from stools of 2 or more ill persons or isolation of 10^5 organisms per gram from epidemiologically implicated food.

5. Occurrence—A well-recognized cause of foodborne disease throughout the world.

6. Reservoirs—Ubiquitous organism in soil and the environment.

7. Incubation period—From 1 to 6 hours for the emetic illness and 6 to 24 hours for the diarrheal illness.

8. Transmission—Through ingestion of contaminated foods. *B. cereus* spores are heat resistant and can survive cooking and boiling, so when food is kept at ambient temperatures after cooking surviving spores can germinate and produce enterotoxins. Reheating of food does not destroy the toxins that cause the emetic illness. Ingested spores can germinate in the gastrointestinal tract and produce toxin that can cause the diarrheal illness. Outbreaks of the emetic illness have been most commonly associated with cooked rice held at room temperature. A wide variety of foods have been implicated in outbreaks of the diarrheal illness.

9. Treatment—Supportive treatment for approximately 24 hours.

10. Prevention—Food should not be kept at ambient temperature for more than 2 hours. Food should be held at above 60°C (140°F) or refrigerated at below 4°C (39.2°F) to inhibit spore germination. Cooked food should be refrigerated in wide, shallow containers in order to cool quickly.

11. Special considerations—See Foodborne Staphylococcal Intoxication in this chapter.

SEAFOOD POISONING

IV. SCOMBROID POISONING (histamine poisoning)

1. Clinical features—A syndrome of tingling and burning sensations around the mouth, facial flushing and sweating, nausea and vomiting, headache, palpitations, dizziness, and rash (especially of face and upper torso).

2. Risk groups—Most people are likely susceptible. This is not an allergic reaction but a reaction to histamine. Symptoms may be markedly worse in patients taking isoniazid or other drugs interfering with histamine metabolism.

3. Causative agents—Biogenic amines, particularly histamine, at concentrations higher than 500 ppm. Histamine poisoning is caused by eating improperly stored fish that have accumulated high levels of histamine in the muscle (dark flesh). Histamine is formed by decarboxylation by predominantly Gram-negative bacteria of histidine into histamine. Implicated species include fish from the Scombroidea fish group (e.g., mackerel and tuna), mahi-mahi, sardine, anchovy, herring, bluefish, amberjack, and marlin. Cheese has also been implicated.

4. Diagnosis—Based on clinical signs and symptoms and history of eating certain foods, particularly fish from the Scombroidea fish group (e.g., mackerel and tuna). Detection of histamine in epidemiologically implicated food confirms the diagnosis.

5. Occurrence—Worldwide problem.

6. Reservoirs—Not applicable.

7. Incubation period—Symptoms occur within minutes to hours after eating food containing high levels of free histamine.

8. Transmission—Not applicable.

9. Treatment—Supportive treatment. In severe cases, antihistamines, either through inhalators or intravenously, may be effective in relieving symptoms. There have been no long-term follow-up studies. Symptoms resolve spontaneously within 12 hours and no long-term sequelae have been identified.

10. Prevention—Good food management principles and rapid refrigeration prevent microbial spoilage and decarboxylation of histadine to histamine.

11. Special considerations—The contaminated fish often reportedly taste peppery or bubbly, not normal. Histamines can be present in raw, smoked, or cooked fish.

V. PUFFER FISH POISONING (TETRODOTOXIN)

1. Clinical features—Puffer fish poisoning is characterized by onset of neurologic symptoms (e.g., ataxia, dizziness, paresthesias) often progressing to paralysis, including of the diaphragm muscles, leading to death within several hours after eating. Symptoms may include gastrointestinal distress.

2. Risk groups—Most people are likely susceptible.

3. Causative agents—Tetrodotoxin, a heat-stable, nonprotein neurotoxin, thought to be produced by bacteria in the gut, then concentrated in the skin and viscera of puffer fish, porcupine fish, ocean sunfish, and species of newts and salamanders.

4. Diagnosis—Based on clinical signs and symptoms and history of eating puffer fish. Evidence of tetrodotoxin in epidemiologically implicated shellfish confirms the diagnosis.

5. Occurrence—Most cases occur in Japan.

6. Reservoirs—Not applicable.

7. Incubation period—Hours.

8. Transmission—Not applicable.

9. Treatment—Supportive treatment. There have been no long-term follow-up studies.

10. Prevention—Japan implements control measures such as species identification and adequate removal of toxic parts (e.g., ova, intestine) by qualified cooks.

11. Special considerations—Case-fatality rates from 10% to 60% have been reported. Implicated puffer fish should also be tested for the presence of paralytic shellfish poisoning (PSP) toxins.

VI. CIGUATERA FISH POISONING

1. Clinical features—Gastrointestinal symptoms (diarrhea, vomiting, abdominal pain) occur usually within 12 to 24 hours of consumption. In severe cases, patients may also become hypotensive, with a paradoxical bradycardia. Neurologic symptoms, including pain and weakness in the lower extremities and circumoral and peripheral paresthesias, may occur at the same time as the acute symptoms or follow within 1 to 2 days later; they may persist for weeks or months. Symptoms such as abnormal temperature sensations (a cold tile floor seems hot when stepped on), burning feet, and aching teeth are frequently reported. In very severe cases, neurologic symptoms may progress to coma and respiratory arrest within the first 24 hours of illness.

2. Risk groups—Most people are likely susceptible, but spear fishers and subsistence fishers harvesting near reefs are more likely to be exposed if they consume contaminated fish.

3. Causative agents—Ciguatoxins found in reef fish (e.g., groupers, barracudas).

4. Diagnosis—Based on clinical signs and symptoms and history of eating reef fish. Evidence of ciguatoxin in epidemiologically implicated fish confirms the diagnosis.

5. Occurrence—Ciguatera is widespread in tropical and subtropical waters, usually between the latitudes of 35°N and 35°S; it is particularly common in the Pacific and Indian Oceans and the Caribbean Sea. The incidence and geographic distribution of ciguatera poisoning are increasing. Newly recognized areas of risk include the Canary Islands, the eastern Mediterranean, the western Gulf of Mexico, and Africa. Travelers to these areas may become ill after returning home to areas where ciguatera is not known.

6. Reservoirs—Not applicable.

7. Incubation period—Hours.

8. Transmission—Not applicable.

9. Treatment—

Drug	• Supportive treatment. • Mannitol has been demonstrated to have an effect on acute musculoskeletal symptoms of ciguatera poisoning based on a double-blind study; another follow-up double-blind study did not confirm this, which may be attributable at least partly to methodologic limitations. • Administration of brevenal may relieve symptoms.
Dose	Not applicable
Route	IV infusion (mannitol 1 g/kg)
Alternative drug	Not applicable
Duration	Most patients recover completely within a few weeks; intermittent recrudescence of symptoms can occur over a period of months to years. There have been no long-term follow-up studies.
Special considerations and comments	None

Note: IV = intravenous(ly).

10. Prevention—The consumption of large reef fish should be avoided. It is especially important to avoid eating the heads, viscera, and roe of reef fish. Where laboratory-based assays for toxic fish are available, screening all large high-risk fish before consumption can reduce risk.

11. Special considerations—The occurrence of toxic fish is sporadic and not all fish of a given species or from a given locale will be toxic. Cooking and preserving foods (e.g., freezing, boiling) do not destroy the toxin and the fish reportedly taste delicious. Recommendations to prevent recurrence of symptoms include avoiding certain foods (fish [including freshwater species], caffeine, nuts, chicken, and pork), alcohol, and physical overexertion or dehydration.

VII. PARALYTIC SHELLFISH POISONING

1. Clinical features—PSP is a characteristic syndrome that is predominantly neurologic. Initial symptoms can begin from 15 minutes to 10 hours after eating and include paresthesias of the mouth and extremities accompanied by gastrointestinal symptoms. In severe cases, ataxia, dysphonia, dysphagia, and muscle paralysis with respiratory arrest and death may occur within 12 hours.

2. Risk groups—Most people are likely susceptible.

3. Causative agents—Saxitoxins or other toxins produced by *Alexandrium* spp. and other dinoflagellates that accumulate in shellfish.

4. Diagnosis—Based on clinical signs and symptoms and history of eating shellfish. Evidence of saxitoxins in epidemiologically implicated shellfish confirms the diagnosis.

5. Occurrence—PSP occurs worldwide but is most common in temperate waters, especially off the Pacific and Atlantic coasts of North America, including Alaska. Cases have also been reported from countries such as the Philippines, China, Chile, Scotland, Ireland, New Zealand, and Australia.

6. Reservoirs—Not applicable.

7. Incubation period—Within minutes to several hours after eating bivalve mollusks.

8. Transmission—Not applicable.

9. Treatment—Supportive treatment. Symptoms usually resolve completely within hours to days after shellfish ingestion. There have been no long-term follow-up studies.

10. Prevention—Surveillance of high-risk shellfish harvest areas is routine in Canada, the EU, Japan, and the USA. Shellfish harvest closures occur when the shellfish saxitoxin levels equal or exceed the international standard action level of 80 μg/100 g of shellfish meat or when a positive result on the qualitative Jellett Rapid Test (Jellett Rapid Testing, Nova Scotia, Canada) occurs based on screening standards from the Interstate Shellfish Sanitation Conference.

11. Special considerations—Shellfish can remain toxic for several weeks after the bloom subsides. Most cases occur in individuals or small groups who gather shellfish for personal consumption. Cooking and preserving foods (e.g., freezing, boiling) do not destroy the toxin and the shellfish taste normal.

VIII. NEUROTOXIC SHELLFISH POISONING (and associated illnesses)

1. Clinical features—Foodborne: symptoms include circumoral paresthesias and paresthesias of the extremities, dizziness and ataxia, myalgia, and gastrointestinal symptoms. Aerosol exposures to toxins in sea breezes: respiratory and eye irritation. People with asthma may experience exacerbations.

2. Risk groups—Most people are likely susceptible. People with asthma are more susceptible to the aerosolized toxins.

3. Causative agents—Brevetoxins produced by the dinoflagellate *Karenia brevis* and that accumulate in shellfish or are aerosolized and incorporated into sea breezes.

4. Diagnosis—Foodborne: based on clinical signs and symptoms and history of eating shellfish or visiting the beach during a Florida red tide. Evidence of brevetoxins in epidemiologically implicated shellfish confirms the diagnosis. Aerosol exposures: based on clinical signs and symptoms of respiratory irritation or asthma exacerbation and a history of visiting a beach during a *K. brevis* bloom (also called a Florida red tide) with onshore breezes.

5. Occurrence—Neurotoxic shellfish poisoning (NSP) and respiratory brevetoxin exposure are associated with algal blooms (Florida red tides) of *K. brevis*, which produce brevetoxin. NSP has been reported from the southeastern coast of the USA, the Gulf of Mexico, the Caribbean, and New Zealand.

6. Reservoirs—Not applicable.

7. Incubation period—Minutes to hours.

8. Transmission—Not applicable.

9. Treatment—

Drug	Supportive treatment
Dose	Not applicable
Route	Not applicable
Alternative drug	Not applicable
Duration	• NSP symptoms tend to be mild and resolve quickly and completely in most people but there have been no long-term follow-up studies. • Those with asthma after aerosol exposure may experience symptoms for a few days after initial exposure. There have been no long-term follow-up studies.
Special considerations and comments	None

Note: NSP: neurotoxic shellfish poisoning.

10. Prevention—Avoid recreational shellfish harvesting along the Florida coast. Commercial shellfish-harvesting areas are monitored for brevetoxins and commercially available shellfish are safe to eat. Persons with asthma should avoid the coast during active Florida red tides with onshore winds. They may be able to prevent symptoms from aerosol exposures using asthma medications.

11. Special considerations—Red tides have long occurred along the Florida coast, where the syndrome has been most studied, with associated mortality in fish, seabirds, and marine mammals. Cooking and preserving foods (e.g., freezing, boiling) do not destroy the toxin and the contaminated seafood reportedly tastes delicious.

IX. DIARRHETIC SHELLFISH POISONING

1. Clinical features—Symptoms include diarrhea, nausea, vomiting, and abdominal pain.

2. Risk groups—Most people are likely susceptible.

3. Causative agents—Shellfish contaminated with okadaic acid (OA) and derivative toxins produced by *Dinophysis* spp. and other dinoflagellates.

4. Diagnosis—Based on clinical signs and symptoms and history of eating shellfish. Evidence of OA in epidemiologically implicated shellfish confirms the diagnosis.

5. Occurrence—It occurs worldwide and outbreaks have been reported from China, Japan, Scandinavia, France, Belgium, Spain, Chile, Uruguay, Ireland, the USA, and Canada.

6. Reservoirs—Not applicable.

7. Incubation period—Hours.

8. Transmission—Not applicable.

9. Treatment—Supportive treatment. Duration is days, but there have been no long-term follow-up studies.

10. Prevention—Shellfish-harvesting areas are monitored. The USA established the action level for diarrhetic shellfish poisoning at 0.2 ppm OA plus 35-methyl OA.

11. Special considerations—Cooking and preserving foods (e.g., freezing, boiling) do not destroy the toxin and reportedly the shellfish taste good.

X. AMNESIC SHELLFISH POISONING

1. Clinical features—Symptoms include vomiting, abdominal cramps, diarrhea, headache, and possibly short-term memory loss. When tested several months after acute intoxication, some patients reportedly showed antegrade memory deficits with relative preservation of other cognitive functions together with clinical and electromyographic evidence of pure motor or sensorimotor neuropathy and axonopathy. There were mortalities in members of the original group of patients who had existing chronic diseases. There may be a memory deficit with long-term low-dose exposure.

2. Risk groups—Most people are likely susceptible.

3. Causative agents—Amnesic shellfish poisoning results from ingestion of shellfish containing domoic acid produced by the diatom *Pseudonitzschia pungen.*

4. Diagnosis—Based on clinical signs and symptoms and history of eating shellfish. Evidence of domoic acid in epidemiologically implicated shellfish confirms the diagnosis.

5. Occurrence—Amnesic shellfish poisoning has been reported from Canada, Scotland, Ireland, France, Belgium, Spain, Portugal, New Zealand, Australia, and Chile. Toxic mussels, scallops, razor clams, and crustaceans were responsible in those outbreaks.

6. Reservoirs—Not applicable.

7. Incubation period—Hours.

8. Transmission—Not applicable.

9. Treatment—Supportive treatment for possibly years. There have been no long-term follow-up studies.

10. Prevention—Canadian authorities now analyze mussels and clams for domoic acid and close shellfish beds to harvesting when levels exceed 20 ppm domoic acid. European Community (EC) directive 91/492/EEC and amendments for the safety of shellfish (Amendment 97/61/EC) state that "total Amnesic Shellfish Poison (ASP) content in the edible parts of molluscs (the entire body or any part edible separately) must not exceed 20 micrograms of domoic acid per gramme using the HPLC [high-pressure liquid chromatography] method."

11. Special considerations—None.

XI. AZASPIRACID POISONING

1. Clinical features—Severe diarrhea and vomiting with abdominal pain and occasional nausea, chills, headaches, and stomach cramps from eating shellfish contaminated with azaspiracid. Azaspiracid poisoning can cause necrosis in the intestine, thymus, and liver.

2. Risk groups—Most people are likely susceptible.

3. Causative agents—Azaspiracids produced by the dinoflagellate *Azadinium spinosum* in contaminated shellfish.

4. Diagnosis—Based on clinical signs and symptoms and history of eating shellfish. Evidence of azaspiracid in epidemiologically implicated shellfish confirms the diagnosis.

5. Occurrence—Azaspiracid poisoning incidents have been identified in several European countries and the toxin has been isolated from mussels in European waters as well as in North Africa and Canada.

6. Reservoirs—Not applicable.

7. Incubation period—12 to 24 hours.

8. Transmission—Not applicable.

9. Treatment—Supportive treatment for up to 5 days. There have been no long-term follow-up studies.

10. Prevention—A regulatory limit of 160 mg azaspiracid per kilogram whole-shellfish flesh has been established by the EU.

11. Special considerations—None.

[S. Crowe, L. Backer]

FUNGAL DISEASES OF THE SKIN, HAIR, AND NAILS

(tinea, ringworm, dermatophytosis, dermatomycosis, epidermophytosis, trichophytosis, microsporosis, superficial mycosis)

DISEASE	ICD-10 CODE	CAUSATIVE AGENTS	SITE	OCCURRENCE
TINEA BARBAE TINEA CAPITIS	ICD-10 B35.0	Various species of *Microsporum*, *Trichophyton*, and *Epidermophyton*	Beard, scalp	Common in urban areas worldwide. Tinea barbae occurs primarily in bearded adult males.

(Continued)

(Continued)

DISEASE	ICD-10 CODE	CAUSATIVE AGENTS	SITE	OCCURRENCE
BLACK PIEDRA	ICD-10 B36.3	*Piedraia hortae*	Hair shaft	Tropical areas of South America, south-eastern Asia, and Africa
WHITE PIEDRA	ICD-10 B36.3	*Trichosporon* spp. (*asahii, inkin, ovoides, mucoides, asteroides,* and *cutaneum*)	Hair shaft	Temperate and semitrop-ical climates worldwide
TINEA CRURIS, TINEA CORPORIS	ICD-10 B35.6, ICD-10 B35.4	Most species of *Microsporum* and *Trichophyton* (in particular, *Trichophyton rubrum*); also *Epidermophyton floccosum*	Groin and perianal region; trunk, arms, and legs	Worldwide and relatively frequent. Males are affected more often than females.
TINEA PEDIS	ICD-10 B35.3	*Trichophyton rubrum, Trichophyton mentagrophytes* var. *interdigitale,* and *Epidermophyton floccosum*	Feet	Common worldwide
ONYCHOMYCOSIS DUE TO DERMATOPHYTES	ICD-10 B35.1	Various species of *Trichophyton*; rarely, other dermatophytes	Nails	Common worldwide

I. TINEA BARBAE AND TINEA CAPITIS (ringworm of the beard and scalp, kerion, favus, Majocchi granuloma), BLACK PIEDRA, WHITE PIEDRA

1. Clinical features—A superficial fungal disease that begins as a small area of erythema and/or scaling and spreads peripherally, leaving scaly patches of temporary baldness. Infected hairs become brittle and break off easily. Occasionally, thickened, raised suppurative lesions develop called kerions. Favus of the scalp, a variety of tinea capitis, is characterized by an unpleasant smell and by the formation of small, yellowish, cuplike crusts that amalgamate to form a pale or yellow visible mat on the scalp surface. Affected hairs of a favus do not break off but become gray and lusterless, eventually falling out and leaving baldness that may be permanent. Majocchi granuloma is a deep folliculitis most commonly due to cutaneous infection with *Trichophyton rubrum* and is associated with the use of topical steroids.

Tinea capitis and black piedra both affect the scalp, but they are easily distinguished from each other. Black piedra is characterized by black, hard, gritty nodules on hair shafts, caused by *Piedraia hortae*. White piedra is caused by *Trichosporon* spp., particularly *Trichosporon ovoides* or *Trichosporon inkin*, which produce white, soft, pasty nodules. Infections of the latter are usually seen on the scalp but may also be seen on armpit, facial, or pubic hair.

2. Risk groups—Tinea barbae occurs almost exclusively in adult men with facial hair. Tinea capitis occurs primarily in preadolescent children. Reinfections mainly occur as a result of infections spread among humans.

3. Causative agents—See earlier table. Species and genus identification is important for epidemiologic, prognostic, and therapeutic reasons.

4. Diagnosis—Examination of the scalp under ultraviolet (UV) light (Wood's lamp) for yellow-green fluorescence is helpful in diagnosing tinea capitis caused by *Microsporum* spp. such as *Microsporum canis* and *Microsporum audouinii*; *Trichophyton* spp. do not fluoresce. In infections caused by *Microsporum* spp., microscopic examination of scales and hair in 10% potassium hydroxide or under UV microscopy of a calcofluor white preparation reveals characteristic nonpigmented ectothrix (outside the hair) arthrospores; many *Trichophyton* spp. present an endothrix (inside the hair) pattern of invasion, and *Trichophyton verrucosum*, the cause of cattle ringworm, produces large ectothrix spores. In black piedra, epilated hairs show hard black nodules on the shaft. Confirmation of the diagnosis requires culture of the fungus. Genetic identification methods and direct polymerase chain reaction (PCR) detection assays are a useful supplement to traditional morphology-based methods of identification.

5. Occurrence—Tinea capitis caused by *Trichophyton tonsurans* has been epidemic in urban areas in Australia, the UK, eastern USA, and Puerto Rico, as well as in Mexico and many developing countries. *M. canis* infections occur in rural and urban areas wherever infected cats and dogs are present. *M. audouinii* is endemic in western Africa and was formerly widespread in Europe and North America, particularly in urban areas. *T. verrucosum* and *Trichophyton mentagrophytes* var. *mentagrophytes* infections occur primarily in rural areas where the disease exists in cattle, horses, rodents, and wild animals. Black piedra occurs in tropical areas of South America, southeastern Asia, and Africa.

6. Reservoirs—Humans for *T. tonsurans*, *Trichophyton schoenleinii*, and *M. audouinii*; animals, especially dogs, cats, and cattle, harbor the other organisms noted above. Most cases of white piedra are endogenous in origin. The natural habitat of the black piedra agent is likely in soil and stagnant water.

7. Incubation period—Usually 10 to 14 days.

8. Transmission—Tinea barbae and tinea capitis are transmitted through direct skin-to-skin or indirect contact, especially from the backs of seats, barber clippers, toiletries (combs, hairbrushes), clothing, and hats that are contaminated with hair from infected people or animals. Infected humans can generate considerable aerosols of infective arthrospores. Viable fungus and infective arthrospores may persist on contaminated materials for long periods. Black piedra and white piedra are also spread by common use of combs, hairbrushes, and cosmetics; it is not thought these agents are transmitted directly from person to person.

9. Treatment—In mild cases, daily washing of scalp removes loose hair. Selenium sulfide or ketoconazole shampoo helps remove scale. In severe cases, wash scalp daily and cover hair with a cap, which should be boiled after use.

Topical agents (e.g., topical imidazoles, 2% selenium sulfate) can be helpful in control, although relapse is common. Oral antifungal therapy is often required. The following table details pharmacologic considerations.

Drug	Griseofulvin	Terbinafine	Itraconazole
Dose (adult)	500 mg daily	250 mg daily	200 mg daily
Route	PO	PO	PO
Duration	4–6 weeks	2 weeks	4 weeks
Special considerations and comments	• Better for *Microsporum* infections. • Not recommended for patients with active or chronic liver disease.	• Better for *Trichophyton* infections. • Higher doses should be used for *Microsporum* infections. • Not recommended for patients with active or chronic liver disease.	Better for *Trichophyton* infections.

Note: PO = oral(ly).

10. Prevention—Measures include educating the public, especially parents, about the danger of acquiring infection from infected individuals, dogs, cats, and other animals. Additionally, in the presence of epidemics or in hyperendemic areas where non-*Trichophyton* spp. are prevalent, survey of heads of young children by UV light (Wood's lamp) before school entry should be performed.

11. Special considerations—

1) Reporting: report to local health authority of epidemics is obligatory in some countries. Outbreaks in schools should be reported to school authorities.

2) Epidemic measures: in school or other institutional epidemics, educate children and parents on mode of spread, prevention, and personal hygiene. If more than 2 infected children are present in a class, examine the others. Enlist services of physicians and nurses for diagnosis and carry out follow-up surveys.

II. TINEA CRURIS (ringworm of groin and perianal region, jock itch), TINEA CORPORIS (ringworm of the body)

1. Clinical features—A fungal disease of the skin other than of the scalp, bearded areas, and feet, characteristically appearing as flat, spreading, ring-shaped or circular lesions with a characteristic raised edge around all or part of the lesion. This periphery is usually reddish, vesicular, or pustular and may be dry and scaly or moist and crusted. As the lesion progresses peripherally, the central area often clears, leaving apparently normal skin. Patients report pruritus. Differentiation from inguinal candidiasis, often distinguished by the presence of satellite pustules outside the lesion margins, is necessary because treatment differs. Lesions are aggravated by friction and excessive perspiration in axillary and inguinal regions and when environmental temperatures and humidity are high. All ages are susceptible.

2. Risk groups—All humans are susceptible. Tinea cruris is seen mostly in men. Other forms of dermatophytosis (e.g., tinea pedis) commonly occur concurrently.

3. Causative agents—See earlier table.

4. Diagnosis—Presumptive diagnosis is made by taking scrapings of scales from the advancing lesion margins, clearing in 10% potassium hydroxide, and examining microscopically or under UV microscopy of calcofluor white preparations for segmented, branched, nonpigmented fungal filaments. Final identification is through culture or direct PCR analysis.

5. Occurrence—Commonly occurring worldwide but more frequent in hot humid climates.

6. Reservoirs—Humans, farm animals, household pets, and soil.

7. Incubation period—Usually 4 to 10 days.

8. Transmission—Direct or indirect contact with skin and scalp lesions of infected people or lesions of animals or by fomites, such as contaminated floors, towels, shower stalls, benches, and similar articles. Communicable for as long as lesions are present and viable fungus persists on contaminated materials.

9. Treatment—Consider topical therapy with topical azoles (e.g., ketoconazole, clotrimazole, miconazole) or allylamines (e.g., terbinafine) for localized infection. Agent should be applied to the lesion and approximately 2 cm beyond once or twice daily for at least 2 weeks.

For extensive skin infection, immunosuppression, or failure of topical therapy, a systemic agent is required. See the following table for pharmacologic considerations.

Drug	Griseofulvin	Terbinafine	Systemic azoles (fluconazole, itraconazole)
Dose (adult)	10 mg/kg daily	250 mg daily	Fluconazole 50–100 mg daily or 150 mg once weekly Itraconazole 100 mg daily
Route	PO	PO	PO
Duration	4 weeks	2–4 weeks	2 weeks
Special considerations and comments	Not recommended for patients with active or chronic liver disease.	Not recommended for patients with active or chronic liver disease.	None

Note: PO = oral(ly).

10. Prevention—Launder towels and clothing with hot water and/or fungicidal agent; discourage close contact and stop the sharing of fomites (e.g., towels) between infected and noninfected persons. Prevention of reinfection or spreading infection to other body sites includes attention to drying crural folds after bathing and wearing breathable clothing. Maintain general cleanliness in public showers and dressing rooms (repeated washing of benches; frequent hosing and rapid draining of shower rooms). A fungicidal agent should be used to disinfect benches and floors.

11. Special considerations—

1) Reporting: reporting to the local health authority of epidemics is obligatory in some countries. Infections in children should be reported to school authorities.
2) Epidemic measures: educate children and parents about the infection, its mode of spread, and the need to maintain good personal hygiene. Outbreaks are common among military personnel.

3) Atypical presentations: consider further evaluation for human immunodeficiency virus (HIV) infection or an immunocompromised state.

III. TINEA PEDIS (ringworm of the foot, athlete's foot)

1. Clinical features—Presents with characteristic scaling or cracking of the skin, especially fissures between the toes (interdigital), diffuse scaling over the sole of the foot (dry type), or blisters containing a thin watery fluid; commonly called athlete's foot. Patients may report pruritus and/or pain. In severe cases, vesicular lesions appear on various parts of the body, especially the hands; these dermatophytids do not contain the fungus but are an allergic reaction to fungus products. Other organisms can cause similar-appearing lesions, including bacteria (e.g., Gram-negative organisms) as well as other fungi (e.g., *Candida* and *Scytalidium*); they can also complicate the infection as secondary pathogens.

2. Risk groups—Common in industrial workers, schoolchildren, athletes, and military personnel who share shower or bathing facilities. Repeated attacks and chronic infections are frequent.

3. Causative agents—See earlier table.

4. Diagnosis—Presumptive diagnosis is verified by microscopic examination of potassium hydroxide- or calcofluor white-treated scrapings from lesions that reveal septate branching filaments. Clinical appearance is not diagnostic; final identification is through culture or direct PCR.

5. Occurrence—Considered the most common dermatophytosis worldwide. Adults are more often affected than children and males more than females. Infections are more frequent and more severe in hot weather.

6. Reservoirs—Humans.

7. Incubation period—Unknown.

8. Transmission—Direct or indirect contact with skin lesions of infected people or with contaminated floors, shower stalls, and other articles used by infected people. Communicable as long as lesions are present and viable spores persist on contaminated materials.

9. Treatment—Can be treated with topical and/or oral systemic antifungal therapy. Topical imidazoles (e.g., clotrimazole, ketoconazole) and allylamines (e.g., terbinafine) are available over the counter with varying instructions depending on formulation.

Systemic antifungal therapy is summarized in the following table.

Drug	Terbinafine	Itraconazole
Dose (adult)	250 mg daily	100 mg daily
Route	PO	PO
Duration	2–6 weeks	2 weeks
Special considerations and comments	Not recommended for patients with active or chronic liver disease.	None

Note: PO = oral(ly).

10. Prevention—See Tinea Corporis in this chapter. Educate the public about maintaining strict personal hygiene; consider wearing protective footwear in communal bath or pool areas. Take special care in drying between toes after bathing; consider using a dusting powder or cream containing an effective antifungal on the feet and particularly between the toes. Occlusive shoes may predispose to infection and can be a source of reinfection; wearing cotton socks may be helpful.

11. Special considerations—

1) Reporting: reporting to the local health authority of epidemics is obligatory in some countries. Infections in children should be reported to school authorities.

2) Epidemic measures: thoroughly clean and wash floors of showers and similar sources of infection; disinfect with a fungicidal agent. Educate the public about the mode of spread.

IV. ONYCHOMYCOSIS DUE TO DERMATOPHYTES
(tinea unguium, ringworm of the nails, onychomycosis, toenail fungus)

1. Clinical features—A chronic fungal disease involving one or more nails of the hands or feet; it may involve any part of the nail, including the matrix, bed, or plate. Presentation with dystrophic nails and no other symptomatic complaints is common; however, pain and discomfort can occur. The nail gradually becomes detached from the nail bed, thickens, and becomes discolored and brittle; an accumulation of soft keratinous material forms beneath the nail or the nail becomes chalky and disintegrates.

2. Risk groups—All humans are susceptible.

3. Causative agents—See earlier table.

4. Diagnosis—By microscopic examination of potassium hydroxide preparations of the nail and of detritus beneath the nail for hyaline fungal elements. Etiology should be confirmed by culture, which seeks to differentiate infection by dermatophytes from that by nondermatophytes (by using culture medium with and without cycloheximide, which, when present, is selective for dermatophytes).

5. Occurrence—See earlier table.

6. Reservoirs—Humans; rarely, animals or soil.

7. Incubation period—Unknown.

8. Transmission—Presumably through extension from skin infections acquired by direct contact with skin or nail lesions of infected people or from indirect contact (contaminated floors and shower stalls). Low rate of transmission, even to close family associates. Communicable for as long as an infected lesion is present.

9. Treatment—Nonpharmacologic therapy can be combined with pharmacologic therapy; these approaches include mechanical, chemical, or surgical removal of nails, laser treatment, or photodynamic therapy.

Drug	Terbinafine	Itraconazole
Dose (adult)	250 mg daily	200 mg daily
Route	PO	PO
Duration	6–12 weeks	12 weeks
Special considerations and comments	• Fingernails, 6 weeks; toenails, 12 weeks. • Not recommended for patients with active or chronic liver disease.	Alternative regimen (fingernails): 2 treatment pulses with 200 mg every 12 hours for 1 week.

Note: PO = oral(ly).

10. Prevention—Cleanliness and use of a fungicidal agent for disinfecting floors in common use; frequent hosing and rapid draining of shower rooms.

11. Special considerations—

1) Patients with HIV infection may have more severe presentations, including more prevalent proximal subungual involvement.
2) Patients with diabetes may have bacterial colonization and vascular insufficiency that could complicate treatment.

[S. Tsay, N. Chow]

GIARDIASIS
(*Giardia duodenalis*)

DISEASE	ICD-10 CODE
GIARDIASIS	ICD-10 A07.1

1. Clinical features—A protozoan infection, principally of the upper small intestine; it can remain asymptomatic. When symptomatic, it may manifest with some combination of the following signs, symptoms, and complications: gradual onset of 2 to 5 loose stools per day and gradually increasing fatigue, self-limited in 2 to 4 weeks; other intestinal symptoms such as chronic diarrhea; steatorrhea; abdominal cramps; bloating; flatulence; frequent loose and pale greasy stools that tend to float; nausea, anorexia, dehydration; malabsorption (of fats and fat-soluble vitamins); and weight loss. Uncommon symptoms include fever, vomiting, pruritus, hives, and swelling of the eye and joints. Chronic sequelae have been recognized, including reactive arthritis and irritable bowel syndrome; in children, in particular, severe giardiasis may cause stunting, developmental delay, failure to thrive, and malnutrition.

2. Risk groups—People in child care settings; people who are in close contact with someone who has the disease; travelers to countries where giardiasis is common; people who have contact with feces during sexual activity; backpackers or campers who drink untreated water from springs, lakes, or rivers (i.e., surface water); people who have a shallow well as a residential source of water; and people who have contact with infected animals or animal environments contaminated with feces.

3. Causative agents—*Giardia duodenalis* (*Giardia intestinalis*, *Giardia lamblia*), a flagellate protozoan.

4. Diagnosis—Detection of *Giardia* cysts or trophozoites, antigen, or deoxyribonucleic acid in stools, intestinal fluid, or tissue. For increased diagnostic sensitivity, at least 3 stool specimens should be examined over several days. Because *Giardia* infection can be asymptomatic, the presence of *G. duodenalis* does not necessarily indicate that *Giardia* is the cause of illness. Diagnostic techniques include microscopy with direct fluorescent antibody testing (considered the gold standard), rapid immunochromatographic cartridge assays, enzyme immunoassay kits, microscopy with trichrome staining, and molecular assays. Only molecular testing (such as polymerase chain reaction) can be used to identify the genotypes and subtypes of *Giardia*. Retesting is only recommended if symptoms persist after treatment.

5. Occurrence—Worldwide. Prevalence of giardiasis is much higher in developing countries, with an infection rate of about 1% to 8% in industrialized countries and about 8% to 30% in developing countries. Children are much more susceptible to infection by *Giardia* and tend to have higher infection rates than adults. In the USA, *Giardia* infection is the most common intestinal parasitic disease affecting people, with an estimated more than 1 million cases occurring annually and a cost of US $62 million in hospitalizations per year.

6. Reservoirs—Humans. While animals can be infected with *Giardia*, their importance as a reservoir is unclear. *Giardia* cysts are hardy and can survive several months in cold water or soil.

7. Incubation period—Signs and symptoms may vary and usually develop 1 to 2 weeks following exposure. Generally, giardiasis spontaneously resolves within 2 to 4 weeks; sometimes, however, symptoms may appear to resolve, only to recur after several days or weeks. In cases that become chronic, subsequent complications may include reactive arthritis, irritable bowel syndrome, and intermittent diarrhea that can last for years.

8. Transmission—Most reported giardiasis outbreaks have been associated with consumption of fecally contaminated water. Other routes of transmission include person-to-person, animal-to-person, or consumption of contaminated food. Drinking untreated water from lakes and rivers, swimming in natural waters, having contact with some animal species, and sexual activity involving fecal contact can increase risk for giardiasis. *Giardia* infection rates often rise in late summer and children are more commonly infected. Giardiasis is often diagnosed in international travelers and among internationally adopted children.

Giardia cysts are infectious when passed in the stools, making person-to-person transmission possible in the absence of frequent handwashing. While both cysts and trophozoites can be found in the feces, only cysts can be transmitted and can cause disease, partly because their outer shell allows them to survive for weeks to several months in the gastric tract or the environment and also because the shell makes them moderately chlorine-tolerant.

While animals such as cats, dogs, cattle, deer, and beavers can host *Giardia*, their role in infecting humans or contaminating the environment with human-pathogenic *Giardia* is unclear. The risk of humans acquiring *Giardia* infection from dogs or cats is low. The *Giardia* genotypes that are pathogenic to humans usually differ from those that are pathogenic to dogs and cats. *G. duodenalis* can be subdivided—based on molecular analysis—into what are known as genetic assemblages (A, B, C, D, E, F, G, and H). Some of these assemblages can be classified even further into subtypes (e.g., A-I, A-II, A-III).

9. Treatment—

Preferred therapy	Adults:
	• Metronidazole 250 mg PO TID for 5–7 days OR • Tinidazole 2 g PO single dose OR • Nitazoxanide 500 mg PO BID for 3 days
	Children:

	• Metronidazole 15 mg/kg/day PO in 3 doses for 5–7 days
	OR
	• Tinidazole > 3 years, 50 mg/kg PO single dose ($\leq$ 2 g)
	OR
	• Nitazoxanide:
	   ○ 1–3 years: 100 mg PO BID for 3 days
	   ○ 4–11 years: 200 mg PO BID for 3 days
	   ○ > 12 years: 500 mg PO BID for 3 days

Alternative therapy options	Adults:
	• Paromomycin 25–35 mg/kg/day PO in 3 doses for 5–10 days OR • Furazolidone 100 mg PO QID for 7–10 days OR • Quinacrine 100 mg PO TID for 5 days
	Children:
	• Paromomycin 25–35 mg/kg/day PO in 3 doses for 5–10 days OR • Furazolidone 6 mg/kg/day PO in 4 doses for 7–10 days OR • Quinacrine 6 mg/kg/day PO in 3 doses for 5 days ($\leq$ 300 mg/day)
Special considerations and comments	• Metronidazole is not FDA-approved for this indication. • Trinidazole, nitazoxanide, and paromomycin should be taken with food. • Paromomycin may be useful for treatment in pregnancy. • Due to availability issues, contact the manufacturer for availability of paromomycin, furazolidone, and quinacrine. • Quinacrine should be taken with liquids after a meal; not available commercially in the USA but may be obtained via compounding pharmacies such as Expert Compounding Pharmacy (6744 Balboa Boulevard, Lake Balboa, CA 91406; 1-800-247-9767 or 1-818-988-7979); other compounding pharmacies may be found via the Professional Compounding Centers of America (www.pccarx.com; 1-800-331-2498).

Note: BID = twice daily; PO = oral(ly); QID = 4 times daily; TID = thrice daily.

10. Prevention—

1) Use of safe water, appropriate sanitation, and handwashing are the most important measures to avoid giardiasis. Avoid drinking and recreational water that may be contaminated. If the safety of drinking water is in doubt (e.g., during travel to a location with poor sanitation or lack of water treatment systems), do one of the following:

   - Drink commercially bottled water from an unopened factory-sealed container.
   - Disinfect tap water by heating it to a rolling boil for 1 minute.
   - Use a filter that has been certified for cyst and oocyst removal.

2) Avoid swallowing water while swimming or recreating in pools, hot tubs, interactive fountains, lakes, rivers, springs, ponds, streams, or the ocean or drinking untreated water from lakes, rivers, streams, springs, ponds, or shallow wells.

3) Wash hands frequently with soap and clean, running water for at least 20 seconds; hands should be rubbed together to make a lather; backs of hands, between fingers, and under nails should also be scrubbed. Handwashing should occur at specific times:

   - before, during, and after preparing food
   - before eating
   - before and after caring for someone who is sick
   - after using the toilet, changing diapers, or cleaning a child who has used the toilet
   - after touching an animal, animal waste, or animal environments.

4) Prevent contact and contamination with feces during sex:

   - Use a barrier during oral-anal sex.
   - Properly wash hands immediately after handling a condom used during anal sex and after touching the anus or rectal area.

5) For additional prevention guidance, visit the CDC *Giardia* website at: https://www.cdc.gov/parasites/giardia.

11. Special considerations—

1) In the USA, giardiasis is a nationally notifiable disease.
2) Outbreaks of giardiasis affecting multiple people should be reported to CDC by state health departments. It is important to inform local, state, and federal health authorities about cases of

giardiasis so that appropriate public health responses can be taken to help control the spread of this disease.

[K. Benedict, D. Roellig]

GONOCOCCAL INFECTIONS

DISEASE	ICD-10 CODE
GENITOURINARY GONOCOCCAL INFECTION	ICD-10 A54.0–A54.2
GONOCOCCAL OPHTHALMIA NEONATORUM	ICD-10 A54.3

I. GENITOURINARY GONOCOCCAL INFECTION
(gonorrhea, gonococcal urethritis, gonococcal vulvovaginitis, gonococcal cervicitis, gonococcal bartholinitis, clap, strain, gleet, dose, GC)

1. Clinical features—A bacterial disease, limited to columnar and cuboidal epithelium, that has a varied clinical course. In males, gonococcal infection generally presents as an acute purulent urethral discharge with dysuria within 2 to 7 days after exposure. However, some gonococcal infections in males are asymptomatic. In females, infection may be asymptomatic or can manifest as abnormal vaginal discharge, vaginal bleeding after intercourse, or cervicitis. Subsequent complications of infection can include endometritis, salpingitis, pelvic peritonitis infertility, and ectopic pregnancy.

Pharyngeal and anorectal infections also occur and are often asymptomatic. However, in some instances anorectal infections may cause pruritus, tenesmus, and rectal discharge. Conjunctivitis can occur in newborns born to mothers with gonorrhea and can result in blindness if not rapidly and adequately treated.

Disseminated gonococcal infection occurs in 0.5% to 3% of untreated gonococcal infections and can result in arthritis, skin lesions, and (rarely) endocarditis and meningitis. Arthritis can produce permanent joint damage if appropriate antibiotics are not used. Recurrent disseminated infections are uncommon but can occur in persons with complement deficiency.

2. Risk groups—Men who have sex with men, commercial sex workers, socioeconomically marginalized groups, and sexually active youths, especially when sexual contact is unprotected. Individuals deficient in complement components are uniquely susceptible to recurrent disseminated infections. Infection with gonorrhea increases risk of both acquisition and transmission of human immunodeficiency virus (HIV) infection.

3. Causative agents—*Neisseria gonorrhoeae.*

4. Diagnosis—A presumptive diagnosis is made by Gram stain of urethral discharge. A definitive diagnosis is based on a bacteriologic culture on selective media (e.g., modified Thayer-Martin agar) or tests that detect gonococcal nucleic acid. Gram-negative intracellular diplococci can be considered diagnostic in male urethral smears but a culture or nucleic acid amplification test is recommended to diagnose *N. gonorrhoeae* infection in women. Culture is highly dependent on adequate specimen collection, optimal transport conditions, and proficient laboratory procedures. Nucleic acid amplification tests (NAATs) are more sensitive than culture since viable bacteria are not required and additional specimen types, such as urine, can be utilized. In cases with potential legal implications, specimens should be cultured and isolates confirmed as *N. gonorrhoeae* by biochemical as well as enzymatic tests and preserved to enable additional or repeated testing.

5. Occurrence—Worldwide, the disease affects both men and women, especially sexually active adolescents and younger adults. Prevalence is highest in communities of lower socioeconomic status. In most industrialized countries, incidence has decreased for more than 20 years, but in recent years incidence has increased and is still at unacceptably high levels. *N. gonorrhoeae* readily develops resistance to antimicrobials, through either chromosomal mutations or acquisition of plasmids. Resistance to penicillin, tetracycline, and quinolones is widespread. Isolates resistant to azithromycin have been identified in some countries and decreased susceptibility to azithromycin has been demonstrated in Europe, South America, Asia, and the western Pacific. Decreased gonococcal susceptibility to cefixime has been observed in some countries and treatment failures associated with decreased in vitro susceptibility have been documented in Japan and several countries in Europe. There have been some isolates reported with decreased susceptibility to ceftriaxone in Japan and some countries in Europe.

6. Reservoirs—Humans.

7. Incubation period—Generally 1 to 14 days; can be longer.

8. Transmission—Through contact with exudates from mucous membranes, often as a result of sexual activity. Can be transmitted perinatally. Gonorrhea in children older than 1 year is considered indicative of sexual abuse. Effective treatment ends communicability within hours. Transmission by fomites is extremely rare.

9. Treatment—

Preferred therapy	Dual therapy: • Ceftriaxone 250 mg IM as a single dose PLUS • Azithromycin 1 g PO as a single dose
	If ceftriaxone is not available[a]: • Cefixime 400 mg PO as a single dose PLUS • Azithromycin 1 g PO as a single dose
Alternative therapy options	Persons with cephalosporin or IgE-mediated penicillin allergy: • Dual therapy with gemifloxacin 320 mg PO as a single dose PLUS azithromycin 2 g PO as a single dose OR • Dual therapy with gentamicin 240 mg IM as a single dose PLUS azithromycin 2 g PO as a single dose
	Pregnant women with *Neisseria gonorrhoeae*: • Ceftriaxone 250 mg IM as a single dose PLUS • Azithromycin 1 g PO as a single dose
	Persons with DGI: • Arthritis and arthritis-dermatitis syndrome: ceftriaxone: 1 g IM or IV every 24 hours PLUS azithromycin 1 g PO daily for ≥ 7 days; can switch to PO therapy guided by antimicrobial susceptibility testing 24–48 hours after clinical improvement • Meningitis and endocarditis: ceftriaxone 1–2 g IV every 12–24 hours PLUS azithromycin 1 g PO daily (meningitis for 10–14 days; endocarditis for ≥ 4 weeks)
Special considerations and comments	• For persons with pharyngeal gonorrhea treated with an alternative therapy, a test of cure is recommended 14 days after treatment. • Reinfections are more likely than actual treatment failures. If treatment failure is suspected, retest and collect specimen for NAAT, culture, and antibiotic susceptibility testing prior to retreating; and consult an infectious diseases specialist or STI treatment expert for additional antibiotic options. • Refer recent sex partners (≤ 60 days of symptom onset) for evaluation, testing, and presumptive dual treatment; if > 60 days, treat the most recent sex partner. • DGI frequently results in petechial or pustular acral skin lesions, asymmetric polyarthralgia, tenosynovitis, or oligoarticular septic arthritis; the infection is complicated occasionally by perihepatitis and rarely by endocarditis or meningitis.

Note: DGI = disseminated gonococcal infection; IgE = immunoglobulin class E; IM = intramuscular(ly); IV = intravenous(ly); NAAT = nucleic acid amplification test; PO = oral(ly); STI = sexually transmitted infection.

[a]Not recommended for pharyngeal gonorrhea.

10. Prevention—

1) Prevention is based primarily on safe sexual practices: consistent and correct use of condoms with all partners, avoiding multiple sexual encounters or anonymous/casual sex, and mutual monogamy with a noninfected partner.

2) Patients with gonococcal infections are at increased risk of HIV infection and should be offered confidential counseling and testing.

11. Special considerations—

1) Treatment: on clinical, laboratory, or epidemiologic grounds (contacts of a diagnosed case). In the USA and Europe, the only recommended treatment regimen for uncomplicated gonococcal infections of the cervix, rectum, and urethra in adults is dual treatment that includes intramuscular (IM) therapy. In the USA, the recommended regimen is ceftriaxone 250 mg IM plus azithromycin 1 g orally (PO). In Europe, the recommended regimen is ceftriaxone 500 mg IM plus azithromycin 1 g PO. Dual treatment provides effective treatment for chlamydial coinfection, which is common among patients diagnosed with gonorrhea, and may also inhibit the emergence of antimicrobial-resistant gonococci. When ceftriaxone is not readily available, a single dose of cefixime 400 mg PO may be used in the dual treatment regimen in lieu of ceftriaxone. Patients who cannot take cephalosporins may be treated with dual treatment with single doses of gemifloxacin 320 mg PO, plus azithromycin 2 g PO or (alternatively) dual treatment with single doses of gentamicin 240 mg IM plus azithromycin 2 g PO. Gonococcal infections of the pharynx are more difficult to eliminate than infections of the urethra, cervix, or rectum. Recommended treatment for this infection includes dual treatment with ceftriaxone IM and azithromycin PO. Treatment failure following a ceftriaxone-based regimen is rare. If an alternative regimen is used for gonorrhea treatment, a test of cure should be considered. If symptoms persist, reinfection is most likely, but specimens should be obtained for culture and antimicrobial susceptibility testing to rule out treatment failure. Retesting of high-risk patients after 3 months is advisable owing to the increased risk of reinfection.

2) Reporting: case report to local health authority is required in many countries.

II. GONOCOCCAL OPHTHALMIA NEONATORUM

1. Clinical features—Acute redness and swelling of conjunctiva in 1 or both eyes, with mucopurulent or purulent discharge, typically occurring within 1 to 5 days of birth. Corneal ulcer, perforation, and blindness may occur if antimicrobial treatment is not given promptly. The gonococcus is the most serious, but not the most frequent, infectious cause of ophthalmia neonatorum. The most common infectious cause is *Chlamydia trachomatis*, which produces inclusion conjunctivitis that tends to be less acute than gonococcal conjunctivitis and usually appears 5 to 14 days after birth. Any purulent neonatal conjunctivitis should be considered gonococcal unless proven otherwise.

2. Risk groups—Newborns whose mothers are infected with *N. gonorrhoeae*.

3. Causative agents—*N. gonorrhoeae*, the gonococcus.

4. Diagnosis—Gonococci may be identified by microscopy, NAAT, or culture.

5. Occurrence—The disease is an important cause of blindness throughout the world. Occurrence varies widely according to prevalence of maternal infection, prenatal screening coverage, and use of infant eye prophylaxis at delivery.

6. Reservoirs—Infection of the maternal cervix.

7. Incubation period—Usually 1 to 5 days.

8. Transmission—Contact with the infected birth canal during childbirth. It is communicable while discharge persists if untreated and for 24 hours following initiation of specific treatment.

9. Treatment—

Preferred therapy	<ul><li>Ceftriaxone 25–50 mg/kg IV as a single dose OR</li><li>Ceftriaxone 25–50 mg/kg IM as a single dose (≤ 125 mg)</li></ul>
Alternative therapy options	Not available
Special considerations and comments	<ul><li>Ceftriaxone should be administered cautiously to hyper-bilirubinemic infants, especially those born prematurely.</li><li>Topical antibiotic therapy alone (used for prophylaxis) is inadequate and unnecessary for treatment if systemic antibiotic is administered.</li><li>Mothers of infected infants and their sexual partners should be evaluated, tested, and presumptively treated for gonorrhea.</li></ul>

Note: IM = intramuscular(ly); IV = intravenous(ly).

10. Prevention—

1) Ocular prophylaxis of all infants at birth is warranted because it can prevent sight-threatening gonococcal ophthalmia and because it is safe, easy to administer, and inexpensive (see point 3 later).

2) Prevent maternal infection (see Genitourinary Gonococcal Infection in this chapter; see also "Syphilis"). Diagnose gonorrhea in pregnant women and treat the woman and her sexual partners. Routine screening of the cervix and rectum for gonococci (by NAAT or culture) should be considered prenatally, especially in the third trimester in populations where infection is prevalent.

3) Use an established effective preparation for protection of babies' eyes within 1 hour of birth, regardless of whether they are delivered vaginally or by cesarean section. Erythromycin (0.5%) and tetracycline (1%) ophthalmic ointments are both effective options. Single-use tubes or ampoules are preferable to multiple-use tubes. Instillation of 1% silver nitrate aqueous solution is also effective and widely used but may be associated with an increased risk of chemical irritation. Silver nitrate and tetracycline ointments are no longer manufactured in the USA. Prophylaxis with 2.5% ophthalmic solution of povidone-iodine has not yet been studied adequately.

4) Infants born to mothers who have untreated gonorrhea are at high risk for infection. The recommended regimen for such infants in the absence of signs of gonococcal infection is a single dose of ceftriaxone 25–50 mg/kg intravenously or IM, not to exceed 125 mg.

11. Special considerations—Reporting: case report to local health authority is required in many countries.

Bibliography

CDC. Sexually transmitted diseases (STDs). 2015. Available at: http://www.cdc.gov/std/treatment. Accessed November 14, 2019.

International Union against Sexually Transmitted Infections. Guidelines. Available at: https://www.iusti.org/sti-information/guidelines/default.htm. Accessed November 14, 2019.

WHO. Sexual and reproductive health. Available at: http://www.who.int/topics/sexually_transmitted_infections/en. Accessed November 14, 2019.

[B. Kirkcaldy, S. St. Cyr]

GRANULOMA INGUINALE
(donovanosis)

DISEASE	ICD-10 CODE
GRANULOMA INGUINALE	ICD-10 A.58

1. Clinical features—A chronic and progressively destructive bacterial disease of the skin and mucous membranes of the external genitalia and inguinal and anal regions. One or more indurated nodules or papules lead to slowly spreading, nontender, hypertrophic, granulomatous, ulcerative, or sclerotic lesions. The lesions are characteristically nonfriable, beefy-red granulomas and extend peripherally with characteristic rolled edges that eventually form fibrous tissue. Lesions occur most commonly on warm, moist surfaces, such as the folds between the thighs, the perianal area, the scrotum, or the labia and vagina. The genitalia are involved in close to 90% of cases, the inguinal region in close to 10%, the anal region in 5% to 10%, and distant sites in 1% to 5%. Lymphadenopathy is not commonly associated with disease in adults but may be seen in children. Cervical lesions are uncommon. If neglected, the process may result in extensive destruction of genital organs and may spread by autoinoculation to other parts of the body, including bones and intra-abdominal organs. Lesions may mimic or be complicated by carcinoma.[1]

2. Risk groups—More frequently seen among males than females and among persons of lower socioeconomic status. It is predominantly seen in those aged 20 to 40 years; pediatric cases are rare. Immunity does not appear to follow infection.

3. Causative agents—The causal agent is *Klebsiella granulomatis* (*Donovania granulomatis, Calymmatobacterium granulomatis*), a Gram-negative bacillus.[2]

4. Diagnosis—Laboratory diagnosis is based on demonstration of intracytoplasmic Gram-negative, rod-shaped organisms (Donovan bodies) in Wright- or Giemsa-stained smears of granulation tissue or biopsy specimens. The presence of large infected mononuclear cells filled with deeply staining Donovan bodies is pathognomonic. Culture is not routinely available. Serologic tests are unreliable and polymerase chain reaction is available only in research settings. Syphilis should be excluded through serologic testing. *Haemophilus ducreyi* should be excluded by culture on appropriate selective media.[1]

5. Occurrence—Rare in industrialized countries but cluster outbreaks occasionally occur. Endemic in tropical and subtropical areas, such as central and northern Australia, southern India, Papua New Guinea, Guyana, and

Vietnam; occasionally in Latin America, the Caribbean islands, and central, eastern, and southern Africa.[1,2,3]

6. Reservoirs—Humans.

7. Incubation period—Variable; between 1 and 16 weeks.

8. Transmission—Poorly communicable with transmission occurring presumably by direct contact with lesions during vaginal and anal sexual activity (less commonly by oral sex); in various studies, only 20% to 65% of sexual partners were infected. Donovanosis occurs in sexually inactive individuals and the very young, suggesting that some cases are transmitted nonsexually. The period of communicability is unknown but probably lasts for the duration of open lesions. Vertical transmission may occur.[3]

9. Treatment—includes pharmacologic and surgical measures[1,2,3]:

Preferred therapy	Azithromycin 1 g PO once per week or 500 mg PO daily for ≥ 3 weeks and until all lesions have resolved completely
Alternative therapy options	• Doxycycline 100 mg PO BID for ≥ 3 weeks and until all lesions have resolved completely • Ciprofloxacin 750 mg PO BID for ≥ 3 weeks and until all lesions have resolved completely • Erythromycin base 500 mg PO QID for ≥ 3 weeks and until all lesions have resolved completely • TMP/SMX 1 double-strength (160 + 800 mg) tablet PO BID for ≥ 3 weeks and until all lesions have resolved completely
Special considerations and comments	• Addition of an aminoglycoside to the above regimens as an adjunct for lesions that are slow to respond (e.g., gentamicin 1 mg/kg IV every 8 hours). Daily IV gentamicin dosing should be considered to increase adherence given the need to treat until lesions are completely healed. • Relapse and reinfection may occur. Confirmed lesions that do not resolve with treatment should be evaluated for carcinoma. • Risk of HIV acquisition is increased. Lesions may mimic those of syphilis. Patients with suspected or confirmed disease should receive HIV and syphilis testing. • Macrolides (azithromycin or erythromycin) should be prioritized for treatment of pregnant women.

Note: BID = twice daily; HIV = human immunodeficiency virus; IV = intravenous(ly); PO = oral(ly); QID = 4 times daily; TMP/SMX = trimethoprim-sulfamethoxazole.

10. Prevention—Preventive measures should include barrier methods during sexual activity, particularly during vaginal or anal contact. Educational programs in endemic areas should stress the importance of early diagnosis and treatment. Sexual partners should be examined and considered for treatment.[1,2,3]

11. Special considerations—Reporting: a reportable disease in most states and countries.

References

1. O'Farrell N, Moi H. European guideline on donovanosis. *Int J STD AIDS.* 2016;27 (8):605–607.
2. CDC. Sexually transmitted diseases treatment guidelines. 2015. Available at: www. cdc.gov/std/treatment. Accessed November 10, 2019.
3. Australasian Society for HIV, Viral Hepatitis and Sexual Health Medicine. Australian STI management guidelines for use in primary care. Donovanosis. 2016. Available at: http://www.sti.guidelines.org.au/sexually-transmissible-infections/donovanosis. Accessed November 10, 2019.

Bibliography

CDC. Sexually transmitted diseases. Available at: www.cdc.gov/std/treatment. Accessed 14 November, 2019.
WHO. Sexual and reproductive health. Available at: https://www.who.int/reproductivehealth/topics/rtis/en. Accessed 14 November, 2019.

[M. Taylor]

HANTAVIRAL DISEASES

DISEASE	ICD-10 CODE
HEMORRHAGIC FEVER WITH RENAL SYNDROME	ICD-10 A98.5
HANTAVIRUS PULMONARY SYNDROME	ICD-10 B33.4

HEMORRHAGIC FEVER WITH RENAL SYNDROME (epidemic hemorrhagic fever, Korean hemorrhagic fever, nephropathia epidemica, HFRS), HANTAVIRUS PULMONARY SYNDROME (hantavirus cardiopulmonary syndrome, HCPS, HPS)

1. Clinical features—An acute zoonotic disease with 2 similar syndromes, which share febrile prodrome, thrombocytopenia, leukocytosis, and capillary leakage.

1) Hemorrhagic fever with renal syndrome (HFRS): characterized by abrupt onset of fever, lower back pain, varying degrees of hemorrhagic manifestations, and renal involvement. Disease is characterized by 5 clinical phases that frequently overlap: febrile, hypotensive, oliguric, diuretic, and convalescent.

   The febrile phase, which lasts 3 to 7 days, is characterized by high fever, headache, malaise, and anorexia, followed by severe abdominal or lower back pain, often accompanied by nausea and vomiting, facial flushing, petechiae, and conjunctival injection. Most cases show an elevated hematocrit, thrombocytopenia, and elevated creatinine. The hypotensive phase lasts from several hours to days and is characterized by abrupt onset of hypotension, which may progress to shock and more apparent hemorrhagic manifestations. Blood pressure returns to normal or is high in the oliguric phase (3–7 days); nausea and vomiting may persist; severe hemorrhage may occur and urinary output falls dramatically. The case-fatality rate ranges from 5% to 15% with Hantaan and Dobrava viruses and the majority of deaths occur during the hypotensive and oliguric phases. Diuresis heralds the onset of recovery in most cases, with polyuria of 3 to 6 liters per day. Convalescence takes weeks to months. Infections caused by Puumala, Saaremaa, and Seoul viruses are clinically milder with case-fatality rates of 1% or less.

2) Hantavirus cardiopulmonary syndrome (HCPS) is characterized by 4 phases: the febrile prodrome, the cardiopulmonary stage, diuresis, and convalescence. The febrile prodrome is characterized by fever, severe myalgias, back pain, headache, and gastrointestinal complaints. After several days, the febrile prodrome is followed by the abrupt onset of the cardiopulmonary stage with cough and shortness of breath secondary to noncardiogenic pulmonary edema. In severe disease, this stage progresses rapidly to severe respiratory failure and cardiogenic shock with low cardiac index. In survivors, recovery from acute illness is rapid, but full convalescence may require weeks to months. Restoration of normal lung function generally occurs, but pulmonary function abnormalities may persist in some individuals. Renal and hemorrhagic manifestations are usually absent, except in some severe cases. Milder infections without frank pulmonary edema have occurred, and antibody prevalence studies have detected serologic-positive people with no recollection of the typical disease. Sin Nombre virus and Andes virus have case-fatality rates of about 35%, and mild infections without frank pulmonary edema are uncommon. In contrast, case-fatality rates with Choclo virus infection are low

even with pulmonary involvement, and most infections appear to result in a mild febrile illness without pulmonary edema or shock.

2. Risk groups—The main human groups at risk are persons in rural populations who come into contact with rodents as part of their occupation (forestry workers, farmers) and outdoor enthusiasts (who have been found to have elevated risk of hantavirus exposure); laboratory workers processing clinical specimens or working in research laboratories; and close contacts (usually sex partners or close household contacts of persons with Andes virus infection).

3. Causative agents—Hantaviruses (a genus of the family Bunyaviridae: 3-segmented ribonucleic acid [RNA] viruses with spherical-to-oval particles, 95–110 nm in diameter). More than 25 antigenically distinguishable viral species exist, each associated primarily with a single rodent species. Very few virus isolates from humans or rodents exist, however.

1) HFRS: Hantaan, Dobrava, Puumala, Saaremaa, and Seoul viruses
2) HCPS: Andes (Argentina, Chile), Laguna Negra (Bolivia, Paraguay), Juquitiba (Brazil), Choclo (Panama), Black Creek Canal and Bayou (southeastern USA), New York-1 and Monongahela (eastern USA), and Sin Nombre (North America)

4. Diagnosis—In HCPS, most patients are hospitalized after onset of the cardiopulmonary phase, and most deaths occur within 24 to 48 hours of hospital admission and before results of serologic testing are available. Fortunately, in HCPS a presumptive clinical diagnosis may be established after onset of bilateral pulmonary infiltrates through evaluation of the complete blood count and peripheral blood smear when 4 or more of the following 5 criteria are present: (a) thrombocytopenia, (b) leukocytosis with left shift, (c) increased immunoblasts (>10% of lymphocytes), (d) lack of toxic granulation in neutrophils, and (e) hemoconcentration. In both HFRS and HCPS, almost all patients have immunoglobulin class M and most immunoglobulin class G antibodies (detectable by immunofluorescence assay, enzyme-linked immunosorbent assay, or Western blot) at the time of hospitalization.

Viral RNA may be detected in blood (preferably in the buffy coat) by conventional or real-time PCR for 1 to 3 weeks before onset of symptoms during the acute illness and for 2 to 3 months after onset of the acute illness. Virus isolation is rarely successful from humans and should not be attempted in a routine clinical laboratory (biosafety level 2). Immunohistochemistry on formalin-fixed tissues is the method of choice for diagnosis when other samples are unavailable in fatal human cases.

5. Occurrence—The availability of newer diagnostic techniques has led to increasing recognition of hantaviruses and hantaviral infections.

1) HFRS: the disease is considered a major public health problem in China and South Korea but is likely to occur more widely. Occurrence is seasonal, with most cases occurring in late fall and early winter, primarily among rural populations. In the Balkans, a severe form of the disease due to Dobrava virus affects a few hundred people annually, with case-fatality rates at least as high as those in Asia (5%–15%). Most cases there are seen during spring and early summer. Nephropathia epidemica, due to Puumala virus, is found in most of Europe, including the Balkans, and Russia west of the Ural Mountains. It is often seen in summer and in the fall and early winter. Saaremaa viruses are detected in rodents from Croatia to Estonia but human cases have mostly been described in Estonia and western Russia. Among medical research personnel and animal handlers in Asia and Europe, the disease has been traced to laboratory rats infected with Seoul virus, which has been mostly identified in captured urban rats worldwide, including in Argentina, Brazil, Thailand, and the USA; only in Asia has it been regularly associated with human disease.

2) HCPS: first recognized in the spring and summer of 1993 in southwestern USA populations, caused by Sin Nombre virus; cases have been confirmed in Canada and in many eastern and western regions of the USA. A large number of cases have been reported in South America (Argentina, Bolivia, Brazil, Chile, Panama, and Paraguay). The disease is not restricted to any age, gender, or ethnic groups. Incidence appears to coincide with the geographic distribution and population density of carrier rodents and with their level of infection.

6. Reservoirs—Each hantavirus species is generally associated with one primary rodent species, but there is evidence for host-switches without epidemiologic implications. Recently, hantaviruses have been detected in several insectivore (order Soricomorpha) species but without any evidence of human-associated diseases. Humans are accidental hosts.

1) HFRS: field rodents—*Apodemus* spp. for Hantaan, Dobrava, and Saaremaa viruses in Asia and the central European areas; *Myodes* (formerly *Clethrionomys*) spp. for Puumala virus in Western Europe and Scandinavia; *Rattus* spp. for Seoul virus (worldwide).

2) HCPS: in North America, the major reservoir of Sin Nombre virus appears to be the deer mouse, *Peromyscus maniculatus*. Antibodies have also been found in other *Peromyscus* spp., pack rats, chipmunks, and other rodents. In other regions, other hantavirus strains have been associated mainly with rodent species of the subfamily Sigmodontinae.

7. Incubation period—From 1 to 8 weeks, usually 2 to 4 weeks for HFRS. For HCPS, the usual incubation period is 3 to 4 weeks, with a range of 9 days to 8 weeks.

8. Transmission—The presumed route is through aerosol transmission from rodent excreta, although this does not explain all human cases or all forms of inter-rodent transmission. Virus occurs in urine, feces, and saliva of persistently infected asymptomatic rodents, with maximal virus concentration in the lungs. Indoor exposure in closed, poorly ventilated homes, vehicles, and outbuildings with visible rodent infestation is especially important. Seasonal occupational and recreational activities probably influence the risk of exposure to Puumala virus and other hantaviruses, as do climate and other ecologic factors, on rodent population densities. Household transmission (between close contacts including sex partners) and rare nosocomial transmission of Andes virus have been documented in Argentina and Chile and are associated with close, direct contact. In other settings no human-to-human transmission has been recorded. The protection and duration of immunity conferred by previous infection is unknown but antibodies seem to persist for several years. Reinfection has never been shown to occur in confirmed recovered patients.

9. Treatment—Treatment is supportive and may include hemodialysis in HFRS and venoarterial extracorporeal membrane oxygenation (ECMO) in HCPS. Inotropes such as epinephrine and norepinephrine should be used for hypotension, and fluid resuscitation should be avoided. Venoarterial ECMO appears to reduce mortality in patients with severe cardiogenic shock and/or refractory respiratory failure. Whenever feasible, patients with suspected HCPS should be transferred immediately to an ECMO center, where patients with a presumptive (see criteria above) or confirmed diagnosis should have elective insertion of venous and arterial vascular sheaths concurrent or prior to intubation. Intravenous ribavirin is ineffective in HCPS, but one controlled trial in China showed benefit in patients with HFRS.

10. Prevention—

1) Exclude rodents from houses and other buildings.
2) Store human and animal food in rodent-proof containers.
3) Minimize exposure to wild rodents and their excreta in enzootic areas.
4) Disinfect rodent-contaminated areas by spraying a disinfectant solution (e.g., diluted bleach) prior to cleaning. Do not sweep or vacuum rat-contaminated areas; use a wet mop or towels moistened with disinfectant. As far as possible, ventilate potentially rodent-infected buildings that have been closed for some time prior to entry; avoid inhalation of dust by using approved respirators when cleaning previously unoccupied areas. People working

with potentially infected rodents during ecologic studies should wear appropriate protective equipment (based on risk assessment).

5) Trap rodents and dispose of them using suitable precautions. Live trapping is not recommended.

6) Laboratory rodent colonies, particularly *Rattus norvegicus*, must be tested to ensure freedom from asymptomatic hantavirus infection.

7) Health care workers should always use universal protection when managing patients.

8) Formalin-inactivated vaccines available in South Korea and China against Hantaan and Seoul viruses may have some preventive effect, but their efficacy has not been rigorously evaluated.

11. Special considerations—Reporting: suspected cases should be reported to the local health authorities and confirmed cases are notifiable in several countries. Hantaviruses are not listed as agents that must be assessed in terms of the potential to cause public health emergencies of international concern under the International Health Regulations.

[G. Mertz]

HELICOBACTER PYLORI INFECTION

DISEASE	ICD-10 CODE
HELICOBACTER PYLORI INFECTION	ICD-10 B96.81

A bacterial infection by *Helicobacter pylori* causing acute and chronic gastritis, primarily in the antrum of the stomach, and peptic ulcer disease.

1. Clinical features—Most of those infected with *H. pylori* remain asymptomatic, and without treatment infection is often lifelong. The key pathophysiologic event in *H. pylori* infection is initiation and continuance of an inflammatory response. Development of atrophy and intestinal metaplasia of the gastric mucosa is strongly associated with *H. pylori* infection. Only a minority of those infected develop duodenal ulcer disease. Although individuals infected with the organism have histologic evidence of gastritis, most are asymptomatic. *H. pylori* infection is usually acquired during childhood and atrophy of the gastric mucosa progresses during aging. Cross-sectional serologic studies demonstrate increasing prevalence with increasing age.

Common symptoms include burning discomfort in the upper abdomen, accompanied by bloating and abdominal pain, which may be more intense when the stomach is empty. Patients complain of loss of appetite and there may be unintentional weight loss. *H. pylori* infection can lead to gastritis, peptic ulcer disease, and atrophy of the gastric endothelium transitioning to metaplasia, leading to gastric carcinoma and mucosa-associated lymphoid tissue (MALT).

Epidemiologic and eradication studies have demonstrated a causal relationship between *H. pylori* infections and endothelial dysfunction, leading to vascular diseases. *H. pylori* infection has also been associated with iron deficiency and iron deficiency anemia. There is evidence, from small randomized and nonrandomized trials, for sustained improvement in platelet counts after eradication of *H. pylori* infection in a population of adult patients with idiopathic thrombocytopenic purpura (ITP). The evidence is less compelling for children with ITP. *H. pylori* infection is also an independent risk factor for nonsteroidal anti-inflammatory drug (NSAID)-induced ulcers. Eradication of *H. pylori* infection before starting NSAIDs may reduce the development of ulcers and risk of bleeding. *H. pylori* is also implicated in the development of adenocarcinoma of the esophagus and nonulcer dyspepsia.

Patients with alarm symptoms should be referred for prompt endoscopy; those without alarm symptoms can be tested for *H. pylori* and, if positive, treated.

2. Risk groups—*H. pylori* causes one of the most common chronic bacterial infections affecting humans. It is prevalent more commonly in certain racial and ethnic groups. *H. pylori* is reported to be genetically extremely variable and this heterogenicity may be involved in its ability to cause different diseases and chronic infections. Low socioeconomic status, especially in childhood, is associated with infection. It is more common in African-Americans, Latinos, and American Indians. Its prevalence in immigrant communities may be between 70% and 80%. It is generally thought that a variety of cofactors may be required for the development of disease. No immunity is apparent after infection. Risk factors for acquiring the infection include low socioeconomic status, increasing number of siblings, and having an infected parent, especially an infected mother. Apart from intrafamilial spread, the infection may also be transmitted through contaminated water supplies, particularly in developing countries.

3. Causative agents—*H. pylori* is a Gram-negative, curved bacterium, which is positive for catalase, oxidase, and urease.

4. Diagnosis—Diagnostic methods are categorized according to whether or not an endoscopy is necessary and whether the diagnosis is to be set before or after an eradication treatment. Biopsy-based tests include histologic evaluation, culture, polymerase chain reaction (PCR), and the rapid urease test, all of which are performed on tissue obtained during endoscopy. Alternatively, the urea breath test, serology, and stool antigen test can be performed as noninvasive procedures. Serum antibody tests may remain positive for months after treatment. The sensitivity and specificity of different tests depend on the age of the patients and the disease they present. Testing for *H. pylori* infection is indicated in patients with dyspeptic symptoms; a past history of documented peptic ulcer disease; gastric cancer; or gastric MALT lymphoma.

Traditionally, detection of antibiotic-resistant *H. pylori* has been performed on agar cultures from gastric biopsies as it is the only method to determine antimicrobial susceptibility to all antibiotics. Unfortunately, this is hampered by limitations such as low sensitivity. Molecular techniques are able to detect the different mutations that can confer resistance to antibiotics. PCR testing is an alternative to conventional *H. pylori* detection because of high sensitivity and accuracy.

5. Occurrence—*H. pylori* was discovered in 1983 and is estimated to have infected more than half of the world's population. However, this varies, with prevalence in lower socioeconomic groups being around 80% while in the USA, Canada, Japan, and Western Europe it may be closer to 25% to 30%. Most people have no symptoms; some people may be born with more resistance to the harmful effects of *H. pylori*.

6. Reservoirs—Mainly humans, though recently *H. pylori* has been found in other primates. Isolation of *H. pylori* from nongastric sites, such as oral secretions and stools, has been reported but is infrequent.

7. Incubation period—Data collected from volunteers who ingested 10^6 to 10^9 organisms indicate that the onset of gastritis occurs within 5 to 10 days. No other information about inoculum size or incubation period is available.

8. Transmission—The mode of transmission has not been clearly established but infection is almost certainly a result of ingesting organisms. Transmission is presumed, but not yet confirmed, to be either oral-oral and/or fecal-oral or from inadequately treated drinking water. As infection may be lifelong, those infected are potentially infectious for life. It is not known whether acutely infected patients are more infectious than those with long-standing infection. There is some evidence that persons with low stomach acidity may be more infectious.

9. Treatment—Once infected, the infection is virtually lifelong in the absence of treatment. All patients with a positive test of active infection with *H. pylori* should be offered treatment, so the critical issue is which patients should be tested for the infection.

At present, all patients with active peptic ulcer disease, a past history of peptic ulcer disease (unless previous cure of *H. pylori* infection has been documented), MALT, or a history of endoscopic resection of early gastric cancer should be tested for *H. pylori* infection. Those testing positive should be offered eradication treatment. In patients with uninvestigated dyspepsia who are younger than 60 years and without alarm features, nonendoscopic testing for *H. pylori* infection is a consideration; if positive, eradication therapy should be offered.

H. pylori antibiotic resistance is the primary hurdle to achieving eradication. Conventional treatment regimens are declining in efficacy as a result of drug-resistant strains and nonadherence to therapy. The most common antibiotics still used in *H. pylori* treatment are metronidazole, clarithromycin, amoxicillin, tetracycline, and levofloxacin. Resistance rates vary widely by geography and therapy should be tailored per regional resistance patterns. Culture-guided therapies are now recommended as they significantly lower risk of treatment failure compared with empiric therapy. Triple standard therapy containing clarithromycin is recommended worldwide as first-line treatment. However, the eradication rate has been declining.

Knowledge of local antibiotic resistance is crucial. In regions with clarithromycin and metronidazole resistance greater than 15%, a regimen including clarithromycin should not be used. Further information, such as culture and susceptibility, should be sought when biopsy specimens are available. Previously, empirically tailored triple therapy was suggested with 2 antibiotics (such as amoxicillin, owing to its low rate of resistance, and either metronidazole or clarithromycin) combined with a proton pump inhibitor (PPI). However, a better outcome can be achieved with clarithromycin, amoxicillin, and metronidazole combined with a PPI for 14 days. For the updated guidelines, see treatment table later.

PPI plus amoxicillin plus metronidazole plus clarithromycin or traditional bismuth quadruple therapy is recommended. In a recent study, patients were treated with a single pill containing bismuth 140 mg, metronidazole 125 mg, and tetracycline 125 mg. Three capsules 4 times a day plus omeprazole 20 mg or 40 mg twice a day, given for 10 days, resulted in an *H. pylori* eradication rate of 94.7%. This new bismuth-containing quadruple therapy appears as, or more, effective than either traditional first-line treatment or rescue therapy. Rifabutin may be used but should be limited to patients who fail at least 3 previous regimens. Probiotics may be added to reduce side effects and increase eradication rates.

A new drug, vonoprazan, a potassium-competitive acid blocker, has recently been approved in Japan for clarithromycin-resistant strains of *H. pylori*. Its use could increase eradication rates by raising the intragastric pH and thus increasing bacterial antibiotic susceptibility.

Drug	Clarithromycin-based therapy:
	• Amoxicillin 1 g PO BID PLUS • Clarithromycin 500 mg PO BID PLUS • Metronidazole 500 mg PO BID PLUS • Omeprazole 20 mg PO BID

(Continued)

(Continued)

Bismuth-based therapy	• Omeprazole 20 mg PO BID PLUS • Bismuth subcitrate (420 mg in the USA as part of the Pylera[a] combination pill) PLUS • Tetracycline 500 mg PO QID PLUS • Metronidazole 500 mg PO TID or QID
Duration	The longer duration of 14 days is now recommended for the above regimens.
Special considerations and comments	• Other regimens are available as well. • Clarithromycin-based triple therapy is similar to the quadruple therapy above but provides a choice of amoxicillin *or* metronidazole.

Note: BID = twice daily; PO = oral(ly); QID = 4 times daily; TID = thrice daily.
[a]Pylera combination pill contains bismuth, tetracycline, and metronidazole.

10. Prevention—Persons living in uncrowded, clean environments are less likely to acquire *H. pylori.* Socioeconomic factors seem to affect the prevalence of the bacterium in the population. Appropriate treatment of drinking water is important, as is proper disinfection of gastroscopes, pH electrodes, and other instruments entering the stomach. Gastric cancer is one of the most common causes of cancer death worldwide, and it is now generally accepted that *H. pylori* is one of the most important underlying causes.

11. Special considerations—None.

[M. Gilani]

HEPATITIS, VIRAL

DISEASE	ICD-10 CODE
HEPATITIS A	ICD-10 B15
HEPATITIS B	ICD-10 B16
HEPATITIS C	ICD-10 B17.1
HEPATITIS D	ICD-10 B17.0
HEPATITIS E	ICD-10 B17.2
HEPATOCELLULAR CARCINOMA	ICD-10 C22.0

Several distinct infections are grouped as the viral hepatitides; they are primarily hepatotrophic and have similar clinical presentations but differ in etiology and in some epidemiologic, immunologic, clinical, and pathologic characteristics. Their prevention and control vary greatly. Each is presented later in a separate section.

I. HEPATITIS A (infectious hepatitis, epidemic hepatitis, epidemic jaundice, catarrhal jaundice, type A hepatitis, HA)

1. Clinical features—The disease varies in clinical severity from asymptomatic illness to a severely disabling disease lasting several months. In most developing countries, infection manifests as an asymptomatic or mild illness in childhood. Onset of illness in adults in nonendemic areas is usually abrupt, with fever, malaise, anorexia, nausea, and abdominal discomfort, followed within a few days by jaundice. Dark urine (bilirubinuria) and pale stools may be observed. Prolonged, relapsing hepatitis for up to 1 year occurs in 15% of cases; no chronic infection is known to occur. Convalescence is often prolonged. In general, severity increases with age but complete recovery without sequelae or recurrences is the rule. Reported case-fatality rate is normally low, at 0.1% to 0.3%; it can reach 1.8% for adults older than 50 years.

2. Risk groups—

1) Children living in high-endemicity areas.
2) Children and adults living in intermediate-endemicity areas.
3) Susceptible persons traveling to, or working in, hepatitis A virus (HAV)–endemic countries.
4) Injection drug users.
5) Close personal contacts (e.g., household, sexual) of hepatitis A patients. Cases have resulted from contact with newly adopted children from HAV-endemic countries.
6) Those working with infected primates or with HAV in research laboratories.
7) Persons with chronic liver disease who have an elevated risk of death from fulminant hepatitis A. Homologous immunity after infection probably lasts for life.

3. Causative agents—HAV, a 27-nm picornavirus (positive-strand ribonucleic acid [RNA] virus). It has been classified as a member of the family Picornaviridae.

4. Diagnosis—Mild infections may be detectable only through laboratory tests of liver function. Demonstration of immunoglobulin class M (IgM) antibodies against hepatitis A virus (IgM anti-HAV) in the serum of acutely or recently ill patients establishes the diagnosis; antibodies become detectable

5 to 10 days after exposure. If laboratory tests are not available, epidemiologic evidence may provide support for the diagnosis. HAV RNA can be detected in blood and stools of most persons during the acute phase of infection through nucleic acid amplification methods but these are not generally used for diagnostic purposes.

5. Occurrence—Worldwide; geographic areas can be characterized by high, intermediate, or low levels of endemicity. In areas of high endemicity, environmental sanitation is generally poor; infection is common and occurs at an early age. In some areas of Africa and Asia, more than 90% of the general population has serologic evidence of prior HAV infection versus a rate of 33% in industrialized countries. In these high-endemicity areas, adults are usually immune and outbreaks are uncommon. In many parts of the world that have formerly been highly endemic, improved sanitation has decreased the rate of HAV infection and endemicity has become intermediate. In these areas, young adults are susceptible and the frequency of outbreaks is increasing. Regions of intermediate endemicity include China and countries in South America, Central and Southeast Asia, and the Middle East. In most industrialized countries, endemicity is low and outbreaks rare.

6. Reservoirs—Humans; rarely, chimpanzees and other primates.

7. Incubation period—Average 28 to 30 days (range, 15–50 days).

8. Transmission—Person to person by the fecal-oral route. Levels of endemicity are related to hygienic and sanitary conditions. The virus is found in feces, reaches peak levels 1 to 2 weeks before the onset of symptoms, and diminishes rapidly after liver dysfunction or symptoms appear, which is concurrent with the appearance of circulating antibodies to HAV. Because most children have asymptomatic or unrecognized infections, they play an important role in HAV transmission and serve as a source of infection for others. Maximum infectivity is believed to occur during the latter half of the incubation period and continues for a few days after onset of jaundice (or during peak aminotransferase activity in anicteric cases). Most cases are probably noninfectious after the first week of jaundice, although prolonged viral excretion (i.e., 6 months) has been documented in infants and children. Chronic shedding of HAV in feces does not occur.

9. Treatment—There is no specific treatment against HAV. The most effective tools to prevent HAV include vaccination and attention to hygienic practices. Passive immunization, though limited by expense, may be indicated for some patients, particularly those at risk of poor outcome after HAV infection (e.g., chronic liver disease) or those incapable of mounting an adequate immune response to vaccine.

10. Prevention—

1) Educate the public about proper sanitation and personal hygiene, with special emphasis on careful handwashing and sanitary disposal of feces.

2) Provide proper water treatment and distribution systems and sewage disposal.

3) If preferred, exposure immunization: both inactivated and live attenuated hepatitis A vaccines are highly immunogenic and generate long-lasting protection against hepatitis A in children and adults. Protection against clinical hepatitis A begins as early as 14 to 21 days after a single dose of vaccine. A second dose is regarded as necessary for long-term protection. Depending on the level of HAV endemicity, it may in some cases be cost-effective to screen for HAV antibody prior to immunization.

   - Hepatitis A vaccination should be integrated into the national immunization schedule for children aged 12 months and older based on hepatitis A incidence, on a change from high to intermediate endemicity (i.e., transitional), or on consideration of cost-effectiveness. WHO does not, however, recommend its routine use in highly endemic countries where almost all persons are infected with HAV in childhood situations.
   - Hepatitis A vaccine should be considered for use in other risk populations as well.
   - All susceptible travelers to intermediate- or high-endemicity areas should be vaccinated prior to departure, possibly together with immunoglobulin (IG) if departure takes place in less than 1 week.

4) Raw oysters, clams, and other shellfish are risky for a variety of infections, including hepatitis. Preferably, these items should be heated to a temperature of 85°C to 90°C (185°F-194°F) for 4 minutes or steamed for 90 seconds before eating. In endemic areas, travelers should consume only boiled and still hot or bottled beverages and well-cooked food served hot.

5) Raw vegetables and fruits washed with contaminated water or prepared by an infectious food handler are also a risk. Raw vegetables and fruits should always be washed with clean water or peeled.

11. Special considerations—

1) Reporting: report to local health authority is obligatory in some countries.

2) Epidemic measures:

- Determine mode of transmission (person-to-person or common vehicle) through epidemiologic investigation; identify the population exposed. Eliminate common sources of infection.
- Make special efforts to improve sanitary and hygienic practices to eliminate fecal contamination of food and water.
- Outbreaks in institutions may warrant mass prophylaxis with hepatitis A vaccine or IG.

3) Disaster implications: hepatitis A is a potential problem in large collections of susceptible people with overcrowding, inadequate sanitation, and access to clean water; if cases occur, increase efforts to improve sanitation and safety of water supplies. Mass administration of hepatitis A vaccine, which should be carefully planned, is not a substitute for environmental measures.

II. HEPATITIS B (type B hepatitis, serum hepatitis, homologous serum jaundice, Australia antigen hepatitis, HB)

1. Clinical features—Fewer than 10% of children and 30% to 50% of adults with acute hepatitis B virus (HBV) infection show icteric disease: disease is often milder and anicteric in children, while in infants it is usually asymptomatic. In those with clinical illness, the onset is usually insidious, with anorexia, vague abdominal discomfort, nausea, and vomiting; sometimes, patients also have arthralgia and rash, often progressing to jaundice. Fever may be absent or mild. Severity ranges from unapparent cases detectable only by liver function tests to fulminant, fatal disease characterized by acute hepatic necrosis. The case-fatality rate is about 1%; higher in those older than 40 years. Fulminant HBV infection may also occur during pregnancy and among newborns of infected mothers.

After acute HBV infection, the risk of developing chronic infection varies inversely with age; chronic HBV infection occurs among about 90% of infants infected at birth, 20% to 50% of children infected between age 1 and 5 years, and 1% to 10% of persons infected as older children and adults. Chronic HBV infection is also common in persons with immunodeficiency. Persons with chronic infection may or may not have a history of clinical hepatitis. Those with active chronic HBV infection have elevated aminotransferases; biopsy findings range from normal to severe necro-inflammatory hepatitis, with or without cirrhosis. An estimated 15% to 25% of persons with chronic HBV infection die prematurely of either cirrhosis or hepatocellular carcinoma (HCC). Approximately 50% of HCC cases globally are attributable to chronic HBV infection.

2. Risk groups—Sexual partners and household contacts of hepatitis B surface antigen (HBsAg)-positive persons, including men who have sex with men; persons with a history of injection drug use; hemodialysis patients; inmates of juvenile detention facilities, prisons, and jails; health care and public safety workers who perform tasks involving contact with blood or blood-contaminated bodily fluids; clients and staff of institutions for the developmentally disabled who are bitten by patients; those diagnosed as having recently acquired a sexually transmitted disease and those who have a history of sexual activity with more than 1 partner in the previous 6 months; international travelers who plan to spend more than 6 months in areas with intermediate-to-high rates of chronic HBV infection (> 2%) and who will have close contact with the local population; and persons with diabetes who require blood glucose monitoring and other chronic conditions requiring frequent injections.

In the past, recipients of blood products were at high risk. In countries where pretransfusion screening of blood for HBsAg is performed and where pooled blood clotting factors (especially antihemophilic factor) are processed to destroy the virus, this risk has been virtually eliminated; however, it is still present in many developing countries.

3. Causative agents—HBV, a hepadnavirus, is a 42-nm partially double-stranded deoxyribonucleic acid (DNA) virus composed of a 27-nm nucleocapsid core (hepatitis B core antigen [HBcAg]), surrounded by an outer lipoprotein coat containing the HBsAg. HBsAg is antigenically heterogeneous, with a common antigen (designated "a") and 2 pairs of mutually exclusive antigens (d, y, w [including several subdeterminants], and r), resulting in 4 major subtypes: adw, ayw, adr, and ayr. The distribution of subtypes varies geographically; because of the common "a" determinant, protection against one subtype appears to confer protection against the other subtypes and no differences in clinical features have been related to subtype. Genotype classification based on sequencing of genetic material has been introduced and is becoming the standard: HBV is currently classified into 8 main genotypes (A–H). HBV genotypes are associated with the modes of HBV transmission (vertical vs. horizontal) and with the risk of certain outcomes of chronic infection, such as cirrhosis and HCC. In the North American Arctic, HBV genotype F is associated with HCC in young children as well as in adults younger than 30 years. In Asia and the Arctic, HBV genotype C has also been associated with a significantly higher risk of HCC than other genotypes.

4. Diagnosis—Demonstration in serum of specific antigens and/or antibodies confirms diagnosis. Three clinically useful antigen-antibody systems have been identified for hepatitis B:

1) HBsAg and antibody to HBsAg (anti-HBs)
2) HBcAg and antibody to HBcAg (anti-HBc)
3) Hepatitis B e antigen (HBeAg) and antibody to HBeAg (anti-HBe)

Commercial kits are available for all markers except HBcAg. HBsAg can be detected in serum from several weeks before onset of symptoms to days, weeks, or months after onset; it is present in serum during acute infections and persists in chronic infections. The presence of HBsAg indicates that the person is infectious. Anti-HBc appears at the onset of illness and persists indefinitely. Demonstration of anti-HBc in serum indicates HBV infection, current or past; high titers of IgM anti-HBc occur during acute infection—IgM anti-HBc usually disappears within 6 months but can persist in some cases of chronic hepatitis. The presence of HBeAg is associated with relatively high infectivity. Protective immunity follows infection if antibodies to HBsAg (anti-HBs) develop and HBsAg is negative.

5. Occurrence—Worldwide; endemic in many countries. WHO estimates that more than 2 billion persons have been infected with HBV globally (including 240 million chronically infected). Each year, approximately 600,000 persons die as a result of HBV infection. In countries where HBV is highly endemic (HBsAg prevalence ≥ 8%), most infections occur during infancy and early childhood. Where HBV endemicity is intermediate (HBsAg prevalence from 2% to 7%), infections occur commonly in all age groups, although the high rate of chronic infection is primarily maintained by transmission during infancy and early childhood. Where endemicity is low (HBsAg prevalence 2%), most infections occur in young adults, especially through sexual contact and injection drug use. Even in countries with low HBV endemicity, a high proportion of chronic infections may be acquired during childhood because the development of chronic infection is age dependent. Almost all of these infections would be prevented by perinatal vaccination against hepatitis B of all newborns or infants.

6. Reservoirs—Humans. Chimpanzees are susceptible but an animal reservoir in nature has not been recognized. Closely related hepadnaviruses are found in woodchucks, ducks, ground squirrels, and other animals, such as snow leopards and German herons; none cause disease in humans.

7. Incubation period—Usually 45 to 180 days; average 60 to 90 days. As short as 2 weeks to the appearance of HBsAg and rarely as long as 6 to 9 months; variation is related in part to amount of virus in the inoculum, mode of transmission, and host factors.

8. Transmission—Occurs by percutaneous and mucosal exposure to infective bodily fluids. Since HBV is stable on environmental surfaces for at least 7 days, indirect inoculation of HBV can occur via inanimate objects. Fecal-oral or vector-borne transmission has not been demonstrated.

Body substances capable of transmitting HBV include blood and blood products; saliva (although no outbreaks of HBV infection due to saliva alone have been documented); cerebrospinal fluid; peritoneal, pleural, pericardial, and synovial fluid; amniotic fluid; semen and vaginal secretions; any other bodily fluid containing blood; and unfixed tissues and organs. The presence of HBeAg or viral DNA (HBV DNA $\times 10^5$ copies/mL) indicates high virus titer and higher infectivity of these fluids.

Major modes of HBV transmission include sexual or close household contact with an infected person, perinatal mother-to-infant transmission, and injection drug use (sharing syringes and needles either directly or through contamination of drug preparation equipment). Contaminated and inadequately sterilized syringes and needles have resulted in outbreaks of hepatitis B among patients; this risk has been decreased as a major mode of transmission worldwide with the introduction of auto-destructing needles and syringes. Nosocomial exposures—such as transfusion of blood or blood products, hemodialysis, use of meters and lancets for glucose monitoring, insulin pens, acupuncture, and needlestick or other sharps injuries sustained by hospital personnel—have all resulted in HBV transmission. Rare transmission to patients from HBsAg-positive health care workers has been documented. Outbreaks have been reported among patients in dialysis centers in many countries through failure to adhere to recommended infection control practices against transmission of HBV and other bloodborne pathogens in these settings. IG, heat-treated plasma protein fraction, albumin, and fibrinolysin are considered safe. In the past, outbreaks have been traced to tattoo parlors, acupuncturists, and barbers.

Perinatal transmission is common, especially when HBV-infected mothers are also HBeAg-positive (rate of transmission 70%) or if they are highly viremic.

All persons who are HBsAg-positive are potentially infectious. Blood from experimentally inoculated volunteers has been shown to be infective weeks before the onset of first symptoms and to remain infective through the acute clinical course of disease. The infectivity of chronically infected persons varies from high (HBeAg-positive, HBV DNA $\times 10^5$ copies/mL) to modest (anti–HBe-positive).

Any parenteral or mucosal exposure to infected blood represents a potential risk for acquisition of hepatitis B and accounts for the 100 times more efficient transmission of HBV compared with human immunodeficiency virus (HIV) after needlestick exposure.

9. Treatment—

Drug	
	• PegIFN α-2a: for patients with chronic infection who desire time-limited therapy; NOT for patients with acute infection or with decompensated or compensated cirrhosis with portal hypertension. • Nucleoside/nucleotide agents (e.g., entecavir monotherapy). For patients with chronic infection, including those with liver disease; current model is prolonged (years) or lifelong therapy.

(Continued)

(Continued)

Dose	• PegIFN α-2a 180 µg SQ once weekly for 48 weeks • Entecavir 0.5 mg PO once daily; for patients with decompensated liver disease, give 1.0 mg PO daily
Route	Not applicable
Alternative drug	• PegIFN α-2a alternative: standard interferon • Entecavir alternative: tenofovir (tenofovir alafenamide preferred over tenofovir dosoproxil fumarate); lamivudine
Duration	PegIFN α-2a for 48 weeks
Special considerations and comments	**Acute infection:** Treatment of acute HBV is mainly supportive. Patients with encephalopathy, coagulopathy, significant comorbidities, and poor functional status are candidates for hospitalization. Rarely, patients with acute HBV are candidates for nucleoside/nucleotide therapy if severe or protracted illness is present.
	Chronic infection: Choice of nucleoside/nucleotide depends upon prior exposure to this class of drugs. Resistance testing may be indicated. Combination therapy, or added therapy based on viral response, may be considered.

Note: HBV = hepatitis B virus; PegIFN = peginterferon; PO = oral(ly); SQ = subcutaneous(ly).

10. Prevention—

1) Vaccination: effective hepatitis B vaccines are available. Vaccines licensed in different parts of the world may have varying dosages and schedules. Among persons vaccinated as children or adults, vaccine-induced immunity lasts for at least 20 years and may be lifelong. Vaccine-induced immunity among persons vaccinated at birth may be less sustained; however, booster injections are not recommended for immunocompetent persons vaccinated at any age. Several combined vaccines (e.g., hepatitis A and B and tetra- and pentavalent vaccines) have been licensed and show comparable efficacy.

- The current WHO hepatitis B prevention strategy is routine universal newborn or infant immunization. The greatest fall in incidence and prevalence of hepatitis B is in countries with high vaccine coverage at birth or in infancy. Immunization of successive infant cohorts produces a highly immune population and suffices to interrupt transmission. Combined passive-active immunoprophylaxis with hepatitis B IG and vaccine to prevent perinatal HBV transmission from HBsAg-positive mothers is preferred to vaccine alone in newly instituted routine vaccination programs but is expensive and not available in all countries.

- In countries with high HBV endemicity, routine infant immunization rapidly eliminates transmission because virtually all chronic infections are acquired among young children. Where HBV endemicity is low or intermediate, immunizing infants alone will not substantially lower disease incidence for about 15 years because most infections occur among adolescents and young adults; vaccine strategies for older children, adolescents, and adults may be desirable. In addition, immunization strategies can be targeted to high-risk groups, which account for most cases among adolescents and adults.
- Testing to exclude adolescents or adults with preexisting anti-HBs or anti-HBc is not required prior to immunization but may be considered as a potential cost-saving method in countries, or among high-risk populations, where the level of preexisting infection is high and screening is less costly than vaccination.
- Persons at high risk should routinely receive preexposure hepatitis B immunization.
- Pregnancy is not a contraindication for receiving hepatitis B vaccine.

2) Single-use, disposable syringes and needles (including acupuncture needles), and lancets for finger puncture, should be used whenever possible. Glucose monitoring equipment and insulin pens should not be shared. A sterile syringe and needle are essential for each individual receiving skin tests, parenteral inoculations, or venipuncture. Aseptic sanitary practices in tattoo parlors, including proper disposal of sharp or cutting tools, should be enforced; traditional tattooing and scarring practices should be discouraged.

3) Blood banks should test all donated blood for HBsAg with sensitive tests and reject as donors all persons with a history of viral hepatitis, those who have a history of injection drug use, those who show evidence of drug addiction, or those who have received a blood transfusion or tattoo within the preceding 6 months. Avoid using paid donors; limit administration of unscreened whole blood or potentially hazardous blood products to those in life-threatening need of such therapeutic measures.

4) Maintain surveillance for all cases of posttransfusion hepatitis; keep a register of all people who donated blood for each case. Notify blood banks of potential carriers so that future donations may be identified promptly.

5) HBV infection alone should not disqualify infected persons from the practice or study of medicine, dentistry, or allied health. Many countries have developed recommendations applicable to HBV-infected health care providers and these should be consulted. For instance, in the USA, recent guidelines from the Advisory Committee on Immunization Practices recommend the following: no pre-notification of patients of the HBV infection status of health care providers or students; use of HBV DNA serum levels rather than HBeAg status to monitor infectivity; and, for those health care professionals performing exposure-prone procedures such as certain types of surgery, counsel and advice should be sought from an expert review panel regarding in what circumstances—if any—they may continue to perform these procedures.

11. Special considerations—

1) Reporting: official report obligatory in some countries.
2) Epidemic measures: institute strict aseptic techniques and universal precautions. When 2 or more cases occur in association with some common exposure, search for additional cases. Consider vaccination of susceptible persons at risk for exposure. If a plasma-derived product is implicated, withdraw the lot from use and trace all recipients of the same lot when searching for additional cases. Information on the investigation and management of hepatitis B outbreaks in particular settings can be found at: http://www.cdc.gov/hepatitis.

III. HEPATITIS C (type C hepatitis; non-A, non-B hepatitis)

1. Clinical features—Onset is usually insidious, with anorexia, vague abdominal discomfort, nausea, and vomiting; progression to jaundice is less frequent than with hepatitis B. While only 20% to 30% of acute infections are symptomatic, 75% to 85% of acute infections become chronic. Reinfection may occur among persons with previous, resolved infections and among those with chronic infection. Of chronically infected persons, about 5% to 20% develop cirrhosis over a period of 20 to 30 years and 1% to 5% will die from the consequence of chronic infection (i.e., from cirrhosis and HCC).

2. Risk groups—

1) People who received injections with nonsterilized needles and syringes in health care settings.
2) Present or past injection drug users.
3) Recipients of unscreened donated blood, blood products, and organs.

4) People who received a blood product for clotting problems made before 1987.

5) Hemodialysis patients or persons who spent many years on dialysis for kidney failure.

6) People who received body piercing or tattoos done with nonsterile instruments.

7) People with known exposures to the hepatitis C virus (HCV), such as:

- Health care workers injured by needlesticks
- Recipients of blood or organs from a donor who tested positive for HCV
- People infected with HIV
- Men who have sex with men
- History of, or current, incarceration
- Children born to mothers infected with HCV.

3. Causative agents—HCV is an enveloped RNA virus classified as a separate genus (*Hepacivirus*) in the Flaviviridae family. At least 6 different genotypes and approximately 100 subtypes of HCV exist. Evidence is limited regarding differences in clinical features, disease outcome, or progression to cirrhosis or HCC among persons with different genotypes. However, differences do exist in responses to antiviral therapy according to HCV genotype.

4. Diagnosis—Detection of antibody to HVC (anti-HCV) and HCV RNA. Tests that detect antibodies include the enzyme immunoassay (EIA), the enhanced chemiluminescence immunoassay, and the recombinant immunoblot assay. These tests do not distinguish between acute, chronic, or resolved infection. EIA tests are suitable for screening at-risk populations. A negative EIA test suffices to exclude a diagnosis of chronic HCV infection in immunocompetent patients. Immunoblot assays are sometimes used as a supplemental assay for persons screened in nonclinical settings and in persons with a positive EIA who test negative for HCV RNA.

Acute or chronic HCV infection in a patient with a positive EIA test should be confirmed by detection of the presence of HCV RNA in the serum using a sensitive assay. Target amplification techniques using polymerase chain reaction (PCR), transcription-mediated amplification, and signal amplification techniques (branched DNA) may be used to measure HCV RNA levels. Among persons with possible recent HCV exposure, a single positive qualitative assay for HCV RNA confirms active HCV replication, but a single negative assay does not exclude viremia and may reflect a transient decline in viral level below the level of detection of the assay. A follow-up HCV RNA detection test should be performed to confirm the absence of active HCV replication in such persons. Among persons without suspicion of recent exposure who are undergoing routine screening, a single negative HCV RNA assay may be sufficient to exclude chronic infection. Quantitative determination of HCV RNA levels and of HCV genotype provides information on the likelihood of response to treatment among patients undergoing antiviral therapy. Liver biopsy can provide direct histologic assessment of liver injury due to HCV but cannot be used to diagnose HCV infection. Noninvasive serum markers (e.g., aspartate aminotransferase-to-platelet ratio index) may sometimes be used to provide an indirect histologic assessment.

In some countries, HCV point-of-care assays have been licensed that can provide results in less than 1 hour, using venous and finger-stick blood specimens.

5. Occurrence—Worldwide. HCV prevalence is directly related to the prevalence of persons who routinely share injection equipment and to the prevalence of unsafe parenteral practices in health care settings. WHO estimates that some 130 to 170 million people (2%-3% of the world's population) are chronically infected with HCV globally and more than 350,000 deaths are attributed to HCV infection annually. Approximately 25% to 50% of global cases of cirrhosis and HCC are attributable to HCV infection. Most populations in Africa, the Americas, Western Europe, most of the Middle East, and South Asia have anti-HCV prevalence rates of less than 2%. Prevalence rates in Eastern Europe, most of Asia, and the Western Pacific Region countries average 2.0% to 2.9%. In North and sub-Saharan Africa and the Middle East, the prevalence of anti-HCV ranges from 1% to more than 12%.

6. Reservoirs—Humans; the virus has been transmitted experimentally to chimpanzees.

7. Incubation period—Ranges from 2 weeks to 6 months; commonly 6 to 9 weeks. Chronic infection may persist for several decades before the onset of cirrhosis or HCC.

8. Transmission—HCV transmission is primarily parenteral, including injection drug use; exposure to blood contaminating inadequately sterilized instruments and needles used in medical and dental procedures; unsterilized objects for rituals (e.g., circumcision, scarification), traditional medicine (e.g., blood-letting), or other activities that break the skin (e.g., tattooing, ear or body piercing); and transfusion of blood or blood products from unscreened donors or blood products that have not undergone viral inactivation. Sexual transmission between heterosexual partners is considered an inefficient mechanism of transmission but does occur. Prosmicuity is considered a risk factor. Infection is more efficiently transmitted between men who have sex with men practicing receptive anal intercourse, particularly in the setting of HIV. Maternal-fetal transmission is estimated to occur at a rate of 3% to 10%, more commonly in HIV coinfection. It is estimated that 10% of cases have no discernable risk factor. The period of communicability is from 1 or more weeks before onset of the first symptoms and may persist indefinitely among persons with chronic infection. Peaks in virus concentration appear to correlate with peaks in alanine aminotransferase activity.

9. Treatment—

Drug	• Drugs vs. HCV are called direct-acting agents. There are 4 basic classes, each targeting steps in the HCV life cycle. Classes include NS3/4A protease inhibitors (e.g., simeprevir); NS5A inhibitors (e.g., daclatasvir); NS5B nucleoside RNA polymerase inhibitors (e.g., sofobuvir); and the NS5B non-nucleoside RNA polymerase inhibitors (e.g., dasabuvir). • Therapy is always offered in combination (usually 2 agents) from complementary classes to prevent emergence of resistance.
Dose	Dependent upon agent selected, viral, and host considerations.
Route	PO
Alternative drug	Interferon products; ribavirin may be used in special situations.
Duration	Usually 8–12 weeks, dependent upon genotype, viral response, and host considerations.
Special considerations and comments	The goal of therapy in chronic HCV infection is eradication of HCV RNA. When virologic goals are met, cure rate with modern agents approaches 100%.
	Acute infection:
	Because of the high cure rate in chronic infection, safety of therapy, the benign nature of acute disease, and the chance for spontaneous clearance, therapy is not offered for acute infection.
	Chronic infection:
	• Choice of regimen is highly dependent upon HCV genotype (1–6), baseline viral load, prior treatment history and resistance testing, status of liver disease (e.g., degree of fibrosis), comorbidities, insurance coverage, and availability of agents. • Because of the complexity of HCV treatment and potential for DAA-drug interactions, therapy should only be offered by experienced caregivers.

Note: DAA = direct-acting agent; HCV = hepatitis C virus; PO = oral(ly); RNA = ribonucleic acid.

10. Prevention—General control measures are similar to those that apply to HBV infection (see Hepatitis B in this chapter). A vaccine is not available and prophylactic IG is not effective. In blood bank operations, all donors should be routinely screened for anti-HCV; all donor units with elevated liver enzyme levels should be discarded. Routine virus inactivation of plasma-derived products, risk-reduction counseling for persons uninfected but at high risk (e.g., injection drug users, health care workers), and nosocomial control activities must be maintained.

11. Special considerations—

1) Reporting: official report obligatory in some countries.
2) Epidemic measures: similar to hepatitis B. Information on the investigation and management of hepatitis C outbreaks in particular settings can be found at: https://www.cdc.gov/hepatitis/hcv/index.htm.
3) International measures: ensure adequate virus inactivation for all internationally traded biologic products.

IV. HEPATITIS D (viral hepatitis D, hepatitis delta virus, delta agent hepatitis, delta-associated hepatitis, HDV infection)

1. Clinical features—Onset is usually abrupt, with signs and symptoms resembling those of hepatitis B; may be severe and is always associated with a coexistent HBV infection, either as acute coinfection or as superinfection among persons with chronic HBV infection. In the former case, the infection is usually self-limited; in the latter, it usually progresses to chronic hepatitis. Acute hepatitis D can be misdiagnosed as an exacerbation of chronic hepatitis B. As the outcome of hepatitis D virus (HDV) infection is associated with the host response to HBV, children with acute coinfection may have a severe clinical course with greater likelihood of progression to chronic hepatitis. In studies throughout Europe and the USA, 25% to 50% of fulminant hepatitis cases thought to be caused by HBV were associated with concurrent HDV infection.

2. Risk groups—All persons susceptible to HBV infection, or who have chronic HBV, can be infected with HDV. High-risk populations include injection drug users, hemophiliacs, and others who come into frequent contact with blood or blood products; persons in institutions for the developmentally disabled; and sexually active adults including men who have sex with men.

3. Causative agents—HDV is a virus-like particle of diameter 35–37 nm consisting of a coat of HBsAg and a unique internal antigen, the delta antigen. Encapsulated with the delta antigen is the genome, a single-stranded RNA that can have a linear or circular conformation. HDV is unable to infect a cell by itself and requires coinfection with HBV to undergo a complete replication cycle. Synthesis of HDV, in turn, results in temporary suppression of synthesis of HBV components. About 70% to 90% of patients with HDV coinfection are HBeAg-negative and most have low serum HBV DNA. HDV is best considered a defective RNA virus that is related more to plant viroids than to other human pathogens. Eight genotypes (1–8) and 2 subgenotypes (1a and 1b) of HDV have been identified.

4. Diagnosis—Through detection of total antibody to HDV (anti-HDV) by EIA; immunoglobulin class G (IgG) anti-HDV persists after HDV infection has cleared. A positive IgM titer indicates ongoing replication; reverse transcription PCR is the most sensitive assay for detecting HDV viremia.

5. Occurrence—Worldwide, but prevalence varies widely. An estimated 5% of the 240 million people infected with HBV globally have serologic evidence of exposure to HDV. HDV occurs epidemically or endemically among populations at high risk of HBV infection in areas where hepatitis B is endemic (highest in Africa and South America, Romania, and parts of Russia). Severe epidemics have been observed in tropical South America (Brazil, Colombia, Venezuela), in the Central African Republic, and among injection drug users in the USA. Since HDV requires a concomitant HBV infection, the recent decrease in prevalence of chronic HBsAg carriers in the general population in the Mediterranean area (Greece, Italy, Spain), and in many other parts of the world, has led to a rapid decline in both acute and chronic hepatitis D. Better sanitation and social standards may also have contributed. New foci of high HDV infection prevalence continue to appear in countries such as Albania, areas of China, northern India, and Japan (Okinawa).

6. Reservoirs—Humans. The virus can be transmitted experimentally to chimpanzees and woodchucks infected with HBV and woodchuck hepatitis virus, respectively.

7. Incubation period—Approximately 2 to 8 weeks.

8. Transmission—The mode of transmission is thought to be similar to that of HBV—via exposure to infected blood and serous bodily fluids, contaminated needles, syringes, and plasma derivatives such as antihemophilic factor and via sexual transmission. Blood is potentially infectious during all phases of active infection. Peak infectivity probably occurs just prior to onset of acute illness, when particles containing the delta antigen are readily detected in the blood. Following the onset of infection, viremia falls rapidly to low or undetectable levels; HDV has been transmitted to chimpanzees from the blood of chronically infected patients in whom particles containing the HDV antigen could not be detected.

9. Treatment—

Drug	PegIFN α-2a[a]
Dose	180 µg SQ weekly
Route	SQ
Alternative drug	PegIFN α-2b[a] 1.5 µg/kg SQ weekly

(Continued)

(Continued)

Duration	1 year
Special considerations and comments	• Candidates for therapy have both elevated levels of HDV RNA and active liver disease. • Nucleoside/nucleotide therapy is not of benefit vs. HDV but is used for HBV coinfection.

Note: HBV = hepatitis B virus; HDV = hepatitis D virus; PegIFN = peginterferon; RNA = ribonucleic acid; SQ = subcutaneous(ly).

[a]Data show superiority of either IFN product to be lacking.

10. Prevention—For persons susceptible to HBV infection, same as for hepatitis B. Prevention of HBV infection with hepatitis B vaccine prevents infection with HDV. A vaccine for HDV infection is not available. Among persons with chronic HBV, the only effective measure is avoidance of exposure to any potential source of HDV. Studies suggest that measures to decrease sexual exposure and needle sharing are associated with a decline in the incidence of HDV infection.

11. Special considerations—Epidemic measures: as for hepatitis B.

V. HEPATITIS E (enterically transmitted non-A, non-B hepatitis [ET-NANB]; epidemic non-A, non-B hepatitis; fecal-oral non-A, non-B hepatitis)

1. Clinical features—Clinical course similar to that of hepatitis A, with a short prodromal phase and a period of symptoms or jaundice lasting days to several weeks. Clinical and epidemiologic characteristics differ according to genotype.

2. Risk groups—Infection with genotype 1 or 2 is common in developing countries and is associated with fecal-waterborne transmission, high rates of icteric disease, and a higher attack rate among adolescents and young adults. Mortality is high among pregnant women (20%). Development of chronic disease has not been reported.

In contrast, infection with genotypes 3 or 4 is associated with endemic disease in developed countries, foodborne transmission, a low rate of icteric disease, and high rates of illness and greater mortality among older adults. Neurologic complications and chronic disease among immunocompromised persons have been reported and infections can become chronic.

Women in the third trimester of pregnancy are especially susceptible to fulminant disease and death (typically with genotype 1 or 2 infection). Among endemic cases, elderly adults appear particularly susceptible to infection with genotypes 3 and 4. The occurrence of major epidemics among young adults in regions where other enteric viruses are highly endemic and most of the population acquires infection in infancy remains unexplained.

3. Causative agents—The hepatitis E virus (HEV), the only known hepevirus, is a spherical, nonenveloped, single-stranded RNA virus approximately 32 to 34 nm in diameter, classified in the Hepeviridae family. There are 4 HEV genotypes.

4. Diagnosis—Depends on clinical and epidemiologic features and exclusion of other causes of hepatitis, especially hepatitis A, by serologic means. Commercial assays are available in some countries. Viremia occurs during the incubation period and antibodies (IgM and IgG) appear just before elevations in serum aminotransferase levels and symptoms. Acute hepatitis E is diagnosed if IgM antibody to HEV (anti-HEV) is present. Tests for HEV RNA in serum and stools are confirmatory but currently still experimental. Recovery is marked by viral clearance and by increase in IgG (which may persist for years) and decrease in IgM levels (which disappear after 3–12 months).

5. Occurrence—HEV is the most common cause of acute hepatitis and jaundice in the world. In developing countries, hepatitis E occurs sporadically and as epidemic disease and is largely due to genotype 1 (genotype 2 is more common in Mexico and parts of Africa); anti-HEV prevalence ranges from 30% to 80%. Outbreaks often occur as waterborne epidemics but sporadic cases and epidemics not clearly related to water have been reported. Outbreaks have been reported from Algeria, Bangladesh, Chad, China, Côte d'Ivoire, Egypt, Ethiopia, Greece, India, Indonesia, Iran, Jordan, Libya, Mexico, Myanmar, Nepal, Nigeria, Pakistan, southern areas of Russia, Somalia, Sudan and South Sudan, Uganda, and The Gambia.

Anti-HEV prevalence is lower in Europe and the USA than in Asia and Africa. Previous surveys in the USA (during 1988–1994) showed relatively high rates (21%) in the general population.

6. Reservoirs—Humans are natural hosts for HEV; some nonhuman primates (e.g., chimpanzees, cynomolgus monkeys, rhesus monkeys, pigtail monkeys, owl monkeys, tamarins, and African green monkeys) are reported to be susceptible to infection with HEV. HEV strains have been detected in domestic and wild pigs, deer, elk, sheep, cattle, rats, and rabbits. Thus, they are possibly sources of zoonotic infections of humans.

7. Incubation period—The range is 15 to 64 days; the mean incubation period has ranged from 26 to 42 days in various epidemics.

8. Transmission—Primarily by the fecal-oral route; fecally contaminated drinking water is the most commonly documented vehicle of transmission. Person-to-person transmission probably also occurs through the fecal-oral route; secondary spread among household cases has been described during outbreaks. Studies suggest that hepatitis E may, in fact, be a zoonotic infection with coincident introduction in areas of high human infection. The period of communicability is not known. HEV has been detected in stools 14 days after the onset of jaundice and approximately 4 weeks after oral ingestion of contaminated food or water, where it persists for about 2 weeks. Blood transfusion is a potential but rare route of HEV transmission.

9. Treatment—

Drug	Ribavirin (not to be used in pregnant women owing to the risk of teratogenicity)
Dose	600–1,000 mg daily in 2 divided doses
Route	PO
Alternative drug	No alternative drugs have been established.
Duration	12 weeks
Special considerations and comments	Acute infection: Treatment is supportive. The role of antiviral therapy has not been established.
	Chronic infection: • Since chronic infection occurs almost exclusively in immunocompromised hosts, reduction in immunosuppressive agents (e.g., antirejection drugs after organ transplantation) is an important principle of therapy. • Benefit of ribavirin is largely derived from case series.

Note: PO = oral(ly).

10. Prevention—

1) Provide educational programs to highlight sanitary disposal of feces and careful handwashing after defecation and before handling food; follow basic measures to prevent fecal–oral transmission.
2) Boiling and chlorination of water inactivates HEV.
3) Administration of IG, though in endemic areas this has not decreased infection rates during epidemics.
4) Thorough cooking of pork and avoidance of raw shellfish may be advisable.
5) No HEV vaccine is available.

11. Special considerations—

1) Reporting: report to local health authority is obligatory in some countries.
2) Epidemic measures: determine mode of transmission through epidemiologic investigation; investigate water supply and identify populations at increased risk of infection; make special efforts to

improve sanitary and hygienic practices in order to eliminate fecal contamination of foods and water.

3) A potential problem where there is mass crowding and inadequate sanitation and water supplies. If cases occur, increased effort should be exerted to improve sanitation and the safety of water supplies.

VI. HEPATOCELLULAR CARCINOMA (HCC, primary liver cancer, primary hepatocellular carcinoma, hepatoma)

1. Clinical features—A small proportion of persons with chronic HBV or HCV infection may eventually develop HCC. HCC rarely occurs before age 40 years and peaks at approximately age 70 years. Cirrhosis is present in 80% to 90% of HCV-associated HCC cases (70%–80% of persons with HBV-associated HCC). The progression to cirrhosis is often clinically silent and some patients are not known to have underlying viral hepatitis until they present with HCC. Symptoms—including anorexia, weight loss, right upper quadrant abdominal pain or tenderness, ascites, and jaundice—commonly appear later in the course of the illness. Depending on lesion size and cancer stage at diagnosis, 5-year survival may range from high (75%–90%) among persons with limited disease to very low (10% 1-year survival) among persons with extrahepatic spread or vascular involvement.

2. Risk groups—Rates of HCC among men are 2 to 4 times higher than among women. Among persons with chronic HBV infection, risk of HCC further increases by male sex, older age, infection of long duration, family history of HCC, coinfection with HIV or HDV, exposure to aflatoxin, use of alcohol or tobacco, high levels of HBV DNA, or infection with genotype C. Among persons with chronic HCV infection, risk of HCC increases by older age at time of infection, male sex, coinfection with HIV or HBV, alcohol, and probably diabetes or obesity.

3. Causative agents—Approximately 50% of cases of HCC are attributable to chronic HBV infection, a slightly lower percentage to chronic HCV infection, and a small proportion to noninfectious causes. Aflatoxin, alcohol, and nonalcoholic fatty liver disease (with or without obesity, metabolic syndrome, and type 2 diabetes) may serve as important cofactors in the development of HCC.

4. Diagnosis—Often made using noninvasive imaging tests, particularly with cirrhotic patients with focal hepatic masses greater than 2 cm in diameter and elevated α-fetoprotein levels. Image-guided biopsy is reserved for focal masses with atypical imaging features.

5. Occurrence—HCC is the fifth most common cancer in men and the seventh most common in women worldwide, with an estimated 0.5 to 1 million new cases per year (5% of all cancers worldwide). Most of the burden of disease (85%) occurs in developing countries; however, HCC related to infection with HCV has become the fastest-rising cause of cancer in the USA (where incidence has tripled in the last 20 years) and some other industrialized countries. HCC is one of the most common malignant neoplasms in many parts of Asia and Africa and its occurrence correlates with rates of chronic HBV and HCV infection in the population. Thus, it occurs with high frequency in areas with high prevalence of HBV carriers, including most of Asia, Africa, the South Pacific, and parts of the Middle East. Rates are intermediate on the Indian subcontinent and relatively low in North America and Western Europe. In industrialized countries, including Japan, and other countries such as Pakistan, Egypt, and Mongolia, HCV infection is considered the dominant viral etiology of HCC.

6. Reservoirs—See Hepatitis B and Hepatitis C in this chapter.

7. Incubation period—The duration from infection with HBV or HCV to development of HCC, when it does occur, typically takes several decades, depending on the presence of cofactors (see Risk Groups under Hepatocellular Carcinoma in this chapter). In the presence of cirrhosis, the 5-year cumulative risk of HCC ranges from 5% to 30%.

8. Transmission—See Hepatitis B and Hepatitis C in this chapter.

9. Treatment—Reactivation of HBV may occur in patients receiving immunosuppressive therapy for HCC. Therefore, it is important to maintain antiviral therapy in this setting.

10. Prevention—Vaccination to prevent HBV infection. There is moderately strong evidence that antiviral treatment controls HBV replication among HBsAg-positive patients and that eradicating HCV among persons with viremia substantially reduces, but does not eliminate, the risk of HCC. Periodic screening of carriers of HBV for α-fetoprotein and ultrasonography can, in some cases, detect the tumor at an early, resectable stage. Newer technologies, such as computed tomography or magnetic resonance imaging scanning, are being evaluated as screening strategies for HCC but currently are too costly for most populations.

11. Special considerations—HCC cases should be reported to a tumor registry according to standard cancer registration procedures.

[D. Cohen]

HERPESVIRUS DISEASE

DISEASE	ICD-CODE
HERPESVIRAL INFECTIONS (herpes simplex, genital herpes, alphaherpesviral diseases, herpesvirus hominis, human herpesviruses 1 and 2)	ICD-10 A60 (anogenital herpesviral infection), B00 (herpesviral infection), P35.2 (congenital herpesviral infection)
HERPESVIRAL ENCEPHALITIS, SIMIAN B	ICD-10 B00.4
KAPOSI'S SARCOMA	ICD-10 C46.0–C46.9

1. Clinical features—Infections with herpes simplex virus (HSV) type 1 (HSV-1) or type 2 (HSV-2) are characterized by neurovirulence, latency, and a tendency to localized recurrence. Most HSV-1 and HSV-2 infections are asymptomatic. After primary infection, herpesviruses establish latency and persist for life. Reactivation of latent virus results in viral shedding, which may be accompanied by symptoms but is usually asymptomatic. When present, symptoms may be localized or systemic. The clinical syndrome and course of infection depend on the anatomic site of infection, age, and immune status of the host and on the infecting viral type. However, either viral type may infect the genital tract or oral mucosa or cause systemic disease. Severe and extensive spread of infection may occur in those who are immunocompromised and may also result in fatal, generalized infections in newborn infants (neonatal herpes).

Oral herpes infection is usually caused by HSV-1. Infection may be mild and unapparent and often occurs in early childhood. However, approximately 10% of newly acquired (primary) infections result in overt disease, with illness of varying severity, marked by fever and malaise lasting a week or more. HSV-1 gingivostomatitis is manifested by vesicular and ulcerative lesions in the oropharynx.. HSV-1 causes about 2% of acute pharyngotonsillitis, usually as a primary infection. Symptomatic reactivations commonly result in herpes labialis (fever blisters, cold sores), classically manifested as single or grouped perioral vesicles, often on the vermilion border of the lips. Reactivation is precipitated by various forms of trauma, fever, physiologic changes, or intercurrent disease and may also involve other body tissues; it occurs in the presence of circulating antibodies, which are seldom elevated by reactivation. Symptomatic reactivation is heralded by tingling prior to the onset of vesicles; if patients learn to identify this sign, they can prevent or shorten the clinical course of the reactivated infection through the use of antivirals. HSV-1 can also cause severe keratoconjunctivitis, encephalitis, or a generalized cutaneous eruption complicating chronic eczema.

Central nervous system (CNS) involvement may appear in association with primary or recurrent disease with either HSV-1 or HSV-2 and may manifest as aseptic meningitis, transverse myelitis, sacral radiculopathy, or encephalitis.

Findings in herpes encephalitis may include fever, headache, leukocytosis, meningeal irritation, drowsiness, confusion, stupor, coma, and focal neurologic signs, frequently referable to the temporal region. The condition may be confused with other intracranial lesions, including brain abscess and tuberculous meningitis. Because antiviral therapy can reduce mortality, suspected encephalitis infections should be treated presumptively for herpes with antiviral therapy.

Genital herpes occurs mainly in adults. Newly acquired, symptomatic infections often include systemic symptoms such as fever and malaise and are classically characterized by bilateral vesiculopustular or ulcerative lesions on the cervix or external genitalia in women and on the external genitalia in men. Men or women engaging in anal sex may become infected at the anus and/or rectum. All people with first clinical episodes of genital herpes should receive antiviral therapy. However, the classical findings are often absent and the clinical diagnosis of genital herpes has both low sensitivity and low specificity. Recurrent disease can involve areas other than the site of initial infection, typically in related dermatomes, such as the perineum, legs, and buttocks. Primary lesions may last 2 to 3 weeks. Recurrent disease is usually unilateral and has a much smaller area of involvement and shorter duration than that of primary infection.

Many people with genital herpes do not have recognized symptoms of infection but still shed virus intermittently in the genital tract. Symptomatic primary infection with HSV-1 cannot be distinguished clinically from that caused by HSV-2; however, recurrences and subclinical shedding are less common with genital HSV-1 than with genital HSV-2 infection. Clinical manifestations of genital herpes may be more severe in immunocompromised persons.

Neonatal infections can be divided into 3 clinical presentations: disseminated infections involving organs such as the liver or lungs; CNS infection (encephalitis); and infections limited to the skin, eyes, or mouth. Disseminated infection is often fatal and survivors of CNS infection often have significant neurologic morbidity. Because skin lesions are present in only 70%, and fever in only 40%, of babies with HSV, clinicians must maintain a high index of suspicion for HSV infection, especially in the first month of life. Infections are due to either HSV-1 or HSV-2. Newborn infants exposed to HSV during birth, as documented by virologic testing of maternal lesions at delivery or presumed by observation of maternal lesions, should be followed carefully in consultation with a pediatric infectious-disease specialist.

2. Risk groups—Persons engaging in unprotected sexual intercourse or oral or anal sex with an infected partner and neonates born to women with genital HSV infection.

The risk of transmission to the neonate from an infected mother depends mainly on whether the maternal infection is new (primary or nonprimary first episode) or recurrent. The risk for transmission is high (25%–50%)

among women who acquire infection in late pregnancy; administration of acyclovir might be considered for neonates born to women who acquired HSV near term because the risk for neonatal herpes is high for these infants. Risk for neonatal infection is much lower (2%) among women with recurrent genital herpes at term or women who have acquired genital HSV infection during the first half of pregnancy, or earlier, in part because maternal immunity confers a degree of protection.

Persons with anogenital herpes are at increased risk for acquiring human immunodeficiency virus (HIV) infection.

3. Causative agents—HSV, which is in the virus family Herpesviridae, subfamily Alphaherpesvirinae. Historically, genital herpes was caused by HSV-2 and oral herpes by HSV-1; however, HSV-1 is now a common cause of primary genital herpes in some populations and causes a substantial proportion of neonatal herpes infections.

4. Diagnosis—Can be confirmed by viral isolation, HSV deoxyribonucleic acid (DNA) detection by polymerase chain reaction (PCR), or HSV antigen detection by enzyme immunoassay or direct fluorescent antibody assay. Cytologic detection of cellular changes (e.g., Tzanck preparation) is insensitive and nonspecific for diagnosis and should not be relied upon.

Viral culture isolates can be typed to determine whether HSV-1 or HSV-2 is the cause of infection. HSV types 1 and 2 can be differentiated immunologically (when type-specific serologic assays are used) and differ with respect to their growth patterns in cell culture, embryonated eggs, and experimental animals.

HSV DNA PCR on spinal fluid is the test of choice for diagnosing herpes CNS infection. Neuroimaging, preferably by magnetic resonance imaging, should be done early during the diagnostic workup. Brain biopsy may be considered in atypical cases when other diagnostic testing is not definitive. Accurate type-specific HSV serologic tests based on glycoprotein G can reliably distinguish HSV-1 and HSV-2 antibodies. Antibodies to HSV may take several weeks to develop after initial infection but then persist indefinitely; false-negative serologic results may occur at early stages of infection. Herpes immunoglobulin class M antibody tests are not reliable in determining whether infection is newly acquired.

Neonates being evaluated for possible herpes infection should have surface cultures of the mouth, nasopharynx, conjunctivae, and anus; culture or PCR of skin vesicles; PCR of cerebrospinal fluid; and HSV PCR of whole blood. Neonates should also have whole blood tested for alanine aminotransferase; elevated transaminase values can suggest HSV hepatitis, or disseminated infection, which can occur even in an afebrile infant.

5. Occurrence—Worldwide; an estimated 67% of the population aged 0 to 49 years possess circulating antibodies against HSV-1. Initial, oral infection with HSV-1 usually occurs before age 10 years; however, more primary infections in adults are now being reported. HSV-2 infection usually begins with sexual activity and is rare before adolescence, except in sexually abused children. HSV-2 seroprevalence is estimated to be 11% among 15- to 49-year-olds worldwide but is much higher in some low-income countries. Seroprevalence increases with age and is higher among females, men who have sex with men, certain racial/ethnic groups, and persons with multiple sexual partners. The majority (~90%) of persons infected with HSV-2 have not been diagnosed with genital herpes.

6. **Reservoirs**—Humans.

7. **Incubation period**—From 2 to 12 days; may be longer for neonatal infections.

8. **Transmission**—Contact with HSV-1 or HSV-2 in saliva or genital secretions is the most important mode of spread. Both types 1 and 2 may be transmitted to various sites by genital-genital, oral-genital, oral-anal, or genital-anal routes. Herpes transmission via a shared towel has not been documented. Ungloved health care personnel (e.g., dentists) may acquire infection on the hands (herpetic whitlow) from patients shedding HSV from the oral cavity.

Transmission to the neonate usually occurs during transit through an infected birth canal (85% of cases) and, less commonly, in utero or post partum. Most cases of neonatal herpes occur in infants born to women with no known history of genital herpes. There have been numerous instances of postnatal transmission to male neonates during direct orogenital suction performed as part of some Jewish ritual circumcisions.

Transmission of HSV can occur during asymptomatic periods. HSV may be shed intermittently from mucosal sites for years and possibly lifelong, in the presence or absence of clinical manifestations. Viral shedding can be detected by PCR on 18% of days that HSV-2 seropositive people are swabbed in the genital area; viral shedding is more common among those with a history of symptomatic genital herpes (20%) than among those with no history of symptoms (10%), lasts longer with symptomatic reactivations than with subclinical reactivations, and is of shorter duration with recurrent versus primary lesions.

9. **Treatment**—

Gingivostomatitis and Pharyngitis: Children 1–6 Years

Preferred treatment	Acyclovir 15/mg/kg PO 5 times a day (≤ 200 mg 5 times daily) within 3 days of onset of lesions and continued for 1 week
Alternative drug	Not applicable
Special considerations and comments	• Adjuvant therapy with topical or oral analgesics; rehydration may be required for children with painful swallowing. • Painful lesions can be treated with viscous lidocaine and with over-the-counter topical medications.

Note: PO = oral(ly).

Gingivostomatitis and Pharyngitis: Adults

Preferred treatment	• Acyclovir 400 mg PO TID for 7–10 days OR • Acyclovir 200 mg PO 5 times a day for 7–10 days OR • Valacyclovir 1 g PO BID for 7–10 days OR • Famciclovir 250 mg PO TID for 7–10 days
Alternative drug	Not applicable
Special considerations and comments	• Treatment can be extended if healing is incomplete after 10 days of therapy. • Treatment for adults with gingivostomatitis has been derived from recommendations for treating first-episode genital herpes. • Placebo-controlled trials have shown that short courses of oral antivirals can shorten the duration of lesions if taken within 1 hour of prodromal symptoms. People with frequently recurrent lesions may benefit from chronic suppressive therapy.

Note: BID = twice daily; PO = oral(ly); TID = thrice daily.

Recurrent Herpes Labialis: Children > 12 Years and Adults

Preferred treatment	Immunocompetent patients: • Children > 12 years: valacyclovir 4 g/day PO in 2 divided doses for 1 day • Adults: acyclovir 400 mg PO 5 times a day for 5 days OR famciclovir 1,500 mg PO as a single dose Immunocompromised/HIV-infected patients (adults): • Valacyclovir 1 g PO BID for 5–10 days OR • Acyclovir 5 mg/kg (ideal body weight) IV every 8 hours for 7 days OR 400 mg PO 5 times a day for 14–21 days OR • Famciclovir 1,000 mg/day PO in 2 divided doses for 7 days
Alternative drug	• Penciclovir 1% cream OR • Acyclovir 5% cream[a]
Special considerations and comments	• Decision to treat recurrent herpes labialis should be made on a case-by-case basis, taking into account symptom severity, frequency or recurrence, patient preference, and cost. • Treatment should be initiated as soon as possible after diagnosis.

Note: BID = twice daily; HIV = human immunodeficiency virus; HSV = herpes simplex virus; IV = intravenous(ly); PO = oral(ly).
[a]Foscarnet can be used for acyclovir-resistant HSV.

Keratoconjunctivitis

Preferred treatment	Herpes simplex virus infections that involve the eye (adult, child, or infant) should be managed in consultation with an ophthalmologist. Treatment agents include topical and oral antivirals (trifluridine and acyclovir) and adjuvant topical corticosteroids.
Alternative drug	<ul><li>Ganciclovir 0.15% ophthalmic gel</li><li>Vidarabine ointment</li></ul>
Special considerations and comments	High recurrence rate (~30%) within 1 year. Consider prophylaxis with acyclovir 400 mg PO BID for 12 months to prevent recurrences.

Note: BID = twice daily; PO = oral(ly).

Encephalitis and Other Severe Disease

Preferred treatment	Acyclovir: <ul><li>Encephalitis (adults): 10 mg/kg IV every 8 hours for 14–21 days</li><li>Encephalitis (children > 12 years): 10 mg/kg IV every 8 hours for 14–21 days</li><li>Encephalitis (children 3 months to 12 years): 10–15 mg/kg IV every 8 hours for 14–21 days (FDA approved for 60 mg/kg/day IV but nephrotoxicity may be increased at this higher dose)</li><li>Other severe herpes disease necessitating hospitalization (adults): 5–10 mg/kg IV every 8 hours for 2–7 days or until clinical improvement is observed, THEN PO antiviral therapy to complete ≥ 10 days of total therapy</li></ul>
Alternative drug	Foscarnet
Special considerations and comments	<ul><li>Early diagnosis and treatment is imperative.</li><li>Infuse doses over 1 hour to lessen risk of nephrotoxicity.</li><li>Generally dosed based on ideal body weight. Adjusted body weight may be considered in patients who are morbidly obese (BMI ≥ 40 kg/m^2) for severe infections.</li><li>Lumbar puncture should be repeated before stopping treatment for herpes encephalitis; if HSV DNA is detected by PCR of the cerebrospinal fluid, treatment should be continued. Repeat lumbar puncture at 7-day intervals with HSV PCR testing until HSV can no longer be detected.</li></ul>

Note: BMI = body mass index; DNA = deoxyribonucleic acid; HSV = herpes simplex virus; IV = intravenous(ly); PCR = polymerase chain reaction; PO = oral(ly).

Genital Herpes: First Clinical Episode

Preferred treatment	• Acyclovir 400 mg PO TID for 7–10 days OR • Acyclovir 200 mg PO 5 times a day for 7–10 days OR • Valacyclovir 1 g PO BID for 7–10 days OR • Famciclovir 250 mg PO TID for 7–10 days
Alternative drug	Not applicable
Special considerations and comments	• All patients with first episodes of genital herpes should receive antiviral therapy. • Treatment can be extended if healing is incomplete after 10 days of therapy.

Note: BID = twice daily; PO = oral(ly); TID = thrice daily.

Genital Herpes: Suppressive Therapy for Recurrent Episodes

Preferred treatment	• Acyclovir 400 mg PO BID OR • Valacyclovir 500 mg PO once daily OR • Valacyclovir 1 g PO once daily OR • Famiciclovir 250 mg PO BID
Alternative drug	Not applicable
Special considerations and comments	Valacyclovir 500 mg once daily might be less effective than other valacyclovir or acyclovir dosing regimens in persons who have very frequent recurrences (i.e., ≥ 10 episodes/year).

Note: BID = twice daily; PO = oral(ly).

Genital Herpes: Episodic Therapy for Recurrent Episodes

Preferred treatment	• Acyclovir 400 mg PO TID for 5 days OR • Acyclovir 800 mg PO BID for 5 days OR • Acyclovir 800 mg PO TID for 2 days OR • Valacyclovir 500 mg PO BID for 3 days OR • Valacyclovir 1 g PO once daily for 5 days OR • Famciclovir 125 mg PO BID for 5 days OR • Famciclovir 1 g PO BID for 1 day OR • Famciclovir 500 mg single dose, THEN 250 mg BID for 2 days

(Continued)

Genital Herpes: Episodic Therapy for Recurrent Episodes (Continued)

Alternative drug	Not applicable
Special considerations and comments	Effective episodic treatment of recurrent herpes requires initiation of therapy within 1 day of lesion onset or during the prodrome that precedes some outbreaks. The patient should be provided with a supply of drug or a prescription for the medication with instructions to initiate treatment immediately when symptoms begin.

Note: BID = twice daily; PO = oral(ly); TID = thrice daily.

Persons with HIV Infection: Daily Suppressive Therapy

Preferred treatment	• Acyclovir 400–800 mg PO BID or TID OR • Valacyclovir 500 mg PO BID OR • Famciclovir 500 mg PO BID
Alternative drug	Not applicable
Special considerations and comments	• Suppressive or episodic therapy with oral anti-viral agents is effective in decreasing the clinical manifestations of HSV among persons with HIV infection. • In HIV patients, acyclovir 400 mg PO BID is usually the starting dose and can be increased to 800 mg PO BID if breakthrough recurrences occur.

Note: BID = twice daily; HIV = human immunodeficiency virus; HSV = herpes simplex virus; PO = oral(ly); TID = thrice daily.

Persons with HIV Infection: Episodic Therapy

Preferred treatment	• Acyclovir 400 mg PO TID for 5–10 days OR • Valacyclovir 1 g PO BID for 5–10 days OR • Famciclovir 500 mg PO BID for 5–10 days
Alternative drug	Not applicable
Special considerations and comments	For severe HSV disease, initiating therapy with acyclovir 5–10 mg/kg IV every 8 hours might be necessary.

Note: BID = twice daily; HIV = human immunodeficiency virus; HSV = herpes simplex virus; PO = oral(ly); TID = thrice daily.

Pregnant Women With Genital Herpes: Suppressive Antiviral Therapy at 36 Weeks

Preferred treatment	• Acyclovir 400 mg PO TID OR • Valacyclovir 500 mg PO BID
Alternative drug	Not applicable
Special considerations and comments	• Suppressive antiviral therapy starting at 36 weeks' gestation can reduce the need for cesarean delivery among women with active recurrent genital herpes but does not eliminate the risk for transmission to the neonate. • Because the risk for herpes is highest in newborn infants of women who acquire genital HSV during late pregnancy, these women should be managed in consultation with maternal-fetal medicine and infectious-disease specialists.

Note: BID = twice daily; HSV = herpes simplex virus; PO = oral(ly); TID = thrice daily.

Neonatal Herpes: Treatment

Preferred treatment	Acyclovir 20 mg/kg IV every 8 hours for 14–21 days
Alternative drug	Not applicable
Special considerations and comments	• Duration of therapy is 21 days for patients with disseminated or CNS infection and 14 days for patients with HSV infections limited to the skin, eyes, or mucous membranes. • All patients with HSV infection of the CNS should have a repeat lumbar puncture performed at the end of 21 days of therapy. If HSV DNA is detected by PCR, therapy should be continued until a negative PCR is obtained. • Administration of acyclovir might be considered for neonates born to women who acquired HSV near term because the risk for neonatal herpes is high for these infants.

Note: CNS = central nervous system; DNA = deoxyribonucleic acid; HSV = herpes simplex virus; IV = intravenous(ly); PCR = polymerase chain reaction.

Neonatal Herpes: Suppressive Therapy

Preferred treatment	Acyclovir 300 mg/m^2 PO TID for 6 months
Alternative drug	Not applicable
Special considerations and comments	Oral suppressive therapy after completion of treatment has been demonstrated to improve neuro-developmental outcomes and to reduce recurrence of HSV.

Note: HSV = herpes simplex virus; PO = oral(ly); TID = thrice daily.

10. Prevention—

1) Health education and personal hygiene should be directed toward minimizing the transfer of infectious material.

2) Avoid contaminating the skin of eczematous patients with infectious material.

3) Health care personnel should wear gloves when in direct contact with mucous membranes or potentially infectious lesions.

4) Correct and consistent use of latex condoms in sexual practice may decrease the risk of genital infection. Persons with known genital herpes infection should disclose their infection status to sex partners.

5) For sexual partnerships in which 1 member is known to have genital herpes infection, type-specific serologic testing can be used to determine whether the other partner is at risk for acquiring herpes infection.

6) A daily regimen of valacyclovir treatment can decrease the rate of HSV-2 transmission in discordant, heterosexual couples in which 1 partner has a history of genital HSV-2 infection. Sexual activity should be avoided when lesions are present.

7) Suppressive antiviral therapy starting at 36 weeks' gestation can reduce the need for cesarean delivery among women with active recurrent genital herpes but does not eliminate the risk for transmission to the neonate. Some specialists recommend type-specific HSV serologic testing for pregnant women and their sex partners to identify women at risk for acquiring herpes (due to HSV-1 or HSV-2) from a sex partner during pregnancy; however, this approach needs further study.

Cesarean delivery reduces the risk of herpes transmission to the neonate. Recommendations for managing pregnant women with genital herpes lesions in the third trimester may differ by country. In the USA, cesarean section is recommended only if prodromal signs or genital lesions are present at the time of delivery, regardless of whether infection is primary, nonprimary first episode, or recurrent. In some other countries, professional organizations recommend cesarean section for women who present with first-episode genital herpes infection (primary or nonprimary) at any time during the third trimester. Moreover, some specialists recommend that, in addition to cesarean delivery, women with a primary or nonprimary first-episode lesion during the third trimester should continue antiviral treatment through delivery.

8) The management of asymptomatic infants born to women with active genital lesions is the subject of detailed recommendations. In settings with access to viral culture, PCR, and type-specific serologic testing, women with active genital lesions at either cesarean or vaginal delivery should have lesions tested by PCR or culture with typing; if there is no history of genital herpes before pregnancy, then type-specific serologic testing should be performed at the same time. Asymptomatic infants born by vaginal or cesarean delivery to women with active genital lesions should have HSV testing of surface swab specimens (mouth, nasopharynx, conjunctivae, and anus), blood, and cerebrospinal fluid performed at 24 hours after birth, with infant treatment with parenteral acyclovir starting immediately after specimen collection if the mother has no history of genital lesions before pregnancy. If the infant remains asymptomatic, decisions regarding the duration of treatment for neonates born to mothers with no previous history of genital herpes depend on the results of both infant and maternal test results. When mothers have a history of genital herpes, decisions on initiating treatment for the neonate depend on the neonatal virologic test results. The risk for neonatal infection is much higher for infants born to women with a first-time genital herpes infection during pregnancy.

11. Special considerations—

1) Reporting: neonatal infections are reportable in some areas.
2) HIV-infected persons: HSV infection can be more severe and prolonged in persons with HIV infection; recommended treatment regimens differ. Treatment of HSV infection in persons with HIV infection can reduce HIV viral load.

[J. Schillinger]

HISTOPLASMOSIS

DISEASE	ICD-10 CODE
ACUTE PULMONARY HISTOPLASMOSIS CAPSULATI	B39.0
CHRONIC PULMONARY HISTOPLASMOSIS CAPSULATI	B39.1
PULMONARY HISTOPLASMOSIS CAPSULATI, UNSPECIFIED	B39.2
DISSEMINATED HISTOPLASMOSIS CAPSULATI	B39.3
HISTOPLASMOSIS CAPSULATI, UNSPECIFIED	B39.4
HISTOPLASMOSIS DUBOISII	B39.5
HISTOPLASMOSIS, UNSPECIFIED	B39.9

Two clinically different mycoses are designated as histoplasmosis; the pathogens that cause them cannot be distinguished morphologically when grown on culture media as molds. Detailed information is given for the infection caused by *Histoplasma capsulatum* var. *capsulatum* and a brief summary is given for that caused by *Histoplasma capsulatum* var. *duboisii*. The taxonomy of *Histoplasma* is under debate as some phylogenetic analyses suggest that *H. capsulatum* var. *capsulatum* and *H. capsulatum* var. *duboisii* could be considered separate species.

I. HISTOPLASMOSIS DUE TO *HISTOPLASMA CAPSULATUM* VAR. *CAPSULATUM* (American histoplasmosis)

1. Clinical features—Most infections are asymptomatic but a small proportion result in clinical illness that ranges from a self-limited respiratory infection to life-threatening disease. Clinical infection typically manifests in 1 of the following forms.

1) Acute pulmonary: ranges from mild to severe, depending on host status and inoculum size. Symptoms and clinical findings include fever, cough, fatigue, chills, headache, myalgia, chest pain, and general malaise; occasional erythema multiforme; and erythema nodosum. Multiple small, scattered calcifications in the lung, hilar lymph nodes, spleen, and liver may be late findings.

2) Chronic pulmonary: clinically and radiologically resembles chronic pulmonary tuberculosis with cavitation; occurs most often in middle-aged and elderly men with underlying emphysema. Progresses over months or years, with periods of quiescence and sometimes spontaneous cure.

3) Acute disseminated: with debilitating fever, gastrointestinal symptoms, evidence of bone marrow suppression, hepatosplenomegaly,

lymphadenopathy, and a rapid course; most frequent in infants and young children and immunocompromised patients, including those with human immunodeficiency virus infection. Usually fatal unless treated.

4) Chronic disseminated: with low-grade intermittent fever, weight loss, weakness, hepatosplenomegaly, mild hematologic abnormalities, and focal manifestations of disease (e.g., endocarditis, meningitis, mucosal ulcers of mouth, larynx, stomach, or bowel, and Addison's disease). Subacute course progressing over 10 to 11 months and usually fatal unless treated.

Other complications and manifestations of histoplasmosis include mediastinal fibrosis, broncholithiasis, pericarditis, endocarditis, and central nervous system infection.

2. Risk groups—Immunosuppressed persons are at risk for opportunistic infection. Susceptibility is general. Inapparent infections are common in endemic areas and usually result in increased resistance to infection.

3. Causative agents—*H. capsulatum* (teleomorph *Ajellomyces capsulatus*), a dimorphic fungus that grows as a mold in soil and as a yeast in animal and human tissue.

4. Diagnosis—Definitive diagnosis can be obtained by culture of tissue of bodily fluids and confirmed with a chemiluminescent deoxyribonucleic acid (DNA) probe. Cultures can take up to 6 weeks to become positive. Histopathology will show oval, narrow-based budding yeasts 2 to 4 μm long; however, other organisms can appear morphologically similar. Serology is a vital diagnostic method, particularly for nonimmunocompromised patients. The immunodiffusion test is the most specific and reliable of available serologic tests. A rise in complement fixation (CF) titers in paired sera may occur early in acute infection; a titer of 1:32 or higher is suggestive of active disease. Low levels of CF antibodies can be detected in approximately 10% of healthy persons in endemic regions. False-negative tests are common, particularly in immunocompromised patients, and negative serology does not exclude the diagnosis. Detection of antigen in serum, urine, or other bodily fluids is useful in making the diagnosis and following the results of treatment for disseminated histoplasmosis; however, there is a high degree of cross-reactivity with patients with blastomycosis, paracoccidioidomycosis, or talaromycosis (formerly penicilliosis). DNA-based direct detection assays for fluids and tissues are available on a research basis.

5. Occurrence—Commonly occurs in geographic foci over wide areas of the Americas, Africa, eastern Asia, Australia, and Europe. Exposure is common in endemic pockets of these areas. Older adults and males are most commonly affected. Outbreaks have occurred following exposure to bird or bat droppings or following disruption of contaminated soil or other environmental material. Histoplasmosis occurs in many animals, often with a clinical picture comparable to that in humans.

6. Reservoirs—Soil with high organic content and undisturbed bird and bat droppings, in particular that around and in old chicken houses, in caves, and around starling, blackbird, and pigeon roosts.

7. Incubation period—Range of 3 to 17 days, with an average of 12 to 14 days; may be shorter with heavy exposure.

8. Transmission—Growth of the fungus in soil produces microconidia and tuberculate macroconidia; infection results from inhalation of airborne microconidia. Person-to-person transmission is extremely uncommon but can occur through transplantation of infected organs, transplacentally, or from inoculation of material from cutaneous lesions.

9. Treatment—Refer also to the Infectious Diseases Society of America's *Clinical Practice Guidelines for the Management of Patients with Histoplasmosis* for complete recommendations.

Acute and Chronic Pulmonary Histoplasmosis

Preferred therapy	Mild-to-moderate acute pulmonary histoplasmosis: • Treatment is usually unnecessary. • Itraconazole 200 mg PO TID for 3 days, THEN itraconazole 200 mg once daily or BID for 6–12 weeks is recommended in patients who have symptoms for > 1 month.
	Moderately severe to severe acute pulmonary histoplasmosis: • Lipid formulation AMB 3–5 mg/kg IV once daily for 1–2 weeks, THEN itraconazole 200 mg PO TID for 3 days, THEN itraconazole 200 mg BID for a total of 12 weeks. PLUS • Methylprednisolone 0.5–1 mg/kg IV once daily during the first 1–2 weeks of antifungal therapy for patients who develop respiratory complications, including hypoxemia or significant respiratory distress.
	Chronic cavitary pulmonary histoplasmosis: • Itraconazole 200 mg PO TID for 3 days, THEN itraconazole 200 mg PO once daily or BID for ≥ 1 year.

(Continued)

Acute and Chronic Pulmonary Histoplasmosis (Continued)

Alternative therapy options	• Fluconazole is not active against *Histoplasma capsulatum* in vitro and has produced less favorable treatment results in clinical trials. Fluconazole should only be considered in patients not able to tolerate itraconazole or who cannot achieve adequate serum concentrations. These patients should be monitored closely for relapse. The recommended dose is 400–800 mg IV or PO daily. • Posaconazole has in vitro activity against *H. capsulatum* and may be considered as salvage therapy in patients who have failed other regimens. • Voriconazole has in vitro activity against *H. capsulatum* and has been shown to be effective in a small number of patients. • Isavuconazole has in vitro activity against *H. capsulatum* but has not been studied in patients with histoplasmosis.
	Moderately severe to severe acute pulmonary histoplasmosis: • Liposomal amphotericin can be replaced with AMB deoxycholate 0.7–1 mg/kg IV once daily (if low risk for nephrotoxicity).
Special considerations and comments	• Chronic cavitary pulmonary histoplasmosis: blood levels of itraconazole should be obtained after ≥ 2 weeks of therapy if available. Because itraconazole has a long half-life, blood concentration variability is minimal during a 24-hour period. Therefore, the timing of blood collection is not important. A random concentration ≥ 1 µg/mL is recommended. • Itraconazole oral solution and capsules are not bioequivalent (PO solution has higher bioavailability) and thus are not interchangeable. Generally, oral solution is the preferred formulation because of improved absorption. Capsules should be taken with food. Solution should be taken on an empty stomach. • Azoles have been associated with significant drug interactions, in particular with cytochrome P450. Itraconazole can be an inhibitor and substrate. Perform drug interaction check prior to prescribing. • Salvage therapy for those who have failed standard therapy is complex with limited data to support an evidence-based recommendation. Consult with infectious diseases expert.

Note: AMB = amphotericin B; BID = twice daily; IV = intravenous(ly); PO = oral(ly); TID = thrice daily.

10. Prevention—

1) Minimize exposure to soil, dust, and bird or bat droppings in a contaminated environment, such as chicken coops, caves, and old buildings. Spray with water to reduce dust; use protective masks. Bird or bat droppings should be professionally remediated.

2) Management of contacts and the immediate environment: investigate household and occupational contacts for evidence of infection from a common environmental source.

11. Special considerations—

1) Reporting: report to local health authority may be required in some endemic areas.

2) Occurrence of grouped cases of acute pulmonary disease in or outside of a known endemic area, particularly with a history of exposure to soil or dust within a closed space (such as caves or construction sites), should arouse suspicion of histoplasmosis. Suspected sites such as attics, basements, caves, or construction sites with large amounts of bird or bat droppings must be investigated.

3) Possible hazard if large groups, especially from nonendemic areas, are forced to move through, live in, or disturb soil in areas where *Histoplasma* is prevalent.

II. HISTOPLASMOSIS DUE TO *HISTOPLASMOSIS CAPSULATUM* VAR. *DUBOISII* (African histoplasmosis)

This usually presents as a subacute granuloma of skin or bone. Thus far, the disease has been recognized only in Africa and Madagascar. Infection, though usually localized, may be disseminated in the skin, subcutaneous tissue, lymph nodes, bones, joints, lungs, and abdominal viscera. Disease is more common in males and may occur at any age but especially in the second decade of life. Diagnosis is made through culture or demonstration of yeast cells of *H. capsulatum* var. *duboisii* in tissue by smear or biopsy. These cells are much larger than the yeast cells of *H. capsulatum* var. *capsulatum*. The true prevalence of *H. duboisii*, its reservoir, mode of transmission, and incubation period are unknown. It is not communicable from person to person. Treatment is the same as for histoplasmosis due to *H. capsulatum*.

Bibliography

Wheat LJ, Freifeld AG, Kleiman MB, Baddley JW, McKinsey DS, Loyd JE, et al. Clinical practice guidelines for the management of patients with histoplasmosis: 2007 update by the Infectious Diseases Society of America. *Clin infect dis.*1;45(7):807–825.

[O. Z. McCotter]

HIV INFECTION AND AIDS

DISEASE	ICD-10 CODE
HIV INFECTION AND AIDS	ICD-10 B20–B24

1. Clinical features—Acquired immunodeficiency syndrome (AIDS) refers to the late clinical stage of infection with the human immunodeficiency virus (HIV). Within 2 to 4 weeks of infection with HIV, 10% to 60% of individuals develop an acute self-limiting infectious mononucleosis-like illness lasting for 1 to 2 weeks. The disease then proceeds to a clinically latent or asymptomatic phase of chronic infection, the duration of which may vary significantly depending on viral and host characteristics. In the absence of antiretroviral therapy (ART), the infection proceeds to early symptomatic HIV infection and then to AIDS. This is characterized by a depletion of cluster of differentiation 4 (CD4+) T-helper lymphocytes (CD4+ cells) to a level of fewer than 200 cells/μL or by the development of any AIDS-defining conditions (ADCs), which may be infectious, noninfectious, or malignant in etiology. The frequency and severity of HIV-related opportunistic infections (OIs) or cancers is, in general, directly correlated with the degree of immune system dysfunction, as reflected by the CD4+ count. The clinical features of these ADCs and OIs vary widely, depending on the organ system involved. Common OIs include pneumocystis pneumonia, cryptococcosis (meningitis most commonly), cerebral toxoplasmosis, cytomegalovirus infection, and tuberculosis (TB) (pulmonary and extrapulmonary); AIDS-associated malignancies include Kaposi's sarcoma, non-Hodgkin's lymphoma, and cervical carcinoma.

2. Risk groups—At the population level, the frequency of unprotected sex and injection drug use, the mixing of sexual and drug-using networks, and concurrent sex partners (multiple partners in the same time period) are important determinants of HIV infection rates. In addition, antiretroviral coverage and rates of HIV viral suppression in various settings play an important contributory role.

Sexual transmission of HIV remains the major driver for new HIV infections worldwide. The risk of HIV transmission varies widely and is dependent on the nature of sexual exposure. Sexual practices that result in injury to mucosa and/or mucosal bleeding are associated with higher risk. Unprotected receptive anal intercourse is likely to confer the highest risk of sexual transmission of HIV, followed by insertive anal intercourse, receptive vaginal intercourse, insertive vaginal intercourse, and oral sex. Behavioral factors influencing risk (besides the use of barrier protection such as condoms) include the number of sexual partners and having sex under the influence of alcohol or recreational drugs. Biologic factors implicated in HIV transmission risk include being uncircumcised or having an uncircumcised male partner and having concomitant sexually transmitted infections (STIs).

In the absence of preventive interventions, the transmission rate from infected mothers to their children is about 25% in the absence of breastfeeding and about 35% in breastfeeding populations. The majority of in utero transmission is likely to occur in the third trimester; transmission during labor and delivery likely occurs through the contact of blood and other secretions carrying HIV in the infant's mucosal membranes. Breastfeeding remains an important mode of transmission among HIV-infected mothers not virally suppressed or not on treatment as breast milk contains both HIV-infected cells and detectable levels of HIV ribonucleic acid (RNA), both of which have been implicated in transmission of infection.

In health care workers, after direct exposure to HIV-infected blood through injury with needles and other sharp objects, the rate of seroconversion is less than 0.5%, much lower than the risk of hepatitis B virus or hepatitis C virus infection after similar exposures (30% and 3%, respectively). The risk to health care workers after mucous membrane exposure has been estimated to be 0.09%; the risk after exposure of nonintact skin has not been quantified but is estimated to be lower than for mucous membrane exposure. Other important determinants of infection in the health care setting include the degree of viremia in the source or in the HIV-infected patient.

HIV coinfection with *Mycobacterium tuberculosis* is of major public health importance. Persons with latent TB coinfected with HIV develop clinical TB at an increased rate, with a lifetime risk of developing TB multiplied by a factor of 6 to 8. This increased risk and the resulting increased TB transmission have contributed to parallel epidemics of HIV and TB: in some urban sub-Saharan African populations where 10% to 15% of the adult population have dual TB/HIV infections, annual incidence rates for TB increased 5- to 10-fold during the latter half of the 1990s. HIV infection may increase rates and severity of malarial infection and antimalarial treatment may be less effective in HIV-infected individuals. Other common and significant OIs and coinfections with HIV include genital herpes, pneumococcal infection, nontyphoidal salmonellosis, visceral leishmaniasis, pneumocystis pneumonia, cryptococcosis, and viral hepatitis. Infections such as TB, malaria, and genital herpes may increase HIV viral load and the rate of decline of CD4+ cells. However, the long-term clinical implications of these laboratory findings are less well understood.

3. Causative agents—AIDS was first recognized in the early 1980s; in 1983 a retrovirus, later named HIV, was first isolated. Two serologically and geographically distinct species, HIV-1 and HIV-2, have since been identified. This chapter refers to HIV-1 except where specified. Four distinct groups of HIV-1 have been identified: M, N, O, and P. Group M is the most prevalent and is subdivided into 9 subtypes or clades (A–D, F–H, J, K). Recombinants of these subtypes arise through viral mixing and circulating recombinant forms reflect ongoing geographically bounded epidemics. Subtype C constitutes nearly half of all infections worldwide; subtype B is the predominant form in North and Latin America, Western and Central Europe, and the Caribbean. The primary clinical implication of the difference in viral subtypes is the difference in the rate of transmission and speed of disease progression.

4. Diagnosis—HIV infection is defined by laboratory criteria, usually based on detection of HIV-1/2 antibodies and/or HIV-1 p24 antigen; molecular tests for HIV deoxyribonucleic acid (DNA) and/or RNA may also be included. For diagnostic purposes, HIV testing algorithms should comprise a 2-step algorithm. Newer guidelines recommend the use of a fourth-generation antigen/antibody combination HIV-1/2 immunoassay as a first step; to be followed by a confirmatory HIV-1/2 differentiation immunoassay if the first test is positive. This algorithm takes into account the increased sensitivity and specificity of the fourth-generation combination immunoassays and supersedes older 2-step algorithms that employ an initial enzyme-linked immunosorbent assay followed by Western blotting as the confirmatory test. In resource-limited settings, WHO recommends testing with a combination of 2 different rapid antibody tests, with the initial test being the most sensitive assay available.

Selection of tests depends on such factors as performance characteristics (accuracy), potential for cross-reactivity, and local operational characteristics. DNA and RNA nucleic acid testing plays an important role in early infant HIV diagnosis because the presence of passively transferred maternal antibody can result in positive HIV serology in infants 18 months or younger in the absence of HIV infection. The WHO guidelines for assuring the accuracy and reliability of HIV rapid testing provide more detailed information and can be found at: http://whqlibdoc.who.int/publications/2005/9241593563_eng.pdf?ua51.

All HIV testing and screening should be voluntary; the patient's knowledge and understanding that HIV testing is being planned and undertaken must be obtained. HIV testing should, ideally, also be provided in concert with counseling for risk reduction. HIV testing services should be implemented with strict attention to maintaining the confidentiality of patients. Linkage to HIV care for individuals testing positive should be prompt.

5. Occurrence—An estimated 37.9 million persons worldwide were living with HIV at the end of 2018. Globally, there were an estimated 770,000 AIDS-related deaths in 2018. The number of new HIV infections worldwide is declining, with an estimated 1.7 million new infections in 2018 compared with 3.2 million in 2001. At the end of 2018, 1.7 million children younger than 15 years were living with HIV. HIV-1 is the most prevalent HIV species throughout the world; HIV-2 has been found primarily in western Africa, with infections also in countries linked epidemiologically to western Africa. Eastern/southern Africa is the most affected region, accounting for 54% of people living with HIV worldwide. The Caribbean region is also heavily affected, especially the Dominican Republic and Haiti, which account for most infections in the Caribbean region.

Prevalence has stabilized or is decreasing in most countries, along with some evidence of decreasing risk behavior. The greatest declines in HIV incidence have been in sub-Saharan Africa, with 33% fewer new HIV infections in 2013 than in 2005. In Asia, prevalence is highest in Southeast Asia, with considerable variation in trends—declining in some countries (e.g., Thailand) while continuing to grow in others (e.g., Pakistan and the Philippines). In Eastern Europe and Central Asia, Russia and Ukraine account for most new HIV diagnoses but rates are also rising in other countries.

In 2013, 16 million women aged 15 years and older were living with HIV, representing almost half of people living with HIV globally; in sub-Saharan Africa the percentage is higher—it is estimated that 58% of all infections are in women.

6. Reservoirs—Humans. HIV-1 appears to have evolved from chimpanzee simian immunodeficiency viruses that crossed over to humans, presumably from blood exposure during hunting and butchering of bushmeat. There is some evidence to suggest that this transspecies crossing occurred at multiple times in history. HIV-2 appears to have evolved from cross-species transmission events of sooty mangabey simian immunodeficiency viruses.

7. Incubation period—Variable. Although the time from infection to the development of detectable antibodies is generally less than 1 month, the time from HIV infection to diagnosis of AIDS has an observed range of less than 1 year to 15 years or longer. The median time to development of AIDS in infected infants is shorter than that in adults. There is some evidence that disease progression from HIV infection to AIDS is more rapid in developing countries than in other populations. One factor that has been consistently shown to affect progression from HIV infection to AIDS is age at initial infection: adolescents and adults who acquire HIV infection at an early age progress to AIDS more slowly than those infected at an older age. Disease progression may also vary by viral subtype. In addition, the presence of symptoms and a prolonged duration of illness (> 14 days) during acute infection seem to correlate with more rapid progression to AIDS.

8. Transmission—Person-to-person transmission through unprotected penile-vaginal or penile-anal intercourse; the use of HIV-contaminated injection and skin-piercing equipment, including sharing of needles and syringes by people who inject drugs; vertical transmission from mother to infant during pregnancy, delivery, or breastfeeding; and transfusion of infected blood or its components. Heterosexual sexual transmission is the predominant mode of HIV transmission in sub-Saharan Africa as well as in Southeast Asia, with young women being particularly vulnerable. However, most epidemics in the region are mixed with epidemics also occurring among key populations at higher risk, including sex workers and men who have sex with men (MSM). Injection drug use is the major mode of transmission in Eastern Europe and Central Asia. In Latin America, transmission occurs primarily in higher risk populations such as sex workers and MSM. In North America, Western and Central Europe, Australia, and New Zealand, HIV continues to be transmitted mainly through unprotected sex between men and unsafe injection practices among people who inject drugs. Less common modes of transmission include contact of abraded skin or mucosa with infectious body secretions, the transplantation of HIV-infected tissues or organs, and tattooing or skin-piercing procedures with improperly sterilized needles. The risk of transmission from oral sex is not easily quantifiable but is presumed to be low. While the virus has occasionally been found in saliva, tears, urine, and bronchial secretions, transmission after contact with these secretions in the absence of blood has not been reported. No laboratory or epidemiologic evidence suggests that biting insects have transmitted HIV infection. The period of communicability begins early after onset of HIV infection and presumably extends throughout life if viral suppression is not achieved through the use of effective ART. Infectiousness is related to viral load. The risk of transmission may be high in the first months after infection when viral load is high, even before immune suppression has occurred, and while the high-risk behaviors that led to infection may still be ongoing. Viral load also increases in late symptomatic infection when immunosuppression is present. The use of antiretroviral drugs reduces HIV viral load in blood and genital secretions, hence reducing the infectiousness of HIV-infected individuals who are on treatment. Susceptibility is presumed to be general: race, gender, and pregnancy status do not appear to affect susceptibility to HIV infection or progression to AIDS. Male circumcision significantly reduces the risk of female-to-male transmission. The presence of other STIs, especially if ulcerative, increases risk of transmission and infection.

9. Treatment—

Drug	
	• HIV treatment involves the use of combination antiretroviral therapy, previously referred to as highly active antiretroviral therapy. Typically, a regimen comprising 3 antiretroviral drugs from any of 6 major classes is used; for most individuals, this will be a dual nucleoside reverse transcriptase inhibitor combination plus a third agent from a different class.
	• The 6 classes of drugs are as follows:
	○ NRTIs, including tenofovir, abacavir, lamivudine, emtricitabine, and zidovudine
	○ Non-NRTIs, including efavirenz, rilpivirine, nevirapine, and etravirine
	○ PIs, such as ritonavir (used as a pharmacologic booster in concert with another PI), darunavir, atazanavir, tipranavir, and lopinavir
	○ Integrase strand transfer inhibitors, such as dolutegravir, raltegravir, elvitegravir, bictegravir, and cabotegravir
	○ CCR5 coreceptor antagonist: maraviroc
	○ Fusion inhibitor (enfuvirtide)
	• The exact choice of drug regimen is dependent on host factors, such as coinfections (especially with hepatitis B virus), comorbid conditions such as renal disease, cardiovascular disease, or osteoporosis, and disease-specific factors, such as the presence of transmitted or acquired drug resistance.
	• Despite the number of antiretroviral drugs available, only a small number in combination are recommended for use by international guideline panels.

(Continued)

(Continued)

Dose	Not applicable
Route	All currently available drugs used for ART are taken PO; however, treatment regimens involving long-acting inject-ables are in development.
Alternative drug	Not applicable
Duration	In the absence of reliable curative therapies, suppressive ARTs should be given for life.
Special considerations and comments	<ul><li>The goals of ART are to reduce HIV-associated morbidity and mortality, which may arise from both infectious and noninfectious causes, as well as to reduce the risk of onward transmission of HIV to others.</li><li>This is accomplished through the sustained suppression of viral replication, such that the plasma viral load is lower than the level of detection by commercially available assays. Viral suppression also allows for immune recon-stitution (with CD4+ cell count recovery) and prevents the selection of drug-resistant mutations.</li><li>Current guidelines recommend that ART be initiated for all HIV-infected individuals regardless of CD4+ cell count or immune function, including in asymptomatic individuals. In addition, treatment should be initiated early, unless there are contraindications to this, such as with certain OIs affecting the central nervous system.</li><li>Adherence to treatment is important and adherence counseling should be a central aspect of all treatment provision protocols.</li></ul>

Note: ART = antiretroviral therapy; CCR5 = C-C chemokine receptor 5; CD4+ = cluster of differentiation 4; HIV = human immunodeficiency virus; NRTI = nucleoside/nucleotide reverse transcriptase inhibitor; OI = opportunistic infection; PI = protease inhibitor; PO = oral(ly).

10. Prevention—HIV prevention programs can be effective only with full community and political commitment to facilitate change and/or reduce HIV risk behaviors. Health education efforts should include both broad-based campaigns to raise awareness of risk, modes of transmission, and prevention measures as well as targeted campaigns to reduce risk among high-risk groups such as sex workers, people who inject drugs, transgender people, and MSM. They should also strive to reduce stigmatization and discrimination in all aspects of HIV prevention and education as HIV-associated stigma is a major barrier to at-risk individuals seeking early and/or regular HIV testing, accessing HIV care services, and retention in long-term care.

1) Abstaining from sexual intercourse prevents sexual transmission. Engaging in sex with an uninfected, mutually monogamous part-ner is also effective, although ensuring mutual monogamy and absence of infection may be challenging. Correct and consistent

use of male and female condoms is highly effective in preventing transmission. The promotion of abstinence and monogamy must, however, be in the context of pragmatic, comprehensive prevention programs incorporating other risk-reduction strategies, as they are unlikely to work on their own.

2) Prevention of injection drug use and effective drug dependence treatment, especially the use of opioid substitution therapy for opioid users, reduce HIV transmission. Programs that provide clean injection equipment and risk-reduction counseling for people who inject drugs are very effective in preventing both HIV transmission and the transmission of other bloodborne infections, including viral hepatitis B and C.

3) Postexposure prophylaxis with combination antiretroviral drugs is available and recommended in some settings after exposure to HIV, such as occupational exposure, and after sexual assault. If indicated, treatment should begin within hours of exposure and is usually recommended to continue for 28 days. The combination of drugs used depends on the setting and the prevalence of transmitted resistance as well as the presence of any known resistance mutations in the source patient.

4) Preexposure prophylaxis (PrEP) with antiretroviral drugs (at present, the combination of tenofovir disoproxil fumarate [TDF] and emtricitabine [FTC]) has been shown to be highly effective in the prevention of HIV infection when used by individuals at risk of infection. Efficacy has been demonstrated in heterosexual men, MSM, and women, especially when adherence is high. PrEP is taken as a single tablet of coformulated TDF and FTC; however, it can also be taken on demand in specific circumstances by MSM. Topical antiretrovirals have not been shown to be efficacious in PrEP. PrEP should be provided as part of a comprehensive sexual health and STI-prevention strategy.

5) HIV testing and counseling are important to identify individuals with HIV for referral for care and treatment and, for pregnant women, to prevent vertical transmission of HIV. HIV testing also provides a setting for condom distribution and delivery of prevention messages for HIV-negative persons. In many settings, the emphasis is on universal, opt-out testing for all individuals, especially in high-prevalence communities. All HIV testing must follow the 5 Cs principles: consent, confidentiality, counseling, correct test results, and linkage to care.

6) Treatment as prevention refers to the strategy of treating HIV-diagnosed individuals with combination ART to achieve sustained viral suppression with viral loads lower than the levels of

detection, with the goal of reducing their infectiousness. Several large, robust observational cohorts involving heterosexual and same-sex male serodiscordant couples have demonstrated that linked HIV transmission does not occur when the HIV-infected partner has an undetectable viral load, a paradigm now known as undetectable = untransmissible or U=U. The success of such a strategy is dependent on high uptake of regular HIV testing, linkage to care, initiation of ART, attainment of viral suppression, and long-term retention in care—which represents the HIV care cascade.

7) Mother-to-child transmission of HIV can be minimized through primary prevention of HIV infection in women of childbearing age, prevention of unintended pregnancy in women with HIV, and universal HIV screening of pregnant women. An additional HIV test in the third trimester of pregnancy may identify women who seroconverted during pregnancy. Vertical transmission rates can be reduced by 50% to 90% or more with the use of maternal and infant antiretrovirals in accordance with national guidelines. WHO recommends that all HIV-infected pregnant and breastfeeding women be initiated on lifelong combination ART to prevent HIV transmission to their infants and for their own health. If lifelong treatment is not provided, mothers who are breastfeeding should use antiretrovirals until 1 week after the complete cessation of breastfeeding in association with the infant being provided with antiretroviral prophylaxis for the first 6 weeks of life. Replacement feeding should only be used when infant formula is acceptable, feasible, affordable, sustainable, and safe. Elective cesarean section may also play a role in resource-rich settings but is only recommended for obstetric and other medical indications in resource-limited settings.

8) Blood donations should only be sought from unpaid volunteer donors. The use of autologous transfusions should be encouraged when feasible. All donated units of blood must be tested for HIV; only donations testing negative should be used. Organizations that collect plasma, blood, or other bodily fluids or organs should inform potential donors of this recommendation and test all donors. Testing for HIV antigen or nucleic acid can further reduce the risk of contamination, taking into account the possibility that donors may be in the window period during which time antibody testing may be unreliable. Patients, their sexual partners, and others who have engaged in behaviors that place them at increased risk of HIV infection should not donate plasma, blood, organs, tissue, or cells (including semen for artificial

insemination). However, criminalization of individuals unaware of their HIV-positive serostatus at the time of blood donation should be discouraged. Some centers have reported safe impregnation of women by HIV-infected male partners through semen processing or viral suppression in the men with antiretroviral treatment. When possible, donations of sperm, milk, or bone should be frozen and stored for 3 to 6 months before use. Donors who test negative after that interval can be considered free of infection at the time of donation. Only clotting factor products that have been screened and treated to inactivate HIV should be used.

9) Only medically necessary injections should be given. Care must be taken in handling, using, and disposing of needles or other sharp instruments. Medical waste should be safely stored and destroyed. Health care workers should be provided with and instructed on the proper use of latex gloves, eye protection, and other personal protective equipment as needed in order to avoid contact with blood or fluids. Universal precautions must be taken in the care of all patients and in all laboratory procedures.

10) Universal precautions should be taken by services that provide tattooing and skin-piercing procedures, including the appropriate sterilization of any equipment that is reused.

11. Special considerations—

1) Reporting: reporting of HIV/AIDS diagnoses is obligatory in most countries. Whether or not name-based reporting is the rule, the utmost care must be taken to protect patient confidentiality.

2) The criminalization of inadvertent HIV transmission or failure to disclose one's HIV serostatus, especially when the HIV-infected individual is virally suppressed and poses no risk of onward transmission to others, is not recommended.

3) Requiring foreign travelers to undergo HIV testing or examinations prior to entry into a country is not recommended.

4) HIV-infected children can safely be given routine childhood immunizations, except for Bacillus Calmette-Guérin vaccine.

5) For case definitions, see: http://www.who.int/hiv/pub/guidelines/HIVstaging150307.pdf?ua51.

[C. S. Wong, S. Archuleta]

❖

HOOKWORM
(ancylostomiasis, uncinariasis, necatoriasis)

DISEASE	ICD-10 CODE
HOOKWORM	ICD-10 B76

1. Clinical features—A common chronic helminth infection of the intestine that causes anemia with a variety of symptoms, usually in proportion to the degree of iron deficiency. In heavy infections, the bloodletting activity of the nematode leads to iron deficiency and hypochromic microcytic anemia, the major cause of disability. Children with heavy long-term infection may have hypoproteinemia and delayed mental and physical development. Occasionally, severe acute pulmonary and gastrointestinal reactions follow exposure to infective larvae. Light hookworm infections generally produce few or no clinical effects. Some species of the causative helminths are unable to survive in the skin and do not cause intestinal infection.

Exposure of humans to larvae of some animal hookworms may lead to self-limited subcutaneous migration of infective larvae (cutaneous larva migrans) with associated pruritus and erythema, which may persist for several months. Humans may also be aberrant hosts for the canine hookworm (*Ancylostoma caninum*). This species does not reach maturity in the human gut but it may cause eosinophilic enteritis characterized by severe abdominal pain, diarrhea, weight loss, and melena.

2. Risk groups—People (especially children) living in warm, moist climates where sanitation and hygiene are poor, particularly those who walk barefoot or in other ways allow their skin to have direct contact with contaminated soil.

3. Causative agents—Patent hookworm infection: *Ancylostoma duodenale, Ancylostoma ceylanicum, Necator americanus*. Eosinophilic enteritis: *A. caninum*. Cutaneous larva migrans: *Ancylostoma braziliense, Uncinaria stenocephala*, possibly other zoonotic hookworm species.

4. Diagnosis—Hookworm infection is usually diagnosed based on characteristic laboratory findings, such as eosinophilia, in combination with detection of hookworm eggs on microscopic examination of stools. The eggs of *Ancylostoma* and *Necator* cannot be differentiated microscopically. Hookworm larvae may be cultured by Baermann sedimentation, Harada-Mori cultures, or Koga agar plates. Adult worms are rarely seen, except via endoscopy, surgery, or autopsy, but, if found, allow for definitive species identification. Fecal polymerase chain reaction is increasingly used for surveillance.

5. Occurrence—Endemic in tropical and subtropical countries where facilities for sanitary disposal of human feces are not available and soil, moisture, and temperature conditions favor development of infective larvae. Also occurs in temperate climates under similar environmental conditions (e.g., in mines). Both *Necator* and *A. duodenale* occur in many parts of Asia, Australia, East Africa, and South America. *N. americanus* is the prevailing species throughout southeastern Asia, most of tropical Africa, and the Americas; *A. duodenale* prevails in North Africa, including the Nile Valley, northern India, northern parts of eastern Asia, and the Andean areas of South America. Human infection *A. ceylanicum* occurs in Southeast Asia, Australia, and the Pacific Islands but is less common than *N. americanus*, which is the predominant hookworm in this region. *A. caninum* has been described in Australia as a cause of eosinophilic enteritis syndrome.

With regard to species causing cutaneous larva migrans, *A. braziliense* is most common in coastal tropical and subtropical regions. *U. stenocephala* is most common in temperate regions.

6. Reservoirs—Humans for *A. duodenale* and *N. americanus*; humans, cats, and dogs for *A. ceylanicum*; cats and dogs for *A. caninum*.

7. Incubation period—Hookworms reach sexual maturity in the host approximately 5 to 8 weeks after first infection with filariform larvae. Pulmonary infiltration, cough, and tracheitis may occur early in infection during the lung migration phase, particularly in *Necator* infections. After entering the body, *A. duodenale* may become dormant in the tissue (arrested development) for up to 8 months, after which development resumes, with evidence of infection (stools containing eggs) 1 month later.

8. Transmission—Eggs in feces are deposited on the ground, embryonate, and hatch; under favorable conditions of moisture, temperature, and soil type, larvae develop and become infective in 7 to 10 days. Human infection usually occurs when infective larvae penetrate the skin, usually of the foot; in so doing, they produce a characteristic dermatitis (ground itch). Normally, the larvae of *Necator*, *A. duodenale*, and *A. ceylanicum* enter the skin and pass via lymphatics and bloodstream to the lungs, enter the alveoli, migrate up the trachea to the pharynx, are swallowed, and reach the small intestine, where they attach to the intestinal wall, developing to maturity in 6 to 7 weeks (3–4 weeks in the case of *A. ceylanicum*). Female *A. duodenale* produce up to 10,000 to 25,000 eggs per day and may live for 8 years or longer, though the normal life span is 3 to 5 years. *N. americanus* produces up to 5,000 to 10,000 eggs per day and may live for up to 14 years, though the normal life span is 3 to 5 years. There is only very limited information on the life span and egg production of *A. ceylanicum* in humans. Infection with *Ancylostoma* may also be acquired by ingesting infective larvae; possible transmammary transmission (transmission of infective larvae from mother to child via breast milk) has been reported for *A. duodenale*. Infected people can contaminate soil for several years in the absence of treatment. Under favorable conditions, larvae remain infective in soil for several weeks.

9. Treatment—

Drug	• Albendazole • Mebendazole
Dose	• Albendazole 400 mg as a single dose[a] OR • Mebendazole 100 mg BID for 3 days or 500 mg as a single dose[a]
Route	PO
Alternative drug	Pyrantel 11 mg/kg ($\leq$ 1 g) PO daily for 3 days
Duration	• Albendazole once • Mebendazole over 3 days (usual dose) or once (higher dose)
Special considerations and comments	Available evidence suggests these drugs are safe for use among women during the second and third trimesters of pregnancy, among those who are lactating, and among children $\geq$ 2 years. Although these drugs are generally considered safe, limited data exist on the risk of treatment in pregnant women during the first trimester or in young children < 2 years; thus, risk of treatment needs to be balanced with the risk of disease progression in the absence of treatment. If very young children (1–2 years) are treated, they should be given tablets that are crushed and mixed with water; treatment should be supervised by trained personnel.

Note: BID = twice daily; PO = oral(ly).
[a]A half dosage is recommended for children < 24 months.

10. Prevention—

1) Educate the public about the dangers of soil contamination by human, cat, or dog feces and about preventive measures, including the use of footwear in endemic areas.

2) Prevent soil contamination by installation of sanitary disposal systems for human feces, especially sanitary latrines in rural areas. Human feces and sewage effluents are hazardous, especially when used as fertilizer.

3) Examine and treat people migrating from endemic to nonendemic areas, especially those who work barefoot in mines, construct dams, or work in the agricultural sector.

4) WHO recommends a preventive chemotherapy strategy focused on mebendazole or albendazole treatment annually or every 6 months in high-risk groups (preschool or school-aged children, adolescents not in school, women of reproductive age); treatment should also be carried out at regular intervals for the control

of morbidity owing to the soil-transmitted helminths causing ascariasis, trichuriasis, and hookworm disease (https://www. who.int/intestinal_worms/en). See "Ascariasis."

11. Special considerations—Epidemic measures: prevalence surveys in highly endemic areas; provide periodic mass treatment. Educate people in environmental sanitation and personal hygiene and provide facilities for excreta disposal. Prevent the use of human excreta as fertilizer.

[R. S. Bradbury, M. Kamb]

HUMAN PAPILLOMAVIRUS INFECTIONS

DISEASE	ICD-10 CODE
VIRAL WARTS	ICD-10 B07
ANOGENITAL (VENEREAL) WARTS	ICD-10 A63
CERVICAL CANCER	ICD-10 C53
VULVAR CANCER	ICD-10 C51
VAGINAL CANCER	ICD-10 C52
PENILE CANCER	ICD-10 C60
ANAL CANCER	ICD-10 C21
OROPHARYNGEAL CANCER	ICD-10 C10

Human papillomaviruses (HPVs) are small, nonenveloped, double-stranded deoxyribonucleic acid (DNA) viruses in the family Papillomaviridae. More than 200 types have been identified. HPV infections are very common but are usually asymptomatic and self-limited. Persistent infections can cause warts or invasive cervical, vaginal, vulvar, penile, anal, and oropharyngeal cancers. HPV types are tissue-tropic; types that cause warts do not cause cancers. Since HPV vaccines were first licensed in 2006, they have been added to national immunization programs in more than 71 countries; to date, significant declines have been observed in HPV prevalence, anogenital warts, and cervical precancers caused by HPV types targeted by the vaccines.

I. HUMAN PAPILLOMAVIRUS INFECTIONS

1. Clinical features—Asymptomatic, self-limited. About 70% resolve within a year and about 90% within 2 years.

2. Risk groups—It is estimated that more than 80% of sexually active adults will acquire a genital HPV infection; however, most infections clear without intervention. People with certain immunocompromising conditions, including human immunodeficiency virus (HIV), are at particularly high risk for persistent HPV infections and related diseases.

3. Causative agents—About 40 HPV types infect mucosal tissue and can be classified as nononcogenic or oncogenic. Other types infect keratinized epithelium.

4. Diagnosis—May be identified as part of cervical cancer screening. HPV screening is not recommended for men.

5. Occurrence—Worldwide.

6. Reservoirs—Humans only.

7. Incubation period—Not applicable.

8. Transmission—Mucosal HPV transmission occurs during direct contact with infected skin during intimate activity, including vaginal, penile, oral, or anal sex.

9. Treatment—No specific treatment is recommended or required for asymptomatic HPV infection.

10. Prevention—Condoms may decrease sexual transmission of mucosal HPV types. Three prophylactic vaccines are available to prevent new HPV infections; vaccination does not treat existing infection or disease. A 9-valent vaccine (Gardasil 9, Merck, Whitehouse Station, NJ) targets HPV types 6, 11, 16, 18, 31, 33, 45, 52, and 58. A quadrivalent vaccine (Gardasil, Merck, Whitehouse Station, NJ) targets HPV types 6, 11, 16, and 18. A bivalent vaccine (Cervarix, GlaxoSmithKline, Rixensart, Belgium) targets HPV types 16 and 18. All available HPV vaccines have high efficacy against the targeted HPV types. These are virus-like particle vaccines; they contain no viral DNA and are noninfectious. Countries that include HPV vaccination in their routine immunization program recommend vaccination in early or preadolescence, either for girls only or for girls and boys. Some countries also recommend catch-up vaccination for older adolescents and/or young adults who were not vaccinated on time when they were younger. In the USA, routine HPV vaccination is recommended for girls and boys at age 11 to 12 years (can be given starting at age 9 years); catch-up vaccination is recommended for adults through age 26 years. Number of recommended doses varies by age at initiation: 2 doses are recommended for persons initiating vaccination before their 15th birthday and 3 doses are recommended for persons with certain immunocompromising conditions or who initiate vaccination on or after their 15th birthday. HPV vaccination is most effective when given before exposure to mucosal HPV types (before sexual activity). There are no recommendations for postexposure vaccination; however, if contacts have not been vaccinated and are in the recommended age group, vaccine can be administered.

11. Special considerations—Additional information is available at:

- https://www.cdc.gov/hpv
- https://www.who.int/immunization/diseases/hpv/en

II. WARTS (verruca vulgaris, common wart, palmar wart, plantar wart, periungual wart, condyloma acuminatum, recurrent respiratory papillomatosis)

1. Clinical features—Skin and mucous membrane lesions characterized by benign growths or changes in the epithelium (verruca vulgaris, common warts). Commonly located on the skin of the hands or feet (palmar warts, plantar warts, periungual warts) or on anogenital areas, such as the anus, vagina, vulva, cervix, penis, or scrotum (condyloma accuminata). Less common in oral, nasal, or conjunctival areas or in the upper respiratory tract (recurrent respiratory papillomatosis). Some examples of clinical types of warts include the following:

1) Hyperkeratotic: well-circumscribed, rough-textured papules 2 mm to 1 cm in size; can be found anywhere on the mucocutaneous surface, sometimes in groups.
2) Filiform: elongated, pointed, delicate lesions that may reach 1 cm in length.
3) Flat: smooth and flat or slightly elevated; may be hypopigmented or hyperpigmented; usually multiple lesions varying in size from 1 mm to 1 cm.
4) Condyloma acuminata: seen in the anogenital area; can present as hyperkeratotic, filiform, flat, or cauliflower-like.

Recurrent respiratory papillomatosis is generally a benign condition but it can result in vocal changes and respiratory tract obstruction.

2. Risk groups—Cutaneous warts are common among children; genital warts are common among sexually active young adults. Incidence is higher among people who are immunosuppressed, including those with HIV or organ transplantation; rarely, malignant transformation of a benign lesion to squamous cell carcinoma can occur.

3. Causative agents—A variety of cutaneous HPV types can infect keratinized epithelium and can cause common skin warts. Nononcogenic, or low-risk, HPV types can cause benign mucosal warts and respiratory papillomatosis. These types include HPV 6 and 11, which cause 90% of anogenital warts and almost all respiratory papillomas.

4. Diagnosis—Usually based on visual examination. If the lesion is atypical, pigmented, indurated, fixed, bleeding, or ulcerated or if the lesion does not respond to therapy or worsens during therapy, particularly in immunocompromised patients, the lesion should be biopsied and examined histologically. Recurrent respiratory papillomatosis can be diagnosed by laryngoscopy.

5. Occurrence—Worldwide.

6. Reservoirs—Humans exclusively.

7. Incubation period—Range of 1 to 20 months.

8. Transmission—Transmission of cutaneous HPV types is usually by direct contact but may also be via fomites. Mucosal HPV transmission occurs during direct contact with infected skin during intimate activity, including vaginal, penile, oral, or anal sex. The period of communicability is unknown but is probably at least as long as visible warts persist. HPV may still be transmitted after warts are treated or no longer present or visible. Recurrent respiratory papillomatosis in children is presumably transmitted vertically during delivery by a mother infected with low-risk HPV.

9. Treatment—Recommended regimens for treating external anogenital warts may be patient-applied or provider-administered.

Preferred therapy	Patient-applied options: • Imiquimod 3.75% or 5% cream • Podofilox 0.5% solution or gel • Sinecatechins 15% ointment • Salicylic acid
	Provider-administered options: • Cryotherapy • Surgical removal by tangential scissor excision, tangential shave excision, curettage, laser, or electrosurgery • Trichloroacetic acid 80%–90% solution • Bichloroacetic acid 80%–90% solution
Route	Topical
Alternative therapy options	There is no definitive evidence to suggest that any one recommended treatment is superior to another.[a]
Duration	Treatment may take months and require several different combinations of therapy. In immunocompetent patients, warts usually regress spontaneously within months to years.

(Continued)

(Continued)

Special considerations and comments	• Many agents used for treatment of warts have not been tested for safety and efficacy in children and some are contraindicated in pregnancy. Cesarean delivery solely to prevent transmission of HPV infection to a newborn is not recommended.
	• Treatment of visible warts may not eradicate HPV infection from the surrounding tissue.
	• People with anogenital warts and their partners can benefit from additional testing for sexually transmitted infections.
	• For recurrent respiratory papillomatosis, repeated surgeries may be required to relieve airway obstruction and/or to preserve speech.
	• Sinecatechins are not recommended for persons with HIV infection, other immunocompromising conditions, or genital herpes, because safety and efficacy have not been evaluated
	• It is unknown whether treatment reduces future transmission.

Note: HIV = human immunodeficiency virus; HPV = human papillomavirus.
[a]Alternatives for treating external genital warts are discussed in detail at: https://www.cdc.gov/std/tg2015/warts.htm.

10. Prevention—Avoid direct contact with lesions on another person; however, because most HPV infections are asymptomatic or subclinical, most people with the infection will not have visible lesions. Condoms may decrease sexual transmission of mucosal HPV types. Prophylactic HPV vaccination is most effective when given before exposure to mucosal HPV types (before sexual activity). Both quadrivalent HPV vaccine (Gardasil) and 9-valent HPV vaccine (Gardasil 9) are highly efficacious in preventing warts and HPV infections due to low-risk HPV types 6 and 11 in males and females. Vaccines do not prevent common skin warts or plantar warts caused by cutaneous types of HPV.

11. Special considerations—Additional information is available at:

- https://www.cdc.gov/std/treatment
- https://www.who.int/topics/sexually_transmitted_infections/en

III. HUMAN PAPILLOMAVIRUS–RELATED CANCERS
(cervical, vulvar, vaginal, penile, anal, and oropharyngeal cancers)

1. Clinical features—High-risk mucosal HPV types can cause cervical, vaginal, and vulvar cancers in women; penile cancers in men; and anal and oropharyngeal cancers in women and men. Clinical presentation of cancer varies by anatomic site. In most of these cancers, invasive cancer is preceded by a preinvasive phase recognized histologically as intraepithelial neoplasia. Clinically, intraepithelial neoplasia can present as atypical warts or skin changes, with pigmentation, erythema, or warts that are fixed to, or show induration of, the underlying skin or mucosa. Histologically, vaginal, vulvar, penile, anal, and cervical intraepithelial neoplasias are categorized by increasing severity or grades of dysplastic changes.

2. Risk groups—People with certain immunocompromising conditions, including HIV, are at particularly high risk for persistent HPV infections and related diseases. In addition, immunosuppressed people are at higher risk for progression of HPV infection to cancer. Epidermodysplasia verruciformis is a rare inherited disorder that predisposes patients to widespread HPV infection and cutaneous squamous cell carcinomas.

3. Causative agents—Oncogenic, or high-risk, HPV types (16, 18, and others) can cause precancers and cancers, including cervical, vulvar, vaginal, penile, anal, and oropharyngeal cancer. Together, HPV types 16 and 18 account for more than 70% of cervical cancers and the majority of other cancers caused by HPV.

4. Diagnosis—Cancer screening recommendations vary by country. HPV tests may be used for cervical cancer screening. Other established cervical cancer screening methods include conventional or liquid-based cytology examination following a Papanicolaou test (Pap smear) or, in certain low-resource settings, direct visual inspection with acetic acid. Characteristic changes on the cervix may lead to colposcopic evaluation and biopsy with histologic examination of the tissue specimen. There are no formal screening programs for other cancers caused by HPV.

5. Occurrence—Globally, about 5% of all cancers are attributable to HPV.

6. Reservoirs—Not applicable.

7. Incubation period—The usual time between initial HPV infection and development of HPV-related cancer is decades.

8. Transmission—Mucosal HPV transmission occurs during direct contact with infected skin during intimate activity, including vaginal, penile, oral, or anal sex.

9. Treatment—For HPV-related cancers, treatment options depend on various factors, including the type of cancer and its stage and grade; these may include surgery, radiation therapy, and/or chemotherapy.

10. Prevention—Detection and treatment of cervical precancers can prevent progression to invasive cervical cancer. Cervical cancer screening programs have reduced cervical cancer incidence and mortality in many high-income countries. However, many countries with the greatest burden of disease do not have cervical cancer screening programs in place; the resources and infrastructure needed for these programs can be substantial.

11. Special considerations—Unlike HPV infections, HPV-related cancers are reportable in many countries. Population-based cancer registries record incidence of malignancy for a specific catchment area, according to the International Classification of Diseases for Oncology. Additional information is available at:

- https://www.cdc.gov/cancer/hpv/index.htm
- https://hpvcentre.net
- https://www.iarc.fr

[E. Meites, L. Markowitz]

HUMAN T-LYMPHOTROPIC VIRUS TYPE 1 INFECTION

DISEASE	ICD-10 CODE
HUMAN T-LYMPHOTROPIC VIRUS TYPE 1 INFECTION (asymptomatic carrier)	ICD-10 Z22.6
ADULT T-CELL LYMPHOMA/LEUKEMIA (acute, chronic, lymphomatoid, smoldering)	ICD-10 C91.5
HUMAN T-LYMPHOTROPIC VIRUS TYPE 1 INFECTION–ASSOCIATED MYELOPATHY/TROPICAL SPASTIC PARAPARESIS	ICD-10 G04.1
POLYMYOSITIS	ICD-10 B97.3
UVEITIS	ICD-10 B97.3
INFECTIVE DERMATITIS	ICD-10 B97.3
BRONCHIECTASIS	ICD-10 B97.3

I. HUMAN T-LYMPHOTROPIC VIRUS TYPE 1

1. Clinical features—Human T-lymphotropic virus type 1 (HTLV-1) causes a lifelong infection that chiefly persists by driving mitotic proliferation of infected cluster of differentiation 4 (CD4+) T lymphocytes. HTLV-1 causes \a number of manifestations in 5% to 10% of HTLV-1–infected individuals while

90% remain lifelong healthy asymptomatic carriers. The 2 most common diseases are an aggressive T-cell malignancy known as adult T-cell lymphoma/leukemia (ATL) and HTLV-1–associated myelopathy (formerly known as tropical spastic paraplegia [HAM/TSP]), which clinically resembles primary progressive multiple sclerosis. In addition, HTLV-1 may cause inflammatory diseases such as polymyositis, uveitis, and infective dermatitis. It is recognized that there is a high incidence of bronchiectasis among HTLV-1 carriers. The mechanisms by which HTLV-1 causes diverse manifestations are unknown; since no viral genotype is associated with clinical disease and there is a strong antiviral immune response, the currently accepted hypothesis is that the efficiency of the host immune response is the main determinant of disease.

2. Risk groups—Since clinical disease occurs several decades after asymptomatic infection, the major risk groups for ATL or HAM/TSP comprise those infected during infancy from breastfeeding and those infected via sexual transmission in endemic regions. Several countries, including many wealthy nations, still do not routinely screen blood products or organs, increasing the risk of HTLV-1 infection within low-prevalence regions.

3. Causative agents—There are 3 genotypes of HTLV-1 (Melanesian, Central African, and Cosmopolitan) but there is no clear association between the viral genotype and disease. HTLV-2, which targets $CD8^+$ T lymphocytes, is not associated with clinical disease.

4. Diagnosis—HTLV-1 antibody detection by enzyme immunoassay or Western blotting. Since HTLV-1 and HTLV-2 antibodies cross-react, any positive results should be confirmed by a second assay that can distinguish HTLV-1 and HTLV-2. Polymerase chain reaction (PCR) can resolve untypeable or indeterminate results. Quantitative real-time PCR to quantify the HTLV-1 proviral load—the proportion of HTLV-1–infected mononuclear cells—is important for determining risk of clinical disease (disease risk highest with proviral load > 4% in Japan and > 10% in the Caribbean). In ATL tumor cells, demonstration of monoclonal integration of HTLV-1 provirus by Southern blotting or inverse/linker-mediated PCR (to distinguish ATL from other incidental T-cell malignancies in asymptomatic HTLV-1 carriers).

5. Occurrence—Worldwide. Endemic within regions of southern Japan, sub-Saharan Africa, the Caribbean, Brazil, Peru, and Iran.

6. Reservoirs—Humans. A genotypically similar simian virus (STLV-1) is found in nonhuman primates (e.g., Japanese monkey); historical transmission from nonhuman to human primates via animal bites is thought to be the origin of HTLV-1.

7. Incubation period—50 to 60 years for disease manifestations.

8. Transmission—In endemic countries mother-to-child transmission via prolonged breastfeeding is the major route (30%–40% risk of transmission). HTLV-1 can also be contracted through infected cellular blood product transfusions, sexual contact, and solid organ transplantation.

9. Treatment—There is no specific treatment for HTLV-1 carriers or those with active infection.

10. Prevention—Antibody screening of pregnant women and known HTLV-1 carriers to avoid breastfeeding; condoms to prevent sexual transmission; antibody screening of blood products and organs for transplantation. In established HTLV-1 infection, there are no means to prevent the onset of clinical disease.

11. Special considerations—The risk of HTLV-1 transmission following a needlestick injury to a health care worker is unknown. Immediate postexposure prophylaxis with antiretrovirals (e.g., raltegravir and zidovudine) to prevent integration of the provirus and chronic infection should be considered.

II. ADULT T-CELL LYMPHOMA/LEUKEMIA

ATL is an aggressive CD4+CD25+ T-cell malignancy with 4 distinct clinical subtypes (Shimoyama classification) defined according to absolute lymphocyte count, percentage of abnormal lymphocytes (flower cells) on a blood smear, corrected calcium, lactate dehydrogenase (LDH), and presence of enlarged lymph nodes and organ infiltration. The acute and lymphoma subtypes are regarded as aggressive while chronic or smoldering subtypes are regarded as indolent, although transformation from indolent to aggressive subtypes is frequent.

For acute subtypes, lymphocyte count is at least 4×10^9/L, with at least 5% abnormal lymphocytes; LDH is typically high; corrected calcium is usually high, often with widespread lymphadenopathy (not essential) and organ infiltration (skin, lung, liver, spleen, central nervous system [CNS], bone, ascites, pleural effusions, gastrointestinal [GI] tract).

For lymphoma subtypes, histology has proven lymphadenopathy with no peripheral blood involvement (lymphocyte count $< 4 \times 10^9$/L, $\leq 1\%$ abnormal lymphocytes); LDH is typically high; corrected calcium is usually high, often with organ infiltration (skin, lung, liver, spleen, CNS, bone, ascites, pleural effusions, GI tract).

For chronic subtypes, there is peripheral blood and/or lymph node involvement (lymphocyte count $\geq 4 \times 10^9$/L, $\geq 5\%$ abnormal lymphocytes) but with LDH less than 2 times the upper limit of normal and normal corrected calcium. Skin and lung may be involved but no CNS, GI tract, or bone infiltration. For smoldering subtypes, there is increased abnormal lymphocytes on peripheral blood smear ($\geq 5\%$) but with a normal absolute lymphocyte count ($< 4 \times 10^9$/L); LDH is less than 1.5 times the upper limit of normal; corrected calcium is normal. There is no associated lymphadenopathy, although skin and lung infiltration may be observed.

For aggressive ATL subtypes, the prognosis of aggressive ATL is extremely poor mainly because of tumor resistance to steroids and cytotoxic agents combined with significant immune suppression and susceptibility to opportunistic infection. In aggressive subtypes, the best clinical trial results to date using combination chemotherapy report complete response rates in only 25% to 40% patients, with median progression-free survival of 5 to 7 months and overall survival of 13 months. In the few cases of acute ATL that do not involve lymph nodes, the disease can respond to treatment with zidovudine and interferon. More recently, the monoclonal antibody mogamulizumab—which targets CC chemokine receptor type 4, which is widely expressed on ATL tumor cells—has been licensed in Japan for clinical use in salvage therapy. The only curative treatment is allogeneic bone marrow transplantation but this is only an option for those who are young enough, fit enough, and have achieved a response to induction treatment.

For indolent ATL subtypes that are untreated, the median survival of chronic ATL is approximately 5 years, with death due to transformation to aggressive disease or opportunistic infection. In the USA and Europe combination with zidovudine and interferon alfa is the standard of care for those patients who can tolerate the treatment.

III. HTLV-1–ASSOCIATED MYELOPATHY/TROPICAL SPASTIC PARAPARESIS

HAM/TSP is characterized by a gradual symmetric paraparesis of the lower limbs with signs of pyramidal tract involvement, which slowly progresses without remissions. Early in the disease the symptoms are weakness of the lower limbs and lumbar pain. Patients frequently describe urinary and sexual problems. Dizziness is common (with normal clinical examination). The weakness in the lower limbs is associated with moderate-to-severe spasticity. As the disease progresses, the weakness and spasticity increase and gait deteriorates. Neuropathic pain becomes common and autonomic dysfunction of the bladder and bowel are a common cause of significant morbidity. There has been a lack of large clinical trials and treatment remains largely palliative, although some patients respond to immune suppression with methotrexate or cyclosporine.

Bibliography

Gonçalves DU, Proietti FA, Ribas JGR, et al. Epidemiology, treatment, and prevention of human T-cell leukemia virus type 1-associated diseases. *Clin Microbiol Rev.* 2010;23 (3):577-589.

[O. A. Khan]

INFLUENZA

DISEASE	ICD-10 CODE
SEASONAL INFLUENZA	ICD-10 J10, J11
OTHER INFLUENZA	ICD-10 J09

I. SEASONAL INFLUENZA

1. Clinical features—An acute viral infection of the respiratory tract characterized by symptoms of fever, cough, headache, myalgia, malaise, coryza, and sore throat. The cough is usually nonproductive but can be severe; along with constitutional symptoms the cough may last for 2 or more weeks (postviral asthenia). Fever and other symptoms generally resolve in less than 5 days. Gastrointestinal (GI) tract manifestations (nausea, vomiting, diarrhea) may accompany the respiratory phase and have been reported in up to 25% of children in school outbreaks of influenza A and B. GI manifestations are uncommon in adults. Infants may present with atypical symptoms or a sepsis-like syndrome. Older patients may not present with typical influenza-like symptoms and less frequently report systemic complaints and fever. Complications of influenza may be due to the virus directly or a secondary bacterial infection. This includes lower respiratory tract involvement such as bronchitis and pneumonitis; viral pneumonia; sinusitis; otitis media; febrile seizures; encephalitis/encephalopathy; myositis and rhabdomyolysis; myocarditis; Reye syndrome in association with use of salicylates (aspirin); and a bacterial pneumonia typically due to *Streptococcus pneumoniae* or *Staphylococcus aureus* (associated with higher mortality and a significant proportion being methicillin-resistant *S. aureus*). Influenza may also exacerbate underlying medical conditions such as congestive heart failure and chronic obstructive pulmonary disease.

2. Risk groups—Yearly seasonal influenza epidemics impose a substantial health burden on all age groups. Outbreaks can be explosive and overwhelm health care services. The highest risk of severe influenza and complications occurs among children younger than 2 years, pregnant women, adults 65 years or older, and persons of any age with chronic medical conditions including cardiovascular, pulmonary, renal, hepatic, hematologic, or metabolic disorders (e.g., diabetes); immunodeficiency; and neurologic/neuromuscular conditions that can compromise respiratory function or ability to expectorate respiratory secretions. Tobacco smoking and obesity are also associated with an increased risk of influenza-associated complications. More than 90% of influenza deaths occur among those aged 65 years and older. Population estimates of influenza-associated global mortality are highest in Africa and Southeast Asia, suggesting that malnutrition and poor access to health care contribute to higher rates of complications and death. Age-specific attack rates during seasonal influenza epidemics reflect immune memory (primarily antibody) from past exposure to circulating viruses and vaccines. The incidence of infection is often highest in children, who have fewer prior influenza infections and hence less preexisting immunity.

3. Causative agents—Four types of influenza virus are known: A, B, C, and D. Influenza A viruses are further divided into subtypes based on 2 viral surface glycoproteins: hemagglutinin (HA) and neuraminidase (NA). There are 18 different HA subtypes and 11 different NA subtypes currently recognized. Influenza circulates among birds and animals in a wide variety of HA and NA combinations. Since 1977, 2 subtypes of influenza A viruses have cocirculated among humans as seasonal influenza: A/H1N1 and A/H3N2. The host range of influenza B is largely restricted to humans, although natural infection of other mammals (e.g., dogs, seals, swine) has been reported. Influenza B viruses can be distinguished as 2 antigenically and genetically distinct lineages (B/Victoria and B/Yamagata). Both influenza A and B viruses cause seasonal epidemics and sporadic outbreaks. Infections with influenza C are generally associated with only a mild respiratory illness; this virus does not cause epidemics. Influenza type D was identified in 2011 and primarily affects cattle. It is currently unknown whether this virus can also cause disease in humans. Influenza viruses are named based on their type, geographic site of detection, laboratory number, year of isolation, and subtype (e.g., A/Michigan/45/2015 [H1N1], A/Switzerland/8060/2017 [H3N2], and B/Colorado/06/2017 [B/Victoria/2/87 lineage]).

HA and NA change continuously during viral replication owing to an error-prone viral ribonucleic acid (RNA)–dependent RNA polymerase. This results in the emergence of new antigenic variants able to escape host immunity in a process termed antigenic drift. The constant emergence of new influenza viruses results in the need for review and replacement of A/H1N1, A/H3N2, and B viruses that are contained in vaccines. This is currently performed biannually by WHO 6 months in advance of northern and southern hemisphere influenza seasons. The constant emergence of drifted viruses is the main reason for yearly epidemics of seasonal influenza and for individuals sometimes being infected with influenza multiple times over their lifetime. Infection induces robust immunity to the same strain and offers some protection against antigenically similar viruses. The duration and breadth of cross-immunity depend, in part, on the degree of antigenic similarity between viruses inducing immunity and those causing disease. Short-lived heterosubtypic protection has also been observed. During seasonal epidemics, much of the population has partial protection because of earlier infections from related viruses.

In addition to antigenic drift, influenza A viruses can also undergo a dramatic change in their surface HA and NA proteins; this is called antigenic shift. This typically refers to the emergence through recombination of a novel influenza A virus capable of causing infection in humans and bearing a HA protein or a combination of HA and NA proteins that have not been in circulation among humans in recent years. The majority of the world's population will have no immunity against this virus; consequently, it may cause a global pandemic if the virus becomes capable of sustained human-to-human transmission (see Other Influenza in this chapter).

4. Diagnosis—Influenza is clinically indistinguishable from disease caused by other respiratory viruses, such as rhinovirus, respiratory syncytial virus, parainfluenza, and adenovirus. In temperate climates, recognition of potential influenza is commonly based on clinical presentation during winter months with a syndrome consistent with influenza-like illness. Clinical diagnosis accuracy improves when influenza surveillance information is available to indicate that influenza viruses are in circulation.

The primary clinical test for laboratory confirmation of influenza infection is reverse transcription polymerase chain reaction (RT-PCR) of virus-specific RNA sequences from throat, nasal, and nasopharyngeal secretions or tracheal aspirate or washings. Results from conventional RT-PCR can be available within 4 to 8 hours from a central laboratory, but batching and processing of tests may result in substantial delay. Molecular assays intended for point-of-care testing have also been developed. These detect influenza viral RNA from upper respiratory tract samples, yield results within 30 minutes, and offer sensitivities of 66% to 100%.

Other rapid tests are available. These are typically immunoassays that screen for viral antigens in nasopharyngeal cells and fluids (fluorescent antibody test or enzyme-linked immunosorbent assay). Commercially available point-of-care tests have variable sensitivity (50%–70%) but good specificity (90%–95%). Thus, in the setting of a known influenza epidemic, negative results from patients with symptoms consistent with influenza must be interpreted cautiously. If excluding a false-negative result is important, then more sensitive testing such as RT-PCR should be considered.

Other diagnostic methods that are not part of routine clinical practice include viral isolation using cell culture or embryonated eggs and demonstration of a 4-fold or greater rise in strain-specific antibody titers between acute and convalescent sera using hemagglutination-inhibition (HAI) or neutralization assays.

Ideally, respiratory specimens should be collected as early into the illness as possible. Virus shedding starts to wane by the third day of onset of symptoms and lasts on average for 5 days in healthy adults. Virus shedding can occur for 7 to 10 days in children and even longer in immunocompromised individuals.

5. Occurrence—The epidemiology of influenza varies with climate. In temperate climates seasonal influenza results in yearly epidemics of varying severity. The timing of epidemics is closely correlated with the winter decline in temperature and absolute humidity. Outside the winter season, only sporadic cases or outbreaks are observed. Within the tropics epidemics are associated with the onset of the rainy season, which may occur twice a year. In equatorial regions, where temperatures are above 18°C year round, epidemics still occur once or twice a year, but the timing is more variable and some degree of continuous year-round transmission is also observed. In temperate areas, local epidemics generally last from 8 to 10 weeks. One or more subtypes and/or types of influenza can circulate within a single influenza season in the same area.

Clinical attack rates during annual epidemics can range from 5% to 20% in the general community to more than 50% in closed populations (e.g., nursing homes, schools). Seroepidemiologic studies suggest that up to 75% of infections may be asymptomatic. During yearly epidemics in industrialized countries, influenza illness often appears first among school-aged children or young adults. The highest illness rates generally occur in children, with accompanying increases in school absences, physician visits, and pediatric hospital admissions. Influenza illness among adults is associated with increases in workplace absenteeism, adult hospital admissions, and mortality, especially among the elderly.

The severity and relative impact of epidemics and pandemics depend upon several factors, including natural or vaccine-induced levels of protective immunity in the population, the age and health condition of the population, the property of the influenza viruses, including antigenicity and pathogenicity, as well as the transmissibility of novel influenza viruses.

6. Reservoirs—Influenza A viruses have a diverse host range, from aquatic birds and bats to swine and horses. However, viruses from 1 species—even when of the same HA/NA subtype—do not replicate efficiently in another. Thus for the influenza strains circulating as seasonal influenza, humans are considered the only reservoir. The impact of zoonotic influenza infections at the human-animal interface will be considered in Other Influenza in this chapter.

7. Incubation period—Average 2 days (range, 1-4 days).

8. Transmission—All routes (droplet, droplet nuclei, and contact) have a role in influenza transmission. Contact with large droplets expelled during coughing and sneezing is likely to be the major route of transmission; face masks and good hand hygiene are effective at reducing the risk of infection. Climate is thought to determine the efficiency of different transmission routes and influences the timing of outbreaks. Cold dry weather appears to support virus stability and transmission in aerosols, whereas warm humid weather may prolong viral stability on surfaces. In adults, virus shedding and communicability is greatest in the first 3 to 5 days of illness. Virus levels are typically low prior to the onset of symptoms.

9. Treatment—

Drug, dose, route	Oseltamivir phosphate (NA inhibitor) 75 mg PO BID (renal dose adjustment is required)
Alternative drug	Other NA inhibitors: • Peramivir 600 mg as a single IV dose for acute, uncomplicated influenza; 600 mg IV once daily for 5–10 days in hospitalized patients • Zanamivir 10 mg PO inhalation BID for 5 days
	Cap-dependent endonuclease inhibitor: • Baloxavir marboxil 40 to < 80 kg (40 mg as single PO dose) and ≥ 80 kg (80 mg as a single PO dose) for acute, uncomplicated influenza
Duration	5 days; longer durations may be used in patients who are critically ill or immunocompromised
Special considerations and comments	• These 4 FDA-approved treatments are effective against influenza A and B. • Treatment should be started as soon as possible—ideally within 48 hours of symptom onset. • Patients with mild illness who are not at increased risk of complications are unlikely to benefit from treatment beyond 48 hours. • The H275Y mutation in A/H1N1 confers resistance to oseltamivir and reduces susceptibility to peramivir. • Baloxavir is only licensed for nonsevere influenza.

Note: BID = twice daily; IV = intravenous(ly); NA = neuraminidase; PO = oral(ly).

10. Prevention—Detailed recommendations for the prevention and control of seasonal influenza epidemics are provided by national health agencies and WHO.

1) Educate the public and health care personnel in basic personal hygiene, including hand hygiene, cough etiquette (especially transmission via unprotected coughs and sneezes), and transmission from hand to mucous membranes.

2) Vaccination: immunization with recommended multivalent (3 or 4 strains) inactivated influenza vaccines (IIVs) and live attenuated influenza vaccines (LAIVs) offers good protection in children and healthy adults when the vaccine viruses closely match the circulating viruses. LAIVs are applied intranasally while IIVs are injected intramuscularly. A single dose of IIV suffices for those who have received seasonal influenza vaccine before or who have had prior exposures to influenza A and B viruses. Two doses at least 4 weeks apart are essential for children younger than 9 years

who have not previously been vaccinated against influenza. LAIVs have been used in Russia for many years for individuals aged 3 years and older. An LAIV has been licensed in the USA for individuals aged 2 to 49 years and is used in many countries.

IIVs primarily stimulate strain-specific HA antibody, titers of which are measured by the traditional HAI assay or by microneutralization. While the HAI titer predicts protection against infection by human influenza viruses, the commonly used seroprotection threshold of 1:40 correlates with only approximately 50% protection against infection. Antibody to NA is also an independent mediator of protection, and cell-mediated immunity inversely correlates with the risk of severe infection. Both are poorly stimulated by IIVs. In older adults, the standard IIV has reduced immunogenicity and may be less effective in preventing illness. Several vaccines have been developed for this population; these vaccines significantly improve immune responses and in some cases also offer modest improvements in vaccine efficacy. FDA-approved options include the high-dose influenza vaccine, which contains 4 times the regular amount of HA; adjuvanted vaccines, which include MF-59 to form an oil-in-water emulsion; and the recombinant vaccine, which contains 3 times the regular amount of HA. Recombinant influenza vaccines do not use eggs in the manufacturing process. The influenza virus adapts to culture in eggs with changes in the HA protein; these changes may reduce vaccine effectiveness. Currently none of these enhanced vaccines is recommended in preference to the standard dose IIV by the Advisory Committee on Immunization Practices (ACIP).

Routine immunization programs should focus efforts on vaccinating those at greatest risk of serious complications or death from influenza (see Risk Groups earlier in this chapter) and those who might spread influenza (health care personnel and household contacts of high-risk persons) to high-risk persons. Immunization of children on long-term salicylate treatment is also recommended to prevent development of Reye syndrome after influenza infection. The vaccine should be given each year before influenza is expected in the community; the timing of immunization should be based on a country's seasonal patterns of influenza circulation (i.e., winter months in temperate zones; often the rainy season in tropical regions). Biannual recommendations for vaccine virus are based on the viruses currently circulating, as determined by WHO through global surveillance.

Contraindications are as follows. The risk of severe allergic reactions to influenza vaccines is extremely low, with an anaphylaxis rate of approximately 1 per million vaccine doses.

Allergic hypersensitivity to vaccine components is a contraindication for that specific vaccine. Most influenza vaccines contain a small amount of egg protein from the manufacturing process; current recommendations from ACIP are that people with an egg allergy of any severity can continue to receive any of the recommended influenza vaccines. People with a history of a severe allergic reaction to egg (such as angioedema or respiratory distress) should receive the vaccine in a medical setting. During the swine influenza vaccine program in 1976, the USA reported an increased risk of developing Guillain-Barré syndrome within 6 weeks after vaccination. Subsequent vaccines produced from other viruses in other years have not been clearly associated with an increased risk of Guillain-Barré syndrome. However, prior Guillain-Barré syndrome is a contraindication for receiving an LAIV. The development of Guillain-Barré syndrome within 6 weeks after a dose of IIV is considered a precaution for future IIV use.

3) Prophylaxis: antiviral agents are supplemental to vaccine when immediate maximal protection is desired in situations such as institutional outbreaks or household settings to protect persons at increased risk of complications due to influenza. Antiviral agents are effective at reducing transmission in facilities during outbreaks, such as among residents of nursing homes for the elderly. The drugs will not interfere with the response to ILVs and should ideally be continued throughout the period of likely exposure to influenza. However, antivirals should not be administered for 2 weeks after receipt of an LAIV and should be stopped for 2 days prior to vaccination with an LAIV.

Inhibitors of influenza NA (oseltamivir and zanamivir) have been shown to be safe and effective for both prophylaxis and treatment of influenza A and B. Oseltamivir is an orally administered medicine; zanamivir is a powder administered via an inhaler. Oseltamivir may be used for persons of all ages and zanamivir is approved for treatment and prophylaxis for persons aged 5 years and older. Dosing is twice a day for 5 days for treatment and once a day for prophylaxis, with dosing for oseltamivir adjusted by body weight for children. Serious cases of bronchospasm have been reported with zanamivir use in patients with and without underlying airways disease. Zanamivir use should be administered carefully in patients with underlying lung disease or reactive airways disease. Wherever available, clinicians should take local antiviral susceptibility information into account when prescribing antivirals.

11. Special considerations—

1) Reporting: weekly reporting from influenza sentinel surveillance sites to monitor disease activity (influenza-like illness and severe respiratory disease). Severe respiratory infection, especially when involving health care workers, should be immediately notified and investigated. Influenza A viruses that cannot be subtyped or new subtypes of influenza infections should be further tested by qualified laboratories in the country or WHO Collaborating Centres of the WHO Global Influenza Surveillance and Response System. Meanwhile, immediately notify public health authorities.

2) Epidemic measures:

- The severe and often disruptive effects of epidemic seasonal influenza on community activities may be reduced in part by effective health planning and education, particularly locally organized immunization programs for high-risk patients, their close contacts, and health care providers. Community surveillance for influenza illness, use of outbreak control measures, adherence to infection control recommendations, and reporting of surveillance and outbreak findings to the community are all important.

- Closure of individual schools can be a useful intervention during influenza outbreaks, with the greatest benefits occurring among school-aged children when applied early in the course of the outbreak. The benefit has to be weighed against the cost of disruption.

- Hospital administrators should anticipate increased demand for medical care during epidemic periods and possible absenteeism of health care personnel as a result of influenza. Health care personnel should be immunized annually to minimize absenteeism and transmission of seasonal influenza from health care personnel to patients.

- Maintaining adequate supplies of appropriate antiviral drugs would be desirable to treat high-risk patients, persons hospitalized with influenza, and essential personnel in the event of the emergence of a new pandemic virus for which no suitable vaccine is available in time for the initial wave.

II. OTHER INFLUENZA

1. Clinical features—Infection with avian, swine, and other zoonotic influenza viruses causes a wide range of symptoms from a mild upper respiratory tract infection to a severe acute respiratory syndrome with pneumonia, shock, and death. Some infections may be asymptomatic.

In recent years, the clinical course has been most severe following infections with the avian influenza subtypes A/H5N1 and A/H7N9. Common initial symptoms are fever (usually $\geq 38°C$) and cough, with sore throat and coryza less prominent. Symptoms of lower respiratory tract involvement such as dyspnea often develop early in the course of illness, and clinically apparent pneumonia with radiologic changes is usually found at presentation to medical care. The disease may progress rapidly to an acute respiratory distress syndrome. Complications of infection include severe pneumonia, secondary bacterial infections, septic shock, and multiorgan dysfunction. The incubation period, severity of symptoms, and clinical outcome vary by the virus causing infection. GI symptoms, including nausea, vomiting, and diarrhea, have been frequently reported with A/H5N1 infection, while conjunctivitis has been described following A/H7N9 infection.

Symptoms following human infection with other avian viruses (such as A/H7N7 and A/H9N2) and the variant viruses (A/H1N1v, A/H1N2v, A/H3N2v) that circulate in swine are typically mild and similar to seasonal influenza. Subclinical infections are common. Similar to seasonal influenza, however, hospitalizations and deaths will sometimes occur.

2. Risk groups—The majority of human cases with zoonotic influenza virus infection have a history of contact with infected animals. The highest risk for exposure to avian influenza is direct exposure to infected live or dead poultry or their environment. This includes poultry workers, persons involved in mass culling operations, live-animal market workers and customers, and children and adults in households with backyard poultry. Consumption of properly cooked poultry or eggs is not thought to be a risk for infection, although a few influenza A/H5N1 cases have been linked to ingestion of dishes made with raw contaminated poultry blood. Familial clustering as well as the relative absence of nonfamilial clusters suggest the existence of a host genetic influence on susceptibility to severe infection. For swine variant influenza viruses, most human cases report close proximity to infected pigs or visiting locations where pigs are exhibited, such as country fairs.

3. Causative agents—New subtypes of influenza A can emerge among humans through direct transmission of an animal influenza virus to humans, or through reassortment of genes derived from an animal influenza virus and a human influenza virus. Such genetic reassortment can create a new virus that combines human and animal influenza properties. Animal influenza A virus subtypes that have infected humans include the avian viruses H5N1, H5N6, H7N2, H7N3, H7N7, H9N2, H10N7, and H7N9 and the swine variant H1 and H3 viruses, which are antigenically distinct from human H1 and H3 viruses. Other types of influenza (B, C, D) have not been clearly associated with zoonotic infection, although the potential exists for swine-to-human transmission and vice versa.

4. Diagnosis—The first laboratory suggestion of a novel influenza A infection from an animal source is the inability of available tests to subtype the detected influenza A virus. Diagnosis of animal influenza viruses often requires specialized laboratories, since these viruses cannot be typed by reagents used for seasonal influenza viruses. Detection of viral RNA in respiratory and other clinical specimens by means of conventional or real-time RT-PCR remains the best method for the initial presumptive diagnosis, which should then be confirmed by other methods such as virus isolation. Infection can also be confirmed by demonstration of seroconversion based upon a rise in antibody titer between an acute and a convalescent serum. Commercially available point-of-care rapid testing (also sometimes called rapid tests) used for human influenza viruses has shown variable sensitivities for animal influenza viruses. It may be useful to support clinical judgment for antiviral treatment during outbreak situations when access to specialized laboratories is limited. However, rapid methods are generally not recommended for definitive diagnosis. If an animal influenza virus infection is suspected, a negative test result by a point-of-care test does not exclude the presence of the virus infection.

5. Occurrence—Avian influenza viruses that have caused most human infections are of the H5, H7, or H9 subtypes, with viruses of the Asian lineages of A/H5N1 and A/H7N9 most common. Of other HA subtypes, A/H10N8, A/H10N7, and A/H6N8 have also been detected in people. The first avian influenza A/H5N1 outbreak among chickens with spillover to humans occurred in Hong Kong in 1997. From 2003 to 2015, there were a large number of A/H5N1 outbreaks, first among poultry in Southeast Asia with subsequent spread to other parts of the world. The viruses are now endemically circulating in poultry populations in parts of Eurasia, Africa, and the Middle East. Avian influenza A/H5N1 virus infections have been associated with high levels of animal mortality among poultry farms and result in substantial economic losses. In 2005, outbreaks in migratory birds in China preceded the spread of A/H5N1 through Mongolia and Russia to many European, Middle Eastern, and African countries. More than 800 confirmed A/H5N1 cases were reported to WHO up to 2015 (with a case-fatality rate of ~50%), but only a handful were reported in the following 3 years. Most human cases occurred in Southeast Asia (Cambodia, Indonesia, Thailand, Vietnam), China, and Egypt.

A number of human infections with subtype A/H5N6 were reported in China in 2014, and circulation of A/H5N8 among migratory birds and poultry has occurred in recent years but with no identified human infection. Sporadic human infection with H7 viruses associated with outbreaks in poultry have been reported, such as influenza A/H7N3 in Canada, Italy, the

UK, and Mexico; influenza A/H7N2 in the USA and the UK; influenza A/H7N7 in the UK, the Netherlands, and Italy; and influenza A/H7N9 in China. In addition, human infection with avian influenza A/H9N2 has been reported in Hong Kong and Bangladesh. But since the first reported human A/H7N9 infection in 2013, more than 1,500 human cases, including more than 600 deaths, have occurred. Almost all cases have been in China.

Swine influenza viruses have also caused illness in humans. In 1976, the A/New Jersey/76 (Hsw1N1) influenza virus of swine origin caused severe respiratory illness in 13 soldiers, including 1 death, at Fort Dix, New Jersey, but did not spread beyond Fort Dix. In 2012, the USA reported 315 cases of human influenza infection with a nonseasonal variant of A/H3N2 (designated A/H3N2v) that was circulating in swine in the USA, mostly associated with swine exposure at agricultural fairs. Since then, sporadic human infections with A/H3N2v and other subtypes (A/H1N1v, A/H1N2v, A/H7N9v) have been reported, with the majority of cases in children.

Human infections with influenza viruses of swine or avian origin are regularly collated by WHO, which publishes a monthly risk assessment summary of reported influenza cases at the human-animal interface (see: http://www.who.int/influenza/human_animal_interface/HAI_Risk_Assessment/en). Although human-to-human transmission of these zoonotic influenza viruses is currently limited and not sustained, continued vigilance is needed to detect adaptations that might signal a pandemic.

6. Reservoirs—Aquatic birds are natural reservoirs of influenza A subtypes. For some avian influenza viruses the range of mammals that can be infected with avian influenza viruses from aquatic birds has been wide (including pigs, whales, seals, horses, ferrets, cats, dogs, and tigers). Domestic poultry can also be infected and is likely the main source of human infections. Swine influenza viruses are endemic in pigs. Influenza infections are also known to occur in other animals besides birds and pigs, including A/H7N7 in horses and A/H3N8 in horses and dogs. With the exception of pigs, influenza viruses have not been shown to transmit from these mammals to humans.

7. Incubation period—For A/H5N1 and A/H7N9 infections, incubation may be up to 17 days but is typically 2 to 5 days. For infections with influenza viruses normally circulating in swine, an incubation period of 2 to 7 days has been reported.

8. Transmission—Most human infections by animal influenza viruses are thought to result from direct contact with infected animals. Migratory birds may sometimes spread avian influenza viruses to new geographic regions, but their importance as a vector for spread is uncertain. Similar to seasonal influenza the route of transmission is likely to include inhalation of small particles into the lower respiratory tract, contamination of facial mucous membranes by self-inoculation or by droplet contact, or ingestion. In about one-fourth of patients, the source of exposure is unclear; infection arising from exposure to contaminated environments remains possible. Visiting live-poultry markets is a recognized risk factor. Human-to-human transmission is thought to have occurred in some instances when there had been very close and prolonged contact between a very sick patient and caregivers, who have usually been family members. This observation suggests that near-distance aerosol, droplet, or direct contact may have been the routes of transmission. However, the potential contribution of each route has not been demonstrated. No evidence to support long-distance airborne transmission has been reported to date.

For swine influenza virus infections in humans, close proximity to ill pigs or visiting a place where pigs are exhibited has been reported for most cases. Some human-to-human transmission has occurred, such as among soldiers in the 1976 Fort Dix outbreak and during the outbreak of influenza A/H3N2v in the USA in 2012. Serologic studies show increased prevalence of swine influenza antibody among persons occupationally exposed to pigs compared with controls.

For avian influenza, limited data suggest that patients may remain infectious for as long as 3 weeks, and perhaps even longer in immunosuppressed patients (e.g., those using corticosteroids). The longest documented period has been 27 days after the onset of illness, based upon detection of virus antigen in a patient's respiratory specimens.

9. Treatment—

Drug	Oseltamivir phosphate (NA inhibitor)
Dose	75 mg BID (renal dose adjustment is required)
Route	PO
Alternative drug	Other neuraminidase inhibitors: • Peramivir 600 mg as a single IV dose for acute, uncomplicated influenza; 600 mg IV once daily for 5–10 days in hospitalized patients • Zanamivir 40 to < 80 kg (40 mg as single PO dose) and ≥ 80 kg (80 mg as a single PO dose) for acute, uncomplicated influenza
Duration	5 days; longer durations may be used in patients who are critically ill or immunocompromised.
Special considerations and comments	• Treatment should be started as soon as possible for all avian influenza virus infections. • While most viruses isolated are susceptible to NA inhibitors, resistance has been reported among the Asian lineage A/H5N1 and A/H7N9 viruses.

Note: BID = twice daily; NA = neuraminidase; PO = oral(ly).

10. Prevention—

1) Preventing human exposure to infected animals or contaminated environments and controlling spread of infection among domesticated animal populations are critical elements for protecting humans from animal influenza virus infections. Guidelines for controlling outbreaks in domesticated animals have been issued by relevant national and international agencies (e.g., the Food and Agriculture Organization of the United Nations and the World Organisation for Animal Health).

2) Rapid information sharing among animal and/or agricultural sectors and human health authorities is essential for timely implementation of public health actions. Social mobilization and risk communication targeting high-risk populations in affected areas are important measures for raising disease awareness and initiating protective behavioral changes.

3) Use of appropriate personal protective equipment and proper training is recommended for those at high risk of exposure to infected birds. Following a probable exposure, asymptomatic persons should be followed for signs of illness for at least 1 week, while symptomatic persons should be tested for infection, administered antiviral medicines, and monitored closely.

4) Immunization: several avian influenza vaccines have been licensed as part of pandemic preparedness, including an A/H5N1 vaccine (approved by FDA in 2007) and an AS03 adjuvanted A/H5N1 vaccine (approved by FDA in 2013). Production of avian influenza vaccines is complicated by a number of factors. These include the difficulties with achieving adequate immunogenicity, the technical issues with culturing highly pathogenic viruses in biocontainment facilities when the wild-type virus is also lethal in eggs, and genetic evolution among circulating avian influenza viruses such that numerous subtypes exist; in addition, within each subtype there are antigenically diverse clades/subclades. Because of inadequate immunogenicity with standard vaccine preparations of inactivated avian influenza virus, booster doses administered 3 weeks or more after priming are necessary. In addition to booster doses, a range of different immune adjuvants have been tested, including Alum, AS03, and MF59, although not all have been successful; concern about reactogenicity and other side effects persists. While some countries are stockpiling these vaccines as part of their pandemic preparedness measures, the effectiveness of these vaccines in preventing avian influenza infection and their ability to reduce disease severity are

unknown. Use of seasonal influenza vaccination in certain high-risk occupational groups with animal exposure is recommended in some countries for reducing influenza-like illness caused by seasonal influenza viruses. Such vaccines will not provide direct protection against animal influenza virus infections but may prevent seasonal and animal influenza coinfections. These coinfections can lead to reassortment, which may generate potential viruses with pandemic potential. WHO maintains a list of candidate vaccine viruses that have passed relevant safety testing and serologic testing (see: https://www.who.int/influenza/vaccines/virus/en).

11. Special considerations—

1) Reporting: laboratory-confirmed human infection with a novel subtype of influenza A virus or influenza A infection where the virus cannot be subtyped should be reported immediately to the national authority and then to WHO. Reporting to WHO is mandatory under the International Health Regulations (IHR). Under IHR, human influenza caused by a new subtype is considered to be an event that may constitute a public health emergency of international concern. Human infection with a novel influenza A virus has been a nationally notifiable condition in the USA since 2007.

2) Any specimen from a patient suspected of novel influenza A virus infection should be immediately tested and forwarded to a national reference laboratory or WHO Collaborating Centre/Reference Laboratory for confirmatory testing. WHO Collaborating Centres provide technical support for influenza surveillance, preparedness, and response. More information on the Centres can be found at: https://www.who.int/influenza/gisrs_laboratory/collaborating_centres/list/en.

3) Continued viral and disease surveillance is critical for identifying human infections caused by influenza viruses of animal origin, including H5N1, and determining their ability to transmit efficiently among humans.

4) Pandemic influenza: the response to an influenza pandemic must be planned at the local, national, and international levels; guidance is provided on the WHO website at: http://www.who.int/influenza/preparedness/pandemic/en. Similar information is available on the websites of many governments, including that of the USA at: https://www.cdc.gov/flu/pandemic-resources/index.htm.

5) **Epidemic measures:**

- Clinicians and local public health officers should be aware that human infections may occur in countries with outbreaks of avian influenza among poultry. The clinical presentation of influenza is nonspecific and has often resulted in an initial misdiagnosis, especially in circumstances in tropical countries where endemic acute febrile diseases are common. Infection with a zoonotic influenza virus should be considered in the differential diagnosis for patients who present with fever, rapidly progressing atypical pneumonia, and epidemiologic risk factors.

- Develop or use a case definition and undertake active surveillance in the appropriate epidemiologic setting for early detection of human cases. If an infection occurs or is strongly suspected, family members and close contacts should be placed under medical observation with daily temperature monitoring and tested if they develop symptoms.

- Establish a mechanism for rapidly obtaining reliable laboratory testing results. Characterization of the virus and its susceptibility to antivirals is an important factor in disease control.

- Establish good communication between human and animal health sectors.

- Provide information about the disease and preventive measures to at-risk populations. Social mobilization, including sensitization campaigns, may be required for effective message penetration. Timely provision of information to the public is essential.

- Collect epidemiologic, clinical, and other information to assess the situation. If efficient human-to-human transmission is observed, a large-scale operation should be considered to stop or limit further spread of the infection.

[B. Young]

JAPANESE ENCEPHALITIS

DISEASE	ICD-10 CODE
JAPANESE ENCEPHALITIS	ICD-10 A83.0

1. Clinical features—The majority of human infections with Japanese encephalitis virus (JEV) are asymptomatic. Fewer than 1% of people infected with JEV develop clinical disease, of which acute encephalitis is the most common clinical presentation. Milder forms of disease such as aseptic meningitis or a febrile illness could also occur. Among persons who develop clinical disease, initial symptoms are nonspecific and may include fever, rigors, myalgias, coryza, diarrhea, headache, and vomiting; these usually precede the onset of neurologic symptoms by 3 to 5 days. During the acute phase of the infection, hepatomegaly with hepatitis and splenomegaly have also been reported. Pulmonary edema and a capillary-leak syndrome have been described in severe pediatric cases.

The most common neurologic presentation of JEV infection is an acute encephalitis syndrome marked by mental status changes, including psychosis or decreased consciousness, lethargy, generalized weakness, or focal neurologic deficits (e.g., paresis and cranial nerve palsies). Seizures are very common and occur in around one-third of infected persons. In adults, the seizures are usually generalized tonic-clonic seizures; in children with advanced disease they can be subtle motor findings (e.g., twitching of a digit, eye deviation, or irregular breathing).

A distinctive clinical presentation is a Parkinsonian syndrome resulting from extrapyramidal system involvement; findings include a flat, mask-like face with wide unblinking eyes, tremor, cogwheel rigidity, and choreoathetoid movements. Other neurologic presentations include a poliomyelitis-like acute flaccid paralysis due to anterior horn cell damage. A flaccid paralysis occurs in 1 or more limbs, usually asymmetric and more common in the lower extremities. About 30% of these patients subsequently develop encephalitis. JEV-associated Guillain-Barré syndrome has been described, similar to other *Flavivirus* infections.

Clinical laboratory findings in JEV infection include leukocytosis with neutrophilia, hyponatremia, elevated liver transaminases (aspartate transaminase and alanine transaminase). Thrombocytopenia can occasionally occur, although it is not a prominent feature of JEV infection. Cerebrospinal fluid (CSF) findings can include a lymphocytic pleocytosis, normal or elevated protein, and normal glucose. Magnetic resonance imaging is the most sensitive modality to detect changes in the brain in JEV infection. Thalamic enhancement is almost always present. The hippocampus, midbrain, and basal ganglia are usually enhancing as well; meningeal enhancement can also be observed. Electroencephalogram abnormalities may also be present.

The course of the illness can last several days to weeks; it generally resolves 7 days after resolution of fever, although recovery can be prolonged for severe illness. The case-fatality rate varies but is generally 20% to 30% for those who develop encephalitis. About 30% to 50% of survivors have long-term neurologic, cognitive, or psychiatric sequelae. Japanese encephalitis should be considered in patients with evidence of a neurologic infection (e.g., meningitis, encephalitis, or acute flaccid paralysis) who have recently traveled to or resided in an endemic country in Asia or the western Pacific. The differential diagnosis includes other causes of acute encephalitis, infectious or noninfectious.

2. Risk groups—The risk for JEV infection is related to exposure to infected mosquitoes and is highest in rural agricultural or surrounding urban areas, often those where rice production is common. In endemic areas, the majority of Japanese encephalitis cases occur in children younger than 15 years. However, in areas with childhood Japanese encephalitis immunization programs, a shift in age distribution occurs with similar numbers of cases observed in children and adults. In unvaccinated, nonimmune travelers, Japanese encephalitis infection can occur at any age. Infection generally results in lifelong immunity.

3. Causative agents—JEV, of the family Flaviviridae and genus *Flavivirus*.

4. Diagnosis—Diagnosis is based on clinical presentation and suspicion in at-risk patients; it is confirmed through serologic testing by measurement of immunoglobulin class M (IgM) and/or immunoglobulin class G in serum and CSF. Acute-phase specimens should be tested for JEV-specific IgM antibodies using an enzyme-linked immunosorbent assay (ELISA), of which there are several commercially available kits. JEV-specific IgM antibodies can be measured in CSF of most patients by 4 days after onset of symptoms and in serum by 7 days after onset. If JEV infection is suspected and acute specimens collected within 10 days of illness onset lack detectable IgM, a convalescent specimen should be collected and tested. Detection of Japanese encephalitis IgM in CSF is diagnostic of neuroinvasive disease and can help distinguish clinical disease attributable to JEV infection from recent vaccination.

Plaque-reduction neutralization tests can be performed to measure virus-specific neutralizing antibodies and to discriminate between cross-reacting antibodies in primary *Flavivirus* infections. A 4-fold or greater rise in virus-specific neutralizing antibodies between acute- and convalescent-phase serum specimens collected 2 to 3 weeks apart may be used to confirm evidence of recent infection. Vaccination history, date of symptom onset, and information regarding other flaviviruses known to circulate in the geographic area that might cross-react in serologic assays should be considered when interpreting results. In patients who have been immunized against or infected with another *Flavivirus* previously (i.e., who have secondary flavivirus infections), cross-reactive antibodies in both ELISA and neutralization assays may make confirmatory diagnosis difficult. Viral isolation from fluid or tissue is low yield because viremia has usually resolved by the time clinical symptoms are recognized; therefore, detection of JEV in blood or CSF with polymerase chain reaction is rare. These tests are not routinely recommended for diagnosis of JEV infection. However, in fatal cases, nucleic acid amplification, histopathology with immunohistochemistry, and virus culture of autopsy tissues can be useful.

5. Occurrence—The distribution of JEV is broad and encompasses East, South, and Southeast Asia as well as parts of Oceania. An estimated 67,900 cases occur annually in endemic countries and disease can present in rolling epidemic forms as well. JEV transmission occurs primarily in rural agricultural areas, often associated with rice production and flooding irrigation. In some areas of Asia, these conditions can occur near urban centers. Determining the overall incidence of infection is difficult owing to the high percentage of asymptomatic cases but is estimated at 1.8 per 100,000 in endemic areas. Among travelers from nonendemic areas, the estimated incidence is less than 1 case per 1 million travelers. There are 2 general seasonal patterns of JEV transmission. In temperate areas of Asia, most cases occur over a period of several months (late summer) when the weather is warmest. By contrast, transmission is often year-round in the tropics and subtropics but can intensify during the rainy season.

6. Reservoirs—Similar to other flaviviruses such as West Nile and St. Louis encephalitis viruses, JEV is transmitted in an enzootic cycle between mosquitoes and vertebrate amplifying hosts, primarily pigs and wading birds. Domestic pigs are the most important source of infection for mosquitoes that transmit JEV to humans because they have high viremia levels and rapid population turnover with a large number of susceptible offspring. Infection is usually asymptomatic in pigs but gestational infection can result in abortions and stillbirths. Humans are incidental and dead-end hosts in the JEV transmission cycle as concentrations of the virus in blood are generally not high enough to infect feeding mosquitoes. Similar to humans, horses are also susceptible to infection and encephalitis but are considered dead-end hosts. Other animals have the capacity for JEV infection but there is little evidence that they contribute to viral transmission.

7. Incubation period—5 to 15 days.

8. Transmission—JEV is transmitted to humans through the bites of infected *Culex* mosquitoes, especially *Culex tritaeniorhynchus*. *C. tritaeniorhynchus* commonly breeds in rice fields, marshes, and other shallow pools of water. It is an evening- and nighttime-biting mosquito that mainly feeds outdoors, preferentially on large animals such as pigs and wading birds, and only infrequently on humans.

Direct person-to-person spread of JEV does not occur, except rarely through intrauterine transmission. Based on experience with other flaviviruses, blood transfusion and organ transplantation are possible modes of transmission. Laboratory-acquired JEV infections have been reported. In a laboratory setting, JEV might be transmitted through needlesticks and, theoretically, through mucosal or inhalational exposures.

9. Treatment—There are currently no approved pharmacotherapeutics for the treatment of JEV infection and only a small number of randomized clinical trials have evaluated potential therapeutic agents. To date, clinical trials evaluating ribavirin, interferon alfa, intravenous immunoglobulin, and minocycline have not shown benefit. The standard treatment for JEV infection is supportive care and should focus on the management of complications from encephalitis, such as seizures. High-dose corticosteroids (dexamethasone 0.6 mg/kg for 5 days) did not show therapeutic benefit in the management of Japanese encephalitis in a randomized controlled trial, although they are often used as an adjunct in the management of increased intracranial pressure. Adjunctive supportive care including physical and occupational therapy, neurologic rehabilitation, and potentially wound care should be implemented to aid in long-term recovery.

10. Prevention—

1) Vector prevention measures (see Arboviral Encephalitides in "Arboviral Diseases").

2) Vaccine: several inactivated and live attenuated Japanese encephalitis vaccines are available worldwide. Inactivated Vero cell culture–derived Japanese encephalitis vaccine (IXIARO Valneva Austria GmbH, Vienna) is the only vaccine licensed and available in the USA. This vaccine was approved in March 2009 for use in people aged 17 years and older and in May 2013 for use in children aged 2 months through 16 years. Other Japanese encephalitis vaccines are manufactured and used in other countries but are not licensed for use in the USA. JEV immunization is considered the most effective prevention strategy in endemic regions and childhood vaccination is routine in many countries in Asia. Japanese encephalitis vaccination may be advised for those traveling to endemic areas. Recommendations should be based on evaluation of an individual traveler's risk of exposure, taking into account the person's planned itinerary, trip duration, activities, and season. More detailed recommendations can be found at: http://www.cdc.gov/mmwr/pdf/rr/rr5901.pdf. Vaccination is recommended for laboratory workers with a potential for exposure to infectious JEV.

3) Other prevention measures: to prevent laboratory infections, precautions should be taken when handling viruses in the laboratory at the appropriate biosafety level.

11. Special considerations—Reporting: local health authorities may be required to report cases in residents in endemic areas or in travelers from nonendemic countries.

[E. Ewers, C. F. Decker]

KAWASAKI DISEASE

(Kawasaki syndrome, mucocutaneous lymph node syndrome, acute febrile mucocutaneous lymph node syndrome)

DISEASE	ICD-10 CODE
KAWASAKI SYNDROME	ICD-10 M30.3

1. Clinical features—An acute, febrile, mostly self-limited, systemic vasculitis of early childhood, presumably of infectious origin. Clinically characterized by a high, spiking fever, unresponsive to antibiotics, associated with pronounced irritability and mood change; usually solitary and frequently unilateral nonsuppurative cervical lymphadenopathy; bilateral nonexudative bulbar conjunctival injection; and an enanthem consisting of a strawberry tongue, injected oropharynx, or dry, fissured, or erythematous lips. Also present are limb changes consisting of edema, erythema, or periungual/generalized desquamation and a generalized polymorphous erythematous exanthem that can be truncal or perineal, ranging from a morbilliform maculopapular rash to an urticarial rash or vasculitic exanthem. Vasculitis occurs throughout the body and causes a range of cardiac complications, including myocarditis, pericarditis, valvular damage, and coronary artery abnormalities. In the USA and Japan, it is the leading cause of acquired heart disease in children. Although it affects all races and ethnicities, the incidence is highest among Asian populations, particularly in children of Japanese ancestry.

Typically there are 3 phases:

1) Acute febrile phase of about 10 days' duration, characterized by a high, spiking fever, rash, adenopathy, peripheral erythema or edema, conjunctival injection, and enanthem.
2) Subacute phase lasting about 2 weeks, with thrombocytosis, desquamation, and resolution of fever.
3) Lengthy convalescent phase, during which clinical signs fade.

The case-fatality rate is less than 0.1%, with half the deaths occurring within 2 months of illness onset. Coronary artery vasculitis leading to lumen dilatation and aneurysm are serious complications.

2. Risk groups—Children younger than 5 years old, male sex, and Asian ancestry seem to be risk factors for Kawasaki disease. In the USA, the incidence is highest among children of Asian origin, followed by African-American and white patients. Recurrences appear infrequent (~3% of reported patients).

3. Causative agents—Unknown. Postulated to be a virus or a superantigen bacterial toxin secreted by *Staphylococcus aureus* or group

A streptococci. However, this has been neither confirmed nor generally accepted.

4. Diagnosis—There is no pathognomonic laboratory test for Kawasaki disease, but an elevated erythrocyte sedimentation rate, C-reactive protein, and platelet counts higher than 450,000/mm^3 (SI units 450×10^9/L) are common laboratory features. The following 6 principal clinical signs are part of the diagnostic criteria for Kawasaki disease:

1) Fever persisting 5 days or more (including patients in whom the fever has subsided before the fifth day in response to treatment).
2) Bilateral conjunctival redness without exudate.
3) Changes of lips and oral cavity: reddening of lips, strawberry tongue, and diffuse injection of oral and pharyngeal mucosa.
4) Polymorphous exanthema.
5) Changes of peripheral extremities: reddening of palms and soles, indurative edema in the initial stage, and membranous desquamation from fingertips in the convalescent stage.
6) Acute nonpurulent cervical lymphadenopathy.

In the USA, the presence of fever and at least 4 of the remaining 5 clinical signs are required for the diagnosis of Kawasaki disease. By contrast, the Japan Kawasaki Disease Research Committee recommends the presence of at least 5 of the 6 principal clinical signs to diagnose the illness; fever is not a required criterion. However, when evidence of coronary artery aneurysm or dilatation is present, Kawasaki disease can be diagnosed with fewer clinical signs. Because some children, particularly those younger than 1 year, may not manifest with the complete signs and symptoms in the early phase of illness, a strong clinical suspicion is required to initiate treatment to reduce the risk of cardiac complications.

5. Occurrence—Worldwide; the reported incidence per 100,000 children younger than 5 years is highest in Japan (309 in 2016) followed by South Korea (195 in 2014), Taiwan (75 in 2011), and Shanghai, China (56 in 2012). The incidence in Japan has shown a steady increase since the 1970s, more than doubling during the last 2 decades. In the USA, the incidence appears to be stable at around 20 cases per 100,000 children younger than 5 years. European countries generally have a much lower incidence than the USA. Cases are more frequent in the winter and spring.

6. Reservoirs—Unknown, perhaps humans.

7. Incubation period—Unknown.

8. Transmission—Mode of transmission is unknown; there is no firm evidence of person-to-person transmission, even within families. Seasonal variation, limitation to the pediatric age group, and outbreak occurrence in communities are all consistent with an infectious etiology.

9. Treatment—

Preferred therapy	• IVIG 2 g/kg as a single dose administered over 10–12 hours, with treatment starting as soon as possible before 10 days of illness onset AND • High-dose aspirin 80–100 mg/kg/day in 4 divided doses until patient is afebrile for 48–72 hours THEN • Low-dose aspirin (3–5 mg/kg/day as a single dose; ≤ 81–325 mg/day) is given until a follow-up echocardiogram confirms no coronary changes by 6–8 weeks after onset of illness
Alternative therapy options	High-risk patients with acute Kawasaki disease: • Adjunctive initial treatment recommendation with a combination of IVIG 2 g/kg as a single dose administered over 10–12 hours PLUS a longer course corticosteroid regimen such as prednisolone 2 mg/kg/day IV divided every 8 hours until afebrile, THEN prednisone PO until CRP normalized, THEN taper over 2–3 weeks
	High-risk patients with IVIG resistance: • Retreatment with IVIG 2 g/kg as a single dose administered over 10–12 hours and a continuation of high-dose aspirin • A longer course corticosteroid regimen such as prednisolone 2 mg/kg/day IV divided every 8 hours until afebrile • Infliximab 5 mg/kg IV as a single infusion given over 2 hours
Special considerations and comments	• IVIG is most useful when initiated before the tenth day of illness and should be started as soon as diagnosis is suspected. • Low-dose aspirin can be continued indefinitely in children who develop coronary artery abnormalities. • Persistent fever beyond 36 hours after IVIG completion is reported in 10%–20% of patients considered to be IVIG-resistant. • More details on the treatment of IVIG resistance and adjunctive therapies for primary treatment in high-risk patients are available in the 2017 consensus recommendations of the American Heart Association.

Source: McCrindle et al.[1]
Note: CRP = C-reactive protein; IV = intravenous(ly); IVIG = intravenous immunoglobulin; PO = oral(ly).

10. Prevention—Unknown.

11. Special considerations—

1) Reporting: clusters and epidemics should be reported immediately to the local health authority.

2) Investigate outbreaks and clusters to elucidate etiology and risk factors.

References

1. McCrindle BW, Rowley AH, Newburger JW, et al. Diagnosis, treatment, and long-term management of Kawasaki disease: a scientific statement for health professionals from the American Heart Association. *Circulation.* 2017;135(17): e927–e999.

[E. Belay]

LARVA MIGRANS

DISEASE	ICD-10 CODE
VISCERAL LARVA MIGRANS	ICD-10 B83.0
GNATHOSTOMIASIS	ICD-10 B83.1
CUTANEOUS LARVA MIGRANS (CREEPING ERUPTION)	ICD-10 B76.9
OCULAR LARVA MIGRANS	ICD-10 B83.9
NEURAL LARVA MIGRANS	ICD-10 B83.9

I. VISCERAL LARVA MIGRANS (larva migrans visceralis, visceral larva migrans, ocular larva migrans, *Toxocara canis* and *Toxocara cati* infections)

1. Clinical features—Usually a chronic infection and insidious disease, predominantly of young children but increasingly recognized in adults. It is caused by migration of larval forms of nematodes in several organs and tissues, including the eye (in this case the term ocular larva migrans [OLM] is used; see Ocular Larva Migrans in this chapter). *Toxocara* spp. (*Toxocara canis* and *Toxocara cati*) are the most common causes of visceral larva migrans (VLM) and OLM and these are the primary agents covered in this section. While infection with few larvae is usually asymptomatic, clinical VLM can result from high-intensity infections.

VLM is characterized by hypereosinophilia of variable duration, hepato-megaly, hyperglobulinemia, pulmonary symptoms, and fever. With an acute and heavy infection, the white blood cell (WBC) count may reach 100,000/mm^3 or higher (SI units $> 100 \times 10^9$/L) with 50% to 90% eosino-phils. Symptoms may persist for a year or longer; symptomatology is related to total parasite load. Pneumonitis, chronic abdominal pain, a generalized rash, and focal neurologic disturbances may occur. VLM is rarely fatal; differential diagnosis includes larval ascariasis (which has a shorter duration) and strongyloidiasis (longer duration).

Larvae may also enter the eye, thus causing an endophthalmitis that can result in loss of vision in the affected eye (OLM); see Ocular Larva Migrans in this chapter for discussion.

2. Risk groups—The greatest risk group includes children, particularly those who play in areas with soil or sand contaminated by host feces, those who have poor hand hygiene, or those who exhibit geophagy. The lower incidence in older children and adults may be the result of a lack of these behaviors.

3. Causative agents—Larvae of the zoonotic nematodes *T. canis* and *T. cati*, predominantly the former. *Baylisascaris procyonis* (raccoon roundworm) is capable of causing VLM, but the associated clinical syndrome is poorly characterized.

VLM might also be caused by other animal ascarids such as *Ascaris suum*, *Baylisascaris columnaris*, *Parascaris equorum*, *Toxascaris leonina*, *Toxocara* (= *Neoascaris*) *vitulorum*, and other zoonotic nematodes that can produce larva migrans in animal hosts. Information is limited regarding the ability of these species to induce VLM in humans.

4. Diagnosis—Although biopsy of affected tissues has revealed *Toxocara* larvae in a small number of cases, this approach is invasive and has poor sensitivity. Diagnosis of VLM requires consideration of clinical mani-festations in conjunction with serologic results. The standard method for serologic diagnosis is by indirect *Toxocara* excretory-secretory (TES) antigen enzyme-linked immunosorbent assay (ELISA); any specimen with a positive result should be tested by Western blot (to improve specificity). Currently, recombinant TES antigen immunoglobulin class G ELISA kits are available from several commercial manufacturers and detect antibodies to *Toxocara* spp. larvae in humans with similar sensitivities and specificities, estimated to be 86% and 91%, respectively, though the absence of a gold standard makes definitive assessment of performance difficult. Cross-reactions can occur with sera from strongyloidiasis, trichinellosis, and ascariasis cases; these nonspecific reactions can be avoided by using TES Western blot to detect *Toxocara* low-molecular-weight antigenic fractions (24, 28, 30, and 35 kDa). Note that a detectable antibody response may be absent in OLM cases: because OLM typically results after a light infection (vs. a heavy infection for

VLM), negative serologic results should not be the sole reason for excluding the diagnosis. If *Baylisascaris* VLM is suspected, a *B. procyonis*-specific Western blot should be performed. This Western blot is based on a 37-kDa recombinant antigen and has a sensitivity of 89% and a specificity of 98%. The test is offered by CDC.

5. Occurrence—*Toxocara* spp. occur worldwide in domestic dogs and cats and also in many wild canids and felids. Therefore, *Toxocara* VLM also has a global occurrence. Severe disease occurs sporadically and affects mainly children aged 14 to 40 months but also older children. Siblings often have eosinophilia or other evidence of light or residual infection. Serologic studies detecting anti-*Toxocara* antibodies reveal a wide range of prevalence among different populations; this variability is also subject to assay performance characteristics.

6. Reservoirs—Dogs and cats, for *T. canis* and *T. cati*, respectively; raccoons and rarely dogs for *B. procyonis*; and a wide range of other animals for other possible causative agents. Hypobiotic *T. canis* larvae arrested in somatic tissues may become reactivated in pregnant bitches and pass transplacentally to puppies. Puppies may pass eggs in their stools by the time they are 3 weeks old. *T. cati* can also be vertically transmitted but transmission occurs mostly by the transmammary route to kittens. Similar though less marked differences apply for cats; older animals are less susceptible than young ones.

7. Incubation period—In children, weeks or months, depending on intensity of infection, reinfection, and sensitivity of the patient. Ocular manifestations may occur as late as 4 to 10 years after initial infection. In infections through ingestion of raw liver, very short incubation periods (hours or days) have been reported.

8. Transmission—For most infections in children, infective *Toxocara* eggs are transmitted from contaminated soil to the mouth, directly by contact with infected soil or indirectly by eating unwashed raw vegetables. Foodborne transmission is via ingestion of larvae in undercooked poultry, duck, cattle, and sheep meat (especially liver).

Fecal contamination by pet dogs and cats and urban populations of wild canids and felids presents a risk for transmission. Once passed in the environment, eggs require 1 to 3 weeks' incubation to become infective; eggs can remain infective in soil for extended periods and are resilient towards adverse conditions such as freezing. Environmental contamination with *Toxocara* eggs has been noted in many parks, sandpits, and backyards in many different regions. Eggs may also adhere to pet hair, presenting a potential exposure risk to pet owners.

B. procyonis transmission is via ingestion of eggs shed by infected raccoons and rarely dogs. It is not known whether the foodborne route can occur as in *Toxocara* spp.

After ingestion, embryonated eggs hatch in the intestine; larvae penetrate the wall and migrate to the liver and other tissues via the lymphatic and circulatory systems. From the liver, larvae spread to other tissues, particularly the lungs and abdominal organs (VLM) or the eyes (OLM), and induce granulomatous lesions. The parasites cannot replicate in the human or other end-stage hosts but reinfection can occur. Direct person-to-person transmission does not occur.

9. Treatment—Treatment of asymptomatic ELISA-positive individuals is not indicated. Treatment with oral albendazole (400 mg twice daily for 5 days) or mebendazole (100–200 mg twice daily for 5 days) is indicated for symptomatic visceral toxocariasis, although optimal duration of treatment is undefined. Prolonged use of albendazole (weeks to months) has led to development of pancytopenia in some patients with compromised liver function. Patients on long-term treatment should be monitored by serial blood cell counts.

10. Prevention—

1) Educate the public, especially pet owners, concerning sources and origin of the infection; the need for removal of pet feces from public areas such as parks and beaches and proper collection and disposal of pet feces in the immediate vicinity of the house; the particular danger of pica; the danger of exposure to areas contaminated with feces of untreated puppies; and the danger of ingestion of raw or undercooked liver from animals exposed to dogs or cats. Parents of toddlers should be made aware of the risk associated with pets in the household and how to minimize them.

2) Prevent contamination of soil and sand by dog and cat feces in areas immediately adjacent to houses and children's play areas, especially in urban areas and multiple housing projects. Encourage cat and dog owners to practice responsible pet ownership, including prompt removal of pets' feces from areas of public access, particularly play areas. Children's sandboxes/sandpits offer an attractive site for defecating cats; cover when not in use. Control stray dogs and cats; ensure that raccoons do not live in close proximity to human dwellings.

3) Deworm dogs and cats, beginning at 3 weeks old, repeated 3 times at 2-week intervals, and every 6 months thereafter. Also treat lactating bitches. Dispose of feces passed as a result of treatment, as well as other stools, in a sanitary manner. A variety of

monthly preventives in chewable or spot-on preparations are effective in preventing infection in pets.

4) Always wash hands after handling soil and sand and before eating.

5) Teach children not to put dirty objects into their mouths.

6) Management of contacts and the immediate environment: search for geographic site of infection of index case; identify others exposed. Intensify preventive measures.

11. Special considerations—None.

II. GNATHOSTOMIASIS (larva migrans profundus)

1. Clinical features—Diverse, depending on which organs are impacted by *Gnathostoma* spp. larvae. Shortly after infection, larval penetration of the gastrointestinal wall and migration through the liver can create acute, non-specific symptoms (vomiting, diarrhea, malaise, myalgias, fever, arthralgia, epigastric pain) that may subside after 2 to 3 weeks. Chronic manifestations most commonly involve subcutaneous tissue (cutaneous gnathostomiasis) with transient migratory swellings and motile erythematous or urticarial tracks, which can move approximately 1 cm/hour. A painless, migrating, intermittent edema can occur. Larvae may also invade the brain, producing focal cerebral lesions associated with eosinophilic pleocytosis. Other sites that may be impacted include the eyes (OLM; see Ocular Larva Migrans in this chapter), lungs, gastrointestinal wall, and genitourinary tract. Peripheral eosinophilia nearly always occurs, which can be extreme (> 50% of total WBC count). Eosinophilia of the cerebrospinal fluid (CSF), with reported levels of 5%–94%, has also been noted in neural involvement.

2. Risk groups—Travelers to and immigrants from endemic regions, particularly habitual consumers of raw meat products.

3. Causative agents—Larval and subadult stages of some *Gnathostoma* spp. nematodes. *Gnathostoma spinigerum* is the most commonly reported in human infections; other zoonotic species include *Gnathostoma hispidum*, *Gnathostoma doloresi*, *Gnathostoma nipponicum*, *Gnathostoma binucleatum*, and possibly *Gnathostoma malaysiae*. It is not known whether the several other *Gnathostoma* spp. found in animal hosts are zoonotic. Many of these species share similar clinical and epidemiologic features.

4. Diagnosis—Usually by a combination of case history, clinical presentation, and laboratory findings (i.e., eosinophilia). Travel history and culinary habits may prompt diagnosis, including a history of eating raw meat, particularly fish (e.g., sashimi in Japan, somfak in Thailand, or ceviche in Central and South America) and poultry. This information in conjunction with the presence of migratory lesions or urticarial tracts is suggestive of gnathostomiasis. Diagnosis can be confirmed by various serologic tests (ELISA or immunoblot), although these are not widely available. Species can be identified morphologically by experienced parasitologists via histologic sections or examination of recovered worms. If worms are recovered, polymerase chain reaction and sequencing of some genes may also allow for species identification.

5. Occurrence—*G. spinigerum* is common throughout Asia (including Thailand, Vietnam, China, and the Indian subcontinent) and has also been reported in China, tropical Australia, and sub-Saharan Africa. *G. hispidum* infection has occurred in Southeast Asia and India. *G. doloresi* somewhat overlaps with the former, identified in parts of Southeast Asia, the Philippines, Papua New Guinea, and Japan. *G. nipponicum* seems to be restricted to Japan. Two cases of possible (but not confirmed) *G. malaysiae* infection acquired in Myanmar have been reported. The sole identified species in the Americas is *G. binucleatum*, which is endemic in many parts of Latin America, including Mexico. Note that geographic distribution of these species in animal hosts is wider than their reported recovery in human infections but many human infections are not identified to the species level.

6. Reservoirs—Definitive hosts (harboring adult worms) are primarily canids, felids, other carnivores, and swine. These hosts pass eggs into water sources; eggs develop and release larvae infective to copepods (first intermediate host). Many species of fish, reptiles, amphibians, and some fowl serve as second intermediate and/or paratenic hosts following ingestion of copepods. These second intermediate/paratenic hosts harbor the *Gnathostoma* spp. larval stage infective to humans.

7. Incubation period—Nonspecific; acute symptoms may occur within 48 hours. Dermal and other more specific manifestations caused by migration of larvae throughout the body most commonly occur within 3 to 4 weeks but can be much longer (months to years).

8. Transmission—Through ingestion of undercooked fish, frogs, poultry, or snakes containing third-stage larvae. Other routes include direct percutaneous penetration of larvae from infected host tissue during food handling; waterborne transmission (ingestion of infected copepods) has also been postulated.

9. Treatment—Although no clear recommendation is available, albendazole and ivermectin have produced good cure rates. Mebendazole has also been shown to have some effect. Larvae migrating close to the surface of the skin can sometimes be excised or erupt spontaneously.

10. Prevention—

   1) Thorough cooking of potentially infected meat. Salting, pickling, marinating, and fermentation methods may not reliably kill larvae.

2) Management of contacts and the immediate environment: search for geographic site of infection of index case; identify others exposed to the same raw meat source. Intensify preventive measures.

11. Special considerations—None.

III. CREEPING ERUPTION/CUTANEOUS LARVA MIGRANS/LARVA CURRENS

1. Clinical features—A dermatitis in which each larva causes a serpiginous, reddish track, advancing several millimeters to a few centimeters a day, with intense itching, especially at night. Most common locations include feet and buttocks (i.e., areas exposed to the ground). The disease is self-limited, with spontaneous cure after weeks or months. *Ancylostoma caninum* larvae may migrate to the small intestine, where they cause eosinophilic enteritis.

2. Risk groups—Utility workers, gardeners, children, seabathers, and others who come into contact with damp sandy soil or sand contaminated with dog or cat feces. Infections have also been noted in travelers returning from tropical countries.

3. Causative agents—Cutaneous larva migrans (CLM) is typically caused by the hookworm species *Ancylostoma braziliense* and possibly *A. caninum*; more rarely by *Uncinaria stenocephala. Bunostomum phlebotomum* (cattle hookworm) is known to produce CLM following accidental exposure. Other hookworm species of animals may also prove to cause this condition.

Strongyloides CLM (called larva currens) is most commonly caused by skin migration of *Strongyloides stercoralis* and possibly *Strongyloides fuelleborni* infesting the human intestinal tract. However, *Strongyloides* spp. of animals may also cause larva currens (e.g., *Strongyloides procyonis, Strongyloides myopotami, Strongyloides ransomi, Strongyloides westeri,* and *Strongyloides papillosus*) but without intestinal establishment.

Other rarer causes of CLM/larva currens apart from hookworm and *Strongyloides* spp. may occur. A free-living saprophytic nematode found in decaying organic matter, *Pelodera* (= *Rhabditis*) *strongyloides*, may cause larva currens-like infection. An unidentified larva designated Spirurina type X has caused about 50 cases of CLM/creeping eruption in Japan.

4. Diagnosis—Laboratory testing is not used in the diagnosis of CLM but may be used to rule out other causes. Diagnosis is based on the clinical picture and potential exposure history (e.g., soil or sand, especially in areas where dogs are common). Subadult *A. caninum* recovered on colonoscopy may be identified morphologically.

The laboratory confirmation of *S. stercoralis* larva currens is discussed in "Strongyloidiasis."

5. Occurrence—*A. caninum* is common in dogs across the globe. *A. braziliense* mostly occurs in warmer regions of the Americas but sporadic reports exist from Africa and Australia. *U. stenocephala* has a more northern distribution. *S. stercoralis* occurs globally but incidence is highest in resource-poor tropical and subtropical areas.

6. Reservoirs—Canids for *A. caninum* and *U. stenocephala*; both canids and felids for *A. braziliense*. Domestic dogs may also be reservoirs for zoonotic strains of *S. stercoralis*.

7. Incubation period—Creeping eruption usually appears a few days after skin penetration by larvae for the more commonly implicated agents.

8. Transmission—Follows contact of the skin with soil or sand harboring infective (filariform) larvae. The larvae enter the skin and migrate intracutaneously for long periods; eventually they may penetrate to deeper tissues. Direct person-to-person transmission does not occur.

9. Treatment—CLM is self-limiting and larvae typically die within 1 to 2 months, though rare chronic cases may persist up to 14 months. Treatment can relieve some symptoms. Topical interventions, such as freezing the affected area with ethyl chloride spray or application of thiabendazole ointment, can kill individual larvae, although this is difficult as the larvae are usually found centimeters from the advancing end of the inflammatory track. A single dose of albendazole or a single dose of ivermectin is effective systemically. A 7-day course of albendazole prevents recurrence. Eosinophilic enteritis responds to treatment with pyrantel, mebendazole, or albendazole.

10. Prevention—

1) Reduce contact with soil or sand by wearing shoes and appropriate clothing. Treat pet dogs and cats with appropriate anthelmintics to reduce environmental contamination.

2) Management of contacts and the immediate environment: search for geographic site of infection of index case; identify others exposed. Intensify preventive measures.

11. Special considerations—None.

IV. OCULAR LARVA MIGRANS

OLM refers to intraocular invasion and migration within the eye by larval stages of various nematode species. For the purposes of this section, OLM should be distinguished from other ocular nematodiases in which (a) adult worms (not larvae) are implicated, (b) intraocular invasion and/or migration does not occur (e.g., conjunctival or orbital localization), or (c) ocular invasion is solely a result of broadly disseminated infection.

1. Clinical features—Clinical manifestations of OLM and the severity of visual impairment vary depending on the etiologic agent and localization within the eye. The cornea, aqueous humor, vitreous humor, anterior and posterior chamber, and the retina are all potential areas of localization. OLM is typically unilateral and commonly presents with signs such as strabismus, optic nerve atrophy, uveitis, endophthalmitis, and chorioretinitis. In severe cases, these complications can lead to permanent vision loss. Patients may report interference with vision if larvae are of a large species and/or highly motile.

Toxocara and *Baylisascaris* OLM typically present with visual impairment associated with diffuse unilateral subacute retinitis and other inflammatory and degenerative lesions of the retinal and optic nerve. Occasionally, granuloma formation is observed within the anterior or posterior chamber of the eye. In ocular baylisascariasis, ocular signs are typically, but not always, present without concomitant neurologic disease. *Gnathostoma* OLM commonly presents with glaucoma, corneal ulceration, and vitreal hemorrhage. Retinoblastoma and toxoplasmosis should be included in the differential diagnosis in suspected OLM cases.

2. Risk groups—As for VLM. The greatest risk group for *Toxocara* and *Baylisascaris* infection is young children, particularly those who play in areas with soil or sand contaminated by host feces, have poor hand hygiene, or exhibit geophagy. OLM occurs in older children and adults more frequently than VLM does in such age groups.

3. Causative agents—Most commonly *T. canis* and *T. cati* but also *B. procyonis*, *Angiostrongylus cantonensis*, *Dirofilaria* spp., zoonotic *Onchocerca* spp., *Acanthocheilonema* spp., *Gnathostoma* spp., *Loaina* spp., and, rarely, hookworms (*Ancylostoma* spp.) have been implicated.

4. Diagnosis—Ocular examination with visualization of the larvae with a slit lamp is usually required. Diagnosis of OLM is often presumptive based on larval size (e.g., 200–500 μm for *Toxocara* spp. vs. 1,000–1,800 μm for *B. procyonis*) and gross morphology, case/exposure history, clinical signs, and species-specific serologic results. Note that a detectable antibody response may be absent in *Toxocara* OLM cases: because OLM typically results after a light infection (vs. a heavy infection for VLM), negative serologic results should not be the sole reason for excluding the diagnosis.

5. Occurrence—Potential causative agents are found in a wide array of locations and several are globally present, including the most typical cause of OLM, *Toxocara* spp. *B. procyonis* is common in raccoons in North America, particularly in upper midwestern and West Coast states. Known human cases have generally originated from these highly endemic areas. The parasite also occurs in raccoons across much of Europe and also in Japan and China. Distributions of other agents are discussed in their respective chapters.

6. Reservoirs—Dogs and cats, for *T. canis* and *T. cati*, respectively; raccoons and rarely dogs for *B. procyonis*; and a wide range of other animals for other possible causative agents. Hypobiotic *T. canis* larvae arrested in somatic tissues may become reactivated in pregnant bitches and pass transplacentally to puppies. Puppies may pass eggs in their stools by the time they are 3 weeks old. *T. cati* can also be vertically transmitted, but transmission occurs mostly by the transmammary route to kittens. Similar though less marked differences apply for cats; older animals are less susceptible than young ones.

7. Incubation period—Highly variable, between a few months and a few years following potential exposure.

8. Transmission—For *Toxocara*, ingestion of infective eggs from host feces, which may occur directly during contact with contaminated soil or surfaces or indirectly by eating unwashed raw vegetables. Foodborne transmission is via ingestion of larvae in undercooked poultry, duck, cattle, and sheep meat (especially liver).

Fecal contamination by pet dogs and cats and urban populations of wild canids and felids presents a risk for transmission. Once passed in the environment, eggs require 1 to 3 weeks incubation to become infective; eggs can remain infective in soil for extended periods and are resilient towards adverse conditions such as freezing. Environmental contamination with *Toxocara* eggs has been noted in many parks, sandpits, and backyards in many different regions. Eggs may also adhere to pet hair, presenting a potential exposure risk to pet owners.

B. procyonis transmission is also via ingestion of eggs shed by infected raccoons and rarely dogs. It is not known whether the foodborne route can occur as in *Toxocara* spp.

The other less common causative agents have diverse modes of transmission, including arthropod vector-borne (*Dirofilaria* spp., *Onchocerca* spp., *Loaina* spp.) and foodborne (*A. cantonensis*, *Gnathostoma* spp.) routes. No direct person-to-person transmission occurs.

9. Treatment—Measures to prevent progressive damage to the eye are necessary and will vary by localization and causative agent. Laser photocoagulation of the larva is possible if the larva is visible in the retinal space. Topical corticosteroids may be useful in controlling inflammatory damage to the eye. Systemic anthelmintics (albendazole, mebendazole) administered as with VLM may aid in killing larvae.

10. Prevention—

    1) As for VLM. Raise awareness of potential *Toxocara* infection sources and encourage practices that reduce environmental

contamination (e.g., disposing of pet feces properly, deworming pets appropriately, covering sandboxes when not in use). Individuals should always wash hands after handling soil and sand and before eating. Hygiene habits should be taught to children from a young age, including discouraging putting objects into their mouths.

2) For *B. procyonis*, the presence of raccoons around homes should be minimized (e.g., wildlife removal services, not keeping pet food outside, securing garbage sources, avoiding intentional feeding of wild raccoons). Extreme caution must be exercised in removing raccoon feces and latrines. High heat (via steam or torch) is the only method for inactivating potentially infectious eggs.

3) Prevention of other causal agents are discussed in respective sections (for *Gnathostoma*, see Gnathostomiasis in this chapter).

4) Management of contacts and the immediate environment: search for geographic site of infection of index case; identify others exposed. Intensify preventive measures.

11. Special considerations—None.

V. NEURAL LARVA MIGRANS (*Baylisascaris procyonis* infection)

Neural larva migrans (NLM) refers to the invasion of the central nervous system (CNS) by migrating larval stages of nematodes, classically *A. cantonensis* or *B. procyonis*. *B. procyonis* is the primary agent discussed in this section; clinical features of *A. cantonensis* NLM are addressed in "Angiostrongyliasis."

1. Clinical features—Migration of *B. procyonis* larvae through the CNS is associated with serious clinical disease. Neurologic manifestations may include weakness; incoordination; ataxia; torticollis; altered mental status, which can progress to seizures; coma; and death. The onset can initially be subtle, sometimes preceded by nonspecific somatic symptoms, but may rapidly increase in severity because of larval growth during migration. However, slower progression with a more chronic course may also be observed. Eosinophilic meningoencephalitis and peripheral eosinophilia are often present. Survivors often develop permanent neurologic sequelae but full recovery may occur in patients with early diagnosis and treatment. Human baylisascariasis is rare, with approximately 50 cases of ocular and cerebral baylisascariasis having been reported worldwide since 1980. The actual number of cases may be greater, in part because of lack of awareness and diagnostic difficulties. *B. procyonis* and *A. cantonensis* share clinical similarities, notably eosinophilic meningitis; however, peripheral eosinophilia is moderate to high in baylisascariasis and rarely so in angiostrongyliasis.

2. Risk groups—The majority of *Baylisascaris* NLM cases have been reported in young children or developmentally disabled persons, particularly those who play in areas with soil or sand contaminated by host feces, have poor hand hygiene, or exhibit geophagy. Individuals with pet raccoons or those who have extensive contact with raccoons may also be at risk for exposure to eggs within feces.

3. Causative agents—Larvae of *B. procyonis*, the raccoon roundworm. It is not known whether other *Baylisascaris* spp. are capable of infecting humans.

Larvae of other nematodes such as *Gnathostoma* spp., *Toxocara* spp., *S. stercoralis*, and *Lagochilascaris* spp. may occasionally invade the CNS.

4. Diagnosis—Antemortem diagnosis of baylisascariasis NLM is typically based on clinical presentation and detection of antibodies to *Baylisascaris* in serum and/or CSF. Antibody detection is achieved via an immunoblot, which is based on a 37-kDa recombinant antigen and has a sensitivity of 89% and a specificity of 98%. The test is offered by CDC. The patient's exposure history, including possible contact with raccoons and/or raccoon feces, may aid in diagnosis. Larvae recovered on biopsy (e.g., brain) can be identified morphologically; however, obtaining biopsy specimens constitutes a highly invasive, low-sensitivity approach for detecting *Baylisascaris* larvae. The diagnosis of neural angiostrongyliasis is discussed in "Angiostrongyliasis."

5. Occurrence—*B. procyonis* is common in raccoons in North America, particularly in upper midwestern and West Coast states. Prevalence is generally lower in southern states. Known human cases have generally originated from these highly endemic areas. The parasite also occurs in raccoons across much of Europe and also in Japan and China.

6. Reservoirs—For *B. procyonis*, the definitive hosts are raccoons, rarely dogs or other procyonids (e.g. kinkajou). For *A. cantonensis*, the definitive hosts are rats; the intermediate hosts (harboring stages infective to humans) include several genera of mollusks. Various other animals (e.g., frogs, freshwater shrimp, land crabs, planarians) may serve as paratenic (transport) hosts for *A. cantonensis*.

7. Incubation period—Likely variable, but in some cases clinical disease has been noted 2 to 4 weeks after known exposure to raccoon feces (containing large numbers of *B. procyonis* eggs).

8. Transmission—Ingestion of *B. procyonis* infective eggs from host feces, which may occur during contact with contaminated soil or surfaces. Eggs require about 2 to 3 weeks in the environment to become infective following passage by the definitive host.

For *A. cantonensis*, ingestion of third-stage larvae in intermediate (e.g., undercooked snails, accidental ingestion of snail or slug tissue on unwashed produce) or sometimes paratenic hosts (e.g., undercooked freshwater shrimp).

9. Treatment—Early and aggressive treatment is critical in *Baylisascaris* NLM; a full recovery may be possible if successful. Treatment protocols typically consist of albendazole with corticosteroids to control inflammation. Mebendazole and ivermectin have also been used, although the latter has poorer penetration of the blood-brain barrier and thus should not be a first-line drug. The prophylactic use of albendazole in individuals with a high suspicion of exposure (20–50 mg/kg for 10–20 days) mitigates the risk of complications by halting the migration of larvae to the CNS and allowing more time for further diagnostic testing.

The management of neural angiostrongyliasis is discussed in "Angiostrongyliasis."

10. Prevention—

1) For *B. procyonis*, hygiene habits should be taught to children from a young age, including proper handwashing and discouraging putting objects into their mouths. The presence of raccoons around homes should be minimized (e.g., wildlife removal services, not keeping pet food outside, securing garbage sources, avoiding intentional feeding of wild raccoons). Extreme caution must be exercised in removing raccoon feces and latrines. High heat (via steam or torch) is the only method for inactivating potentially infectious eggs. For those who have occupational contact with raccoons, proper infection control practices and personal protective equipment must be used. Though rare, domestic dogs may also carry *B. procyonis* infections and shed eggs; proper deworming and use of monthly preventives mitigates this risk.

2) For *A. cantonensis*, prevention is primarily centered on raising awareness and thorough washing and/or cooking of potentially contaminated food items, particularly during travel to endemic areas.

3) Management of contacts and the immediate environment: search for geographic site of infection of index case; identify others exposed. Intensify preventive measures.

11. Special considerations—None.

[S. G. H. Sapp, R. S. Bradbuy]

LEGIONELLOSIS

DISEASE	ICD-10 CODE
LEGIONNAIRES' DISEASE	ICD-10 A48.1
PONTIAC FEVER	ICD-10 A48.2

1. Clinical features—Two distinct clinical manifestations: Legionnaires' disease and Pontiac fever. Both conditions initially present with fever, myalgia, and headache. Abdominal pain and diarrhea are also common.

1) Legionnaires' disease: characterized by pneumonia and a nonproductive cough. Chest imaging findings are variable and may show patchy or focal areas of consolidation or bilateral involvement. The illness can be quite severe and may ultimately progress to respiratory failure. Extrapulmonary disease is rare. Despite improvements in diagnostics and treatment, case-fatality rates remain at approximately 15% with higher rates of up to 25% in persons with health care–associated infection.

2) Pontiac fever: a self-limited febrile illness, occasionally accompanied by cough, which does not progress to pneumonia or death. Patients recover spontaneously in 2 to 5 days without treatment. The exact etiology of the clinical syndrome remains unknown, although it is suspected to result from an inflammatory reaction to inhaled aerosols containing *Legionella* bacteria or endotoxin rather than true bacterial invasion.

2. Risk groups—Risk factors include male gender, age older than 50 years, cigarette smoking, hot tub exposure, diabetes mellitus, chronic heart or lung disease, end-stage renal failure, malignancy, and compromised immunity, particularly organ transplant recipients and patients receiving corticosteroids. The male-to-female ratio is about 2.5:1. Outbreaks are most commonly recognized among travelers (hotels, resorts, and cruise ships) and in health care settings (hospitals and long-term care facilities). Approximately 10% to 15% of all reported cases of Legionnaires' disease occur in people who have traveled during the 10 days before symptom onset.

3. Causative agents—*Legionella* spp., Gram-negative bacilli. Of the 16 serogroups of *Legionella pneumophila* currently recognized, *L. pneumophila* serogroup 1 is most commonly associated with disease. Related organisms, including *Legionella micdadei*, *Legionella bozemanii*, *Legionella longbeachae*, and *Legionella dumoffii*, have been identified as clinically relevant species and isolated predominately from immunosuppressed patients with pneumonia. Currently, at least 58 species of *Legionella* and 78 distinct serogroups are recognized.

4. Diagnosis—

1) Legionnaires' disease: isolate the causative organism from a lower respiratory specimen, tissue, or pleural fluid using selective medium (buffered charcoal yeast extract); detect *L. pneumophila* serogroup 1 antigens in the urine; or measure a 4-fold rise in immunofluorescent antibody titer to *L. pneumophila* serogroup 1 between acute-phase serum and serum drawn 3 to 6 weeks later. Urine antigen and some serologic tests only detect *L. pneumophila* serogroup 1 (which may account for up to 84% of cases), so disease due to other serogroups or species will be missed, emphasizing the importance of culture. Direct immunofluorescent antibody stain of involved tissue or respiratory secretions may be used but sensitivity and specificity are highly variable and dependent upon the experience of laboratory personnel. Polymerase chain reaction is used in some research laboratories but is not currently commercially available in the USA.

2) Pontiac fever: usually diagnosed by identifying symptoms consistent with the disease in the appropriate epidemiologic setting. If disease is due to *L. pneumophila* serogroup 1, urine antigen and serologic testing can be used to confirm the diagnosis; test sensitivity is lower for Pontiac fever than for Legionnaires' disease.

5. Occurrence—The disease has been identified worldwide. Although cases occur throughout the year, both sporadic cases and outbreaks are recognized more commonly in the summer and fall. The proportion of community-acquired pneumonia cases due to *Legionella* ranges between 0.5% and 5%. Outbreaks of Legionnaires' disease may be difficult to detect owing to low attack rates (0.1%–5%). Pontiac fever often causes explosive outbreaks with attack rates as high as 95% reported.

6. Reservoirs—*Legionella* spp. occurs naturally in freshwater environments. Man-made water supplies that aerosolize water, such as potable water systems (showers), air-conditioning cooling towers, whirlpool spas, and decorative fountains, are the common sources for transmission. Conditions promoting *Legionella* growth include warm water temperatures (25°C–42°C [77°F–108°F]), stagnation, scale and sediment, and low disinfectant levels.

7. Incubation period—For Legionnaires' disease, 2 to 10 days, most often 5 to 6 days; for Pontiac fever, 5 to 72 hours, most often 24 to 48 hours.

8. Transmission—*Legionella* is transmitted by inhalation of infectious aerosol (airborne) or microaspiration of contaminated water. Person-to-person transmission has not been documented.

9. Treatment—

1) Legionnaires' disease:

Drug, dose, route	• Levofloxacin 750 mg IV/PO every 24 hours OR • Moxifloxacin 400 mg IV/PO every 24 hours OR • Azithromycin 1 g IV on day 1, THEN 500 mg IV/PO every 24 hours
Alternative drug	Doxycycline 100 mg PO BID
Duration	7–10 days, 14–21 days for severe disease or immunocompromised
Special considerations and comments	Azithromycin 500 mg PO on first day, THEN 250 mg once daily for 4 days can be considered for out-patients with CAP, normal hosts

Note: BID = twice daily; CAP = community-acquired pneumonia; IV = intravenous(ly); PO = oral(ly).

2) Pontiac fever: no antibiotic treatment; self-limited illness no benefit from antibiotics. Usual recovery within 1 week.

10. Prevention—No vaccine is available. Minimizing *Legionella* growth in complex building water systems and devices, including potable water, hot tubs, decorative fountains, and cooling towers, is key to preventing infection. Proper maintenance and disinfection of whirlpool spas, cooling towers, and supplies of drinking water are the most effective measures for preventing outbreaks. Cooling towers should be drained when not in use and mechanically cleaned periodically to remove scale and sediment. Appropriate disinfectants should be used to limit the growth of *Legionella* and the formation of protective biofilms. Maintaining temperatures of hot-water systems at 50°C (122°F) or higher may reduce the risk of transmission. Point-of-use water filtration (0.2 μm) has been used under some circumstances to prevent health care–associated legionellosis in immunosuppressed patients. Tap water should not be used in respiratory therapy devices. Timely identification and reporting of legionellosis cases is also important because this allows public health officials to quickly identify and stop potential clusters and outbreaks by linking new cases to previously reported ones. Antibiotic prophylaxis may be considered for immunocompromised patients during an active nosocomial epidemic.

11. Special considerations—The threshold for initiating environmental sampling and remediation varies among published guidelines. During an outbreak, identify common exposures and review maintenance logs for water systems that are potential sources of infection. *Legionella* culture of water and biofilm swabs collected from the potential source(s) may be necessary to determine the cause of the outbreak and should be considered for any cluster of health care–associated legionellosis. To optimize detection, at least 250 mL of water should be collected from each site. Remediation usually requires biocide disinfection of the implicated water system.

[S. Wood, C. F. Decker]

LEISHMANIASIS

DISEASE	ICD-10 CODE
CUTANEOUS LEISHMANIASIS	ICD-10 B55.1
MUCOSAL LEISHMANIASIS	ICD-10 B55.2
VISCERAL LEISHMANIASIS	ICD-10 B55.0

I. CUTANEOUS AND MUCOSAL LEISHMANIASIS
(Aleppo evil, Baghdad boil, Delhi boil, chiclero ulcer, oriental sore, espundia)

1. Clinical features—A polymorphic disease of skin and mucous membranes that starts with a macular, papular, or nodular lesion that enlarges and typically becomes an indolent ulcer in the absence of bacterial infection. The lesions can develop on any part of the body where the inoculation of the parasite has occurred; however, lesions usually appear on exposed surfaces of the body such as the face, arms, and legs. Lesions may be single or multiple, occasionally nonulcerative and diffuse. Lesions may heal spontaneously within weeks to months or last for a year or more. After apparent cure cutaneous lesions may recur as ulcers, papules, or nodules at or near the healed original ulcer.

In some individuals, certain strains (mainly from the western hemisphere) can disseminate to cause mucosal lesions (espundia), even years after the primary cutaneous lesion has healed. In the eastern hemisphere, a chronic granulomatous lesion occurs, following anthroponotic cutaneous leishmaniasis (CL) due to *Leishmania tropica*; this is called the recidivans form. These sequelae, which involve nasopharyngeal tissues, are characterized by progressive tissue destruction and often scanty presence of parasites; they can be severely disfiguring if left untreated.

Eventually spontaneous healing occurs in most cases, but the rate of healing varies by species. A small proportion of patients infected with *Leishmania amazonensis* or *Leishmania aethiopica* may develop diffuse parasite-rich cutaneous lesions that do not heal without treatment. Metastatic mucosal lesions may develop months or years later in a small proportion of infections with parasites of the *Leishmania braziliensis* complex.

2. Risk groups—Factors responsible for late mutilating disease are still poorly understood, although nutritional and immunogenetic factors have been implicated; occult infections may be activated years after the primary infection. Lifelong immunity may be present after lesions due to *L. tropica* or *Leishmania major* heal but may not protect against other leishmanial species.

3. Causative agents—*Leishmania* protozoa. These are obligate intracellular parasites in humans and other mammals. Eastern hemisphere: *L. tropica*, *L. major*, *L. aethiopica*, *Leishmania infantum*, and *Leishmania donovani*. *L. tropica* is the usual cause of leishmaniasis recidivans cutaneous lesions. Western hemisphere: *L. braziliensis* and *Leishmania mexicana* complexes. Members of the *L. braziliensis* complex are more likely to produce mucosal lesions; members of the *L. donovani* complex usually cause visceral disease in the eastern hemisphere; in the western hemisphere the responsible organism is *L. infantum/Leishmania chagasi*. Both may cause CL without concomitant visceral involvement. Post–kala-azar dermal leishmaniasis is a condition characterized by hypopigmented or erythematous macules, papules, or nodules that develops usually after apparent cure of visceral leishmaniasis (VL). Post–kala-azar dermal leishmaniasis cases are considered to be residual reservoirs for the maintenance and dissemination of the parasite.

4. Diagnosis—Through microscope identification of the nonmotile intracellular form (amastigote) in stained specimens from lesions and through culture of the motile extracellular form (promastigote) on suitable media. An intradermal (Montenegro) test with leishmanin, an antigen derived from promastigotes, is usually positive in established disease; it is not helpful with very early lesions, anergic disease, or immunosuppressed patients. Serologic (indirect immunofluorescence assay [IFA] or enzyme-linked immunosorbent assay [ELISA]) testing can be done, but antibody levels are typically low or undetectable; this may not be helpful in diagnosis (except for mucosal leishmaniasis [ML]).

Species identification is based on biologic (development in sandflies, culture media, and animals), immunologic (monoclonal antibodies), molecular (deoxyribonucleic acid techniques), and biochemical (isoenzyme analysis) criteria.

5. Occurrence—China; India; Pakistan; Southwest Asia, including Afghanistan and Iran; southern regions of the former Soviet Union; the Mediterranean littoral; the sub-Saharan African savanna; Sudan; the highlands of Ethiopia and Kenya; Namibia; the Dominican Republic, Mexico (especially Yucatan); south-central Texas; all of Central America; and every country of South America except Chile and Uruguay. About 1 million new cases are diagnosed per year.

A nonulcerative, keloid-like form due to *L. infantum/chagasi* (atypical CL) has been observed with increasing frequency in Central America, especially Honduras and Nicaragua. In some areas in the eastern hemisphere, urban population groups, including children, are at risk for anthroponotic CL due to *L. tropica*. In rural areas, people are at risk for zoonotic CL due to *L. major*. In the western hemisphere, disease is usually restricted to special groups, such as those working in forested areas, those whose homes are in or next to a forest, and visitors to such areas from nonendemic countries. CL is generally more common in rural than urban areas, with the exception of *L. tropica*, which can cause large urban outbreaks—such as that in Kabul, Afghanistan, in the late 1990s and mid-2000s.

6. Reservoirs—Locally variable; humans (in anthroponotic CL); wild rodents (gerbils); hyraxes; edentates (sloths); marsupials; and domestic dogs (considered victims more than reservoirs except for *L. infantum*). Unknown hosts in many areas.

7. Incubation period—At least a week, up to many months.

8. Transmission—In zoonotic foci, from the animal reservoir through the bite of infective female sandflies (phlebotomines). Motile promastigotes develop and multiply in the gut of the sandfly after it has fed on an infected mammalian host; in 8 to 20 days, infective parasites develop and are injected during biting. In humans and other mammals, the organisms are taken up by macrophages and transform into amastigote forms, which multiply within the macrophages until the cells rupture, enabling spread to other macrophages. In anthroponotic foci, indirect person-to-person transmission occurs through sandfly bites as long as parasites remain in lesions in untreated cases—usually a few months to 2 years. Person-to-person transmission can occur, very rarely, through blood transfusion.

9. Treatment—Immunocompetent individuals with simple skin lesions healing spontaneously may not need treatment. When treatment is opted for, multiple factors should be considered, including the geography of acquisition, extent of disease, and local treatment patterns. Expert consultation is recommended.

For CL and ML, there is no single treatment of choice. Parenteral options include pentavalent antimonials (e.g., sodium stibogluconate [Pentostam] and meglumine antimoniate, both dosed at 20 mg/kg/day for 20 days) and amphotericin B (off-label per FDA). Oral alternatives include azoles and miltefosine (although its use is off-label per FDA for non-Viannia species in CL).

Pentostam is available in the USA through CDC under an investigational new drug protocol. The CDC Drug Service may be consulted by phone (404-639-3670) or via the website (www.cdc.gov).

10. Prevention—No vaccine is currently available, although candidate vaccines are in development. Control measures vary according to the habits of mammalian hosts and phlebotomine vectors and include the following:

1) Vector control: apply residual insecticides periodically at the beginning of the active season for sandflies. Phlebotomine sandflies have a relatively short flight range and are highly susceptible to control by systematic spraying with residual insecticides. Spraying must cover exteriors and interiors of doorways and other openings if transmission occurs in dwellings. Possible breeding places of eastern hemisphere sandflies, such as stone walls, animal houses, and refuse heaps, must be sprayed. Exclude vectors by screening with a fine mesh screen (10–12 holes/linear cm or 25–30 holes/linear inch, with an aperture of 0.89 mm or 0.035 inches). Insecticide-treated bed nets are additional vector control measures and should be promoted especially in anthroponotic foci.

2) Eliminate refuse heaps and other breeding places for eastern hemisphere phlebotomines.

3) Destroy gerbils (and their burrows) implicated as reservoirs in local areas by deep plowing and removal of the plants they feed on (chenopods).

4) In the western hemisphere, avoid sandfly-infested and thickly forested areas, particularly after sundown; use insect repellents and protective clothing if exposure to sandflies is unavoidable.

5) Apply appropriate environmental management and forest clearance.

11. Special considerations—Epidemic measures: in areas of high incidence, use intensive efforts to control the disease by provision of diagnostic facilities and appropriate measures directed against phlebotomine sandflies and the mammalian reservoir hosts.

II. VISCERAL LEISHMANIASIS (kala-azar)

1. Clinical features—A systemic disease caused by intracellular protozoa of the genus *Leishmania*. The disease is characterized by fever, hepatosplenomegaly, lymphadenopathy, anemia, leukopenia, thrombocytopenia, and progressive emaciation and weakness. Untreated clinically evident disease is usually fatal. Evidence indicates that asymptomatic and subclinical infections are common. Only very few progress to develop full-blown disease. However, the role of asymptomatic infections in transmission is yet to be elucidated. Fever may have gradual or sudden onset, is persistent and irregular, and may alternate with periods of apyrexia or low-grade fever.

Post–kala-azar dermal leishmaniasis consists of macular, papular, and/or nodular skin lesions that occur weeks to years after apparent cure of systemic disease. Post–kala-azar dermal leishmaniasis occurs in up to 50% of VL cases in Sudan and 10% to 20% of cases in the Indian subcontinent. *Leishmania/* human immunodeficiency virus (HIV) coinfection is a serious form of the disease in southern Europe, eastern Africa, and Southeast Asia.

2. Risk groups—Evidence indicates that malnutrition and HIV infection increases the likelihood of progression to clinical disease. Manifest disease occurs among patients with acquired immunodeficiency syndrome, presumably as reactivation of latent infections. Kala-azar apparently induces lasting homologous immunity.

3. Causative agents—Typically *L. donovani*, *L. infantum* (in eastern hemisphere), and *L. infantum/chagasi* (in western hemisphere).

4. Diagnosis—Parasitologic diagnosis, based on invasive methods, is demonstration of intracellular amastigotes in stained smears from bone marrow, spleen, liver, and lymph node aspirates. The polymerase chain reaction technique is the most sensitive but remains expensive. Serologic diagnosis has traditionally been based on IFA and ELISA, tests that are expensive and difficult to decentralize. Recently, inexpensive, reliable rapid tests, such as the recombinant k39 immunochromatographic strip test, have become available for first-line diagnosis and field use, becoming the primary diagnostic modality for uncomplicated cases. An antigen-detection test in urine has shown good specificity but low-to-moderate sensitivity. Serologic testing has poor sensitivity in HIV-coinfected patients; parasitologic diagnosis is recommended.

5. Occurrence—VL occurs in 62 countries, with an estimated annual incidence of 300,000 cases and a population at risk of 120 million. It is usually a rural disease, occurring in foci in Asia, Africa, and the Americas. More than 90% of the global disease burden occurs in India, Bangladesh, Sudan, South Sudan, Brazil, and Ethiopia. In Brazil, many cases now occur in peri-urban areas. Foci also occur in China, Pakistan, southern regions of eastern Europe, the Middle East including Turkey, the Mediterranean basin, Mexico, Central and South America, Kenya, Uganda, and sub-Saharan savanna parts of Africa. In many affected areas, the disease occurs as scattered cases among infants, children, and adolescents but occasionally in epidemic waves. Incidence is modified by the use of antimalarial insecticides. Where zoonotic transmission was predominant and dog populations have been drastically reduced (e.g., China), human disease has also been reduced.

6. Reservoirs—Known or presumed reservoirs include humans, wild Canidae (foxes and jackals), and domestic dogs. Humans are the only known reservoir in Bangladesh, India, and Nepal.

7. Incubation period—Generally 2 to 6 months; range of 10 days to years.

8. Transmission—Through the bite of infected phlebotomine sandflies. In foci of anthroponotic VL, humans with VL or post-kala-azar dermal leishmaniasis (especially the highly infectious nodular form) are the sole reservoir, and transmission occurs from person to person through the sandfly bite. In foci of zoonotic VL, dogs constitute the main source of infection for sandflies. Person-to-person transmission has been reported in *Leishmania*/HIV-coinfected intravenous drug users through exchange of syringes. HIV-coinfected patients are highly infectious to sandflies, acting as human reservoirs even in zoonotic foci. Infectivity for phlebotomines may persist after clinical recovery of human patients.

9. Treatment—Multiple factors should be considered, including the geography of acquisition, extent of disease, and local treatment patterns. Expert consultation is recommended.

For VL, the treatment of choice is amphotericin B (consult local expertise for exact preferred regimens for immunocompetent vs. immunosuppressed individuals). Miltefosine is an alternative for VL caused by *L. donovani* (dosed for 28 days at 50 mg twice daily for persons 30–44 kg and 50 mg thrice daily for those > 44 kg). The pentavalent antimonials sodium stibogluconate and meglumine antimoniate are alternatives as well.

Miltefosine is contraindicated in pregnancy and breastfeeding; additionally, it is not approved for those younger than 12 years. Pentavalent antimonials should also not be used in those who are pregnant or nursing. The safety of amphotericin B in pregnancy and breastfeeding has not been established; it should only be used in these circumstances with expert consultation and joint patient decision-making in situations where benefit outweighs risk.

10. Prevention—See Cutaneous and Mucosal Leishmaniasis in this chapter. Infection in dogs should be monitored, and infected dogs should be treated or managed according to locally acceptable measures. In industrialized countries, dogs are usually treated, but they often relapse. In many developing countries, massive culling of infected dogs has failed, except in China. Insecticide-impregnated collars have proved effective in Iran and southern Europe, reducing the incidence of canine and human VL.

11. Special considerations—

1) Reporting: report to local health authority is required in most endemic areas.
2) Epidemic measures: effective control must include an understanding of the local ecology and transmission cycle, followed by

adoption of practical measures to reduce mortality, stop transmission, and avoid geographic extension of the epidemic, especially in anthroponotic foci. Active case detection and treatment of patients should reduce transmission rate. Institute coordinated programs of control among neighboring countries where the disease is endemic. WHO Collaborating Centres provide support as required. More information can be found at:

- http://www.who.int/collaboratingcentres/database/en
- http://www.who.int/leishmaniasis/en
- http://www.who.int/tdr/diseases-topics/leishmaniasis/en/index.html

Bibliography

Aronson N, Herwaldt BL, Libman M, et al. Diagnosis and treatment of leishmaniasis: clinical practice guidelines by the Infectious Diseases Society of America (IDSA) and the American Society of Tropical Medicine and Hygiene (ASTMH). *Clin Infect Dis.* 2016;63(12):1539–1557.

CDC. Leishmaniasis. 2018. Available at: https://www.cdc.gov/parasites/leishmaniasis/health_professionals/index.html. Accessed July 7, 2020.

[O. A. Khan]

LEPROSY
(Hansen's disease)

DISEASE	ICD-10 CODE
LEPROSY	ICD-10 A30

1. Clinical features—A slowly progressive mycobacterial infection causing lesions in the skin, peripheral nerves, mucous membranes, and eyes. Its clinical manifestations in a given patient appear on a continuum between 2 polar forms of leprosy—tuberculoid and lepromatous—with several intermediate (borderline) forms. Under WHO classification, tuberculoid leprosy is termed paucibacillary and exhibits 1 to 5 hypopigmented or erythematous anesthetic lesions, usually large, flat plaques with irregular borders and asymmetric distribution. Lepromatous leprosy is termed multibacillary by WHO classification; the lesions are more numerous, typically symmetric, and consist of small, smooth hyperpigmented papules and plaques that may or may not show loss of sensation.

Enlargement and/or tenderness of major superficial nerves (see later) is a frequent presenting or persisting finding. Nerve involvement may occur together or separately as sensory, motor, and/or autonomic neuropathies.

Clinical manifestations can include 2 acute adverse events: reversal reactions, also termed type 1, and erythema nodosum leprosum (ENL), often called type 2. Type 1 reactions present with edema and erythema of existing skin lesions, revelation of subclinical skin lesions, and acute neuritis with additional sensory and/or motor loss, often with edema of hands, feet, and face. Type 1 reactions with acute motor nerve involvement represent one of the few true emergencies in clinical leprosy. Treatment should begin immediately (see Special Considerations in this chapter).

Type 2 reactions (ENL) are characterized by new tender, erythematous subdermal nodules on apparently normal skin, often with systemic symptoms such as fever, malaise, anorexia, arthralgia, and edema. ENL may also be associated with acute neuritis; it is therefore considered a medical emergency, necessitating prompt drug and supportive therapy.

Differential diagnosis of the cutaneous manifestations of leprosy includes (among many other skin diseases) tinea corporis, tinea versicolor, psoriasis, vitiligo, pityriasis alba, sarcoidosis, syphilis, mycosis fungoides, neurofibromatosis, miliaria profunda, and streptocerciasis, as well as other mycobacterial and infiltrative skin diseases. Differential diagnosis of the neural aspects of leprosy includes any of many peripheral neuropathies, nerve trauma, syringomyelia, or, rarely, other spinal cord lesions.

2. Risk groups—Persons at highest risk are those living (or who have lived) in endemic areas in close contact with multibacillary cases. The disease is rarely seen in children younger than 3 years (however, cases have been identified in children < 1 year). There is accumulating evidence that genetic factors play a major part in determining risk of disease, leading to varying estimates of the percentage of populations who have innate immunity, the maximum estimate being up to 95% of individuals of northern European descent. Leprosy reactions may be masked in patients with advanced human immunodeficiency virus (HIV) disease. However, HIV-infected individuals may be at risk for reversal reactions (type 1) after immune reconstitution (immune reconstitution inflammatory syndrome), especially when beginning antiretroviral treatment.

3. Causative agents—*Mycobacterium leprae* and *Mycobacterium lepromatosis*. These mycobacteria cannot be grown in bacteriologic media or cell cultures. Both organisms cause the same clinical disease and respond to the same treatment. Clinical findings follow from 3 salient growth characteristics of *M. leprae*: slow growth—a doubling time of approximately 21 days; cool growth—optimum temperature of 28°C (82°F), that is, surface and mucous membrane body temperatures; neurophilic growth—optimum within the peripheral nerves.

4. Diagnosis—Clinical diagnosis is based on complete examination of the skin, eyes, ears, nose, and peripheral nerves.

1) Inspection and palpation of 1 or more chronic skin lesions, typically with reduction or loss of sensation within the lesions. Notably, treatment for other more common diseases (see Clinical Features in this chapter) has failed.

2) Search for signs of peripheral nerve involvement. Sensory hypoesthesia or anesthesia; motor paralysis and/or muscle wasting, with contractures if long-standing. In advanced cases, trophic ulcers may be found, sometimes with secondary bacterial infection or osteomyelitis, often resulting from loss of protective sensation in the limbs.

3) Conduct bilateral palpation of peripheral nerves for enlargement and tenderness: great auricular nerve, ulnar nerve at the elbow, radial nerve in the spiral groove of the humerus, dorsal radial cutaneous nerve and median nerve at the wrist, peroneal nerve below the head of the fibula, and the posterior tibial nerve posterior to the medial malleolus.

4) Test skin lesions and affected nerve trunks for sensation. Loss of hot/cold discrimination is the first sensory loss, followed by light touch. The 10 g monofilament used to test for protective sensation in the diabetic foot is useful (and was derived from leprosy research). Sharp versus dull and 2-point discrimination may be tested but are rarely necessary.

5) Laboratory diagnosis is through microscopic visualization of acid-fast bacilli, stained using the Fite method, in slit-skin smears (incision-scrape method) or in full-thickness 4-mm skin biopsy (preferable). In practice, laboratory studies are not essential for the diagnosis of leprosy. However, confirmation by skin biopsy is recommended if at all possible. In the paucibacillary lesions, bacilli may be rare and difficult to find; in the multibacillary lesions, bacilli are abundant.

6) *M. leprae* and *M. lepromatosis* may also be detected and identified using polymerase chain reaction. Differentiation of these 2 organisms can be accomplished by deoxyribonucleic acid sequencing.

7) Notably, at this time no serologic tests have proven to be sufficiently sensitive and specific to be used for the diagnosis of leprosy, although currently this is an area of vigorous research.

5. Occurrence—Though changes in data reporting make trend analysis difficult, the prevalence of leprosy appears to be declining in most countries, while the incidence (new cases reported) has continued at a similar level for many years. Declines are attributable to a combination of socioeconomic development, early and effective treatment of cases, and widespread vaccination with bacillus Calmette-Guérin against tuberculosis. During 2015, WHO recorded 211,973 new reported cases, more than three-fourths of them in India, Brazil, and Indonesia—nations with large populations.

WHO has targeted the disease for elimination (defined as registered prevalence of <1 case/10,000 population). Currently, the highest prevalences of leprosy in the world are in the Federated States of Micronesia.

In the USA, 150 to 200 new cases are reported each year, 75% in foreign-born individuals. However, the majority of those US cases originated in the USA itself.

6. Reservoirs—Humans and 9-banded armadillos are the only proven reservoirs. *M. leprae*-infected 9-banded armadillos have now been identified in all of the states bordering the Gulf of Mexico. Infected armadillos have also been found in Brazil.

7. Incubation period—Incubation has been reported to be as short as a few weeks to 30 years; however, the average incubation period is between 3 and 10 years.

8. Transmission—*M. leprae* transmission is favored by close contact. The bacterium may be transmitted from nasal mucosa, possibly through respiratory secretions, but the exact mechanism of transmission is not clearly understood. Indirect transmission is unlikely, although the bacillus can survive up to 7 days in dried nasal secretions.

Clinical and laboratory evidence suggests that infectiousness is lost in most instances within a day of beginning treatment with multidrug therapy (MDT).

9. Treatment—

Preferred therapy	For paucibacillary patients: • Dapsone 100 mg daily for 1 year PLUS • Rifampin 600 mg daily for 1 year
	For multibacillary patients: • Dapsone 100 mg daily for 2 years PLUS • Rifampin 600 mg daily for 2 years PLUS • Clofazimine 50 mg daily for 2 years

(Continued)

(Continued)

Preferred WHO therapy	For paucibacillary patients: • Dapsone 100 mg daily for 6 months PLUS • Rifampin 600 mg monthly for 6 months
	For multibacillary patients: • Dapsone 100 mg daily for 1 year PLUS • Rifampin 600 mg monthly for 1 year PLUS • Clofazimine 50 mg daily AND 300 mg monthly for 1 year
Special considerations and comments	• *Mycobacterium leprae* and *Mycobacterium lepromatosis* respond to the same treatment regimens. • The National Hansen's Disease Programs in the USA recommends these same drugs but with rifampin used daily instead of monthly; it recommends treatment of paucibacillary patients for 1 year and multibacillary patients for 2 years. • Relapse after completion of treatment is uncommon; the occurrence of new lesions during or after treatment is usually due to a reaction; drug resistance in *M. leprae* is rare; when this occurs or if individuals are unable to take any of the first-line antimicrobials, any of the following may be used as an alternative: clarithromycin, ofloxacin/levofloxacin, moxifloxacin, or minocycline; note that doxycycline is not effective against *M. leprae*. • See chapter text for initial/urgent drug treatment of type 1 (upgrading) and type 2 (erythema nodosum leprosum) leprosy reactions.

10. Prevention—

1) Public campaigns that raise awareness and reduce stigma by emphasizing curability.
2) Early detection and prompt MDT of cases.
3) Case finding by clinical examination of household contacts, especially of multibacillary index cases.

11. Special considerations—

1) Continuity of care in patients is critical to assure completion of treatment and thus minimize disease progression and disability. This is especially true for patients who move from one state or nation to another. They should be definitively referred prior to moving to a public leprosy program and specific clinician in their destination. This is a chronic disease and patients with sensory, motor, or eye disabilities may require lifelong care.

2) Leprosy reactions (reversal—type 1 or ENL—type 2) can occur prior to, during, or after completion of treatment. As stressed in Clinical Features in this chapter, many patients are first diagnosed with leprosy when they present in reaction.

Reactions do not indicate inadequate anti-leprosy drug treatment but rather immune reaction to antigens of *M. leprae*. As these reactions may result in disability, follow-up with patients should continue for several years after completion of treatment.

3) Treatment of reactions: as noted earlier, reactions—especially type 1 with motor nerve involvement—are relative emergencies in clinical leprosy.

In most cases, both types 1 and 2 respond well to initial treatment with 60 mg prednisone daily but treatment must be individualized to minimize nerve injury.

When available, thalidomide should be used in type 2 (ENL) reactions at 200 to 400 mg daily, with tapering over 5 to 10 days to 100 mg if the ENL is controlled. Tapering of prednisone and/or thalidomide must be individualized and may require several months. All patients in reaction should be referred to a physician experienced in clinical leprosy. In the USA, emergency advice on any clinical leprosy problem can be obtained by contacting the National Hansen's Disease Program by phone (800-642-2477) or via the website (http://www.hrsa.gov/hansens-disease). In the USA, the National Hansen's Disease Program provides free diagnostic and consultation services as well as antimicrobials for leprosy at no cost to patients.

4) Further information from WHO can be found at: http://www.who.int/lep.

[R. Pust, D. Scollard]

LEPTOSPIROSIS
(Weil's disease, canicola fever, hemorrhagic jaundice, mud fever, canefield fever, swineherd disease, rat urine disease)

DISEASE	ICD-10 CODE
LEPTOSPIROSIS	ICD-10 A27

1. Clinical features—A bacterial zoonotic disease that is self-limiting and often clinically inapparent in the majority of cases but can cause fulminant fatal disease. The disease typically presents as 1 of the following 4 clinical categories:

1) Mild influenza-like illness
2) Weil's syndrome, characterized by jaundice, renal failure, hemorrhage, and myocarditis with arrhythmias
3) Meningitis or meningoencephalitis
4) Pulmonary hemorrhage with respiratory failure (leptospirosis-associated pulmonary hemorrhage syndrome).

Clinical illness lasts from a few days to 3 weeks or longer. Generally, there are 2 phases in the illness. The acute, or leptospiremic, phase occurs during the first week of illness and is characterized by the abrupt onset of high fever, myalgias (calves and lumbar region), and headache (retro-orbital and frontal). Other acute manifestations can include nausea, vomiting, abdominal pain, diarrhea, cough, photophobia, and a truncal or pretibial rash. About 30% or more of patients also have conjunctival suffusion (redness of the conjunctiva)—a pathognomonic finding of leptospirosis when observed with scleral icterus. The second, or immune, phase occurs in conjunction with the development of the antibody response and is characterized by prolonged fever and systemic complications, such as jaundice, renal failure, bleeding, respiratory insufficiency with or without hemoptysis, hypotension, myocarditis, meningitis, mental confusion, and depression. The 2 phases can be separated by a 3- to 4-day abatement of fever. However, the distinction between the phases might not be apparent and patients sometimes present only in the second phase. Recovery of untreated cases can take several months.

It is estimated that between 5% and 10% of clinical infections progress to severe illness. The icteric form (Weil's disease) is associated with severe hepatic dysfunction and hemorrhage; cardiac, pulmonary, and neurologic involvement; and high mortality. However, severe complications can also occur in patients without jaundice. Prognostic predictors for death include age older than 40 years, oliguria, respiratory insufficiency, pulmonary hemorrhage, cardiac arrhythmias, and altered mental status. Deaths are mainly due to renal failure, cardiopulmonary failure, widespread hemorrhage, and, rarely, liver failure. Case-fatality rates are estimated to be from 5% to 15% in patients with severe illness to greater than 50% in those with pulmonary hemorrhage syndrome, characterized by massive pulmonary bleeding and acute respiratory distress.

In countries where leptospirosis is endemic, it appears to be a significant cause of undiagnosed aseptic meningitis (between 5% and 40% of cases). Late sequelae can occur, including chronic fatigue; neuropsychiatric symptoms (paresis, depression); and unilateral or bilateral uveitis, characterized by iritis, iridocyclitis, and chorioretinitis, which can develop up to 18 months after acute illness and persist for years.

Cases are often underrecognized or misdiagnosed as dengue, malaria, aseptic meningitis, encephalitis, and influenza due to the nonspecific manifestations of acute leptospirosis. Severe leptospirosis must be differentiated from other causes of acute jaundice and renal failure, such as rickettsial disease, hantaviral infection, enteric fevers, viral hepatitis, and Gram-negative sepsis. During pregnancy infection can result in fetal death, abortion, stillbirth, or congenital infection.

2. Risk groups—Children and adults in areas where infection is endemic in animal reservoirs. An occupational hazard for agricultural workers such as rice and sugarcane field workers; fish workers; miners; veterinarians; workers in animal husbandry, dairies, and abattoirs; sewer workers; and military troops.

3. Causative agents—Organisms from the genus *Leptospira* are classified into 20 named pathogenic and nonpathogenic genomospecies as determined by deoxyribonucleic acid (DNA)-DNA hybridization. They are subdivided into nearly 300 antigenically defined serovars, which are grouped into 26 serogroups based on serologic relatedness. Serologic classification continues to provide useful epidemiologic information, since serogroups and serovars are often associated with specific animal reservoirs. The severity of illness tends to vary with the infecting serovar.

4. Diagnosis—Clinical diagnosis is by isolation of leptospires from blood or cerebrospinal fluid during the first 7 to 10 days of acute illness or from urine beginning in the second week of illness. Immunoglobulin class G assays, enzyme-linked immunosorbent assays (ELISAs), and anti-whole *Leptospira* immunoglobulin class M (IgM) detection kits in ELISA or rapid formats are used to provide presumptive confirmation for leptospirosis. However, sensitivity is low (39%–72%) during acute-phase illness (first 7 days). Immunofluorescence, immunohistochemical, and nucleic acid detection techniques are used for the demonstration of leptospires in clinical and autopsy specimens.

Polymerase chain reaction assays for detection of leptospire DNA have been developed for use on clinical samples, such as blood or urine, and can be used for diagnostic testing on whole blood during the first 4 days of clinical illness and on urine after the first week of illness. These tests are available in reference and research laboratories. Direct examination of blood or urine using dark-field microscopy has poor sensitivity and specificity. Inoculation of experimental animals, such as golden hamsters, guinea pigs, or gerbils, can also confirm diagnosis but is rarely used. Where laboratory capacity is not well established, a positive test by 2 different rapid diagnostic tests could be considered as a laboratory-confirmed case.

Diagnosis is most frequently confirmed by seroconversion, from a negative to a positive value, or is demonstrated by a 4-fold or greater increase in serum agglutination titer on the microscopic agglutination test (MAT)—the confirmatory serologic test—using acute and convalescent specimens obtained at least 10 days apart. Seroconversion can occur as early as 5 to 7 days after disease onset but might not develop until after 10 days or longer, especially if antimicrobial therapy is initiated. Patients can develop cross-reactive antibodies to several serovars during acute infection; these gradually decrease weeks to months later. Different serovars of leptospires can occur in different regions. Therefore, the MAT preferably uses a panel of locally occurring leptospire serovars. However, antibody titer increase can be delayed or absent in some patients, and seroconversion can occur asymptomatically, especially in endemic areas. Antibodies to IgM can remain detectable for months to years at low titers.

Culture and isolation can be very difficult, requiring special media and incubation for up to 16 weeks; the sensitivity of culture for diagnosis is low.

5. Occurrence—Worldwide, except polar regions. The disease is most prevalent in tropical and subtropical regions, with the highest incidence reported in island countries or low-lying countries with frequent flooding. Leptospirosis is an endemic disease in rural subsistence farming areas and urban slum settlements in tropical regions because of the high density of domestic and wild reservoirs and poor sanitation. Rodent-borne leptospirosis exposure appears to be increasing in urban areas, especially during floods.

Outbreaks can occur following excessive rainfall or flooding, especially in endemic areas. They also occur among those exposed to fresh river, stream, canal, and lake water contaminated by the urine of domestic and wild animals and to the urine, bodily fluids, and tissues of infected animals. In recent years, large outbreaks have been reported in Asia, Europe, Australia, and the Americas. Affluent populations are increasingly affected following travel, recreation, and water sports in contaminated waters, especially after immersion or swallowing water.

6. Reservoirs—Approximately half of the pathogenic serovars belong to *Leptospira interrogans* or *Leptospira borgpetersenii*. Pathogenic leptospires are naturally carried in the renal tubules and genital tract of wild and domestic animals, which serve as natural maintenance hosts and can remain asymptomatic shedders for years or even for life. Serovars are adapted to 1 or more reservoir animal species, such as rats (*L. interrogans* serovars Copenhageni and Icterohaemorrhagiae), swine (*L. interrogans* serovar Pomona), cattle (*L. borgpetersenii* serovar Hardjo), dogs (*L. interrogans* serovar Canicola), and raccoons (*L. interrogans* serovar Autumnalis). The leptospires can be shed in infected urine, amniotic fluid, or placental tissue and contaminate soil and water. They can remain viable for weeks or months under favorable conditions in moist soil or water, especially where temperatures are 28°C to 32°C (82.4°F–89.6°F).

A high proportion of both stray and domestic dogs in some urban and suburban areas show evidence of infection and shed leptospires in the urine. Other animal hosts, some with a shorter carrier state, include feral rodents, badgers, deer, squirrels, foxes, skunks, raccoons, and opossums. Reptiles and frogs have been found to carry pathogenic leptospires but are unlikely to play an important epidemiologic role.

7. Incubation period—Usually 5 to 14 days, with a range of 2 to 30 days.

8. Transmission—Contact of the skin (especially if abraded or after prolonged immersion) or mucous membranes with

1) Moist soil or vegetation contaminated with the urine of infected animals
2) Contaminated waters (e.g., through swimming, wading in floodwaters, accidental immersion, or occupational abrasion)
3) Urine, fluids, or tissues of infected animals

Occasionally, transmission can be by consuming water or food contaminated with urine of infected animals (often rats) or through inhalation of droplet aerosols of contaminated fluids.

Direct person-to-person transmission is rare. Leptospires can be excreted in the urine—usually for 1 month, although leptospiruria has been observed in humans for months, even years, after acute illness.

9. Treatment—

Drug	• Penicillin G (for severe leptospirosis) • Doxycycline (for mild leptospirosis)
Dose	• Penicillin G 30 mg/kg ($\leq$ 1.2 g) • Doxycycline 2 mg/kg ($\leq$ 100 mg)
Route	• Penicillin G IV • Doxycycline PO
Alternative drug	• Azithromycin (for pregnant patients allergic to penicillin) 500 mg PO once daily for 3 days • Cefotaxime 1 g IV every 6 hours for 7 days • Ceftriaxone 1–2 g IV once daily for 7 days
Duration	• Penicillin G every 6 hours for 5–7 days • Doxycycline every 12 hours for 5–7 days
Special considerations and comments	Not applicable

Note: IV = intravenous(ly); PO = oral(ly).

10. Prevention—

1) Educate the public on modes of transmission and avoidance of swimming or wading in potentially contaminated waters.
2) Protect workers in hazardous occupations by providing protective clothing and equipment such as boots, gloves, and aprons. Covering wounds with waterproof dressings could reduce the risk of infection in persons with occupational or recreational exposure.

3) Recognize potentially contaminated waters and soil; drain such waters and when possible create physical barriers, such as closing open sewers, to prevent exposures to potential sources. Small environmental areas, such as human habitations that become contaminated, can be cleaned and disinfected; leptospires are rapidly killed by disinfectants and desiccation.

4) Control rodents and reservoir wildlife populations (e.g., raccoons, opossums) in human habitations—urban or rural—and recreational areas. Refuse removal and improved sanitation can also reduce rodent infestation. Management of sugarcane fields, such as through controlled preharvest burning, reduces risks in harvesting.

5) Segregate infected domestic animals. Humans living, working, or playing in potentially contaminated areas must avoid direct or indirect contact with the urine of infected animals. Maintain hygienic measures during care and handling of animals and avoid contact with urine or other bodily fluids.

6) Immunization of farm and pet animals prevents illness from serovars contained within the vaccine but not necessarily from infection and renal shedding. Any vaccine must contain the dominant local strains.

7) Immunization of people has been carried out against occupational exposures to specific serovars with varying degrees of success but is not available in most countries at present. Serovar-specific immunity follows infection or immunization occasionally but may not protect against infection with a different serovar.

8) Doxycycline 200 mg immediately and then weekly for the duration of exposure might provide effective prophylaxis against clinical disease. It could be considered for preventing leptospirosis among high-risk groups with short-term exposure.

11. Special considerations—

1) Reporting: obligatory case report in many countries.

2) Epidemic measures: search for source of infection, such as sewers, contaminated wells, swimming areas, or other contaminated water sources; eliminate the contamination or prohibit use. Investigate industrial and occupational sources, including potential animal exposures.

3) A potential problem in endemic areas following disasters such as heavy rainfall, monsoons, and extreme climactic events (e.g., hurricanes, flooding). Outbreaks can be confused, or occur concurrently, with outbreaks of dengue or other viral hemorrhagic diseases, typhoid, rickettsial infection, malaria, or other febrile illnesses. Difficulties in diagnosis can compromise disease control and result in increased severity and elevated mortality.

4) Surveillance case definitions: the WHO-recommended case definition for leptospirosis can be found at: https://www.who.int/zoonoses/diseases/Leptospirosissurveillance.pdf. The Pan American Health Organization–recommended case definition for leptospirosis can be found at: http://www1.paho.org/english/SHA/be_v21n2-cases.htm.

[H. Badaruddin]

LISTERIOSIS

DISEASE	ICD-10 CODE
LISTERIOSIS	ICD-10 A32

1. Clinical features—A bacterial infection that typically causes invasive disease. In older adults and persons with certain immunocompromising conditions, invasive disease usually presents as septicemia or meningitis. The onset of meningitis can be sudden—with fever, intense headache, nausea, vomiting, and signs of meningeal irritation; subacute meningoencephalitis or rhombencephalitis can also occur. Delirium and coma may appear early; occasionally there is collapse and shock. Endocarditis, granulomatous lesions in the liver and other organs, localized internal or external abscesses, septic arthritis or osteomyelitis, and pustular or papular cutaneous lesions may occur on rare occasions. Surveillance data from the USA indicate that the case-fatality rate among nonpregnant adults with invasive listeriosis is 18%. In otherwise healthy people, *Listeria* infection is often asymptomatic but may cause an acute febrile gastroenteritis.

In pregnant women, symptoms may be mild and nonspecific—fever, headache, myalgia, or gastrointestinal symptoms—or absent. Fortunately, central nervous system infection in pregnancy is rare. However, placental invasion can lead to fetal infection, resulting in stillbirth, preterm delivery, or neonatal infection. Neonatal infection typically presents as septicemia or meningitis; meningitis is more common with late onset of symptoms (> 1 week of age). *Listeria* can also cause spontaneous abortions, although the incidence is difficult to estimate since bacterial cultures are not routinely obtained. Listeriosis has not been associated with recurrent pregnancy loss. The case-fatality rate is 20% to 30% in infected newborns and approaches 50% when onset occurs in the first 4 days after birth.

2. Risk groups—There is a strong association between decreased immunity (particularly cell-mediated) and invasive listeriosis. The population groups at increased risk include pregnant women; persons with debilitating illnesses or conditions such as malignancy, organ and bone marrow transplantation, diabetes, cirrhosis, renal disease, heart disease, and human immunodeficiency virus infection; and persons who take corticosteroids. The normal immunosuppression of pregnancy may account for the higher risk of invasive disease in this population. Among older adults, risk increases with advancing age because of immunosenescence and the higher prevalence of underlying illnesses. There is no evidence of acquired immunity.

3. Causative agents—*Listeria monocytogenes*, a Gram-positive rod-shaped bacterium. Most human infections (95%) are caused by serotypes 1/2a, 1/2b, and 4b.

4. Diagnosis—For symptomatic patients, diagnosis is confirmed only after isolation of *L. monocytogenes* from a normally sterile site, such as blood or cerebrospinal fluid (in the setting of nervous system involvement), or from amniotic fluid/placental or fetal tissue (in the setting of pregnancy). Stool samples are of limited use and are not recommended. *L. monocytogenes* can be isolated readily on routine media but care must be taken to distinguish this organism from other Gram-positive rods, particularly diphtheroids. Selective enrichment media improve rates of isolation from contaminated specimens. The cultures can be expected to take 1 to 2 days to grow. Identification of agent by nucleic acid testing on blood or spinal fluid, where available, can dramatically shorten the time to diagnosis. Importantly, a negative culture does not rule out infection in the presence of strong clinical suspicion. Serologic tests are unreliable and not recommended at the present time.

5. Occurrence—Worldwide, but uncommonly diagnosed and reported in many regions. *Listeria* infections account for a small fraction of all foodborne illnesses. However, listeriosis is an important cause of severe illness and results in a disproportionately high number of hospitalizations and deaths compared with other foodborne pathogens such as *Salmonella*. Most infections are sporadic but numerous outbreaks have been reported. Fewer than 20% of clinical cases are associated with pregnancy. In nonpregnant adults, infections occur mainly after 40 years of age. Outbreaks in health care settings have been reported. Asymptomatic infections probably occur at all ages, although they are only clinically important during pregnancy because of the risk of fetal loss.

6. Reservoirs—Animal reservoirs include domestic and wild mammals, fowl, and humans. *L. monocytogenes* can be detected in soil, water, mud, forage, livestock food, and silage. The seasonal use of silage as fodder is frequently followed by an increased incidence of listeriosis in animals. Unlike most other foodborne pathogens, *Listeria* can multiply in refrigerated foods. *Listeria* can grow and survive in biofilms in production facilities, enabling attachment (e.g., to stainless steel surfaces) and transfer to food products. Bacteria in biofilms can show increased resistance to sanitizers, disinfectants, and antimicrobial agents.

7. Incubation period—Typically 2 or 3 weeks. However, cases have occurred up to 70 days after a single exposure to a contaminated product. Data from some outbreak investigations suggest that the median incubation period is longer among pregnant women than among nonpregnant adults.

8. Transmission—Nearly all cases result from foodborne transmission. Outbreaks have been reported in association with dairy products, especially soft cheeses made from raw (unpasteurized) milk, processed and ready-to-eat meats (e.g., hot dogs, pâté, and delicatessen meats), raw vegetables, and cantaloupe melon. In neonatal infections, *L. monocytogenes* is almost always transmitted from mother to fetus—most likely transplacentally, during passage through the birth canal or perhaps from ascending infection from vaginal colonization. Neonatal clusters in nursery settings have been reported, including 1 attributed to a fomite source (mineral oil).

Asymptomatic fecal carriage is common, even without a known exposure. Carriage rate estimates vary (point prevalence 1%–21%) and can be much higher among slaughterhouse workers, laboratory workers who work with *L. monocytogenes* cultures, and in asymptomatic household contacts of persons with invasive listeriosis. Infected individuals can shed the organisms in their stools for several months. Determination of the infectious dose has been elusive. Newer risk assessment modeling has enabled the preparation of dose-response curves that indicate that the probability of infection varies markedly, depending on the dose and strain ingested and on the susceptibility of the host.

9. Treatment—

Preferred therapy	For meningitis:
	• Ampicillin 2 g IV every 4 hours for 14 days
	For febrile gastroenteritis (when treatment required):
	• Amoxicillin 500 mg PO TID for 5–7 days
Alternative therapy options	For meningitis (penicillin-allergic):
	• A carbapenem (e.g., meropenem 2 g IV every 8 hours); experience with vancomycin limited
	For febrile gastroenteritis:
	• TMP/SMX double-strength BID for 7 days
Special considerations and comments	• Gastroenteritis in the nonpregnant patient is a self-limited illness and does not always require treatment. • In penicillin-allergic pregnant patients with gastroenteritis, TMP/SMX can be used in short course with emphasis on taking prenatal vitamins with the goal of preventing teratogenicity. • In penicillin-allergic patients with invasive disease (bacteremia, meningitis), penicillin desensitization should be considered.

Note: IV = intravenous(ly); PO = oral(ly); BID = twice daily; TID = thrice daily; TMP/SMX = trimethoprim-sulfamethoxazole.

10. Prevention—Preventing listeriosis requires many actions that are similar to those for preventing other foodborne illnesses. However, additional actions to ensure food safety, including avoidance of certain foods and proper preparation and storage, are especially important for groups at higher risk for invasive listeriosis (pregnant women, older adults, and immunocompromised individuals).

1) Higher risk groups should not consume unpasteurized milk or soft cheeses made with unpasteurized milk. They should not consume ready-to-eat meats, hot dogs, other processed meats, or leftover foods unless heated until steaming hot. These groups should not eat refrigerated smoked seafood unless it is part of a dish that is cooked and hot, such as a casserole, or unless it is a canned or shelf-stable product.
2) Thoroughly wash raw vegetables before eating and keep them separate from raw food from animal sources (e.g., beef, pork, or poultry). Thoroughly cook raw food from animal sources. Wash hands, knives, and cutting boards after handling uncooked foods.
3) Use a thermometer to ensure that the refrigerator is at 4.4°C (40°F) or colder and the freezer is at -17.8°C (0°F) or colder.
4) Manufacturers should ensure the safety of all foods of animal origin. Pasteurize all dairy products and irradiate soft cheeses after ripening. Use microbial growth inhibitors in processed meats where possible. Apply hazard analysis critical control points systems and process monitoring (e.g., environmental culturing).
5) Processed, ready-to-eat, and raw foods found to be contaminated by *L. monocytogenes* (e.g., during routine bacteriologic surveillance) should be recalled.
6) Avoid the use of untreated manure on vegetable crops.
7) Veterinarians and farmers must take proper precautions in handling aborted fetuses and sick or dead animals, especially sheep that died of encephalitis. Higher risk groups should avoid contact with possibly infectious materials.

11. Special considerations—

1) Reporting: obligatory case report required in many countries. In others, report of clusters required.
2) WHO risk assessment of *L. monocytogenes* in ready-to-eat food: https://www.who.int/news-room/fact-sheets/detail/food-safety.

[D. Cohen]

LIVER FLUKE DISEASE

DISEASE	ICD-10 CODE
CLONORCHIASIS	ICD-10 B66.1
OPISTHORCHIASIS	ICD-10 B66.0
CHOLANGIOCARCINOMA	ICD-10 C22.1

I. CLONORCHIASIS AND OPISTHORCHIASIS

1. Clinical features—A trematode disease of the bile ducts. Clinical complaints may be slight or absent in light infections; in heavy infections (> 10,000 eggs/g of stool) abdominal symptoms occur in about 10% of patients. These result from local irritation of bile ducts by the flukes. Loss of appetite, diarrhea, and a sensation of abdominal pressure are common early symptoms. Rarely, bile duct obstruction producing jaundice may be followed by cirrhosis, enlargement, and tenderness of the liver, with progressive ascites and edema. Eggs in the gallbladder increase risk of gallstones.

Liver fluke disease can become chronic, sometimes lasting 30 years or longer, but is rarely a direct or contributing cause of death; it is often completely asymptomatic. Chronic symptoms, if present, may include chronic fatigue, abdominal discomfort, dyspepsia, weight loss, and diarrhea. Regardless, it is a significant risk factor (15-fold increase) for the development of cholangiocarcinoma. Other complications of chronic infections include cholangitis and cholangiohepatitis arising from chronic irritation and fibrosis.

2. Risk groups—In most endemic areas, the highest prevalence is among adults older than 30 years.

3. Causative agents—*Clonorchis sinensis* for clonorchiasis; *Opisthorchis felineus* and *Opisthorchis viverrini* for opisthorchiasis. These worms are the leading cause of cholangiocarcinoma throughout the world.

4. Diagnosis—Demonstration of the characteristic eggs in feces or duodenal/bile drainage fluid. Eggs cannot be easily distinguished between these worms. Formalin-ethyl acetate sedimentation concentration technique to count eggs and quantify the intensity of infection is considered the gold standard. Eggs may be absent or scanty in light infections. There may be peripheral eosinophilia with raised levels of serum immunoglobin class E. Serologic diagnosis by enzyme-linked immunosorbent assay can be performed but is not always specific. Immunoblot assays based on antigens have variable sensitivities. Polymerase chain reaction for detection of eggs in stools has been reported to be sensitive for heavier infections and less so in light infections. Scans such as ultrasonography, computed tomography (CT), and magnetic resonance imaging (MRI) may be used as adjunct diagnostic tools. Occasionally adult worms may be found during endoscopy or cholangiopancreatography or passed in stools on initiation of treatment.

Although not transmitted from person to person, family members of persons diagnosed with clonorchiasis or opisthorchiasis should be evaluated with stool microscopy as they may be exposed to common sources. Those with evidence of infection should be treated to avoid the risk of future complications, even if asymptomatic.

5. Occurrence—Clonorchiasis is present throughout China (including Taiwan), except in northwestern areas, and is highly endemic in southeastern China and eastern Russia. It also occurs in Japan (rarely), South Korea, the Mekong River delta region of Vietnam, and probably Cambodia and Laos. In other parts of the world, imported cases may be recognized in immigrants from Asia. Opisthorchiasis occurs in Europe and Asia, especially in Russia and the former USSR, with prevalence rates of 40% to 95% in some areas; *O. viverrini* is endemic in southeastern Asia, with prevalence rates between 24% and 80% in some areas, especially in Thailand, Laos, and possibly Vietnam. It is estimated that the number of people infected with liver fluke are as many as 25 million, with 15 million for *C. sinensis*, 10 million for *O. viverrini*, and about 1 million for *O. felineus*. Up to 700 million people worldwide are at risk of infection.

Parts of North America and Russia are endemic for a liver fluke (*Metorchis conjunctus*) belonging to the same family. Disease is associated with consumption of raw fish and similarly responds to praziquantel.

6. Reservoirs—Humans, cats, dogs, swine, rats, and other animals for clonorchiasis; cats and some other fish-eating mammals for opisthorchiasis.

7. Incubation period—Unpredictable as it varies with the number of worms present; flukes reach maturity within 1 month after encysted larvae are ingested.

8. Transmission—Acquired by eating raw or undercooked freshwater fish containing encysted larvae. During digestion, larvae are freed from cysts and migrate via the common bile duct to biliary radicles. Eggs deposited in the bile passages are excreted in feces. Eggs in feces contain fully developed miracidia; when ingested by a susceptible operculate snail (e.g., *Parafossarulus*), they hatch in its intestine, penetrate the tissues, and asexually generate larvae (cercariae) that emerge into the water. On contact with a second intermediate host (110 species of freshwater fish belonging mostly to the family Cyprinidae), cercariae penetrate the host fish and encyst (metacercariae), usually in muscle and occasionally on the underside of scales. The complete life cycle, from person to snail to fish to person, requires at least 3 months. Infected individuals may pass viable eggs for as long as 30 years; because protective immunity does not develop, repeat infection can occur with cumulative worm burden increasing with age in endemic areas. Infection is not directly transmitted from person to person.

9. Treatment—

Preferred therapy	Praziquantel 25 mg/kg/dose PO TID for 1–2 days
Alternative therapy options	Albendazole 10 mg/kg/day PO for 7 days (efficacy better for clonorchiasis than opisthorchiasis)
Special considerations and comments	<ul><li>Single-dose praziquantel (30–50 mg/kg) was found to be as effective as the standard regimen for treatment of light infection due to opisthorchiasis (< 1000 eggs/g of stool).</li><li>Symptoms may take months to resolve, although eggs disappear from stools within 1 week of starting treatment.</li></ul>

Note: PO = oral(ly); TID = thrice daily.

10. Prevention—

1) Thoroughly cook all freshwater fish at 70°C (158°F) for at least 30 minutes or freeze at -20°C (-4°F) for at least 7 days. Storage of fish for several weeks in a saturated salt solution has also been recommended, but effectiveness remains unproven.

2) In endemic areas, educate the public to the dangers of eating raw or improperly treated fish and the necessity for sanitary disposal of feces to avoid contaminating sources of food fish.

3) Mass treatment of persons living in opisthorchiasis-endemic areas with praziquantel (40 mg/kg as a single dose) was shown to be effective.

11. Special considerations—Epidemic measures: locate source of infected fish. Shipments of dried or pickled fish are the likely source in nonendemic areas, as are fresh or chilled freshwater fish brought from endemic areas. Control fish or fish products imported from endemic areas.

II. CHOLANGIOCARCINOMA

Cholangiocarcinoma is malignancy of the biliary duct system. Incidence is low in Western countries but notably high in Asia, where the prevalence of liver fluke infections is high. It can be divided into 2 types—intrahepatic and extrahepatic—depending on which bile ducts are affected.

The incidence of cholangiocarcinoma, especially of the intrahepatic type, is the highest in the world in the northeastern part of Thailand (78/100,000 population in males and 33/100,000 population in females) and has been associated with high prevalence of *O. viverrini* infection. Consumption of fermented food containing high levels of *N*-nitroso compounds and nitrosamines also accelerates carcinomatous changes of the epithelial cells in the bile duct. Smoking and heavy alcohol intake may also interact with the carcinogenic effects of liver flukes.

Cholangiocarcinoma related to liver fluke infection may appear early in the fourth decade of life. Persons infected with liver flukes may have been carrying infection from as young as 1 year old. Cholangiocarcinoma can manifest as malignant obstructive jaundice or as a nonjaundice type with liver mass. Cholangitis is a common complication.

Alkaline phosphatase level is very high in both types. Tumor marker levels (e.g., carbohydrate antigen [CA] 19-9, CA 125, and carcinoembryonic antigen) are high, but the α-fetoprotein tumor marker is normal. Ultrasonography of the liver may show single or multiple masses with localized dilatation of bile ducts in peripheral type or diffuse intrahepatic/extrahepatic bile duct dilatation. CT scan or MRI/magnetic resonance cholangiopancreatography is useful for staging of the disease and planning surgical intervention. Cholangiography has been replaced with magnetic resonance cholangiopancreatography where available. Surgical resection of the tumor mass can cure the disease in the early stages only. In late cases, palliative biliary bypass with stent using endoscopy or surgery can relieve the symptoms but does not affect survival. Results of chemotherapy are not good.

High levels of alkaline phosphatase in people with a history of liver fluke infection may be an early indication of cholangiocarcinoma and should be followed up with ultrasonography of the liver. After confirming diagnosis, cases should be reported to a tumor registry and specialists should manage the patient.

Bibliography

Hughes T, O'Conner T, Techasen A, et al. Opisthorchiasis and cholangiocarcinoma in Southeast Asia: an unresolved problem. *Int J Gen Med.* 2017;10:227-237.

Liu LX, Harinasuta KT. Liver and intestinal flukes. *Gastroenterol Clin North Am.* 1996; 25(3):627.

Marcos LA, Terashima A, Gotuzzo E. Update on hepatobiliary liver flukes: fascioliasis, opisthorchiasis and clonorchiasis. *Curr Opin Infect Dis.* 2008;21(5):523-530.

Pungpak S, Chalermrut K, Harinasuta T, et al. Opisthorchis viverrini infection in Thailand: symptoms and signs of infection—a population-based study. *Trans R Soc Trop Med Hyg.* 1994;88(5):561-564.

Sayasone S, Meister I, Andrews JR, et al. Efficacy and safety of praziquantel against light infections of Opisthorchis viverrini: a randomised parallel single-blind dose-ranging trial. *Clin Infect Dis.* 2017;64(4):451-458.

[V. Lee, Z. J. M. Ho]

LOIASIS

(*Loa loa* infection, eyeworm disease of Africa, Calabar swelling)

DISEASE	ICD-10 CODE
LOIASIS	ICD-10 B74.3

1. Clinical features—A chronic filarial disease characterized by migration of the adult worm through subcutaneous or deeper tissues of the body, causing episodic angioedema (Calabar swellings) several centimeters in diameter; the swellings can be located on any body part but are most commonly found on the limbs. These swellings may be preceded by localized pain with pruritus. A major symptom is pruritus localized on arms, thorax, face, and shoulders. Infection is also sometimes characterized by subconjunctival migration of the adult *Loa loa* worm, which may be accompanied by pain and edema. Allergic reactions with giant urticaria (large urticaria with severe edema of the skin) and fever may occur occasionally. Infection is often asymptomatic.

2. Risk groups—Individuals living in endemic areas are most at risk of infection. Travelers to endemic areas are also at risk; however, risk is typically higher if travelers stay in endemic areas over the course of many months as there is greater opportunity for repeated exposures to infected vectors. Susceptibility is universal. Immunity has not been demonstrated with repeated infections.

3. Causative agents—*L. loa*, a filarial nematode helminth.

4. Diagnosis—In general, diagnosis should be made with a blood smear. Larvae (microfilariae) are present in peripheral blood during the daytime and can be demonstrated in Giemsa-stained thin or thick blood smears obtained between 10 AM and 4 PM, in stained sediment of blood where erythrocytes and hemoglobin have been separated (laking), or through membrane filtration. Eosinophilia is frequent. *L. loa*–specific deoxyribonucleic acid can be detected in blood from asymptomatic infected individuals. Serologic testing can be used to exclude infection when blood smears are negative but clinical suspicion of infection is high. An adult worm may also be identified either prior to the worm's removal from the eye or after its removal. A travel history is essential for diagnosis in non-African individuals. Infections with other filariae, such as *Wuchereria bancrofti*, *Onchocerca volvulus*, *Mansonella* (*Dipetalonema*) *perstans*, and *Mansonella streptocerca* (common in areas where *L. loa* is endemic), should be considered in the differential diagnosis.

5. Occurrence—The geographic distribution of *L. loa* is constrained by the distribution of the *Chrysops* spp. vectors (tabanid flies). *L. loa* is endemic to Africa and is predominantly found in rain forests in Central Africa. In the Congo River basin, up to 90% of indigenous inhabitants of some villages are infected.

6. Reservoirs—Humans. Simian *L. loa* occurs but is transmitted by a different vector, *Chrysops langi*, which does not commonly bite humans. Therefore, the infection is not believed to be zoonotic.

7. Incubation period—Symptoms usually appear several years after infection but may occur after as little as 4 months. Microfilariae may appear in the peripheral blood as soon as 6 months after infection.

8. Transmission—Transmitted by *Chrysops* tabanid flies. *Chrysops dimidiata*, *Chrysops silacea*, and other species ingest blood that contains microfilariae. The larvae develop to their infectious stage within 10 to 12 days in the fly and migrate to the proboscis, from where they are transferred to a human host by the bite of the infective fly. The larvae then migrate to subcutaneous tissue in the human host (loose connective tissue between fascial layers), where they mature to adults over the course of approximately 1 year. The adult worms mate and shed microfilariae into the blood for up to 17 years. Approximately 10 to 12 days after the fly is infected, the larvae become infective and can be transmitted to humans.

9. Treatment—

Drug	Diethylcarbamazine
Dose, duration	For patients without evidence of microfilariae: • 8–10 mg/kg/day in 3 divided doses daily (recommended dosage is the same for both adults and children)
	For patients with microfilaremia a graded dosing schedule may be used: • Day 1: 50 mg (1 mg/kg) • Day 2: 50 mg (1 mg/kg) TID • Day 3: 100 mg (1–2 mg/kg) TID • Days 4–21: 9 mg/kg/day in 3 divided doses
Route	PO
Alternative drug	Albendazole
Dose, duration	Days 1–21: 200 mg BID

(Continued)

(Continued)

Special considerations and comments	• Treatment of *Loa loa* is highly individualized and decisions should be guided by an expert. • Diethylcarbamazine is the preferred treatment because of its activity against both the microfilariae and adult worm, therefore resulting in quicker resolution of infection. With diethylcarbamazine, hypersensitivity reactions (sometimes severe) are common owing to rapid death of the microfilariae; more severe reactions occur with higher levels of circulating microfilariae. Treatment must be individualized and closely supervised. In symptomatic patients with high levels of circulating microfilariae, apheresis (if available) or pretreatment with albendazole may be indicated prior to initiating diethylcarbamazine. • Surgical excision of migrating adult worms is an effective treatment for symptoms localized to the migrating worm and provides an opportunity for diagnosis. Surgery is not curative. Antiparasitic medication is required for cure. • When diethylcarbamazine is ineffective or unavailable, albendazole may be used for treatment; however, because it does not kill microfilariae repeated courses may be necessary. Albendazole results in death or sterilization of the adult worms, leading to a gradual decline in microfilariae. • Patients who come from a region of Africa coendemic for loiasis, lymphatic filariasis, or onchocerciasis should be screened for *L. loa* infection prior to initiating treatment. This is because when microfilaremia is heavy[a] there is a risk of meningoencephalitis with ivermectin (the drug of choice for lymphatic filariasis and onchocerciasis); the advantages of treatment must be weighed against the risk of life-threatening encephalopathy. Like diethylcarbamazine, ivermectin has microfilaricidal activity against *L. loa* and can result in rapid death of microfilariae and severe adverse events. Ivermectin is not active against adult worms. • Coinfection with loiasis and onchocerciasis requires particular attention because of severe inflammatory responses. If the burden of *L. loa* is low, ivermectin pretreatment is indicated prior to diethylcarbamazine. If the burden of *L. loa* is high, risks and benefits of treatment must be considered; apheresis or albendazole may considered prior to treatment with ivermectin and, later, diethylcarbamazine.

Note: BID = twice daily; PO = oral(ly); TID = thrice daily.

[a]Various thresholds for maximum microfilaremia (mF) counts have been proposed, ranging from 2,500 mF/mL to 8,000 mF/mL blood.

10. Prevention—

1) Diethyltoluamide or dimethyl phthalate applied to exposed skin are effective fly repellents.

2) Protective clothing (long sleeves and trousers) and application of screens to windows and doors of houses are effective to decrease exposure to vectors.

3) For temporary residents of endemic areas whose risk of exposure is high or prolonged, a weekly dose of diethylcarbamazine has been shown to be an effective prophylactic treatment (300 mg once a week).

4) Measures directed against the fly larvae are effective but have not proven practical because the moist, muddy breeding areas are usually too extensive.

11. Special considerations—None.

[S. Guagliardo]

LYME DISEASE
(Lyme borreliosis, tickborne meningopolyneuritis)

DISEASE	ICD-10 CODE
LYME DISEASE	ICD-10 A69.2, L90.4

1. Clinical presentation—Clinical manifestations of this tickborne, spirochetal disease can be divided into 3 phases: early localized, early disseminated, and late disease.

The majority (70%–80%) of patients develop early localized disease within the first month of infection with a red macule or papule at the site of the tick bite that expands slowly in an annular manner, often with central clearing. This lesion is called erythema migrans. To be considered significant for case surveillance purposes, the erythema migrans lesion must reach at least 5 cm in diameter. With or without erythema migrans, early nonspecific constitutional symptoms may include malaise, fatigue, fever, headache, myalgia, arthralgias, or lymphadenopathy, all of which might last several weeks in untreated patients.

Early disseminated disease can develop in untreated patients when the spirochete replicates and spreads beyond the local tick attachment site. Manifestations develop within weeks to months of infection. Multiple erythema migrans lesions may appear. Neurologic manifestations of early disseminated disease include cranial nerve palsies (usually facial; can be bilateral), lymphocytic meningitis, peripheral neuropathy, myelitis, or encephalitis. Cardiac manifestations include atrioventricular block and, rarely, acute myopericarditis or cardiomyopathy.

Late Lyme disease typically manifests months to years after infection in untreated patients. The most common manifestation of late Lyme disease is Lyme arthritis. Patients develop intermittent episodes of swelling and pain in large joints (especially the knees); this may recur for several years. In Europe, cutaneous findings have been described, including acrodermatitis chronica atrophicans. In 1 published case series from Europe, which included patients of all infection stages, 89% had erythema migrans alone, 5% presented with arthritis, 3% with early neurologic manifestations, 2% with lymphocytoma, 1% with acrodermatitis chronica atrophicans, and fewer than 1% with cardiac manifestations. Similar observations on clinical presentation have been reported in the USA.

2. Risk groups—All people are likely susceptible; however, only people exposed to infected ticks can develop Lyme disease. Reinfection can occur.

3. Causative agents—Two spirochetes have been shown to cause Lyme disease in North America. Most cases in North America are caused by *Borrelia burgdorferi* sensu stricto, which was identified in 1982. Recently, the spirochete *Borrelia mayonii* was discovered to cause Lyme disease in a small number of patients in the upper Midwest. The spirochetes associated with most Lyme disease in Europe or Asia are *Borrelia afzelii*, *B. burgdorferi* sensu stricto, and *Borrelia garinii*.

In the USA, people are infected through the bite of the black-legged tick. *Ixodes scapularis* is the primary vector of *Borrelia* spp. that causes Lyme disease in the USA. The tick *Ixodes pacificus* is a competent vector of *Borrelia* spp. that causes sporadic cases of Lyme disease in the western coastal USA.

4. Diagnosis—In a region where Lyme disease is highly endemic, diagnosis of early localized Lyme disease can be made in patients presenting with an erythema migrans rash with or without the knowledge of a tick bite. In later stages of illness, however, diagnosis should be supported by 2-step serologic testing. The first test is typically an enzyme immunoassay (EIA) or, rarely, an indirect immunofluorescence assay (IFA). If this first test is negative, the patient is considered seronegative and no further testing should be done. If the first test is equivocal or positive, it should be followed by a second step test that is FDA-cleared. This second step might be another EIA or a Western immunoblot for Lyme disease immunoglobulin class M (IgM) or immunoglobulin class G (IgG). Positive immunoblot tests require the presence of at least 5 IgG bands or 2 IgM bands (https://www.cdc.gov/lyme/diagnosistesting/labtest/twostep/westernblot/index.html). The IgM results on the Western immunoblot should only be considered for diagnosis if symptom onset is in the prior month; beyond that time period, the IgM results should not be considered owing to relatively high false-positivity outside the acute disease period.

Serologic tests in the early stages of illness should be interpreted with caution as they can be insensitive during the first weeks of infection and may remain negative in people treated very early with antibiotics.

In general, serologic sensitivity increases in patients who have progressed to later stages of illness. Lyme disease serologic tests can cross-react with antibodies from other pathogens. As a result, Lyme disease serologic tests may be falsely positive in patients with other diseases, which include syphilis, herpes simplex, relapsing fever, leptospirosis, Rocky Mountain spotted fever, infectious mononucleosis, lupus, and rheumatoid arthritis. Conversely, antibody levels to Lyme disease can remain elevated for years, and positive serologic tests do not necessarily imply active infection.

5. Occurrence—USA; Canada; northwestern, central, and eastern Europe; and forested areas of Asia. In the USA, the vast majority of Lyme disease cases are acquired in the northeastern and upper midwestern regions of the country, where the disease is considered to be enzootic in ticks and small rodent reservoir hosts. In Canada, the areas of risk include southern parts of Manitoba, Ontario, and Quebec; some parts of New Brunswick and Nova Scotia; and southern British Columbia. In Europe, Lyme disease risk extends from Portugal and the British Isles east to Turkey and north into Scandinavia and Russia. In Asia, disease distribution reaches across Eurasia, extending from Japan to the western part of Russia. Disease more frequently occurs when nymphal ticks are most active in late spring or in the summer, peaking in June and July, but may occur throughout the year, depending on the seasonal abundance of local tick vectors and ground temperatures. Dogs, cattle, and horses develop systemic disease that may include the articular and cardiac manifestations seen in human patients. The explosive repopulation of the eastern USA by white-tailed deer, on which adult black-legged ticks feed, has been linked to the spread of Lyme disease in this region.

6. Reservoirs—The disease is maintained in an enzootic transmission cycle that involves *Ixodes* ticks and wild rodents. A broad range of small rodents, and possibly birds, may serve as reservoir hosts. Of particular importance, however, are *Peromyscus* spp. in northeastern and midwestern USA and *Neotoma* spp. and gray squirrels in western USA. *Ixodes* ticks become infected as larvae or nymphs when they feed on an infected reservoir host; they remain infected for life. Deer serve as important mammalian maintenance hosts for vector tick species but are refractory to infection with Lyme *Borrelia*. Larval and nymphal ticks feed on small mammals and adult ticks feed primarily on deer. The majority of human Lyme disease cases result from bites by infected nymphs.

7. Incubation period—For erythema migrans, 3 to 30 days after tick bite (mean, 7 days). Early stages of the illness may be unapparent and the patient may present later with manifestations of disseminated disease.

8. Transmission—Tickborne; transmission by *I. scapularis* and *I. pacificus* usually does not occur until the tick has been attached for 36 hours or longer. It is possible that *Borrelia* might be transmitted through blood transfusion. Although no such cases have been reported, patients undergoing treatment for Lyme disease should refrain from donating blood. Person-to-person transmission has not been shown. Untreated Lyme disease during pregnancy may lead to infection of the placenta and possible stillbirth. No serious fetal effects have been found in cases where the mother received appropriate antibiotic treatment. Immediate treatment of Lyme disease in pregnant women is recommended to avoid adverse maternal and fetal outcomes.

9. Treatment—

Erythema Migrans: Single or Multiple

Preferred therapy	Adults: • Doxycycline 100 mg PO BID for 10 days OR • Amoxicillin 500 mg PO TID for 14 days OR • Cefuroxime axetil 500 mg PO BID for 14 days
	Children: • Doxycycline 4.4 mg/kg/day PO divided into 2 doses (≤ 100 mg/dose) for 10 days OR • Amoxicillin 50 mg/kg/day PO divided into 3 doses (≤ 500 mg/dose) for 14 days OR • Cefuroxime axetil 30 mg/kg/day PO divided into 2 doses (≤ 500 mg/dose) for 14 days
Alternative therapy options	Adults[a]: • Azithromycin 500 mg PO once daily for 7–10 days
	Children[a]: • Azithromycin 10 mg/kg/day PO for 7–10 days
Special considerations and comments	• For early localized Lyme disease, PO doxycycline, amoxicillin, and cefuroxime have been shown to have equivalent efficacy. • Recent studies have shown that for erythema migrans shorter courses of doxycycline (10 days) have equal treatment efficacy to longer treatment courses. • The added benefit of doxycycline is that it is also effective treatment for anaplasmosis, which can co-occur in patients with Lyme disease.

Note: BID = twice daily; PO = oral(ly); TID = thrice daily.
[a]High rates of clinical failure reported with azithromycin and should be considered last line.

Arthritis: Initial Episode

Preferred therapy	Adults: • Doxycycline 100 mg PO BID for 28 days OR • Amoxicillin 500 mg PO TID for 28 days
	Children: • Doxycycline 4.4 mg/kg/day PO divided into 2 doses (≤ 100 mg/dose) for 28 days[a] OR • Amoxicillin 50 mg/kg/day PO divided into 3 doses (≤ 500 mg/dose) for 28 days
Alternative therapy options	Adults: • Cefuroxime axetil 500 mg PO BID for 28 days
	Children: • Cefuroxime axetil 30 mg/kg/day PO divided into 2 doses (≤ 500 mg/dose) for 28 days
Special considerations and comments	May consider adding nonsteroidal anti-inflammatory drugs to help manage symptoms.

Note: BID = twice daily; PO = oral(ly); TID = thrice daily.
[a]There are limited safety data for use of doxycycline for > 21 days in children < 8 years.

Arthritis: Persistent or Recurrent After First Course of Antibiotics

Preferred therapy	Adults: • Ceftriaxone 2 g IV once daily for 14–28 days OR • Doxycycline 100 mg PO BID for 28 days OR • Amoxicillin 500 mg PO TID for 28 days
	Children: • Ceftriaxone 50–75 mg/kg IV once daily (≤ 2 g/day) for 14–28 days OR • Doxycycline 4.4 mg/kg/day PO divided into 2 doses (≤ 100 mg/dose) for 28 days[a] OR • Amoxicillin 50 mg/kg/day PO divided into 3 doses (≤ 500 mg/dose) for 28 days

(Continued)

Arthritis: Persistent or Recurrent After First Course of Antibiotics (Continued)

Alternative therapy options	Adults:
	• Cefuroxime axetil 500 mg PO BID for 28 days
	Children:
	• Cefuroxime axetil 30 mg/kg/day PO divided into 2 doses (≤ 500 mg/dose) for 28 days
Special considerations and comments	• May consider adding nonsteroidal anti-inflammatory drugs to help manage symptoms.
	• For patients with improved but incomplete resolution of symptoms after 1 course of antibiotics, a second course of 28 days of the same oral antibiotic is recommended.
	• For patients without any improvement after 1 course of antibiotics, a course of 2–4 weeks of IV antibiotics is recommended.
	• For patients without improvement after 2 courses of antibiotics, consider a referral to a rheumatologist for consideration of antirheumatic medications.

Note: BID = twice daily; IV = intravenous(ly); PO = oral(ly); TID = thrice daily.
[a]There are limited safety data for use of doxycycline for > 21 days in children < 8 years.

Carditis: Mild (First-Degree Atrioventricular Block With PR Interval < 300 Milliseconds)

Preferred therapy	Adults:
	• Doxycycline 100 mg PO BID for 14–21 days OR
	• Amoxicillin 500 mg PO TID for 14–21 days OR
	• Cefuroxime axetil 500 mg PO BID for 14–21 days
	Children:
	• Doxycycline 4.4 mg/kg/day PO divided into 2 doses (≤ 100 mg/dose) for 14–21 days OR
	• Amoxicillin 50 mg/kg/day PO divided into 3 doses (≤ 500 mg/dose) for 14–21 days OR
	• Cefuroxime axetil 30 mg/kg/day PO divided into 2 doses (≤ 500 mg/dose) for 14–21 days
Alternative therapy options	Not available

Note: BID = twice daily; PO = oral(ly); TID = thrice daily.

Carditis: Severe (Symptomatic First-Degree Atrioventricular Block With PR Interval ≥ 300 Milliseconds or Second- or Third-Degree Atrioventricular Block)

Preferred therapy	Adults:
	• Ceftriaxone 2 g IV once daily for 14–21 days
	Children:
	• Ceftriaxone 50–75 mg/kg IV once daily (≤ 2 g/day) for 14–28 days
Alternative therapy options	Not available
Special considerations and comments	• For early or late disseminated disease with neurologic or more severe cardiac manifestations, IV therapy is usually recommended. For patients unable to tolerate β-lactam antibiotics, PO doxycycline or penicillin desensitization is recommended.
	• Patients with severe carditis should be hospitalized with cardiac telemetry because of the potential for sudden cardiac death.

Note: IV = intravenous(ly); PO = oral(ly).

Neurologic Disease: Isolated Facial Palsy

Preferred therapy	Adults:
	• Doxycycline 100 mg PO BID for 14 days
	Children:
	• Doxycycline 4.4 mg/kg/day PO divided into 2 doses (≤ 100 mg/dose) for 14 days
Alternative therapy options	Adults:
	• Amoxicillin 500 mg PO TID for 14 days
	Children:
	• Amoxicillin 50 mg/kg/day PO divided into 3 doses (≤ 500 mg/dose) for 28 days
Special considerations and comments	Not applicable

Note: BID = twice daily; CSF = cerebrospinal fluid; PO = oral(ly); TID = thrice daily.

Neurologic Disease: Complicated Disease (e.g., Meningitis, Encephalitis)

Preferred therapy	Adults:
	• Doxycycline 100 mg PO BID for 14 days OR • Ceftriaxone 2 g IV once daily for 14 days
	Children:
	• Doxycycline 4.4 mg/kg/day PO divided into 2 doses ($\leq$ 100 mg/dose) for 14 days OR • Ceftriaxone 50–75 mg/kg IV once daily ($\leq$ 2 g/day) for 14 days
Alternative therapy options	Not available
Special considerations and comments	Not applicable

Note: BID = twice daily; IV = intravenous(ly); PO = oral(ly).

All Types of Lyme Disease

Special considerations and comments	• There are limited safety data on the use of doxycycline for > 21 days in children < 8 years. The 2018 *Red Book* now recommends that doxycycline can be safely used for $\leq$ 21 days in patients of all ages.[1]
	• The majority of patients with early Lyme disease who receive appropriate therapy have complete resolution of illness. Some patients have symptoms, including fatigue, arthralgia, and headache, that persist after treatment. Studies have shown that these symptoms are not due to ongoing *Borrelia* infection and additional antibiotics are not indicated. These symptoms usually spontaneously resolve within months without additional antibiotics.

10. Prevention—

1) Avoid tick-infested areas (wooded areas or areas with high grass or leaf litter) when feasible. Apply EPA-registered insect repellents such as DEET and apply 0.5% permethrin to clothing and gear prior to exposure to tick habitat.

2) If working or playing in an infested area, shower soon after being outdoors. Check for ticks daily, examining the total body area. Do not neglect hairy areas. Remove ticks promptly; these may be very small, especially nymphs. Remove ticks by using gentle, steady traction with forceps (tweezers) applied close to the skin so as to avoid leaving mouth parts in the skin. Protect hands with gloves, cloth, or tissue when removing ticks. Following removal, clean the attachment site with soap and water.

3) Measures designed to reduce tick populations on residential properties (host management, habitat modification, chemical control) are usually impractical on a large scale.

4) No vaccine is currently available in the USA. The vaccine LYMErix was licensed in 1998 but was withdrawn from market in 2002 owing to limited market value.

5) Postexposure prophylaxis: following a high-risk bite by *I. scapularis*, a single prophylactic dose of doxycycline (200 mg for adults or 4.4 mg/kg for children weighing < 45 kg) might be indicated if it can be given within 72 hours of tick removal. A high-risk tick bite is defined as an engorged tick that has fed for ≥ 36 hours in an area of high Lyme disease endemicity. Testing of the tick for spirochete infection has a poor predictive value and is not recommended.

11. Special considerations—

1) Reporting: case report obligatory in some countries. In the USA, states are encouraged to report cases to CDC for surveillance purposes.

2) Epidemic measures: in hyperendemic and infested areas, identify tick species involved, if possible. See Prevention in this chapter.

References

1. *Red Book: 2018–2021 Report of the Committee on Infectious Diseases*. 31st ed. Itasca, IL: American Academy of Pediatrics; 2018:905–906.

[G. Marx]

LYMPHOCYTIC CHORIOMENINGITIS
(LCM, benign [or serous] lymphocytic meningitis)

DISEASE	ICD-10 CODE
LYMPHOCYTIC CHORIOMENINGITIS	ICD-10 A87.2

1. Clinical features—Lymphocytic choriomeningitis virus (LCMV) is a viral infection of rodents, including mice, rats, and hamsters, transmissible to humans, in whom it produces diverse clinical manifestations. There is often a biphasic illness initially with influenza-like symptoms, fever, myalgia, retro-orbital headache, anorexia, nausea, and vomiting. In some cases, the illness begins with meningeal or meningoencephalomyelitic symptoms or these symptoms may appear after a brief remission. Orchitis, parotitis, arthritis, myocarditis, and rash occur occasionally. The acute course is usually short, very rarely fatal, and even with severe manifestations (e.g., coma with meningoencephalitis) prognosis for recovery without sequelae is usually good, although convalescence with fatigue and vasomotor instability may be prolonged. Laboratory findings may include leukopenia, thrombocytopenia, and mildly elevated liver enzymes. The cerebrospinal fluid (CSF) in cases with neurologic involvement typically shows a lymphocytic pleocytosis and CSF white blood cell (WBC) counts of greater than 1,000 WBC/μL may be seen. Low CSF glucose is seen in 20% to 30% of cases and mild elevation of CSF protein may be present. The primary pathologic finding in the rare human fatality is diffuse meningoencephalitis. Fatal cases of hemorrhagic fever-like disease have been reported in immunosuppressed patients after organ transplantation from an infected donor. Transplacental infection of the fetus occurs, leading to hydrocephalus, chorioretinitis, micro- or macrocephaly, intracranial calcifications, and nonimmune hydrops; testing for LCMV should be considered when such findings are present.

2. Risk groups—Individuals of all ages who come into contact with urine, feces, saliva, or blood of the house mouse are potentially at risk for infection. Laboratory workers who work with the virus or handle infected animals are at risk as well as personnel working in breeding colonies of mice or hamsters for laboratory or pet production. Owners of pet mice or hamsters may be at risk for infection if these animals originate from colonies that have become contaminated with LCMV or if the animals become infected from other wild mice or hamsters. Immunocompromised transplant recipients are at risk for acquiring LCMV through an infected donor; human fetuses are at risk for vertical transmission.

3. Causative agents—LCMV is an enveloped ambisense ribonucleic acid (RNA) virus in the genus *Arenavirus*, family Arenaviridae. Among viruses in the *Arenavirus* genus, LCMV is the prototype of the Old World arenaviruses, which include Lassa and Lujo viruses.

4. Diagnosis—Laboratory methods include detection of virus RNA by conventional or real-time polymerase chain reaction or isolation of the virus by inoculation of cell cultures with CSF collected early in the course of illness. Specific immunoglobulin class M (IgM) in serum or CSF, as evidenced by IgM capture enzyme-linked immunosorbent assay, or rising antibody titers by immunofluorescence assay in paired sera are considered diagnostic. Lymphocytic choriomeningitis requires differentiation from other aseptic meningitides and viral encephalitides in young adults and differentiation from other congenital infections that cause central nervous system damage and chorioretinitis (e.g., toxoplasmosis, Zika virus, herpes simplex virus, cytomegalovirus).

5. Occurrence—Underdiagnosed and not uncommon in Europe and the Americas; antibody prevalence of 5% to 10% has been reported among adults from the USA, Argentina, and endemic areas of Germany. Loci of infection among feral mice often persist over long periods and cause sporadic clinical disease. Outbreaks have occurred from exposure to infected laboratory animals and infected breeding colonies of mice and hamsters for the pet industry. Infection acquired from wild rodents peaks during winter, when rodents seek food and shelter in human dwellings.

6. Reservoirs—The house mouse *Mus musculus* is the natural reservoir. Infected females transmit infection to their offspring, which become asymptomatic persistent viral shedders. In laboratories, infection may be present in some mouse and hamster colonies and LCMV has been known to contaminate transplantable tumor lines.

7. Incubation period—Thought to be 8 to 21 days.

8. Transmission—LCMV is excreted in urine, saliva, feces, milk, and semen of infected animals. Transmission to humans is usually from mice and probably through oral or respiratory contact with excreta, food, or dust or through contamination of skin lesions or cuts. Handling articles contaminated by infected mice may place individuals at a high risk of infection. Person-to-person transmission between immunocompetent individuals has not been demonstrated and is unlikely. Vertical transmission is associated with maternal viremia and is usually transplacental; it may occur during intrapartum exposure to maternal blood or vaginal secretions. Transmission to immunosuppressed transplant recipients may occur through an infected donor or via subsequent environmental exposure. Several clusters of transmission through organ transplants have been described with severe, often fatal, clinical outcomes in immunosuppressed recipients. Recovery from the disease probably results in long-term immunity.

9. Treatment—There is no specific antiviral therapy for LCMV. Most immunocompetent older children and adults recover fully with supportive care. Hydrocephalus may warrant CSF shunting. Neonates with congenital infection experience varying degrees of neurologic dysfunction and often require treatment for developmental delay, seizures, spastic quadriparesis, vision abnormalities, and ataxia.

10. Prevention—Keep home and work environments clean. Eliminate wild mice and understand that rodent pets, such as hamsters and mice, could be infected. Wash hands after handling or changing animal bedding and food. Keep foods in closed containers. Pathogen monitoring of commercial rodent-breeding establishments, especially those producing hamsters and mice, is helpful. Colony managers should take measures to ensure that laboratory mice do not come into contact with wild mice and that, within animal facilities, personnel handling mice follow strict biosecurity procedures to prevent transmission from infected animals. Pregnant women and immunosuppressed individuals should avoid rodent exposure.

11. Special considerations—Reporting to local health authority may be required in some areas.

Bibliography

Barton LL, Mets MB. Congenital lymphocytic choriomeningitis virus infection: decade of rediscovery. *Clin Infect Dis*. 2001;33(3):370–374.

Bonthius DJ. Lymphocytic choriomeningitis virus: an under-recognized cause of neurologic disease in the fetus, child, and adult. *Semin Pediatr Neurol*. 2012;19(3):89–95.

Bonthius DJ, Perlman S. Congenital viral infections of the brain: lessons learned from lymphocytic choriomeningitis virus in the neonatal rat. *PLoS Pathog*. 2007;3(11):e149.

Tanveer F, Younas M, Fishbain J. Lymphocytic choriomeningitis virus meningoencephalitis in a renal transplant recipient following exposure to mice. *Transpl Infect Dis*. 2018;20(6):e13013.

[E. Muth, S. Eppes]

LYMPHOGRANULOMA VENEREUM
(lymphogranuloma inguinale, climatic or tropical bubo, LGV)

DISEASE	ICD-10 CODE
LYMPHOGRANULOMA VENEREUM	ICD-10 A55

1. Clinical features—A sexually acquired bacterial infection that, in its classic form, consists of 3 stages. The first stage is characterized by a small, painless, self-limited papule or ulcer at the site of inoculation (e.g., on the penis or within the urethra in men or on the vulva, vaginal wall, or cervix in women), which has often resolved by the time the patient seeks care. The second stage involves extension to the regional lymph nodes draining the area of the primary lesion, where suppuration may occur, typically unilaterally. In men, inguinal and/or femoral buboes (inflamed or purulent lymph nodes) are seen that may become adherent to the skin, fluctuate, and result in sinus formation. In women, these external nodes are less frequently affected and involvement is mainly of the pelvic nodes with extension to the rectum and rectovaginal septum. This stage can be associated with fever and other systemic symptoms. If untreated, some patients progress to a chronic inflammatory stage that can be prolonged and debilitating, with fibrosis and lymphatic obstruction that can lead to formation of colorectal strictures, fistulas, lymphedema, and genital elephantiasis.

Rectal exposure in women or men who have sex with men (MSM) can result in proctocolitis, with mucoid and/or hemorrhagic rectal discharge, anal pain, constipation, fever, and/or tenesmus. Outbreaks of lymphogranuloma venereum (LGV) proctocolitis have been reported among MSM. This syndrome may be difficult to distinguish clinically or histologically from other conditions such as inflammatory bowel disease, colorectal cancer, and lymphoma; if untreated, it can lead to chronic colorectal fistulas and strictures. Rectal LGV can also be asymptomatic.

2. Risk groups—In tropical or subtropical climates: sexually active persons. In temperate climates: MSM, especially those who are infected with human immunodeficiency virus (HIV) and have had unprotected receptive anal intercourse.

3. Causative agents—The invasive *Chlamydia trachomatis* serovars L-1, L-2, and L-3. These are related to, but distinct from, those chlamydial serovars that cause ocular (trachoma) and non-LGV genital infections.

4. Diagnosis—Diagnosis is based on clinical suspicion, epidemiologic information, and the exclusion of other possible etiologies. Direct detection of chlamydial organisms in swabs from lesions or bubo aspirates by direct immunofluorescence, nucleic acid detection, or culture is suggestive of LGV since non-LGV chlamydial infections rarely result in lesion formation or lymphadenopathy. Extragenital nucleic acid amplification testing for *C. trachomatis* was cleared by FDA on May 23, 2019 and is the preferred chlamydia test for patients presenting with proctocolitis. Most tests are not specific for LGV and positive specimens may need additional testing to differentiate LGV from non-LGV chlamydial infections. LGV-specific tests include serotyping, genotyping, and LGV-specific polymerase chain reaction. These tests are not widely available and results are usually not reported in time to influence diagnosis and treatment. Serologic tests, such as complement fixation (CF) and microimmunofluorescence (MIF), can be used in conjunction with clinical presentation to support the diagnosis (CF single titer of >1:64 and MIF single titer of >1:256). However, these tests have not been validated for proctitis presentation and *C. trachomatis* serovar-specific serologic tests are not widely available.

5. Occurrence—LGV occurs worldwide, especially in tropical and subtropical areas. It is endemic in parts of Africa, India, Southeast Asia, Latin America, and the Caribbean. Acute LGV is reported much more frequently in men than in women, whereas late complications, such as hypertrophy of the genitalia and rectal strictures, are reported more frequently in women. Since 2003, LGV infection has been increasingly reported in developed countries, predominantly presenting as proctitis among MSM with HIV infection.

6. Reservoirs—Humans.

7. Incubation period—Variable, with a range of 3 to 30 days for a primary lesion. If a bubo is the first manifestation, incubation ranges from 10 to 30 days to several months.

8. Transmission—Transmitted through anal, vaginal, or oral sex. Neonatal infection can be acquired during passage through an infected birth canal. The period of communicability is variable, from weeks to years.

9. Treatment—Patients with a clinical syndrome consistent with LGV— proctocolitis or genital ulcer disease with lymphadenopathy—should be presumptively treated for LGV.

Preferred therapy	Doxycycline 100 mg PO BID for 21 days
Alternative therapy options	Erythromycin base 500 mg PO QID for 21 days
Special considerations and comments	• Patients should continue to be followed until all signs and symptoms have resolved. • Pregnant and lactating women should be treated with erythromycin. • Azithromycin 1 g PO once weekly for 3 weeks may be effective but clinical data are lacking. • Although optimal duration of treatment has not been evaluated, fluoroquinolone-based treatments might also be effective.

Note: BID = twice daily; PO = oral(ly); QID = 4 times a day.

1) Buboes may require incision and drainage to prevent the formation of inguinal/femoral ulcerations.
2) Partner management: the patient's sexual contacts within 60 days before onset of symptoms should be examined, tested based on anatomic site of exposure, and presumptively treated for *C. trachomatis* (with either azithromycin 1 g orally in a single dose or doxycycline 100 mg orally twice a day for 7 days).

10. Prevention—When used correctly and consistently, condoms prevent the spread of sexual infections transmitted through bodily fluids, such as *C. trachomatis*.

11. Special considerations—

1) Reporting: in the USA, LGV reporting laws vary by state. Few other countries require official notification of LGV cases.
2) Persons who are diagnosed with LGV should be tested for other sexually transmitted diseases, especially HIV and syphilis.
3) Patients should be followed clinically until symptoms have resolved.
4) Persons with HIV infection should receive the same treatment regimen as HIV-negative patients. Prolonged resolution of symptoms and therapy may occur.
5) International measures: see "Syphilis." Further information can be found at:

• http://www.cdc.gov/std/treatment
• http://www.who.int/topics/sexually_transmitted_infections/en

[B. Furness]

❖

MALARIA

DISEASE	ICD-10 CODE
MALARIA	ICD-10 B50–B54

1. Clinical features—Malaria is an acute febrile illness that can present with a wide range of nonspecific signs and symptoms. A person with malaria may initially experience headache, tiredness, abdominal discomfort, and muscle and joint pains, followed by fever paroxysms, anorexia, and vomiting. In young children malaria can present with or without fever, poor feeding, and cough. The progression from uncomplicated malaria to severe malaria is unpredictable and can occur within hours of presentation, highlighting the need for immediate appropriate treatment once malaria is diagnosed. Severe malaria can present with fever and neurologic manifestations, primarily coma, severe anemia, hypoglycemia, renal failure, and pulmonary edema. The mortality from untreated severe malaria approaches 100%.

2. Risk groups—See Special Considerations in this chapter.

3. Causative agents—Malaria is caused by infection with 1 or more of the *Plasmodium* spp. that infect humans: *Plasmodium falciparum*, *Plasmodium vivax*, *Plasmodium ovale* (*Plasmodium ovale curtisi* and *Plasmodium ovale wallikeri*), *Plasmodium malariae*, and *Plasmodium knowlesi*. *P. knowlesi is* transmitted from monkeys to humans when monkeys come into contact with humans in the forested regions of Southeast Asia.

4. Diagnosis—Because of the nonspecific presentation of malaria a clinical diagnosis is not reliable. Malaria should be included in the differential diagnosis of every febrile patient in a malaria-endemic region or returning from such a region. To avoid overtreatment a clinical suspicion of malaria should be confirmed by a diagnostic test. Malaria may be diagnosed by microscopy or rapid diagnostic tests (RDTs). Both microscopy and RDTs can be completed within minutes but microscopy requires a functioning laboratory for the preparation of the blood film and a skilled microscopist to read the slide. *P. falciparum* histidine-rich protein 2 (PfHRP2)–based RDTs are affordable, easy to use, and widely employed. But PfHRP2-based RDTs can remain positive for days after the infection has been cleared by antimalarials. PfHRP2-based RDTs produce false-negative results during infection with *P. falciparum* strains with PfHRP2 deletions, an emerging phenomenon. *P. vivax* infections can be diagnosed with RDTs based on *P. vivax* lactate dehydrogenase (LDH) or pan-malarial antigens (pan-pLDH or aldolase). Molecular techniques including quantitative polymerase chain reaction (qPCR) are available to detect *Plasmodium* infections but have no role in the management of clinical malaria because the turnaround time is too long and the sensitivity is too high. Ultra low-density *Plasmodium* infections, detectable by qPCR but not by RDT or microscopy, are unlikely to be the cause of a febrile disease; other etiologies for fever should be explored.

5. Occurrence—In 2016 an estimated 216 million cases (range, 196–263 million) and 445,000 deaths occurred globally, mostly (>90%) in young children in Africa. Endemic malaria no longer occurs in most temperate-zone countries nor in many areas of subtropical countries. *P. falciparum* and *P. vivax* are the primary causes of malaria in humans, with vivax malaria having the broadest geographic distribution. High falciparum transmission areas can be found throughout tropical Africa (where vivax malaria is rarer), in the southwestern Pacific, in forested areas of South America (e.g., Brazil, Guyana), in southeastern Asia, and in parts of the Indian subcontinent. Malariae malaria has a similar distribution to falciparum malaria but is uncommon. Ovale malaria occurs at a low frequency mainly in sub-Saharan Africa.

6. Reservoirs—Humans are the only reservoir of human malaria, except for *P. malariae* and *P. knowlesi*, which can also infect apes and monkeys. *P. knowlesi* has been documented as a cause of hundreds of human infections and some fatalities in forest fringe areas in Asia where the natural monkey hosts and mosquito vector of this species occur. Nonhuman primates can become infected by a range of *Plasmodium* spp., some of which are closely related to the human malarias and natural transmission to humans occurs sporadically.

7. Incubation period—Approximately 9 to 14 days for *P. falciparum*, 12 to 18 days for *P. vivax* and *P. ovale*, and 18 to 40 days for *P. malariae*. Some *P. vivax* strains in temperate areas can have extended incubation periods of 6 to 12 months. The incubation periods of infections acquired through blood transfusion depend on the number of parasites infused and are usually short but may range up to 2 months.

8. Transmission—Malaria is transmitted by the bite of an infective female *Anopheles* spp. mosquito. A mosquito feeding on an infected human host becomes infected after ingesting gametocytes, the sexual stage of the parasite. An infected female *Anopheles* mosquito injects *Plasmodium* spp. sporozoites contained in her saliva into the bloodstream of a human host while feeding. Most *Anopheles* spp. in sub-Saharan Africa feed typically indoors at night but some important vectors also bite at dusk or in the early morning. The predominant *Anopheles* spp. in Southeast Asia tends to bite outdoors and during day time, preferentially in forested areas.

Induced malaria refers to infection that is passed directly from one individual to another through contaminated blood or blood products, injection equipment, or organ transplant. Transfusion-related transmission may occur as long as asexual forms remain in the circulating blood (with *P. malariae*, 40 years or longer). Stored blood can remain infective for at least a month. Because there is no liver stage with transfusion-transmitted malaria, vivax or ovale relapses cannot occur following transfusion malaria. Congenital malaria refers to infection passed from mother to infant in utero.

9. Treatment—

1) Uncomplicated falciparum malaria: the global first-line treatment for uncomplicated falciparum malaria is artemisinin combination therapy (ACT). The short-acting artemisinin component of this therapy rapidly clears the bulk of the parasites and the longer acting partner drug mops up remaining parasites, prevents resistance, and provides a period of posttreatment prophylaxis.

Five ACTs are currently recommended:

- Artemether and lumefantrine
- Artesunate and amodiaquine
- Artesunate and mefloquine
- Artesunate and sulfadoxine-pyrimethamine (S/P)
- Dihydroartemisinin and piperaquine

Drug	Artemether + lumefantrine tablets (coformulated): • Pediatric: 20 mg + 120 mg • Adult: 40 mg + 240 mg
Dose	• 5 to < 15 kg: 20 mg + 120 mg • 15 to < 25 kg: 40 mg + 240 mg • 25 to < 35 kg: 60 mg + 360 mg • ≥ 35 kg: 80 mg + 480 mg
Duration	BID for 3 days; first 2 doses 8 hours apart, THEN doses 12 hours apart
Special considerations and comments	• A flavored dispersible tablet is available for young children. • Treatment responses need to be closely monitored in young children, pregnant women, large adults, smokers, and patients on mefloquine, rifampicin, or efavirenz because of potentially reduced exposure to lumefantrine. • To optimize lumefantrine absorption, artemether and lumefantrine should be administered with food or milk.

Note: BID = twice daily.

Drug	Artesunate + amodiaquine tablets (coformulated): • 25 mg + 67.5 mg • 50 mg + 135 mg • 100 mg + 270 mg

(Continued)

(Continued)

Dose	• 4.5 to < 9 kg: 25 mg + 67.5 mg • 9 to < 18 kg: 50 mg + 135 mg • 18 to < 36 kg: 100 mg + 270 mg • ≥ 36 kg: 200 mg + 540 mg
Duration	Once daily for 3 days
Special considerations and comments	• Treatment responses in underweight children need to be closely monitored. • Concomitant use with zidovudine, efavirenz, and cotrimoxazole should be avoided.

Drug	Artesunate + mefloquine tablets (coformulated): • Pediatric: 25 mg + 55 mg • Adult: 100 mg + 220 mg
Dose	• 5 to < 9 kg: 25 mg + 55 mg • 9 to < 18 kg: 50 mg + 110 mg • 18 to < 30 kg: 100 mg + 220 mg • ≥ 30 kg: 200 mg + 440 mg
Duration	Once daily for 3 days
Special considerations and comments	• Mefloquine has been associated with nausea, vomiting, dizziness, dysphoria, and sleep disturbances (nightmares). • Rifampicin reduces the exposure to mefloquine. Treatment responses in patients receiving rifampicin must be closely monitored.

Drug	Artesunate + sulfadoxine-pyrimethamine (not available as coformulated fixed dose combination): • Blister-packed 50 mg artesunate + fixed dose 500 mg sulfadoxine with 25 mg pyrimethamine
Dose	• 5 to < 10 kg: 25 mg + 25 mg/55 mg • 10 to < 25 kg: 50 mg + 50 mg/110 mg • 25 to < 50 kg: 100 mg + 100 mg/220 mg • ≥ 50 kg: 200 mg + 200 mg/440 mg
Duration	• Artesunate once daily for 3 days; sulfadoxine-pyrimethamine as a single dose on day 0
Special considerations and comments	• Low-dose folate supplementation (0.4 mg/day) does not reduce the efficacy of sulfadoxine-pyrimethamine but larger doses do. • The spread of sulfadoxine-pyrimethamine–resistant *Plasmodium falciparum* strains limit the usefulness of the combination.

Drug	Dihydroartemisinin + piperaquine tablets (coformulated):
	• 20 mg + 160 mg
	• 40 mg + 320 mg
Dose	• 5 to < 8 kg: 20 mg + 160 mg
	• 8 to < 11 kg: 30 mg + 240 mg
	• 11 to < 17 kg: 40 mg + 320 mg
	• 17 to < 25 kg: 60 mg + 480 mg
	• 25 to < 36 kg: 80 mg + 640 mg
	• 36 to < 60 kg: 120 mg + 960 mg
	• 60 to < 80 kg: 160 mg + 1,280 mg
	• ≥ 80 kg: 200 mg + 1,600 mg
Duration	Once daily for 3 days
Special considerations and comments	• High-fat meals can lead to accelerated piperaquine absorption, which has been associated with cardiotoxicity and should be avoided.
	• Piperaquine is to be avoided in patients with congenital QT prolongation or patients on medications that tend to prolong the QT interval.

ACTs have limited efficacy against *P. falciparum* gametocytes, the infectious stage in the life cycle of the *Plasmodium*. To minimize the risk of transmission all patients diagnosed with falciparum malaria residing in regions where competent *Anopheles* vectors are endemic should receive a single low-dose primaquine (0.25 mg/kg).

Drug	Primaquine with ACT:
	• Single low-dose (0.25 mg/kg) with ACT
Dose	• 10 to < 25 kg: 3.75 mg
	• 25 to < 50 kg: 7.5 mg
	• 50–100 kg: 15 mg
Duration	As early as possible to prevent transmission of *Plasmodium falciparum*
Special considerations and comments	• Low-dose primaquine is safe in G6PD-deficient individuals.
	• Single low-dose primaquine is not recommended for pregnant women, infants < 6 months, and women breastfeeding infants < 6 months.

Note: ACT = artemisinin combination therapy; G6PD = glucose-6-phosphate dehydrogenase.

2) Non-artemisinin-based drugs for uncomplicated falciparum malaria:

Drug	Atovaquone + proguanil tablets (coformulated):
	• Pediatric: 62.5 mg + 25 mg
	• Adult: 250 mg + 100 mg

(Continued)

(Continued)

Dose	Single dose (0.25 mg/kg) with ACT:
	• 5 to < 9 kg: 125 mg + 50 mg
	• 9 to < 11 kg: 187 mg + 75 mg
	• 11 to < 21 kg: 250 mg + 100 mg
	• 21 to < 31 kg: 500 mg + 200 mg
	• 31 to < 41 kg: 750 mg + 300 mg
	• > 41 kg: 1,000 mg + 400 mg
Duration	Once daily for 3 days
Special considerations and comments	Used for prophylaxis and as second-line treatment of uncomplicated malaria in travelers. Because of the rapid emergence of resistant *Plasmodium falciparum* strains, atovaquone + proguanil is not suitable for public health purposes in endemic countries.

Note: ACT = artemisinin combination therapy.

3) Severe falciparum malaria:

Drug	Artesunate (parenteral)
Dose	< 20 kg: 3.0 mg/kg ≥ 20 kg: 2.4 mg/kg
Duration	3 doses every 12 hours daily (0, 12, 24) until patient can take PO medication for ≤ 7 days, THEN prescribe a full 3-day ACT course.
Special considerations and comments	• All patients with severe malaria, including infants and pregnant and lactating women, should be treated with parenteral artesunate to maximize survival. • If parenteral artesunate not available, use parenteral artemether in preference to quinine.

Note: ACT = artemisinin combination therapy; PO = oral(ly).

4) Uncomplicated non-falciparum malaria (*P. vivax*, *P. ovale*, *P. malariae*, or *P. knowlesi*): if the *Plasmodium* spp. is uncertain treat as the worst-case scenario (i.e., assume a *P. falciparum* infection). In areas with chloroquine-susceptible *P. vivax*, *P. ovale*, *P. malariae*, or *P. knowlesi* infections treat with ACTs or chloroquine. ACTs with piperaquine, mefloquine, or lumefantrine are preferred over the use of S/P as there are pockets of S/P-resistant *P. vivax* strains. When unsure about the susceptibility and in regions with potential chloroquine resistance, treat with ACT. (Women in the first trimester of pregnancy should be treated with chloroquine or quinine and not ACT.) Severe vivax malaria is increasingly recognized as a life-threatening emergency and needs to be treated in the same fashion as severe falciparum malaria.

Drug	Chloroquine
Dose, route	Day 1: 10 mg/kg PO Day 2: 10 mg/kg PO Day 3: 5 mg/kg PO
Duration	For 3 days
Special considerations and comments	Chloroquine has an excellent safety record but its usefulness is steadily shrinking owing to the spread of resistant *Plasmodium vivax* strains.

The appropriate treatment of *P. vivax* and *P. ovale* requires not only the administration of a schizontocidal drug such as an ACT but also the administration of a full course of an 8-aminoquinoline for the elimination of the dormant liver stage parasites (hypnozoites). 8-Aminoquinolines are a class of hypnozoitocidal drugs that include primaquine and tafenoquine. Tafenoquine is a more novel 8-aminoquinoline that received FDA approval in 2018; it is administered as a single 300-mg dose in adults. 8-Aminoquinolines have the potential to trigger hemolysis in glucose-6-phosphate dehydrogenase (G6PD)–deficient individuals. The results of a G6PD test should therefore guide the prescription of primaquine or tafenoquine. (A single low-dose primaquine, administered to kill *P. falciparum* gametocytes, does not cause clinically significant hemolysis.)

Drug	Primaquine tablets: • 7.5 and 15 mg
Dose, route	0.25–0.5 mg/kg PO
Duration	Daily for 14 days
Special considerations and comments	• For G6PD-deficient people (or when G6PD status cannot be ascertained), administer 0.75 mg/kg/week for 8 weeks under medical supervision. • A full course should not be administered to pregnant women, infants < 6 months, women breastfeeding infants < 6 months, or people with G6PD deficiency. • Consider chloroquine prophylaxis for women who are pregnant or breastfeeding until they can be safely treated with primaquine.

Note: G6PD = glucose-6-phosphate dehydrogenase.

5) Resistance: the treatment of malaria is complicated by the emergence and spread of antimalarial resistance against every class of antimalarials widely used. The documentation of resistance to artemisinin in 2007 in western Cambodia was followed by multidrug resistance

within a decade. Multidrug-resistant *P. falciparum* strains have by 2020 not yet spread beyond the Greater Mekong subregion. More than half of uncomplicated falciparum cases in some areas of Cambodia and Vietnam fail on first-line ACTs. Three strategies are successfully employed to cure people with multidrug-resistant falciparum malaria:

- A switch in ACT regimen (e.g., from dihydroartemisinin-piperaquine to artesunate-mefloquine).
- The empirical use of triple therapy (e.g., adding mefloquine to dihydroartemisinin-piperaquine). The safety and efficacy of triple therapies are currently systematically explored in a series of trials in Asia and Africa.
- A switch to a different class of antimalarials.

Residents of non–malaria-endemic high-income countries have access to atovaquone-proguanil, to which multidrug-resistant strains remain susceptible. Because of the rapid emergence of resistant falciparum strains atovaquone-proguanil is not recommended for public health purposes in malaria-endemic regions. Oral quinine remains effective in all endemic populations but requires a 7-day course, which is poorly tolerated and rarely adhered to. For all antimalarials, extending treatment courses and increasing doses have not yielded promising results. Severe falciparum malaria cases suspected to be artesunate-resistant should be treated with combined parenteral artesunate and quinine. Utmost medical attention is required to assure adequate dosing and prevention of adverse events (e.g., hypoglycemia).

10. Prevention—

1) Vector control for malaria prevention has 2 goals: protect individual people against infective mosquito bites and reduce the intensity of transmission at the community level. The most powerful and broadly applied interventions are long-lasting insecticide-treated bed nets (LLINs) and indoor residual spraying with insecticides (IRS), which in a few specific settings and circumstances may be complemented by other methods such as larval control and insect repellents. All people living in malaria-endemic regions should have access to LLINs. IRS involves the application of residual insecticides to the inner surfaces of dwellings, where many anopheline vector species tend to rest after taking a blood meal. IRS has no individual protective effect but can rapidly reduce transmission when used as a community public health intervention by treatment of more than 80% of houses and animal

shelters in the target area. IRS requires a complex logistical effort involving teams of sprayers that move from community to community. IRS may need to be carried out at least twice a year. The choice of insecticide is made in a given area based on insecticide resistance, residual efficacy of the insecticide, the type of surface to be sprayed, safety, and costs. LLINs and IRS are less promising in Southeast Asia where vectors bite during the daytime outdoors. Where vector breeding sites are easy to identify, map, and treat, larval control may be a useful complementary intervention. Examples of larval control include filling and draining breeding sites, increasing the speed of water flow in channels, and chemical and biologic control methods (bacterial larvicides, larvivorous fish) applied to water bodies.

2) Preventive chemotherapy can inhibit liver-stage (preerythrocytic) development of the parasite, known as causal prophylaxis, or kill the blood stages of the parasite, known as suppressive prophylaxis. Causal prophylaxis (atovaquone + proguanil, primaquine) can be stopped as soon as leaving a malaria-endemic area while suppressive prophylaxis should be continued for 4 weeks after leaving an area. Chemoprevention of malaria is recommended for special risk groups in malaria-endemic countries, as follows:

- Intermittent preventive treatment of malaria in pregnancy: monthly S/P is provided to women starting in the second trimester with the aim of providing at least 3 doses during the course of pregnancy. The spread of S/P-resistant *P. falciparum* is a major limitation of the success of this strategy.

- Intermittent preventive treatment in infants: intermittent preventive treatment of infants with S/P at the time of the second and third rounds of diphtheria, tetanus toxoids, and pertussis vaccination. With the spread of S/P-resistant *P. falciparum* and a shift of peak malaria incidence to older children the uptake of this strategy is low.

- Seasonal malaria chemoprevention (S/P): the provision of monthly amodiaquine plus S/P for children younger than 6 years during the transmission season in the sub-Sahel region of Africa during each transmission season. This intervention has proven highly successful and popular. The extension of this intervention to older age groups is under discussion.

3) Antimalarial vaccines: there is still no licensed malaria vaccine in 2018. Many vaccine candidates are in clinical trials. The most advanced vaccine, known as RTS,S/AS01, has received a positive

scientific evaluation from the European Medical Agency, the European regulator, following a large trial in 7 sub-Saharan African countries. Owing to the incomplete and short-lasting protection afforded by this vaccine more evidence for a positive cost-benefit ratio is required before WHO will recommend the licensing and rollout of the vaccine in malaria-endemic countries, an essential step for local regulators and international funders.

4) Personal preventive measures for international travelers: all people who visit an endemic area exposed to mosquito bites are at risk of becoming infected with *Plasmodium*. Depending on the malaria risk in the area visited, the recommended prevention method may be mosquito bite prevention only or mosquito bite prevention in combination with chemoprophylaxis or standby emergency treatment (SBET). The choice of malaria prevention will depend on the destination, season, duration and conditions of travel, and individual factors; prevention should be customized for the individual traveler.

- Use of an insect repellent on exposed skin as well as clothing. Choose a repellent containing *N,N*-diethyl-3-methyl-benzamide, IR3535 (3-[*N*-acetyl-*N*-butyl]-aminopropionic acid ethyl ester), or icaridin (1-piperidinecarboxylic acid, 2-[2-hydroxyethyl]-1-methylpropylester).
- As the malaria vectors are generally most active at night, sleeping under an is recommended. The edges of the insecticide-treated bed net (ITN) should be tucked-in under the mattress; ensure that the net is not torn and that there are no mosquitoes inside it; sleep in the middle of the bed; and avoid contact between body and net.
- Well-constructed, air-conditioned rooms provide protection against mosquito entry. Doors and windows should be screened. The protection afforded by air-conditioning disappears during power outages. Sleeping under an ITN even in air-conditioned hotel rooms can prevent unpleasant surprises.
- Anti-mosquito sprays or insecticide dispensers that contain tablets impregnated with pyrethroids in bedrooms at night (or mosquito coils if there is no electricity) can reduce mosquito densities and reduce the risk of infection. Protective measures should be used in combination, especially when staying in areas where there is intense malaria transmission.

5) Chemoprophylaxis for travelers to malaria-endemic areas: the characteristics of the antimalarial drug have to match the characteristics of the traveler and the parasites in the destination country (species, resistance pattern). CDC recommends in 2018 the consideration of the following drugs for chemoprophylaxis for travelers: atovaquone-proguanil, chloroquine (for *P. vivax* prophylaxis in the few remaining countries with susceptible parasites), doxycycline, mefloquine, and primaquine. Travelers should start prophylaxis well ahead of travel, usually 2 weeks to minimize the risk of new onset adverse events while traveling and to build up therapeutic drug levels. Consultation with an expert in travel medicine can be helpful (see: https://www.cdc.gov/malaria/travelers/drugs.html).

6) SBET: considering the limited number of useful drugs available for chemoprophylaxis, the risk for adverse events, and the cost to buy the drugs, travelers may be well advised to consider SBET instead of chemoprophylaxis. Some travelers may be exposed to a high risk of malaria while being more than 12 hours away from competent medical attention. WHO recommends that prescribers issue antimalarial medicines to be carried for self-administration by persons who may be in such situations. Also, in light of the spread of counterfeit medicines, some travelers may opt to buy antimalarial treatment before departure so that they can be confident of drug quality should they become ill. Persons prescribed SBET must understand that SBET is a temporary measure and medical advice is to be sought as soon as possible for complete evaluation and to exclude other serious causes of fever. If several people travel together, the individual dosages for SBET should be specified. Weight-based dosages for children need to be clearly indicated. The drug options for SBET are in principle the same as for treatment of uncomplicated malaria. Artemether-lumefantrine has been registered in some European countries for use as SBET for travelers.

7) Pregnant women are particularly susceptible to mosquito bites. Extra diligence is needed in using protective measures, including ITN/LLIN and insect repellents, without exceeding the recommended repellent usage. If possible pregnant women should avoid travel in malaria-endemic countries.

8) Falciparum malaria in a young child may be rapidly fatal. Early symptoms may be atypical and difficult to recognize; life-threatening complications can occur within hours of the initial symptoms. In infants, fever may be absent. As young children are at an increased risk for a range of febrile diseases constant alertness and

frequent testing may be required. Babies and young children should not be taken to areas with risk of falciparum malaria. If travel cannot be avoided, children must be very carefully protected with preventive measures.

11. Special considerations—Several populations including young children, pregnant women, and patients on enzyme-inducing drugs have altered pharmacokinetics of antimalarial drugs that can result in under-dosing. Closer monitoring and a lowered threshold for treatment changes can be lifesaving in very young children.

The administration of artemisinin derivatives during the first trimester of pregnancy is not considered safe. Women in the first trimester of pregnancy should be treated with quinine plus clindamycin. Artemisinin derivatives are considered safe and are well tolerated during the second and third trimesters of pregnancy. When lactating women are treated with antimalarial drugs their infants receive a small fraction of the drugs. Tetracyclines and prima-quine are not recommended for lactating women.

Artemisinin derivatives are safe and well tolerated in young children but S/P, tetracyclines, and primaquine should be avoided. Infants with uncom-plicated malaria weighing less than 5 kg can be treated at the same mg/kg dose as for children weighing 5 kg. Young febrile children tend to vomit frequently. If an antimalarial dose is vomited within 60 minutes of ingestion the administration of the drug should be repeated. If there are any doubts that adequate doses can be administered in a timely fashion, the switch to parenteral antimalarials should be immediate.

1) Blood donations: people infected with *Plasmodium* parasites can transmit infections for extended periods via transfusion. While the risk for extended transmission is well recognized for *Plasmodium* parasites that include a hypnozoite stage in their life cycle (*P. vivax*, *P. ovale*) *P. falciparum* infections have been transmitted via blood donations by individuals who have been outside of transmission areas for more than 10 years. The rules and regulations for blood donations with previous exposure to malaria differ across countries.

2) Reporting: in nonendemic areas, malaria cases should be reported to the local health authority. Outbreaks of falciparum malaria in a normally malaria-free country should be reported to WHO immedi-ately. Other international measures may include the following:

- Disinsectization of aircraft before takeoff from malaria-endemic areas using insecticide aerosols.
- Disinsectization of aircraft, ships, and other vehicles on arrival if the health authority at the place of arrival has reason to suspect importation of malaria vectors.

- Enforcing and maintaining rigid anti-mosquito sanitation within the mosquito flight range of all ports and airports.

3) Epidemic measures: malaria epidemics must be controlled through rapid and vigorous action and effective treatment of all cases. In confirmed *P. falciparum* epidemics where a large part of the population is infected, a 2-pronged vector control strategy that includes LLIN and IRS as well as universal access to early diagnosis and treatment is required. In some situations the institution of presumptive antimalarial treatment of a high-risk population may be considered.

Bibliography

World Health Organization. *Guidelines for the Treatment of Malaria*. 3rd ed. 2015. Available at: http://www.who.int/malaria/publications/atoz/9789241549127/en. Accessed March 18, 2019.

[L. von Seidlein]

MEASLES
(rubeola, hard measles, red measles, morbilli)

DISEASE	ICD-10 CODE
MEASLES	ICD-10 B05

1. Clinical features—An acute, highly communicable viral disease with prodromal fever, conjunctivitis, coryza, cough, and small spots with white or bluish white centers on an erythematous base on the buccal mucosa (Koplik spots). A characteristic red blotchy rash appears on the face on the third to seventh day, becomes generalized, lasts 4 to 7 days, and sometimes ends in brawny desquamation. Leukopenia is common and serum vitamin A levels are often decreased. Complications, resulting from direct viral replication or bacterial superinfection, may occur up to 4 weeks after rash and include otitis media, pneumonia, laryngotracheobronchitis (croup), diarrhea, febrile seizures, and encephalitis. In malnourished children measles may be associated with hemorrhagic rash, protein-losing enteropathy, otitis media, oral sores, dehydration, diarrhea, blindness, and severe skin infections. Persons with deficiencies of cell-mediated immunity may lack the characteristic rash and may have a progressive measles inclusion-body encephalitis. Occurring more commonly than previously estimated, subacute sclerosing panencephalitis develops in 1:10,000 cases 5 to 10 years after infection; the risk is greater, up to 1:1,400 to 1:2,500, when measles is in the first 5 years of life. In adults, hepatitis, hypocalcemia, and elevated creatinine phosphokinase levels are also seen.

The case-fatality rate is estimated to be less than 1% in developed countries but can be 3% to 5% in developing countries, reaching 10% to 30% in some localities. Both acute and delayed mortality in infants and children have been documented.

2. Risk groups—All persons who have not had the disease or been successfully immunized are susceptible. Acquired immunity after illness is permanent. Successful immunization usually requires 2 doses of vaccine. Those receiving the first dose before 12 months old without a second dose and those receiving only 1 dose at any time may still be susceptible. Infants born to mothers who have had measles are protected against disease for the first 6 to 9 months or more, depending on maternal measles antibody levels at the time of pregnancy and the rate of antibody degradation. Children born to mothers with vaccine-induced immunity receive less passive antibody and may become susceptible to measles at an earlier age. Persons at higher risk of complications with measles include children younger than 5 years, adults, pregnant women, and persons with clinical or subclinical vitamin A deficiency, malnutrition, or congenital or acquired deficiencies of cellular immunity, including human immunodeficiency virus (HIV) infection and immunosuppressive therapy. Children living in more crowded conditions may also be at higher risk of complications. In children with borderline nutritional status, measles often precipitates acute kwashiorkor and exacerbates vitamin A deficiency, sometimes to the point of blindness.

3. Causative agents—Measles virus, a member of the genus *Morbillivirus* of the family Paramyxoviridae.

4. Diagnosis—The WHO clinical case definition for measles is any person with fever, maculopapular rash, and cough, coryza, or conjunctivitis. Confirmation by laboratory testing or epidemiologic linkage is recommended in all cases. Laboratory confirmation is usually by detecting measles-specific immunoglobulin class M (IgM) antibodies or a significant (> 4-fold) rise in immunoglobulin class G (IgG) antibody concentrations between acute and convalescent sera. Reverse transcription polymerase chain reaction (RT-PCR) is often used to confirm the presence of measles ribonucleic acid in urine, blood, or nasopharyngeal mucus and can provide important genotype information. Less commonly used techniques include identification of viral antigen in nasopharyngeal mucosal swabs by fluorescent antibody techniques or virus isolation in cell culture from blood or nasopharyngeal swabs collected before day 4 of rash or from urine specimens before day 8 of rash. In low-incidence settings IgM serology may give false-positive results, often making correlation with epidemiologic data and culture or RT-PCR results necessary. Other causes of febrile rash illness include rubella, dengue, chikungunya, scarlet fever, toxoplasmosis, roseola infantum, erythema infectiosum, mononucleosis, meningococcemia, Kawasaki syndrome, and other viral exanthems.

5. Occurrence—Prior to widespread immunization, measles was common in childhood, with more than 90% of people infected by age 20 and an estimated 100 million cases and 6 million measles deaths occurring each year. Measles, endemic in large metropolitan communities, attained epidemic proportions about every second or third year. In smaller communities and areas, outbreaks tended to be more widely spaced and somewhat more severe. With longer intervals between outbreaks, as in the Arctic and some islands, measles outbreaks often involved a large proportion of the population, with a high case-fatality rate. In temperate climates, measles occurs primarily in the late winter and early spring. In tropical climates, measles occurs primarily in the dry season in the African Sahel and during the cooler rainy season in equatorial areas.

With effective childhood immunization programs, measles cases in many industrialized countries have dropped by up to 99% and generally occur in young unimmunized children or older children, adolescents, or young adults who received only 1 dose of vaccine or missed measles vaccination altogether as a young child. The countries of the Pan American Health Organization (PAHO) have reached the regional goal of elimination of indigenous measles transmission by providing measles vaccine through routine services to at least 95% of children, a second opportunity for measles immunization for all children at an older age, and careful measles surveillance. The second opportunity is designed to immunize children who escaped routine immunization and those who failed to respond immunologically to the first vaccine. The strategy started with a catch-up campaign targeting all children aged 9 months to 14 years regardless of disease history or previous vaccination status and continued with follow-up campaigns conducted every 3 to 4 years, targeting all children aged 9 months to 4 years. In Canada and the USA, a second dose of measles vaccine is provided through routine immunization services, generally at school entry. Though the last indigenous case in the PAHO countries was in 2002, importations continue to occur and require maintenance of very high population immunity through vaccination. Evidence of this is the outbreak of measles in Venezuela, which started in 2017 and continued throughout 2018, resulting in more than 6,000 confirmed measles cases and 76 measles-related deaths with spread to Brazil, Colombia, and Chile. While measles elimination goals have been established in countries in the other 5 WHO regions, progress has been slow, reflecting the challenge of achieving and maintaining high homogeneous vaccination coverage.

Despite the existence of a safe, effective, and inexpensive measles vaccine for the past 50 years, measles remains an important vaccine-preventable killer of children worldwide. WHO estimates that 109,638 children died of measles in

2017, an 80% decrease from the estimated 545,174 deaths in 2000. While the vast majority of measles deaths occur in countries with weak health systems, measles outbreaks continue to occur even in countries with high vaccination coverage, revealing the presence of groups with limited access to health services, the presence of those who are reluctant to vaccinate their children, or an accumulation of susceptible adolescents and adults.

6. Reservoirs—Humans.

7. Incubation period—From exposure to rash onset averages 14 days with a range of 7 to 21 days. Immunoglobulin (Ig) given for passive protection early in the incubation period may extend the incubation period.

8. Transmission—Airborne by droplet spread or by direct contact with nasal or throat secretions of infected persons; less commonly by articles freshly soiled with nose and throat secretions. Measles is one of the most highly communicable infectious diseases. The period of communicability extends from 4 days before rash onset to 4 days after rash appearance. It is minimal after the second day of rash. The vaccine virus has not been shown to be communicable.

9. Treatment—

Drug	Vitamin A
Dose	<ul><li>Infants < 6 months: 50,000 IU</li><li>Infants 6–11 months: 100,000 IU</li><li>Children ≥ 12 months: 200,000 IU</li></ul>
Route	PO
Alternative drug	Not applicable
Duration	Not applicable
Special considerations and comments	<ul><li>Vitamin A should be provided to all patients with an acute case of measles. According to the age of the child, the initial dose of vitamin A (see Dose) should be given immediately on diagnosis and repeated the next day. If the child has clinical signs of vitamin A deficiency (e.g., Bitot's spots) a third dose should be given 2–4 weeks later. Even in countries where measles is not usually severe, vitamin A should be given to all patients with a severe case of measles.</li><li>Nutritional support is recommended because of the risk of malnutrition due to diarrhea, vomiting, and poor appetite associated with measles. Breastfeeding should be encouraged where appropriate. Oral rehydration salts should be used as needed to prevent dehydration.</li><li>Antibiotics are not generally recommended for treatment of measles unless secondary bacterial complications develop such as pneumonia or otitis media.</li></ul>

Note: IU = international units; PO = oral(ly).

10. Prevention—

1) Public education by health departments and private physicians should encourage 2 doses of measles vaccine for all susceptible infants, children, adolescents, and young adults.

2) Immunization: live attenuated measles vaccine is the vaccine of choice. All persons not immune to measles should receive 2 doses of vaccine unless specifically contraindicated (see later). Live measles vaccine, often combined with other live vaccines (mumps, rubella, varicella), can be administered concurrently with other inactivated vaccines or toxoids. Maternal antibody interferes with response to the vaccine in the infant. Vaccination at 12 to 15 months induces immunity in 94% to 98% of recipients and reimmunization increases immunity levels to 99%.

   About 5% to 15% of nonimmune vaccinees may develop malaise and fever to 39.5°C (103°F) within 5 to 12 days after immunization; this reaction lasts 1 to 2 days, with little disability. Rash, coryza, mild cough, and Koplik spots may occasionally occur. Febrile seizures occur infrequently and without sequelae; the highest incidence is in children with a history of previous febrile seizures or seizures in parents or siblings. Encephalitis and encephalopathy occur in fewer than 1 case per million measles immunizations; since this rate is lower than the background rate, it is therefore possible that measles vaccine–associated encephalitis and encephalopathy events may not have been caused by the vaccine. Adverse events after administration of combined vaccines may also involve events associated with the other vaccines (mumps, rubella, varicella).

   WHO recommends that all countries vaccinate children with 2 doses of measles vaccine. In countries with ongoing transmission in which the risk of measles mortality among infants remains high, the first dose should be administered at age 9 months and the routine second dose should be given at age 15 to 18 months with an interval between the first and second dose of at least 1 month. In countries with low rates of measles transmission (i.e., those that are near elimination) and a low risk of measles infection among infants, the first dose may be administered at age 12 months. The optimal age for delivering the routine second dose is based on programmatic considerations that achieve the highest coverage with the second dose and, hence, the highest population immunity. Administration of the second dose at age 15 to 18 months ensures early protection of the individual, slows accumulation of susceptible young children, and may correspond with other routine immunizations (e.g., a diphtheria/tetanus and pertussis vaccine booster). If first dose coverage is high (> 90%) and school enrolment is high (> 95%), administration of the second dose at school entry may prove an effective strategy for achieving high coverage and preventing outbreaks in schools.

In countries where health systems are moderately or weakly functioning, conducting regular measles campaigns is a highly effective strategy for providing a second dose and protecting children who do not have access to routine health services. Because the risk of measles outbreaks is determined by the rate of accumulation of susceptible people in the population, data on vaccination coverage should be used to monitor the accumulation of susceptible people and follow-up campaigns should be conducted before the number of susceptible children of preschool age reaches the size of a birth cohort. During community outbreaks, the recommended age for immunization with measles vaccine can be lowered to 6 months. Children vaccinated in these situations should still receive 2 additional doses when aged 9 months and older according to the routine schedule.

3) Vaccine shipment and storage: immunization may not produce protection if the vaccine has been improperly handled or stored. Prior to reconstitution, freeze-dried measles vaccine is relatively stable and can be safely stored for more than a year in a freezer or at 2°C to 8°C (35.6°F-46.4°F). Reconstituted vaccine must be kept at 2°C to 8°C and discarded after 8 hours; both freeze-dried and reconstituted vaccine must be protected from prolonged exposure to ultraviolet light, which may inactivate the virus.

4) Malnutrition: malnourished children are at higher risk of complications and should be a priority group for measles vaccination. Seroconversion rates after vaccination have been found in several studies to be similar in well-nourished and malnourished children.

5) Revaccinations: in many industrialized countries, measles revaccination is offered at entry to high school and to universities or other institutions and to international travelers and health care workers, unless they have a documented history of measles disease or immunization with 2 doses of vaccine or serologic evidence of measles immunity. In those who have received only inactivated vaccine (available in the late 1960s), revaccination may produce reactions such as local edema and induration, lymphadenopathy, and fever but will protect against the atypical measles syndrome that has been associated with the use of inactivated measles vaccine. Children with HIV on stable highly active antiretroviral therapy (HAART) should be revaccinated after achieving adequate immune reconstitution (i.e., when the cluster of differentiation [CD4+] T-lymphocyte count reaches 20%-25%).

When CD4+ T-lymphocyte monitoring is not available, children should receive an additional dose of measles vaccine 6 to 12 months after initiation of HAART.

6) Contraindications to the use of live virus vaccines:

- Patients with primary immune deficiency diseases affecting T-cell function or acquired immune deficiency due to leukemia, lymphoma, or generalized malignancy or those undergoing therapy with corticosteroids, irradiation, alkylating drugs, or antimetabolites should not receive live virus vaccines. Infection with HIV is not an absolute contraindication: unless severely immunocompromised, WHO recommends measles immunization of HIV-infected infants at 6 months old, followed by an additional dose at 9 months, followed by a another additional dose after at least a 1-month interval. Many industrialized countries recommend measles vaccination only in asymptomatic HIV-positive individuals.

- Low CD4+ counts are a contraindication to measles vaccine because of the risk of viral pneumonia.

- In persons with severe acute illness with or without fever, immunization should be deferred until recovery from the acute phase; minor febrile illnesses such as diarrhea or upper respiratory tract infections are not a contraindication.

- Persons with anaphylactic hypersensitivity to a previous dose of measles vaccine, gelatin, or neomycin should not receive measles vaccine. Egg allergy, even if anaphylactic, is no longer considered a contraindication.

- Purely on theoretical grounds, vaccine should not be given to pregnant women; mothers should be advised of the theoretical risk of fetal damage if they become pregnant within 1 month after receipt of measles-containing vaccine.

- Vaccine should be given at least 14 days before Ig or blood transfusion. Ig can interfere with the response to measles vaccine for varying periods depending on the dose. The usual dose administered for hepatitis A prevention can interfere for 3 months; very large doses of intravenous Ig can interfere for up to 11 months. Other Ig-containing blood products can also interfere.

11. Special considerations—

1) Reporting: obligatory case report in most countries. Early reporting (≤ 24 hours) provides opportunity for better outbreak control.

2) Epidemic measures:

- All potential outbreaks should be rapidly investigated and confirmed with an assessment of the risk of spread and mortality.
- Prompt reporting (≤ 24 hours) of suspected cases and comprehensive programs to immunize all susceptibles are needed to limit spread.
- All children 9 to 59 months old presenting to any health facility who lack prior vaccination should be vaccinated against measles.
- If measles attack rates are high in children younger than 9 months, consideration should be given to temporarily recommending that children be vaccinated beginning at 6 months old. Children vaccinated when younger than 9 months should be revaccinated when 9 months or older according to the routine immunization schedule.
- In day care, school, and university or other institutional outbreaks, all persons without documentation of 2 doses of live virus vaccine at least 1 month apart on or after the first birthday should be immunized unless they have documentation of prior physician-diagnosed measles or laboratory evidence of immunity. In other institutional outbreaks (e.g., military barracks, hospitals), new admissions should receive vaccine or Ig.
- If the risk assessment indicates a high risk of a large outbreak, then a nonselective vaccination campaign should be considered. The campaign target population should be based on the susceptibility profile of the population, as determined by the age distribution of cases, and target areas should include outbreak-affected and adjacent areas where the risk assessment shows a high risk of spread.
- Effective communication to the public and to government authorities is critical to the success of outbreak response efforts.

3) Disaster/conflict implications: introduction of measles into refugee populations with a high proportion of susceptibles can result in devastating epidemics with high fatality rates. Providing measles vaccine to displaced persons living in camp settings within a week of entry is a public health priority.

4) Persons traveling to measles-endemic areas should ensure that they are immune to measles, ideally through receipt of 2 doses of measles vaccine given at least 1 month apart.

[P. Strebel]

❖

MELIOIDOSIS
(Whitmore disease)

DISEASE	ICD-10 CODE
MELIOIDOSIS	ICD-10 A24.1–A24.4
GLANDERS	ICD-10 A24.0

1. Clinical features—Clinical manifestations range from subclinical infection to localized acute or chronic cutaneous or visceral abscesses, necrotizing pneumonia, and/or a rapidly fatal septicemia. Community-acquired pneumonia, often severe, is the most common acute presentation for melioidosis. Chronic melioidosis may simulate typhoid fever or tuberculosis, with pulmonary cavitation, empyema, chronic abscesses, and osteomyelitis. Overwhelming infection can occur, resulting in death from septic shock within 48 hours of generalized symptoms. Infection can become persistent and result in latent, recurrent, and recrudescing infections. A specific syndrome of meningoencephalitis with flaccid paraparesis or peripheral motor weakness occurs in 5% of cases in northern Australia. Cerebral abscess is occasionally reported. Mortality ranges from 15% to 40% despite use of appropriate antimicrobial therapy.

In humans, signs and symptoms of glanders—a highly communicable disease of horses, mules, and donkeys—are similar to those of melioidosis. Human glanders is associated with contact with sick animals, contaminated fomites, tissues, or bacterial cultures.

2. Risk groups—Up to 80% of adult cases have a predisposing medical condition such as diabetes, cirrhosis, alcoholism, or chronic renal disease, which may precipitate disease or recrudescence in asymptomatic infected individuals. Other risk factors for disease include chronic lung disease (such as that associated with cystic fibrosis and chronic obstructive pulmonary disease), thalassemia, and malignancy and glucocorticoid treatment or other non-human immunodeficiency virus (HIV)-related immune suppression; HIV infection is not associated with higher risk for disease. Disease severity and fatality rate are also greater in persons with underlying predisposing disease risk. Highest risk for melioidosis exists for persons living in endemic areas as well as for military service personnel who have served in areas with endemic disease, adventure travelers, ecotourists, construction and resource extraction workers, and persons such as rice farmers, whose contact with contaminated soil and water may expose them to the infectious agent. Laboratory workers who work with isolates of *Burkholderia pseudomallei* are also at risk of infection if proper biosafety procedures are not followed. Melioidosis is likely more common than reported owing to underdiagnosis; as awareness has increased and diagnosis improved over the past decade, areas considered to be endemic have expanded.

Rare and sporadic human glanders infections are reported almost exclusively in those whose occupations involve contact with animals or work in laboratories (e.g., veterinarians, equine butchers, pathologists).

3. Causative agents—*B. pseudomallei* is the causative agent for melioidosis; *Burkholderia mallei* for glanders. *B. pseudomallei* is a saprophytic Gram-negative motile rod; *B. mallei* is a Gram-negative nonmotile rod and is an obligate mammalian zoonotic pathogen, which can survive for only a short period in the environment.

4. Diagnosis—Depends on isolation of the causative agent from clinical specimens (blood, urine, sputum, skin lesions, and throat swab); a rising antibody titer in serologic tests in conjunction with clinical signs and symptoms is highly suggestive. In some highly endemic areas, more than 50% of individuals have demonstrable antibodies but no history of overt disease. Direct immunofluorescent microscopy is 98% specific, but only about 70% sensitive compared with culture. The possibility of melioidosis must be kept in mind in any unexplained suppurative disease and sepsis, especially cavitating pulmonary disease, in patients living in or returned from endemic areas; disease may become manifest many years after exposure. Infection with *B. pseudomallei* cannot be differentiated serologically from infection with *B. mallei*; characterization of the isolated organism alone can lead to specific diagnosis.

5. Occurrence—Disease occurrence varies depending on location; northeast Thailand and northern Australia are considered to be highly endemic, with annual incidence rates of up to 50 cases per 100,000 people. In Thailand, it is considered to be primarily a disease of rice farmers and is the third most common cause of death from infectious disease in the northeast region of that country. As a result of increased recognition and availability of diagnostics, melioidosis is emerging as a significant cause of community-acquired pneumonia and sepsis in the tropics. Although it may manifest with a variety of clinical presentations, 50% of patients present with acute pneumonia. Cases have been recorded in many tropical and subtropical areas of Asia, in Australia/the Pacific Islands, and less commonly in the Middle East, South and Central America, and the Caribbean. Increasing numbers of cases are being reported annually in India and in countries in Central and South America as awareness and diagnostics for the disease have become more widespread. Sporadic cases have been reported in Africa as well but the extent of disease on that continent remains to be determined. Increasing numbers of imported cases in travelers visiting endemic countries are being seen in the USA and Europe. The disease is reported to be highly seasonal, with 75% to 85% of cases presenting during the rainy season when exposure to the organism is believed to be greatest. Following the tsunami of 2004, an increase in the number of melioidosis cases was observed, mainly among repatriated tourists.

Glanders has been eliminated from most areas of the world, although enzootic foci are believed to exist in Asia and some eastern Mediterranean countries.

6. Reservoirs—In endemic areas, *B. pseudomallei* is found in soil and water. Various animals, including sheep, goats, horses, swine, monkeys, and rodents, can become infected, without evidence that they are important reservoirs, except in the transfer of the agent to new foci. *B. mallei* is zoonotic in nature, with equids serving as the primary reservoir.

7. Incubation period—Usual range for both melioidosis and glanders is from 1 to 21 days with a mean of 9 days and can be as short as a few hours with high inoculum. However, for melioidosis, years may elapse between presumed exposure and appearance of clinical disease.

8. Transmission—For melioidosis, transmission usually occurs through contact with contaminated soil or water via overt or inapparent skin wounds, inhalation of soil dust, and aspiration or ingestion of contaminated water. Person-to-person transmission is extremely rare but has occurred through direct or sexual contact in 3 reported cases. Transmission has also been reported in utero and through breastfeeding in mothers with mastitis. Rare nosocomial transmission through contaminated needles has also been reported. Direct zoonotic transmission from animals to humans is not known to occur. Glanders, by contrast, is a zoonotic disease, with humans acquiring disease from direct contact with infected animals.

9. Treatment—

Drug	Intensive phase: • Ceftazidime (drug of choice) • Meropenem
	Eradication phase: • TMP/SMX
Dose	Intensive-phase IV therapy: • Ceftazidime 2 g IV every 6 hours • Meropenem 1 g IV every 8 hours
	Eradication-phase PO therapy: • TMP/SMX 320 + 1,600 mg PO every 12 hours
Route	IV for ≥ 10–14 days, THEN PO for ≥ 3 months
Alternative drug	Intensive phase: • Imipenem
	Eradication phase: • Amoxicillin clavulanate • Doxycycline

(Continued)

(Continued)

Duration	IV for $\geq$ 10–14 days, THEN PO for $\geq$ 3 months
Special considerations and comments	• Meropenem is the drug of choice for neurologic melioidosis and the dose should be doubled. • Consider adding TMP/SMX (which has excellent tissue penetration) in the doses recommended for eradication therapy from the start of the initial intensive therapy in cases of neurologic melioidosis, osteomyelitis, septic arthritis, skin and soft-tissue infections, and genitourinary infection including prostatic abscesses. • Long-term IV intensive therapy ($\geq$ 4–8 weeks) is recommended for complicated pneumonia, deep-seated infection (including prostatic abscesses), neurologic melioidosis, osteomyelitis, and septic arthritis. • Longer eradication therapy ($\geq$ 6 months) is recommended for neurologic melioidosis and osteomyelitis. • Dosages of TMP/SMX should be adjusted by weight: 3 + 30 mg/kg in children ($\leq$ 240 + 1,200 mg); 240 + 1,200 mg for adults 40–60 kg. • For children, folic acid 0.1 mg/kg/day PO ($\leq$ 5 mg) should be given in conjunction with TMP/SMX treatment. • Surgical drainage of abscesses may be of benefit. • In vitro resistance to TMP/SMX may be seen; however, this is not reflective of in vivo efficacy.

Note: IV = intravenous(ly); PO = oral(ly); TMP/SMX = trimethoprim-sulfamethoxazole.

10. Prevention—

1) Persons with predisposing medical conditions, including diabetes, and those with traumatic wounds should avoid exposure to soil or water in endemic areas.

2) In endemic areas, skin lacerations, abrasions, or burns that have been contaminated with soil or surface water should be immediately and thoroughly cleaned.

3) Use of boots and gloves is recommended for occupations that involve contact with soil and water, such as work in rice fields.

4) Foods (vegetables, etc.) should be washed thoroughly with clean water prior to consumption to remove potentially contaminated soil before ingestion; water should be chlorinated or boiled before consumption in endemic areas.

5) Prevention of glanders depends on control of glanders in equine species and care in handling causative organisms.

11. Special considerations—

1) Epidemic measures: usually a sporadic disease. Outbreaks should be investigated to determine if there is a point source.

2) Deliberate use: *B. pseudomallei* is a potential agent for deliberate use that is moderately easy to disseminate and has a high case-fatality rate among symptomatic cases. In the unlikely event of the intentional release of *B. pseudomallei*, the value of prophylactic medication is unproven but may be efficacious. In the event that postexposure prophylaxis is indicated, treatment with trimethoprim-sulfamethoxazole (co-trimoxazole) is recommended. *B. mallei* is also a potential agent for deliberate use, with the same recommendation for postexposure prophylaxis as *B. pseudomallei*.

[D. Blaney]

MENINGITIS

DISEASE	ICD-10 CODE
VIRAL MENINGITIS	ICD-10 A87
NONPYOGENIC MENINGITIS	ICD-10 G03.0
BACTERIAL MENINGITIS	ICD-10 G00
MENINGOCOCCAL MENINGITIS	ICD-10 A39.0
HAEMOPHILUS MENINGITIS	ICD-10 G00.0
PNEUMOCOCCAL MENINGITIS	ICD-10 G00.1
NEONATAL MENINGITIS	ICD-10 P37.8, P35–P37, G00, G03

Meningitis is caused by inflammation of the meninges that cover the brain and spinal cord. The inflammation can be caused by a variety of organisms that include bacteria, fungi, and viruses. It is a serious condition that can be life-threatening.

I. ASEPTIC MENINGITIS (viral meningitis, nonbacterial meningitis)

The term "aseptic meningitis" describes the condition in which patients have clinical and laboratory features of meningitis but without a positive Gram stain or routine bacterial culture. Various diseases caused by nonpyogenic infectious agents may be associated with meningitis. Viruses are by far the most common causes of aseptic meningitis. Other infections include tuberculosis, cryptococcal disease, endemic mycoses, cerebrovascular syphilis, brucellosis, leptospirosis, Lyme disease, rickettsial diseases, and certain parasites and amebae (see relevant chapters). Postinfectious and postvaccinal reactions may also cause central nervous system (CNS) conditions, including meningitis.

1. Clinical features—Viral meningitis, a relatively common but rarely serious clinical syndrome with multiple viral etiologies, characterized by sudden onset of febrile illness with signs and symptoms of headache with meningeal involvement. Viral meningitis must be differentiated from encephalitis, which causes neurologic dysfunction. Cerebrospinal fluid (CSF) findings include pleocytosis (usually mononuclear, but often polymorphonuclear in early stages), increased protein, normal sugar, and absence of bacteria. An exanthem is sometimes associated with certain types caused by enteroviruses, including coxsackieviruses, echoviruses, and the more recently identified numbered enteroviruses (e.g., EV 71). Active illness seldom exceeds 10 days. Residual signs lasting a year or more may include weakness, muscle spasm, insomnia, and personality changes. Recovery is usually complete. Gastrointestinal and respiratory symptoms may be associated with enterovirus infections.

2. Risk groups—Children represent the highest risk age group, particularly for enteroviral meningitis. Exposures to vectors, such as mosquitoes and rodent urine, are associated with some forms of viral meningitis. Sexual activity results in transmission of certain pathogens. Agammaglobulinemia poses a risk for chronic enteroviral meningoencephalitis.

3. Causative agents—A wide variety of causative agents exist, many associated with other specific diseases. Predominant causative agents can vary by geographic location and season. In epidemic periods, mumps may be responsible for more than 25% of cases of established etiology in non-immunized populations. In developed countries, non-polio enteroviruses (coxsackieviruses, echoviruses, and the numbered enteroviruses) and human parechoviruses cause both sporadic cases and epidemics of viral meningitis. Arboviruses, measles, herpes simplex and varicella viruses, lymphocytic choriomeningitis virus (LCMV), adenoviruses, and human immunodeficiency virus may cause sporadic cases of meningitis and meningoencephalitis.

4. Diagnosis—Epidemiologic patterns, patient characteristics (e.g., age, clinical findings, vaccination history), and laboratory information should be used to make a diagnosis and help identify the causative agent. Viral culture of CSF, respiratory specimens, and stools was long the gold standard for precise identification of pathogens but growth in the laboratory is often slow and so is less helpful clinically. Serology is useful for some pathogens, such as mumps and arboviruses. Molecular diagnostic methods often yield a more rapid diagnosis and are available for the detection and characterization of most viruses. Multiplex meningoencephalitis panels are increasingly available in developed countries and allow for identification of many viral, bacterial, and fungal causes of meningitis.

5. Occurrence—Worldwide, as epidemics and sporadic cases; true incidence is unknown. Seasonal increases in late summer and early fall are due mainly to arboviruses and enteroviruses, while late winter outbreaks may be due primarily to mumps.

6. Reservoirs—Humans are the only reservoir for enteroviruses and most other causes of viral meningitis. Rodents often harbor LCMV.

7. Incubation period—For non-polio enteroviruses the incubation period after exposure is 3 to 5 days. For other pathogens it varies according to the causative agent (see relevant chapters).

8. Transmission—Human-to-human transmission via the fecal-oral route is responsible for enteroviral disease. For other pathogens, route of transmission varies according to the causative agent (see the relevant chapters).

9. Treatment—Supportive care is the mainstay of treatment for most forms of viral meningitis.

Drug	For HSV or VZV meningitis/encephalitis: • Acyclovir
Dose	10 mg/kg/dose every 8 hours
Route	IV (treatment of encephalitis requires IV therapy while treatment of meningitis may include step-down PO antiviral therapy)
Alternative drug	Not applicable
Duration	• Encephalitis: 14–21 days • Meningitis: 10–14 days
Special considerations and comments	• No antiviral therapy is presently available for enterovirus infections. • For other causes of meningitis, see the relevant chapters.

Note: HSV = herpes simplex virus; IV = intravenous(ly); PO = oral(ly); VZV = varicella-zoster virus.

10. Prevention—Varies according to the causative agent (see the relevant chapters).

11. Special considerations—

1) Reporting: depends on the causative agent.
2) Epidemic measures: refer to the chapter relevant to the causative agent.

II. BACTERIAL (PYOGENIC) MENINGITIS

Neisseria meningitidis, Streptococcus pneumoniae, and *Haemophilus influenzae* type b (Hib) are thought to cause more than 75% of all cases of bacterial meningitis and 90% of cases of bacterial meningitis in children. Meningitis due to Hib, previously the most common cause of bacterial meningitis, has been dramatically reduced in many industrialized countries through immunization programs. Meningococcal disease is unique among the major causes of bacterial meningitis in that it causes both endemic disease and large epidemics. The less common bacterial causes of meningitis, such as staphylococci, enteric bacteria, group B streptococci, and *Listeria*, occur in susceptible persons (such as neonates and patients with impaired immunity) or as a consequence of head trauma.

Initial empiric antibiotic treatment should be aimed at covering suspected bacterial pathogens (the combination of vancomycin and ceftriaxone is recommended for most age groups). Once the bacterial pathogen is identified treatment should be narrowed to the antibiotic of choice.

Other important principles of management of patients with bacterial meningitis include

1) Management of concomitant complications of sepsis, including hypotension and organ/system failure
2) Treatment of neurologic dysfunction, including seizures if present
3) Infection prevention measures in hospitals, including droplet and standard precautions

A. MENINGOCOCCAL MENINGITIS (cerebrospinal fever)

1. Clinical features—An acute bacterial meningitis, characterized by sudden onset of fever, intense headache, nausea and often vomiting, stiff neck, and photophobia. A petechial and/or purpuric rash is typical and tissue necrosis may occur. Even with antibiotics, case fatality remains high at 8% to 15%. In addition, 10% to 20% of survivors will have long-term sequelae, including neurologic deficits, hearing loss, and limb loss. Invasive disease is characterized by 1 or more clinical syndromes, including meningitis (the most common presentation), bacteremia, and sepsis. Meningococcemia, or meningococcal sepsis, is the most severe form of infection, with petechial rash, hypotension, disseminated intravascular coagulation, tissue gangrene, and multiorgan failure.

2. Risk groups—Travelers to countries where disease is epidemic, Hajj pilgrims, military groups, and individuals with underlying immune dysfunctions, such as asplenia, properdin deficiency, and a deficiency of terminal complement components. Crowding, low socioeconomic status, active or passive exposure to tobacco smoke, and concurrent upper respiratory tract infections also increase the risk of meningococcal disease. Infants are at highest risk but rates decrease after infancy and then increase in adolescence and young adulthood. Group-specific immunity may follow subclinical infections.

3. Causative agents—*N. meningitidis*, also called meningococcus, is a Gram-negative aerobic diplococcus. Meningococci are divided into serogroups according to the immunologic reactivity of their capsular polysaccharide. Groups A, B, and C account for at least 90% of cases worldwide. In most European and North American countries and many Latin American countries, serogroups B, C, and Y cause the majority of disease, while serogroup A is the main cause in Africa and Asia. As countries introduce meningococcal conjugate vaccine programs against the most common circulating serogroups (serogroup C in Europe, serogroup A in Africa), the proportion of disease caused by serogroup B is increasing.

4. Diagnosis—The gold standard for diagnosis is recovery of meningococci from a sterile site, primarily CSF or blood. However, the sensitivity of culture in patients who have received antibiotics may be low. In culture-negative cases, identification of group-specific meningococcal polysaccharides in CSF by latex agglutination can help but false-negative results are common, especially for serogroup B. Polymerase chain reaction (PCR) offers the advantage of detecting meningococcal deoxyribonucleic acid (DNA) in CSF and does not require live organisms; however, it is not yet widely available in many countries. Microscopic examination of Gram-stained smears from petechiae may show Gram-negative diplococci.

5. Occurrence—In Europe and North America the incidence of meningococcal disease is higher during winter and spring; in sub-Saharan Africa the disease classically peaks during the dry season. The highest burden of the disease lies in the African meningitis belt—a large area that stretches from Senegal to Ethiopia and affects all or part of 21 countries. In this region, high rates of sporadic infections (1–20 cases/100,000 population) occur in annual cycles, with periodical superimposition of large-scale epidemics (usually caused by serogroup A). In the countries of the African meningitis belt, epidemics with incidence rates as high as 1,000 cases per 100,000 population have occurred every 8 to 12 years over the course of at least the past 50 years. In addition, major epidemics have occurred in adjacent countries not usually considered part of the African meningitis belt (such as Kenya and Tanzania).

6. Reservoirs—Humans.

7. Incubation period—2 to 10 days, commonly 3 to 4 days.

8. Transmission—Through direct contact, including respiratory droplets from the nose and throat, although this usually causes only a subclinical mucosal infection. Up to 5% to 10% of people may be asymptomatic carriers with nasopharyngeal colonization by *N. meningitidis*. Carrier rates of up to 25% have been documented in some populations in the absence of any cases of meningococcal disease. Fewer than 1% of those colonized will progress to invasive disease. Disease often results when a naive individual acquires the organism from a carrier. Communicability continues until live meningococci are no longer present in discharges from nose and mouth. The concentration of meningococci is reduced within the nasopharynx within 24 hours after institution of antimicrobial treatment to which the organisms are sensitive. Penicillin will temporarily suppress the organisms but does not usually eradicate them from the nasopharynx.

9. Treatment—

Drug	• Penicillin G or ampicillin (if Pen MIC < 0.1 µg/mL) • Ceftriaxone (if Pen MIC 0.1–1.0 µg/mL)
Dose	• Penicillin 4 MU every 4 hours (children: 300,000 units/kg/day divided every 4 hours) • Ceftriaxone 2 g every 12 hours (children: 100 mg/kg/day divided every 12 hours)
Route	IV
Alternative drug	β-lactam–intolerant patients: • Meropenem 2 g every 8 hours (children: 40 mg/kg every 8 hours)
Duration	7 days
Special considerations and comments	Not applicable

Note: IU = international units; IV = intravenous(ly); MIC = minimum inhibitory concentration; MU = million units; Pen = penicillin.

10. Prevention—

1) Several meningococcal polysaccharide conjugate vaccines are available. Different serogroup compositions are licensed in different countries, usually determined by the epidemiology of disease in those countries. In many countries 2 quadrivalent (serogroups A, C, Y, and W) conjugate vaccines and 2 serogroup B vaccines are licensed. There are also monovalent and other combination vaccines. In Africa, a serogroup A conjugate vaccine is licensed. Routine recommendations for targeted age groups have been implemented in many countries. In the meningitis belt in Africa, countries have implemented mass vaccination campaigns with conjugate meningitis A vaccine for persons aged 1 to 29 years as a strategy to eliminate serogroup A epidemic meningitis.

2) Postexposure chemoprophylaxis is an effective strategy to prevent secondary cases after known close exposure and also in an outbreak situation. Oral rifampin, oral ciprofloxacin, and

intramuscular ceftriaxone are all effective. If undertaken, chemoprophylaxis should be administered to all exposed persons at the same time.

11. Special considerations—

1) Reporting: case reporting is obligatory in most countries.
2) Epidemic measures: outbreaks may develop in situations of forced crowding. When an outbreak occurs, major emphasis must be placed on surveillance, early diagnosis and identification of serogroup, vaccination if caused by a vaccine-preventable serogroup, and immediate treatment of suspected cases. A high index of suspicion is necessary. A threshold approach tailored to the epidemiology of the country is used in many countries to differentiate endemic disease from outbreaks. When thresholds are passed and the serogroup causing the outbreak is preventable by vaccine, immunization campaigns should be considered.
3) For specific information regarding management, surveillance, and treatment during an outbreak, see: https://apps.who.int/iris/bitstream/handle/10665/154595/WHO_HSE_GAR_ERI_2010.4_Rev1_eng.pdf?sequence=1.

B. HAEMOPHILUS MENINGITIS (meningitis due to *Haemophilus influenzae*)

1. Clinical features—In industrialized countries, before widespread use of Hib conjugate vaccines, invasive disease due to Hib most commonly presented as meningitis. In developing countries, the primary manifestation of Hib is lower respiratory tract infection.

Onset of meningitis can be subacute but is usually sudden, including fever, vomiting, lethargy, and meningeal irritation, with bulging fontanelle in infants or stiff neck and back in older children. Progressive stupor or coma is common. Occasionally, there is a low-grade fever for several days, with subtler CNS symptoms. Overall mortality rate for Hib meningitis is 5%; 6% of the survivors have permanent sensorineural hearing loss; 25% have significant disability of some type.

2. Risk groups—Children younger than 5 years account for the great majority of cases. Susceptibility is assumed to be universal. Immunity is associated with the presence of circulating bactericidal and/or anticapsular antibodies, acquired transplacentally, from prior infection, or through immunization.

3. Causative agents—*H. influenzae* are Gram-negative coccobacilli that are divided into unencapsulated (nontypeable) and encapsulated strains. The encapsulated strains are further classified into serotypes a through f, based on the antigenic characteristics of their polysaccharide capsules. Type b is the most common and the most highly pathogenic.

4. Diagnosis—May be made through isolation of organisms from blood or CSF. Specific capsular polysaccharide may be identified by latex agglutination techniques. PCR offers the advantage of detecting *H. influenzae* DNA in CSF and does not require live organisms; however, it is not yet widely available in many countries.

5. Occurrence—Worldwide. Most prevalent among children aged 2 months to 3 years; unusual in those older than 5 years. As of the late 2000s, with widespread vaccination in early childhood, Hib meningitis has virtually disappeared in industrialized countries and in developing countries that have introduced Hib vaccine. Invasive disease due to other types still occurs but is uncommon.

6. Reservoirs—Humans.

7. Incubation period—Unknown; probably 2 to 4 days.

8. Transmission—Through droplet inhalation and contact with discharges from nose and throat during the infectious period. The portal of entry is most commonly the nasopharynx. The period of communicability lasts as long as organisms are present, which may be for a prolonged period even without nasal discharge. Transmission stops within 24 to 48 hours of starting effective antimicrobial therapy.

9. Treatment—

Drug	• Ceftriaxone for beta-lactamase–positive organisms • Ampicillin for β-lactamase–negative organisms
Dose	• Ceftriaxone 2 g every 12 hours (children: 100 mg/kg/day divided every 12 hours) • Ampicillin 2 g every 4 hours (children: 300–400 mg/kg/day divided every 4–6 hours)
Route	IV
Alternative drug	β-Lactamase–positive: • Aztreonam • Fluoroquinolone β-Lactamase–negative: • Ceftriaxone • Aztreonam • Fluoroquinolone
Duration	7–10 days

(Continued)

(Continued)

Special considerations and comments	Children have improved hearing outcomes when dexamethasone is administered prior to or with the first dose of antibiotics (dose is 0.6 mg/kg/day divided every 6 hours for 2–4 days).

Note: IV = intravenous(ly).

10. Prevention—Routine childhood immunization. Several protein-polysaccharide conjugate vaccines have been shown to prevent invasive Hib disease in children older than 2 months and are licensed in many countries, both individually and combined with other vaccines. Immunization is recommended, starting at 2 months old, followed by additional doses after an interval of 2 months; dosages vary with the vaccine in use. All vaccines require boosters at 12 to 15 months old. Immunization is not routinely recommended for children older than 5 years. Hib conjugate vaccines have been available since the 1980s and efforts to introduce them are increasing worldwide.

11. Special considerations—

1) Reporting: case report may be required in some endemic areas.
2) Monitor for cases occurring in susceptible population settings, such as day care centers and large foster homes.

C. PNEUMOCOCCAL MENINGITIS

1. Clinical features—Onset is usually sudden with high fever, lethargy or coma, and signs of meningeal irritation. It can be fulminant and occurs with bacteremia but not necessarily with any other focus, although there may be otitis media or mastoiditis. Pneumococcal meningitis has a high case-fatality rate.

2. Risk groups—A sporadic disease especially in young infants, the elderly, and other high-risk groups, including asplenic and hypogammaglobulinemic patients. Predisposing factors are cochlear implantation and basilar skull fracture causing persistent communication with the nasopharynx. Immunity is associated with the presence of circulating anticapsular antibody, acquired transplacentally, from prior infection, or from immunization.

3. Causative agents—*S. pneumoniae,* a Gram-positive diplococcus. Nearly all strains causing meningitis and other severe forms of pneumococcal disease are encapsulated. There are 90 known capsular serotypes. The distribution of serotypes varies regionally and with age. In North America the 13 serotypes in pneumococcal conjugate vaccine are those that cause a substantial proportion of pneumococcal meningitis in children and adults.

4. Diagnosis—May be made by isolation of organisms from blood or CSF. Urine pneumococcal antigen testing can be used to identify disease in adults but is not recommended for children because of poor specificity.

5. Occurrence—Worldwide. Pneumococcal meningitis may occur at any age. Most prevalent among children aged 2 months to 3 years. In developing countries infants are at highest risk; in North America, risk peaks at 6 to 18 months old.

6. Reservoirs—Humans. Pneumococci are often found in the upper respiratory tract of healthy persons. Carriage is more common in children than in adults.

7. Incubation period—Unknown; probably 1 to 4 days.

8. Transmission—Through droplet spread and contact with respiratory secretions; direct contact with a person with pneumococcal disease generally results in nasopharyngeal carriage of the organism rather than in disease. The period of communicability lasts as long as organisms are present, which may be for a prolonged period, especially in immunocompromised hosts.

9. Treatment—

Drug	• Penicillin G OR ampicillin (if Pen MIC ≤ 0.06 μg/mL) • Third-generation cephalosporin (if Pen MIC ≥ 0.12 μg/mL and if ceftriaxone MIC < 1.0 μg/mL)
	• Vancomycin (if ceftriaxone MIC ≥ 1.0 μg/mL) PLUS • Third-generation cephalosporin
Dose	• Penicillin G 4 MU every 4 hours • Ampicillin 2 g every 4 hours • Ceftriaxone 2 g every 12 hours • Vancomycin 2 g initially every 8–12 hours, THEN adjust dose to keep trough concentration between 15–20 μg/mL
Route	IV
Alternative drug	Fully Pen susceptible organisms: • Third-generation cephalosporin • Meropenem
	Ceftriaxone nonsusceptible organisms: • Moxifloxacin
Duration	10–14 days

(Continued)

(Continued)

Special considerations and comments	Typically, vancomycin and ceftriaxone are used as initial empiric theraphy. If susceptibility testing confirms penicillin or ceftriaxone sensitivity, vancomycin can be discontinued. Consider adding rifampin if the MIC of ceftriaxone is > 2 μg/mL. Adults with pneumococcal meningitis in the developed world have improved outcomes when dexamethasone is administered prior to or with the first dose of antibiotics (10 mg every 6 hours for 4 days). For children and in developing countries the benefit of dexamethasone is less clear.

Note: IV = intravenous(ly); MIC = minimum inhibitory concentration; MU = million units; Pen = penicillin.

10. Prevention—Vaccination is the mainstay of prevention. In many industrialized countries, pneumococcal conjugate vaccines are recommended for children younger than 2 years and other children and adults with certain high-risk conditions, such as immunocompromising conditions, sickle cell disease, asplenia, heart or lung disease, or cochlear implantation. The vaccines cover either the 10 or 13 serotypes that often cause pneumococcal meningitis in industrialized countries. Developing countries are introducing pneumococcal conjugate vaccines into their routine infant vaccine schedules. A polysaccharide vaccine containing 23 of the most common serotypes has been available since 1983. This is recommended in several countries for use in persons aged 65 years and older and those aged 2 to 64 years with immunocompromising conditions or certain chronic illnesses (after receiving a conjugate vaccine).

11. Special considerations—

1) Reporting: case report to local health authority may be required in some areas.

2) Epidemic measures: pneumococcal meningitis can occur as part of a cluster of pneumococcal disease in institutional settings. Immunization using either the 23-valent polysaccharide vaccine or a conjugate vaccine, depending on the setting and the serotype, should be used to control outbreaks. Targeted antimicrobial prophylaxis (e.g., penicillin) may be useful in some outbreaks, especially those caused by non–vaccine-type strains and when the outbreak strain is not resistant to antimicrobial agents. Widespread antimicrobial prophylaxis is not always effective and can induce resistance.

D. NEONATAL MENINGITIS

Etiologic agents in the early neonatal period include group B streptococci, *Listeria monocytogenes* (see "Listeriosis"), *Escherichia coli* K1, and other organisms acquired from the birth canal. Infants aged 2 weeks to 2 months may also develop meningitis, with recovery from the CSF of group B streptococci, nosocomial Gram-negative bacilli acquired from the nursery environment, or *Salmonella* acquired perinatally or from the community. Symptoms of meningitis include lethargy, seizures, apneic episodes, poor feeding, hypo- or hyperthermia, and sometimes respiratory distress. The white blood cell (WBC) count may be elevated or depressed. The CSF profile is typical for bacterial meningitis with elevated WBCs with neutrophil predominance, low sugar, and high protein; in the absence of prior treatment with antibiotics, the CSF Gram stain and culture will show the causative organism. PCR is also available for identification of most organisms. Empiric treatment is ampicillin plus a third-generation cephalosporin until the causal organism has been identified and its antimicrobial susceptibilities determined.

Group B *Streptococcus* Meningitis Treatment

Drug	Penicillin G OR ampicillin
Dose	The dose for penicillin varies depending upon the age of the neonate: • Infants ≤ 7 days: 250,000–450,000 U/kg/day divided every 8 hours • Infants > 7 days: 450,000–500,000 U/kg/day divided every 6 hours
Route	IV
Alternative drug	Ampicillin is an acceptable alternative. The dose for ampicillin varies depending upon the age of the neonate: • Infants ≤ 7 days: 100 mg/kg/dose IV every 8 hours • Infants > 7 days: 75 mg/kg/dose IV every 6 hours
Duration	14 days
Special considerations and comments	Severely ill infants should receive 21 days of therapy. Low birth-weight infants may require dose adjustment.

Note: IV = intravenous(ly); U = units.

Listeria monocytogenes Meningitis Treatment

Drug	Ampicillin PLUS gentamicin
Dose	Ampicillin: • Infants ≤ 7 days: 100 mg/kg/dose every 8 hours • Infants > 7 days: 75 mg/kg/dose every 6 hours
	The dose of gentamicin varies according to age as follows; these doses apply to patients with normal renal function: • Infants ≤ 7 days: 4 mg/kg every 24 hours • Infants 8 days to 1 month: 5 mg/kg/dose every 24 hours • Infants > 1 month and children: 7.5 mg/kg/day in 3 divided doses
Route	IV
Alternative drug	Meropemem 120 mg/kg/day divided every 8 hours
Duration	21 days
Special considerations and comments	• When infant has improved clinically and CSF is sterile, gentamicin may be discontinued. • Infants with *Listeria* meningitis are often born prematurely and antibiotic dosages may need adjustment based on birth weight.

Note: CSF = cerebrospinal fluid; IV = intravenous(ly).

Escherichia coli Meningitis Treatment

Drug	• Third-generation cephalosporin (e.g., ceftazidime) for empiric therapy • Ampicillin if proven susceptible
Dose	Ampicillin: • Infants ≤ 7 days: 100 mg/kg/dose every 8 hours • Infants > 7 days: 75 mg/kg/dose every 6 hours
	Ceftazidime: • Infants ≤ 7 days: 100–150 mg/kg/day divided every 8–12 hours • Infants > 7 days: 150 mg/kg/day divided every 8 hours
Route	IV
Alternative drug	Meropenem 120 mg/kg/day divided every 8 hours

(Continued)

Escherichia coli Meningitis Treatment (Continued)

Duration	All infants with Gram-negative meningitis should undergo repeat lumbar puncture to ensure sterility of the CSF after 24–48 hours of therapy. If CSF remains culture-positive, choice and doses of antimicrobial agents should be evaluated and another lumbar puncture should be performed after 48–72 hours. Minimum duration is 21 days.
Special considerations and comments	If _E. coli_ is an ESBL producer, β-lactam antibiotics should not be used and meropenem is the drug of choice.

Note: CSF = cerebrospinal fluid; ESBL = extended spectrum β-lactamase; IV = intravenous(ly).

[P. Donovan, S. Eppes]

MOLLUSCUM CONTAGIOSUM

DISEASE	ICD-10 CODE
MOLLUSCUM CONTAGIOSUM	ICD-10 B08.1

1. Clinical features—A viral infection of the skin resulting in smooth-surfaced, firm, dome-shaped, or hemispherical papules with central umbilication. The lesions may be flesh-colored, white, translucent, or yellow. Most papules are 2 to 5 mm in diameter; giant mollusca (10–30 mm) are occasionally seen in immunocompromised patients. Lesions in adults are most often on the lower abdominal wall, pubis, genitalia, or inner thighs; in children, they are most often on the face, trunk, and proximal extremities. In immunocompetent hosts the course of infection is usually benign, typically resulting in 5 to 30 lesions with no other symptoms. Immunocompromised hosts may develop hundreds of lesions. Occasionally the lesions itch and show a linear orientation owing to autoinoculation by scratching. Lesions may become confluent and form a single plaque. Without treatment, molluscum contagiosum can persist for 6 months to 5 years. Any 1 lesion has a life span of 2 to 6 months. Lesions may resolve spontaneously or as a result of inflammatory response following trauma or secondary bacterial infection. There are rarely any systemic symptoms. Treatment (including curettage of the lesions) can shorten the course of infection.

2. Risk groups—All ages may be affected. Disease is more common in patients infected with human immunodeficiency virus. Little is known about the role of the immune system.

3. Causative agents—Molluscum contagiosum virus (MCV), a member of the Poxviridae family, genus *Molluscipoxvirus*; the genus comprises at least 4 distinct genetic types (MCV-1 to -4). The virus has not been grown in cell culture.

4. Diagnosis—Clinical when multiple lesions are present. Lesions visualized by dermatoscopy showing orifices and vessels (in crown, radial, or punctiform patterns) are suggestive of molluscum contagiosum. For confirmation, the core can be expressed onto a glass slide and examined by ordinary light microscopy for classic basophilic, Feulgen-positive, intracytoplasmic inclusions—the molluscum—or Henderson-Patterson bodies. Histology can confirm the diagnosis. The differential diagnosis includes flat warts (condyloma acuminata), pyogenic granuloma, cryptococcosis, and histoplasmosis.

5. Occurrence—Worldwide. Serologic tests are unreliable. Skin inspection is the only screening technique available. Epidemiologic studies have been limited. Surveys have shown that peak disease incidence occurs in childhood. Molluscum contagiosum is common and about 5% of children will experience this infection.

6. Reservoirs—Humans.

7. Incubation period—For experimental inoculation, 19 to 50 days; clinical reports give 7 days to 6 months.

8. Transmission—Usually through direct skin-to-skin contact, including sexual contact, and through handling objects contaminated with the virus (towels, swimming pool kick boards). Infections have been observed in individuals who have recently undergone tattooing or cosmetic hair removal. Autoinoculation also occurs. Atopic skin disease increases susceptibility to this virus. The period of communicability is unknown but probably exists as long as lesions persist.

9. Treatment—

Preferred therapy	Podophyllotoxin 0.5% solution applied directly to the lesions BID for 3 consecutive days per week for 2 weeks.
Alternative therapy options	Cantharidin product applied directly to lesion by a health care provider. Once dry, cover large lesions with tape for 4–6 hours or 6–8 hours, depending on product. May repeat once weekly for new or resistant lesions.

(Continued)

(Continued)

Special considerations and comments	• Curettage and cryotherapy are equally effective and are considered first-line treatment options. • Treatment should occur early to reduce transmission/ limit number of lesions. • Both podophyllotoxin and imiquimod are not recommended for use in pregnancy or while breastfeeding. • For topical application, each lesion must be targeted because of local treatment effects. • Immunocompromised patients may not respond as well to the traditional therapies listed earlier.

Note: BID = twice daily.

10. Prevention—Avoid skin contact or sharing bathtubs, bath towels, or other fomites with infected patients. No vaccine available.

11. Special considerations—

1) Epidemic measures: suspend direct contact activities. Disinfect surfaces.
2) More information can be found at: https://www.cdc.gov/poxvirus/molluscum-contagiosum/treatment.html.

[A. R. Ronald]

MUCORMYCOSIS
(zygomycosis)

DISEASE	ICD-10 CODE
INFECTIONS DUE TO MUCORALES	ICD-10 B46.0–B46.5
INFECTIONS DUE TO ENTOMOPHTHORALES	ICD-10 B46.8
BASIDIOBOLOMYCOSIS	ICD-10 B46.8
CONIDIOBOLOMYCOSIS	ICD-10 B46.8

I. INFECTIONS DUE TO MUCORALES (mucormycosis)

1. Clinical features—Infections caused by fungi of the order Mucorales are rare; when they do occur, they are typically rapidly progressive, destructive, and associated with high mortality. These fungi have an affinity for blood vessels and can cause thrombosis, infarction, and tissue necrosis. The course is typically acute or subacute. Risk factors include prolonged severe neutropenia, poorly controlled diabetes mellitus, and iron overload. In immunocompromised persons, mucormycosis is the most fulminant fungal infection known.

There are 6 major clinical forms of the disease: (a) rhinocerebral, (b) pulmonary, (c) gastrointestinal, (d) cutaneous, (e) disseminated, and (f) uncommon rare forms, such as osteomyelitis or endocarditis.

Rhinocerebral disease is the most common clinical form of the disease and the most common form in patients with diabetes mellitus. It usually presents as nasal or paranasal sinus infection with rapid extension into adjacent tissues; a black necrotic eschar is the hallmark sign. Necrosis of the turbinates, perforation of the hard palate, necrosis of the cheek or orbital cellulitis, proptosis, and ophthalmoplegia may occur. Infection may invade the internal carotid artery or extend directly to the brain via the orbital apex or cribriform plate.

Pulmonary mucormycosis is the second most common form and occurs most often in patients with severe prolonged neutropenia, recipients of hematopoietic stem cell transplants, and those with graft-versus-host disease. In this form, the fungus causes thrombosis of pulmonary blood vessels and infarctions of the lung.

Gastrointestinal mucormycosis is rare; it has been associated with severe malnutrition and has been reported in preterm neonates. In this form, mucosal ulcers or thrombosis and gangrene of stomach or bowel wall may occur.

Cutaneous mucormycosis results from direct inoculation via trauma or use of contaminated supplies over wounds or burns. Clinical manifestations vary; onset may be gradual or fulminant.

Disseminated mucormycosis usually occurs in severely immunosuppressed patients, such as those with profound neutropenia and/or hematologic malignancy. Deferoxamine therapy for iron overload has been associated with disseminated mucormycosis; however, its use has been discontinued with the introduction of novel iron chelators (e.g., deferasirox and deferiprone) that do not predispose to mucormycosis.

Uncommon forms of mucormycosis include endocarditis (including prosthetic or native valve), osteomyelitis, peritonitis, and pyelonephritis. Intravenous drug use has been shown to be a risk factor.

2. Risk groups—Healthy persons rarely develop disease despite frequent exposure to Mucorales in the environment; this is because neutrophils act as a key host defense. Immunosuppressed individuals, especially those with profound neutropenia or a recent hematopoietic stem cell transplant, are at greatest risk. Those receiving other immunosuppressive therapies (e.g., corticosteroids, biologic agents) are also at risk, as are individuals with diabetes (and diabetic ketoacidosis) and those with iron overload. Malnutrition predisposes to the gastrointestinal form. One exception to this is cutaneous disease, in which healthy individuals develop disease after direct inoculation to a traumatic injury.

3. Causative agents—Rapidly growing molds of the order Mucorales. *Rhizopus* is the genus most commonly implicated in human disease. The

2 most common species causing mucormycosis are *Rhizopus oryzae* and *Rhizopus microsporus*. Other genera known to cause human disease include *Mucor*, *Rhizomucor*, *Lichtheimia* (formerly *Absidia*), *Cunninghamella*, *Apophysomyces*, *Saksenaea*, and *Syncephalastrum*.

4. Diagnosis—Can be challenging. Clinical manifestations in immuno-suppressed hosts may be similar to those caused by other invasive mold infections, such as aspergillosis. Definitive diagnosis is usually made by histopathology specimen through microscopic demonstration of broad, ribbonlike, nonseptate or pauciseptate hyphae in tissue or bodily fluids with an accompanying positive culture. Immunohistochemistry reagents and direct deoxyribonucleic acid–based detection testing are also available for tissue blocks. Wet preparations and smears may be examined. Cultures alone are not diagnostic because Mucorales are found widely in the environment. However, in an immunosuppressed patient with a compatible clinical syndrome, a positive culture for Mucorales should be taken very seriously. Similarly, the diagnosis may be difficult to establish based solely upon histopathology since it may be difficult to appreciate the distinctive characteristics of fungal hyphae that differentiate them from those of other molds, such as *Aspergillus* spp., in tissue.

5. Occurrence—Worldwide. Within populations at risk, incidence may be between 1 and 4 cases per 1,000. Incidence may be increasing owing to higher prevalence of diabetes mellitus and immunosuppression in addition to longer survival of patients with certain hematologic conditions. In recent years, there have been reports of increasing numbers of cases among hematopoietic stem cell transplant recipients in association with the prophylactic use of voriconazole, a broad-spectrum azole antifungal that has potent activity against *Aspergillus* spp. but not against the mucormycetes.

6. Reservoirs—Common saprophytes in the environment. Commonly found in soil and in decaying matter.

7. Incubation period—Unknown. Cutaneous infection after traumatic inoculation appears to have an incubation period of 14 days. Fungus spreads rapidly in susceptible tissues.

8. Transmission—Through inhalation of conidia or ingestion of fungal spores by susceptible individuals. Direct inoculation during intravenous drug use and at sites of intravenous catheters and cutaneous burns may occur. No direct person-to-person or animal-to-person transmission.

9. Treatment—

Preferred therapy	Liposomal AMB 5–10 mg/kg IV every 24 hours for prolonged duration (> 6 weeks)
Alternative therapy options	• Posaconazole delayed-release tablets 300 mg PO BID for 2 doses, THEN 300 mg PO daily OR • Posaconazole suspension 200 mg QID, THEN 400 mg BID after stabilization of disease OR • Posaconazole 300 mg IV for 90 minutes BID for 2 doses, THEN 300 mg IV every 24 hours
	Isavuconazonium sulfate (prodrug of isavuconazole) 372 mg PO/IV for 6 doses, THEN 372 mg PO/IV every 24 hours (372 mg of isavuconazonium sulfate = 200 mg isavuconazole)
	AMB deoxycholate 1 mg/kg IV every 24 hours
Special considerations and comments	• Treatment has not been evaluated in randomized controlled trials because of the rarity of this disease. It can be challenging and mortality is high despite therapy. • Strategy is 3-fold: (a) correction of the underlying abnormality (e.g., glucose control and treatment of acidosis in diabetics, reduction of immunosuppression), (b) prompt initiation of antifungal therapy, and (c) surgical resection of infected tissue, if possible. • Posaconazole has been shown to be effective as salvage treatment in some patients who do not tolerate AMB or whose disease is refractory to AMB. • Isavuconazole is the most recently approved antifungal, is noninferior to AMB in small trials, and has a more favorable side effect profile. • Hyperbaric oxygen has been used as adjunctive therapy but its benefit has not been established. • Could consider combination therapy of AMB plus an echinocandin. • The higher doses of AMB (> 5 mg/kg/day) are not supported by strong clinical evidence but may be considered, especially for patients with CNS involvement. • To minimize the risks of toxicity with AMB, it is recommended to administer normal saline, acetaminophen, and diphenhydramine prior to administration of the IV AMB product. It is also recommended to closely monitor electrolytes (potassium and magnesium) and provide supplementation if/when needed. • Posaconazole has several different dosage forms, as noted earlier, and each has its own dosing strategy. Posaconazole delayed-released tablets achieve better serum levels than the suspension and should be the preferred PO formulation when possible.

Note: AMB = amphotericin B; BID = twice daily; CNS = central nervous system; IV = intravenous(ly); PO = oral(ly); QID = 4 times a day.

10. **Prevention—**

1) Optimal clinical control of diabetes mellitus to avoid acidosis. Minimization of immunosuppression.

2) Management of contacts and the immediate environment: typically, a sporadic disease in a susceptible host. Investigation of contacts and source of infection is not usually beneficial owing to the presence of these fungi widely in the environment. However, outbreaks related to construction in a health care facility and to contaminated medical supplies have occurred and may prompt an investigation.

11. **Special considerations—**None.

II. INFECTIONS DUE TO ENTOMOPHTHORALES

Entomophthoromycosis is a rare disease in the USA, but more commonly occurs in tropical and subtropical parts of Africa, Southeast Asia, and Latin America. Its name derives from the Greek word *entomon* (insect) as the fungi were originally identified as pathogens of insects.

This disease includes 2 histopathologically identical entities: basidiobolomycosis (caused by *Basidiobolus ranarum*) and conidiobolomycosis (caused by *Conidiobolus coronatus* and *Conidiobolus incongruus*). Entomophthoromycosis, unlike infections caused by other Mucorales, is typically subcutaneous and slowly progressive; it affects immunocompetent individuals.

Basidiobolomycosis is a chronic subcutaneous infection of the trunk and limbs. It typically presents as a firm, painless, and sharply circumscribed subcutaneous mass, most often in children and adolescents.

Conidiobolomycosis is a chronic mucocutaneous rhinofacial infection. It originates in the nasal mucosa or sinuses and often presents with nasal obstruction or swelling of the nose or adjacent structures, most often in young men.

Treatment usually involves prolonged (months) systemic antifungal therapy with surgical debridement. Potassium iodide and itraconazole are most often used; high doses are required given relative resistance to antifungals.

Incubation periods and modes of transmission are unknown, although transmission is suspected to be traumatic implantation of plant debris for basidiobolomycosis and inhalation of fungal spores for conidiobolomycosis. The fungi are widely found in decaying vegetation, soil, and the gastrointestinal tract of amphibians and reptiles. Person-to-person transmission does not occur. Systemic involvement is extremely uncommon; however, there are reports of a few cases of gastrointestinal basidiobolomycosis, in addition to disseminated conidiobolomycosis due to *C. incongruus*.

[S. Tsay]

MUMPS
(infectious parotitis)

DISEASE	ICD-10 CODE
MUMPS	ICD-10 B26

1. Clinical features—An acute viral disease characterized by fever, swelling, and tenderness of 1 or more salivary glands—usually the parotid—and sometimes the sublingual or submaxillary glands. Parotitis may be unilateral or bilateral and typically lasts 7 to 10 days in unvaccinated individuals. Prodromal symptoms are nonspecific, consisting of myalgia, anorexia, malaise, headache, and low-grade fever. Not all cases of parotitis are caused by mumps infection but other parotitis-causing agents do not produce parotitis on an epidemic scale. Orchitis, the most common complication of mumps infection, occurs in 3% to 10% of affected postpubertal males. Orchitis is typically unilateral; sterility is extremely rare. Mumps orchitis has been reported to be a risk factor for testicular cancer. Mumps can rarely cause permanent sensorineural hearing loss in both children and adults. Pancreatitis, usually mild, in the prevaccine era occurred in 3.5% of cases.

Symptomatic aseptic meningitis occurs in up to 10% of mumps cases; patients usually recover without complications, though many require hospitalization. Mumps encephalitis is reported by CDC to range from 1 in 6,000 mumps cases (0.02%) to 1 in 300 mumps cases (0.3%) and can result in permanent sequelae, such as paralysis, seizures, and hydrocephalus. The case-fatality rate for mumps encephalitis is about 1%. Mumps infection during the first trimester of pregnancy has been associated with spontaneous abortion but there is no firm evidence that mumps during pregnancy causes congenital malformations. In the postvaccine era, among all persons infected with mumps, as noted by CDC, reported rates of meningitis, encephalitis, pancreatitis, and deafness have all been less than 1%.

2. Risk groups—Immunity is generally long-lasting and develops after either inapparent or clinical infections.

3. Causative agents—Mumps virus, a member of the family Paramyxoviridae, genus *Rubulavirus*.

4. Diagnosis—Acute mumps infection can be confirmed through a positive serologic test for mumps-specific immunoglobulin class M (IgM) antibodies; seroconversion—a significant (4-fold) rise in serum mumps immunoglobulin class G (IgG) titer as determined by a quantitative serologic assay, detection of virus by reverse transcription polymerase chain reaction (RT-PCR), or isolation of mumps virus from an appropriate clinical specimen (buccal swab or cerebrospinal fluid). Diagnosis may be more challenging in vaccinated populations, in which the IgM response may be absent or short-lived and viral load may be lower. There is some evidence that serum collected at least 5 to 10 days after parotitis onset may improve the ability to detect IgM among persons who have received 1 or 2 doses of measles, mumps, rubella (MMR) vaccine. The ability to confirm cases by ribonucleic acid detection using real-time RT-PCR is improved when samples are collected within 2 days after symptom onset, regardless of vaccination status. Absence of a mumps IgM response in a vaccinated or previously infected individual presenting with clinically compatible mumps *does not rule out mumps* as a diagnosis. A positive IgG result is expected among previously vaccinated persons. Older persons with no history of mumps illness or vaccination may have detectable mumps IgG owing to a previous subclinical infection.

5. Occurrence—In unvaccinated populations, about one-third of patients have inapparent or subclinical infections, especially young children. In temperate climates, winter and spring are peak seasons. In the absence of immunization, mumps is endemic, with an annual incidence usually of 100 to 1,000 per 100,000 population and epidemic peaks every 2 to 5 years. In many industrialized countries, mumps was a major cause of viral encephalitis. Serosurveys conducted prior to mumps vaccine introduction found that in some countries 90% of persons were immune by age 15 years, while in other countries a large proportion of the adult population remained susceptible. In countries where mumps vaccine has not been introduced, the incidence of mumps remains high, mostly affecting children 5 to 9 years old. By the end of 2012, 120 of 194 WHO member states included mumps vaccine in their national immunization schedules. In countries where mumps vaccine coverage has been sustained at high levels, the incidence of the disease has dropped markedly.

6. Reservoirs—Humans.

7. Incubation period—About 16 to 18 days (range, 12–25 days).

8. Transmission—By droplet spread; also direct contact with the saliva of an infected person. Virus has been isolated from saliva from 7 days before the onset of parotitis to 9 days afterwards. Maximum infectiousness occurs between 2 days before onset of parotitis and 5 days afterwards. Inapparent infections can be communicable.

9. Treatment—Antibiotics are not effective. Supportive care.

10. Prevention—Public education should encourage mumps immunization for susceptible individuals. Routine mumps vaccination is recommended in countries with an efficient childhood vaccination program and sufficient resources to maintain high levels of vaccine coverage. Mumps vaccination is recommended at age 12 to 18 months as part of the MMR vaccine, though most countries have a 2-dose schedule, with the second dose given at least 1 month after the first dose. In the USA, data from outbreaks reveal that the effectiveness of 2 doses preventing clinical cases of mumps ranged from 80% to 92%.

Live attenuated mumps virus vaccines are available as monovalent vaccines or trivalent MMR vaccines. Hydrolyzed gelatin and/or sorbitol are used as stabilizers in mumps vaccine, along with neomycin as a preservative. Mumps vaccines are cold-chain-dependent and should be protected from light. Different strains of live attenuated mumps vaccine have been developed in Japan, Russia, Switzerland, and the USA. All licensed strains are judged acceptable by WHO for public health programs, except the Rubini strain, which is not recommended because of demonstrated low efficacy; persons who received this strain should be revaccinated with another strain. In most industrialized countries, only the Jeryl-Lynn strain, or strains derived from it, are accepted because they show no confirmed association with aseptic meningitis.

The reported incidence of adverse events depends on the strain of mumps vaccine. The most common adverse reactions are fever and parotitis. Rare adverse reactions include orchitis, sensorineural deafness, and thrombocytopenia. Aseptic meningitis, resolving spontaneously in less than 1 week without sequelae, has been reported at frequencies ranging from 0.1 to 100 cases per 100,000 vaccine doses. This reflects differences in vaccine strains and their preparation as well as variations in study design and case ascertainment. Better data are needed to establish more precise estimates of aseptic meningitis incidence in recipients of different strains of mumps vaccine. The rates of aseptic meningitis due to mumps vaccine are at least 100-fold lower than rates of aseptic meningitis due to infection with wild mumps virus. Jeryl-Lynn or Jeryl-Lynn-derived strains are not likely to cause aseptic meningitis.

Accumulated global experience in industrialized countries shows that 2 doses of vaccine afford better protection against mumps than a single dose. The first dose is usually given as MMR vaccine at the age of 12 to 18 months. The age of administration of the second dose may range from the second year of life to age at school entry, depending on programmatic considerations aimed at optimizing vaccination coverage. Less commonly, the second vaccination may be delivered through supplementary campaigns in developing countries.

Countries intending to use mumps or MMR vaccine during mass campaigns should give special attention to planning. The mumps vaccine strain should be carefully selected and health workers should receive training on expected rates of adverse events following immunization and on community advocacy and health education activities. For the purposes of mass campaigns for measles and rubella (MR) elimination, MR vaccine is preferable over MMR in order to minimize the risk of adverse events and simplify risk communication for health workers in the field.

Mumps vaccine is contraindicated in persons with evidence of severe immunosuppression (e.g., cluster of differentiation 4 [CD4+] glycoprotein percentages < 15% [all ages] and CD4+ < 200 cells/mm^3 [age > 5 years] for ≥ 6 months), including those with human immunodeficiency virus infection, congenital immunodeficiencies, and immunosuppression due to high doses of steroids or chemotherapeutic agents. Treatment with a low dose of steroids on alternate days, topical steroid use, and aerosolized steroid preparations are not, however, contraindications. Pregnant women, or women planning a pregnancy in the next month, should not receive mumps vaccine, although no evidence exists that mumps vaccine causes fetal damage.

11. Special considerations—

1) Reporting: WHO recommends making mumps a notifiable disease in all countries.

2) Epidemic measures: immunize susceptibles, especially those at risk of exposure. Serologic screening to identify susceptibles is impractical and unnecessary since there is no risk in immunizing those who are already immune.

[J. Andrus]

MYCETOMA AND NOCARDIOSIS

DISEASE	ICD-10 CODE
ACTINOMYCETOMA	ICD-10 B47.1
EUMYCETOMA	ICD-10 B47.0
NOCARDIOSIS	ICD-10 A43

Mycetoma has 2 distinct etiologies. Infections caused by fungi are termed "eumycotic mycetoma" or "eumycetoma"; those caused by aerobic actinomycetes (filamentous bacteria) are termed "actinomycotic mycetoma" or "actinomycetoma." The latter manifest either as a mycetoma or as a pulmonary infection of varying severity (nocardiosis).

I. EUMYCOTIC MYCETOMA (eumycetoma)

1. Clinical features—A clinical syndrome characterized by formation of small subcutaneous nodules that enlarge and become fixed to the underlying tissue and the skin, eventually forming sinus tracts that drain purulent material with visible granules (or grains) composed of a matrix component and masses of mycelial fungi; this is considered pathognomonic. Eventually, the lesions result in destruction of structures, deformity, and loss of function. Pain is not a feature; bone invasion is common but pathologic fractures are rare. Mycetoma may spread directly or through the lymphatic system with secondary lesions; hematogenous spread occurs but is uncommon.

Lesions are usually on the foot or lower leg; sometimes on the hand, shoulders, and back; and rarely at other sites. Lesions on the head may invade the brain. It is unusual to have lesions on more than 1 extremity or area of the body.

Eumycetoma may be difficult to distinguish from osteosarcoma, rhabdomyosarcoma, sporotrichosis, chronic osteomyelitis, and botryomycosis (a clinically and pathologically similar entity caused by a variety of bacteria, including staphylococci and Gram-negative bacteria).

2. Risk groups—Disease is most common in those aged 20 to 40 years. Men are 4 times more likely to develop disease, which could be related to more occupational exposure to contaminated soil; alternatively there may be a reporting bias. Disease is more common in agricultural and outdoor laborers. It is also more common in warmer climates where less protective clothing, particularly shoes, is worn. Often there are several cases in 1 family; while genetic factors have been demonstrated, factors related to sharing the same environment may also be important.

3. Causative agents—Eumycetoma is mainly caused by *Madurella mycetomatis*; *Trematosphaeria* (formerly *Madurella*) *grisea*; *Pseudallescheria boydii* spp. complex; *Falciformispora* (formerly *Leptosphaeria*) *senegalensis*.

Some species are more frequent in certain regions depending on the climate (rainfall).

4. Diagnosis—Specific diagnosis depends on visualizing the grains in fresh preparations; the color of the grain may indicate the organism involved. Fine-needle aspiration or a biopsy is often required and identification of the causative bacteria or fungus is best made by culture. Molecular methods such as ribosomal deoxyribonucleic acid internal transcribed spacer region sequencing may be used. Recently infected persons lacking lesions are difficult to diagnose as grains are absent. The extent of a lesion is determined with ultrasonography, computed tomography (CT) scan, or magnetic resonance imaging (MRI); the last may show the individual grain as the dot-in-circle sign.

5. Occurrence—Eumycetoma occurs most commonly in tropical and subtropical regions, in the so-called mycetoma belt between latitudes 15°S and 30°N. Endemic areas typically have a long, hot dry season and a short season of heavy rain. Eumycetoma is more common than actinomycetoma in Africa; it also causes disease elsewhere in the mycetoma belt, albeit less frequently. The highest reported incidences are in Sudan (70% are eumycetoma); however, surveillance is limited or lacking in most endemic areas. Other countries where mycetoma has been reported include the following: in Africa, Senegal, Mauritania, Niger, Mali, Cameroon, Somalia, Kenya, Tunisia, Morocco, Madagascar, Nigeria, and Djibouti; in Asia, mainly India, Yemen, Saudi Arabia, Thailand; in the Middle East, Iran; and in Central and South America, Mexico, Brazil, Venezuela, Argentina, Colombia, and Chile.

6. Reservoirs—Fungi that are etiologic agents of eumycetoma are found in soil and decaying vegetation.

7. Incubation period—Can be months to years from exposure.

8. Transmission—Subcutaneous implantation of organisms from a saprophytic source by penetrating wounds (e.g., thorns, splinters). No person-to-person transmission. Causal agents are widespread in nature; there are no data on the occurrence of subclinical infection.

9. Treatment—

Preferred therapy	• Small lesions are treated with surgical excision alone • Larger lesions require itraconazole 200 mg PO BID for 12 months followed by the possibility of surgical excision after medical therapy
Alternative therapy options	Larger lesions: • Posaconazole ER 300 mg PO BID for the first day, THEN 300 mg daily OR • Posaconazole oral suspension 200 mg PO QID or 400 mg PO BID
	Terbinafine has also been successfully used in some cases of eumycetoma.
Special considerations and comments	• The causative agent should be identified prior to initiation of therapy. • In vitro susceptibility testing does not need to be performed routinely. • Azole antifungals are the drug of choice except fluconazole, which is intrinsically resistant. • Typically 12 months of therapy is appropriate; however, could treat for > 2 years if there is bone involvement. • Recurrence rates are high as the fungus is not eradicated.

Note: BID = twice daily; ER = extended release; PO = oral(ly); QID = 4 times a day.

10. Prevention—Protect against puncture wounds by wearing shoes and protective clothing. Early diagnosis and treatment can prevent the debilitating effect of chronic disease.

11. Special considerations—Medical education on mycetoma: early detection, correct diagnosis, and proper treatment are important for a good therapeutic outcome.

II. NOCARDIOSIS AND ACTINOMYCETOMA

1. Clinical features—Pulmonary infection is the most common clinical presentation of infection with nocardia and can present as pneumonia, lung abscesses, or cavitary lesions. Contiguous spread within the thoracic cavity and hematogenous dissemination, particularly to the central nervous system, are common. Superficial abscess or localized cellulitis also occur following inoculation injuries with contaminated soil. Mycetoma is a specific chronic progressive clinical syndrome involving infection with *Nocardia* spp. (or other aerobic actinomycetes) characterized by swelling and suppuration of subcutaneous tissues and formation of sinus tracts, predominately located in the distal extremities.

2. Risk groups—Immunocompromised status (e.g., due to alcoholism, diabetes, or steroid use) is a risk factor in more than 60% of infections; the incidence in those with acquired immunodeficiency syndrome is lower than expected, even accounting for sulfamethoxazole prophylaxis. Men have a greater risk than women of becoming infected; the male-to-female ratio is 3:1.

3. Causative agents—*Nocardia asteroides* complex (including *N. asteroides, Nocardia farcinica, Nocardia nova,* and *Nocardia carnea*); *Nocardia brasiliensis, Nocardia otitidiscaviarum, Nocardia cyriaci-georgica,* and *Nocardia abscessus.*

4. Diagnosis—Diagnosis of nocardiosis is difficult since clinical manifestations are nonspecific, requiring identification from clinical samples. Preliminary diagnosis may be available from microscopic examination of stained smears of sputum, pus, cerebrospinal fluid, bronchial washings or tissue and may reveal beaded Gram-positive, weakly acid-fast, branched filaments; colonies generally appear as snowballs with aerial hyphae. Culture confirmation is desirable but often difficult and any suspicion of nocardial infection should be passed on to the microbiology laboratory to enhance diagnosis. Biopsy or autopsy usually clearly establishes involvement, although histopathology may be nonspecific. Current serologic tests are nonspecific with an exception of a serologic test for detecting *N. brasiliensis.* The extent of the lesion is determined with ultrasonography, CT scan, or MRI; the last may show the individual grain as the dot-in-circle sign.

5. Occurrence—An occasional sporadic disease in people and animals in all parts of the world. *N. asteroides* complex is the most common cause of nocardial pulmonary and disseminated disease worldwide. *N. brasiliensis* is the most common cause of nocardial cutaneous and lymphocutaneous infections and mycetomas reported predominantly in tropical and subtropical regions of southern USA, Central and South America, and Australia.

6. Reservoirs—Found worldwide as an environmental saprophyte in soil, water, and organic material.

7. Incubation period—Uncertain; probably a few days to a few weeks.

8. Transmission—Typically acquired through inhalation or skin inoculation. Not directly transmitted from humans or from animals to humans. Organism-specific virulence variation and host exposure are important determinants of susceptibility.

9. Treatment—Concurrent disinfection of discharges and contaminated dressings.

Preferred therapy	Mild: • TMP/SMX (5–10 mg/kg PO of TMP component in 2 divided doses)
	Severe: • TMP/SMX 15 mg/kg/day IV in 3 or 4 divided doses PLUS • Imipenem-cilastatin 500 mg IV every 6 hours
Alternative therapy options	Mild: • Minocycline 100 mg PO BID • If susceptible, consider amoxicillin-clavulanate, doxycycline, macrolides, or fluoroquinolones
	Severe: • Linezolid 1,200 mg/day PO or IV in 2 divided doses OR • Amikacin (15–30 mg/kg/day IV once daily) AND imipenem-cilas-tatin (2–3 g/day IV in 3–4 divided doses) or meropenem (3 g IV in 3 divided doses for complicated infections other than nocardial infection) or ceftriaxone (2–4 g/day IV in 1–2 divided doses if CNS involvement) or cefotaxime (6–12 g/day IV in 3–4 divided doses if CNS involvement) OR • Amikacin + TMP/SMX
Special considerations and comments	• Antimicrobial sensitivities should be performed on all isolates and this should be used to guide treatment choice. • Attempts at determining the *Nocardia* spp. should be made as susceptibilities vary. Isolates should be referred to a reference laboratory with expertise in *Nocardia* spp. identification and for susceptibility testing. • Clinical improvement is evident within 3–5 days or at most 10 days after initiation of appropriate therapy. • Surgical excision may be required depending on extent and site of lesions or response to medical therapy. • Because of variable resistance, empiric coverage should include 2 or 3 agents in severe infections. • Treatment duration typically is 3–6 months for mild infections, 6–12 months for severe infections, and ≥ 1 year in immunosup-pressed patients. • For patients with skin or soft tissue infections, consider ≥ 6 months of treatment; for immunocompetent patients with pulmonary or systemic infections not involving CNS, consider ≥ 6–12 months; for immunocompromised patients or those with a CNS infection, consider ≥ 1 year; for actinomycetoma treatment, duration is 2–3 years. • Linezolid has severe hematologic toxicity when used longer term; typically, it is not used. • Primary prophylaxis is not necessary.

Note: BID = twice daily; CNS = central nervous system; IV = intravenous(ly); PO = oral(ly); TMP/SMX = trimethoprim-sulfamethoxazole.

10. Prevention—Not applicable.

11. Special considerations—None.

Bibliography

van de Sande WWJ. Global burden of human mycetoma: a systematic review and meta-analysis. *PLoS Negl Trop Dis.* 2013;7(11):e2550.

[K. Beer]

NIPAH AND HENDRA VIRAL DISEASES

DISEASE	ICD-10 CODE
NIPAH VIRUS INFECTION	ICD-10 B33.8
HENDRA VIRUS INFECTION	ICD-10 B33.8

1. Clinical features—Nipah virus (NiV) manifests primarily as encephalitis. Hendra virus (HeV) has been identified in 7 humans to date and appears to manifest either as a respiratory illness or as a prolonged and initially mild meningoencephalitis.

Symptoms range in severity from mild to coma and/or respiratory failure and death and include fever and headaches, sore throat, dizziness, drowsiness and disorientation, influenza-like symptoms, and atypical pneumonitis. Subclinical infections also occur.

Pneumonitis was prominent in the 2 initial HeV cases—1 of which was fatal—whereas NiV cases have been largely encephalitic and were initially misdiagnosed as Japanese encephalitis. A proportion of patients with NiV display pulmonary involvement with atypical pneumonitis; the majority of patients who survive acute NiV encephalitis make a full recovery but up to 20% have residual neurologic deficits. Mild late-onset disease and relapse encephalitis have been observed several months after initial infection. The case-fatality rate varies between 40% and 75%.

2. Risk groups—All ages are susceptible. People in contact with swine potentially infected with NiV are at increased risk of infection. All recorded cases of HeV infection in humans have been the result of very close contact with infected horses. People at risk are horse owners, animal technicians, and veterinarians. There is the potential for rural populations in contact with *Pteropus* bats to become infected, though infection in bat carers in Australia has not been recorded; ingestion of palm sap contaminated with bat excreta has been documented in South Asia.

3. Causative agents—HeV and NiV are members of a new genus, *Henipavirus*, of the Paramyxoviridae family.

4. Diagnosis—NiV or HeV infection can be confirmed by direct detection of virus by virus isolation or polymerase chain reaction (PCR) in blood, cerebrospinal fluid (CSF), urine, oropharyngeal secretions, nasal or oral swabs, and bronchial washings if collected at the early stage of infection. At a later stage, immunoglobulin class M and immunoglobulin class G antibodies may be detectable in the serum and CSF by enzyme-linked immunosorbent assay or by serum neutralization assays. If death occurs rapidly and only tissues (e.g., brain, spleen) are available, diagnosis should be confirmed by PCR or virus isolation or by immunohistochemistry in formalin-fixed tissues and paraffin embedded blocks.

5. Occurrence—HeV, first recognized in 1994 in Australia, has caused severe respiratory disease in horses in Queensland; in 1994, 3 human cases followed close contact with horses with respiratory or neurologic disease, the first 2 during the initial outbreak and the third occurring 13 months after an initially mild meningitis illness, when the virus reactivated to cause a fatal encephalitis. Sporadic cases of disease in horses have continued to occur in coastal Queensland and northern New South Wales from 1999 to the time of writing, with a spike of outbreaks and cases in 2011. A mild human case occurred in 2004 in a veterinarian following an autopsy on a euthanized horse in Cairns, North Queensland; 2 further human cases occurred during an outbreak in horses at a veterinary clinic in Brisbane, Queensland, in 2008; and a fatal case occurred in August 2009 in Cawarral, Queensland; all presented with a moderate-to-severe influenza-like illness requiring hospitalization. All human infections have been associated with contact with infected horses.

NiV was first identified in 1999 in Malaysia as a cause of severe respiratory disease in domestic swine in the pig-farming provinces of Perak, Negeri Sembilan, and Selangor. Asymptomatic infection in the pigs was common and the case-fatality rate was generally low (5%). The first human case is believed to have occurred in 1996, although most cases were identified in the first months of 1999 (with 105 confirmed deaths). During 1999, 22 abattoir workers in Singapore developed NiV infection following contact with pigs imported from Malaysia, with 1 fatality. In 2001, NiV emerged for the first time in Bangladesh and West Bengal, India. In all, there were 11 outbreaks of NiV infection in Bangladesh between 2001 and 2011, with more than 196 cases and a case-fatality rate of about 77%. In the same period, there were 2 confirmed outbreaks in India, with more than 70 cases and a case-fatality rate of about 70%. The outbreaks in India and Bangladesh differed in a number of significant ways from that in Malaysia: there was no evidence of involvement of the intermediate host, swine; a number of cases presented with an acute respiratory distress syndrome, suggesting that transmission could be by inhalation of large droplets; there was strong suggestive evidence of human-to-human transmission for the first time, including nosocomial infections; and there was evidence to suggest that some of the cases were foodborne, hypothesized as a result of ingestion of date palm juice contaminated with virus from infected bats.

6. Reservoirs—Fruit bats, particularly members of the genus *Pteropus*, are the major reservoir hosts of HeV and NiV, without causing overt disease. HeV has been isolated from all 4 Australian members of the genus *Pteropus*; NiV has been isolated from *Pteropus hypomelanus* in Malaysia and from *Pteropus lylei* in Cambodia. Antibodies to Nipah-like or Hendra-like viruses have been found in sera from fruit bats collected in Timor-Leste, Indonesia, New Guinea, Thailand, India, and Madagascar. Recently, African fruit bats of the genus *Eidolon*, family Pteropodidae, were found positive for antibodies against NiV and HeV, indicating that these or related viruses might be present within the geographic distribution of Pteropodidae bats in Africa. NiV has been isolated from *Pteropus medius* bats in Bangladesh. It is therefore reasonable to assume that related viruses exist throughout the range of pteropid bats, spanning a geographic area stretching from Oceania to the Middle East and including Africa.

Testing of other animals has shown variable susceptibility. Cats, pigs, ferrets, guinea pigs, the golden hamster, and inbred mice can all be infected. Recent work has shown that dogs not only succumb to infection but also shed virus. The risk this shedding poses to humans is unknown.

7. Incubation period—From 4 to 32 days.

8. Transmission—There is clear evidence that transmission occurs through direct contact with infected horses (HeV) or swine (NiV) or contaminated tissues. Oral and nasal routes of infection or infection through contaminated bodily fluid entering into cuts and abrasions are suspected in most cases in Australia and Malaysia. In Bangladesh and India, it is documented that transmission can occur as a result of ingestion of contaminated palm sap. In Bangladesh, human-to-human transmission has been reported and is thought to occur through unprotected close contact with infectious human secretions. The period of communicability is unknown. Recurrent infection appears to occur.

9. Treatment—No specific therapeutic agent is currently available.

10. Prevention—

1) Infection control precautions.

2) Health education about precautionary measures to be taken and the need to avoid contact with fruit bats and their guano as well as infected animals such as pigs and horses. Ensure that fruit bats are not able to roost close to pig pens or stables.

3) As NiV outbreaks in domestic animals have preceded human cases, establishing an animal health surveillance system to detect new cases is essential for providing early warning for veterinary and human public health authorities.

4) Isolate and cull infected horses or swine using appropriate personal protective equipment with burial or incineration of carcasses, taking appropriate biosecurity precautions and under official supervision.

5) Restrict movement of horses or pigs from infected farms to other areas.

6) A recombinant subunit vaccine has shown efficacy in animal models and is cross-protective against HeV and NiV. This vaccine has been made recently available for horses in Australia, both to protect horses and to negate the risk to humans in contact with them, though it is unclear how long protection lasts following horse vaccination.

11. Special considerations—

1) Reporting: case report to health authorities is usually mandatory wherever infections occur in livestock or humans.

2) Epidemic measures:

- Precautions for animal handlers: protective clothing, including boots, gloves, gowns, goggles, and face shields; washing of hands and body parts with soap before leaving pig farms.
- Culling of infected horses or swine with burial or incineration of carcasses under official supervision and with biosecurity precautions.
- Restrict movement of horses or pigs from infected farms to other areas.
- Isolate infected humans if person-to-person transmission appears to be a possibility.

3) International measures: prohibit exportation of horses or pigs and horse/pig products from infected areas.

[J. Hughes]

NOROVIRUS INFECTION
(Norwalk-like virus, winter vomiting disease)

DISEASE	ICD-10 CODE
NOROVIRUS INFECTION	ICD-10 A08.1

1. Clinical features—Usually a self-limited, mild-to-moderate disease that often occurs in outbreaks, with clinical symptoms of nausea, vomiting, diarrhea, abdominal pain, myalgia, headache, malaise, low-grade fever, or a combination of these symptoms. Gastrointestinal symptoms typically last 24 to 72 hours. Dehydration is the most common complication.

2. Risk groups—Older adults (>65 years), young children (<5 years), and immunocompromised patients are at elevated risk for severe disease and death.

3. Causative agents—Noroviruses are small (27–32 nm), structured ribonucleic acid viruses classified within the family Caliciviridae; they are highly contagious and recognized as the most common causal agent of sporadic gastroenteritis across all age groups and of gastroenteritis outbreaks worldwide. Differential diagnoses include other viral agents of gastroenteritis such as sapovirus, rotavirus, astrovirus, and enteric adenovirus.

4. Diagnosis—Real-time reverse transcription quantitative polymerase chain reaction (RT-qPCR) assays are the preferred method for norovirus detection on whole-stool samples and vomitus. These assays are highly sensitive and are able to differentiate between norovirus genogroups I and II. Conventional polymerase chain reaction (PCR) followed by sequencing of PCR products is used for genotyping. A multiplex nucleic acid–based assay for a panel of gastrointestinal pathogens and an enzyme immunoassay (EIA) for the detection of norovirus antigen have been cleared by FDA. However, because the sensitivity of the norovirus EIA is limited, these tests should only be used for testing multiple specimens during outbreaks. EIA-negative samples should be confirmed by RT-qPCR.

5. Occurrence—Worldwide and common; frequently occurs in outbreaks but is also an important cause of sporadic disease. Noroviruses account for 9% to 24% of all sporadic gastroenteritis; all age groups are affected, though rates in children younger than 5 years are elevated and more severe disease occurs in adults older than 65 years. Outbreaks have their source in restaurants, day care centers, cruise ships, hotels, and nursing homes. In industrialized countries, outbreaks are most often associated with health care settings.

6. Reservoirs—Humans are the only known reservoir.

7. Incubation period—In volunteer studies, the range was 10 to 50 hours.

8. Transmission—Fecal-oral route, including direct person-to-person contact and indirect transmission through contaminated food, water, or environmental surfaces. Vomitus-oral transmission can also occur through aerosolization, followed by direct ingestion or environmental contamination. Food is contaminated most often by infected food handlers but also by using contaminated water during production (e.g., shellfish, produce). Secondary household transmission is common. Most communicable during acute stage of disease but virus may be shed for 2 to 3 weeks after symptom resolution.

9. Treatment—There is no specific medicine to treat people with norovirus illness. Fluids are recommended for rehydration. Intravenous fluids may be needed for severe dehydration.

10. Prevention—Use hygienic measures applicable to diseases transmitted via fecal-oral route. In particular, hand hygiene using soap and water, environmental disinfection, and exclusion of ill individuals (until 24-72 hours after symptom resolution) can help prevent spread. Alcohol-based hand sanitizers can be used in addition to handwashing but they should not be used as a substitute for washing with soap.

11. Special considerations—

1) Reporting: obligatory report to local health authority of epidemics in some countries; no individual case report.
2) Large-scale outbreaks could be a potential problem in any situation in which water supplies, sanitation, or food preparation do not meet accepted hygiene standards.
3) More information can be found at: https://www.cdc.gov/norovirus/about/treatment.html.

[O. A. Khan, E. Healy]

ONCHOCERCIASIS
(river blindness)

DISEASE	ICD-10 CODE
ONCHOCERCIASIS	ICD-10 B73

1. Clinical features—A chronic, nonfatal filarial disease. Adult worms are found in superficial fibrous nodules in subcutaneous tissues, particularly in the head and shoulders (Americas) or pelvic girdle and lower extremities (Africa). Nodules also occur in deep-seated bundles lying against the periosteum of bones or near joints. Female worms discharge microfilariae that migrate through the skin, often causing an intense pruritic rash as the microfilariae die, with disfiguring skin lesions, including papular and lichenified dermatitis, altered pigmentation, edema, and atrophy of the skin. Pigment changes result in the condition known as leopard skin, while loss of skin elasticity and lymphadenitis may result in the condition known as hanging groin. Microfilariae frequently reach the eye, causing visual impairment and blindness when the microfilariae die. Symptoms are predominantly due to the inflammatory response to endosymbiotic *Wolbachia* bacteria, which are released upon the death of microfilariae. The greater the body load of microfilariae, the greater the risk of developing skin and eye disease. Microfilariae may be found in organs and tissues other than skin and eyes but the clinical significance is unclear; in heavy infections they may also be found in blood, tears, sputum, and urine. Nodding syndrome and seizures have been associated with onchocerciasis, particularly in meso- and hyperendemic areas, but confirmation of the etiology of this epileptic encephalopathy is still under investigation.

Disease manifestations vary between geographic zones, with onchocercal blindness most prevalent in the African savanna; skin manifestations predominate in forest areas. In Yemen and central Sudan, the major disease manifestation is sowda, a hyperpigmented lichenified dermatitis usually affecting 1 limb. In the Americas, blindness predominates.

2. Risk groups—Those who live or work close to fast-flowing rivers where *Simulium* blackfly vectors breed are at highest risk. Severity of disease is related to the cumulative effects of the repeated infections.

3. Causative agents—*Onchocerca volvulus*, a filarial worm belonging to the phylum Nematoda.

4. Diagnosis—Laboratory diagnosis can be made through microscopic examination of fresh superficial skin biopsies incubated in saline for 24 hours at room temperature with observation of 1 or more emerging microfilariae or through the finding of adult worms in excised nodules. Microscopic or deoxyribonucleic acid (DNA) differentiation of *O. volvulus* microfilariae from *Mansonella streptocerca* microfilariae is required where the latter are also endemic. Because of reductions in microfilarial load in people treated with ivermectin, diagnosis from skin-snip biopsies may rely on DNA methodologies using a probe-specific polymerase chain reaction assay. Other diagnostic clues include evidence of ocular manifestations and slit-lamp observations of microfilariae in the cornea, anterior chamber, or vitreous body. Serum antibody testing (using recombinant antigens) provides evidence of prior exposure.

5. Occurrence—Worldwide. An estimated 17 million people are thought to be infected with *O. volvulus* and 198 million people live in areas with transmission potential. More than 99% of cases occur in sub-Saharan Africa, where the disease is transmitted in an extensive area extending west to east below the Sahara from Senegal to Ethiopia, all the way into southern Africa from Angola in the west to Malawi in the east. It also occurs focally in Yemen and remains active in 1 focus that spans 2 countries in the Americas: Brazil and Venezuela. Regional control programs in both Africa and the Americas have had a major impact on the prevalence of disease and in some areas its transmission has been eliminated. The most recent maps can be found at: http://espen.afro. who.int/diseases/onchocerciasis and http://oepa.net/epidemiologia.html.

6. Reservoirs—Humans. The disease can be transmitted experimentally to chimpanzees and has rarely been found in gorillas in nature.

7. Incubation period—Microfilariae are usually found in the skin only after 1 year or more from the time of the infective bite, though they have been found in children as young as 6 months old. *Simulium* vectors can be infective 7 days after a blood meal; the extrinsic incubation period may be longer when ambient temperatures are below 25°C (77°F).

8. Transmission—Human onchocerciasis can only be acquired through the bite of infected female blackflies of the genus *Simulium*. The most important vectors in Africa and Yemen are the *Simulium damnosum* complex and the *Simulium neavei* complexes, as well as *Simulium albivirgulatum* in the Democratic Republic of Congo; in Central America, transmission is mainly from *Simulium ochraceum*; and in South America, *Simulium metallicum* complex, *Simulium sanguineum/amazonicum* complex, *Simulium quadrivittatum*, *Simulium guianense* sensu lato, *Simulium oyapockense*, and other species. Microfilariae, ingested by a blackfly feeding on an infected person, penetrate thoracic muscles of the fly, develop into infective larvae, migrate to the cephalic capsule, are liberated on the skin, and enter the bite wound during a subsequent blood meal. Adult worms live as long as 10 to 14 years and flies can be infected by biting humans as long as living microfilariae occur in the skin (i.e., 10-14 years after last exposure to *Simulium* bites if untreated). No direct person-to-person transmission occurs. Susceptibility is probably universal. Reinfection of infected people is common.

9. Treatment—

Drug	IVM
Dose	150 µg/kg as a single dose (same dose for adults and children)
Route	PO
Alternative drug	Doxycycline 200 mg PO daily for 6 weeks (same dose for adults and children ≥ 9 years)
Duration	Single dose of IVM every 6 months for as long as there is evidence of a continued infection[a]
Special considerations and comments	• IVM is microfilaricidal and does not kill the adult worms. A single dose provides long-lasting (> 6 months) suppression of microfilaria. Studies suggest that IVM treatment twice annually or more frequently facilitates more rapid sterilization of the female worm and that treating a person who no longer lives in an endemic area more frequently, such as every 3–6 months, could result in a shorter duration of symptoms. Treatment for a patient who will not be returning to live in an endemic area should be given every 6 months (and dosing as frequent as every 3 months could be considered) for as long as there is evidence of continued infection.[a] • Doxycycline does not kill microfilariae, so it does not relieve symptoms initially; treatment with IVM would be needed to result in a more rapid decrease of symptoms. A 6-week course of doxycycline kills > 60% of adult female worms and sterilizes 80%–90% of females 20 months after treatment. Safety of simultaneous administration of IVM and doxycycline is unknown. Treating with IVM to reduce the microfilarial load (and therefore reduce the cause of the symptoms) prior to starting doxycycline would be reasonable.

Note: IVM = ivermectin; PO = oral(ly).
[a]Evidence includes skin symptoms such as pruritus, microfilariae in skin biopsies, and microfilariae on eye examination.

10. Prevention—

1) Individual: avoid bites of *Simulium* flies by wearing protective clothing (long sleeves and long pants) and headgear during the day when blackflies bite, by wearing permethrin-treated clothing, and by using an insect repellent such as N,N-diethyl-meta-toluamide.

2) Community level: provide annual or semiannual ivermectin treatment to the eligible population of all endemic communities in an onchocerciasis focus in order to prevent onchocercal morbidity, reduce—and, where possible, interrupt—transmission and prevent new infections.

3) Community-level control and elimination programs: the African Program for Onchocerciasis Control (APOC) was established in 1995 to implement effective and sustainable annual ivermectin community treatment throughout Africa to prevent disease from onchocerciasis. Prior to closing the program in 2015, APOC transitioned towards an elimination program where feasible. The Expanded Special Project for Elimination of Neglected Tropical Diseases launched in 2016 with the goal of elimination and control of 5 neglected tropical diseases, including onchocerciasis, in Africa. The Onchocerciasis Elimination Program for the Americas uses semiannual to 4 times annual mass distribution of ivermectin to prevent transmission and eliminate the disease. Elimination of transmission has been achieved in 11 of 13 foci in the Americas; the last remaining foci are along the Venezuelan-Brazilian border.

11. Special considerations—Epidemic measures: national onchocerciasis elimination programs in endemic countries are making concerted efforts to identify onchocerciasis-endemic areas and to provide community mass drug administration of ivermectin in these areas, as described in Prevention in this chapter.

[R. Chancey]

PARACOCCIDIOIDOMYCOSIS
(South American blastomycosis, paracoccidioidal granuloma)

DISEASE	ICD-10 CODE
PARACOCCIDIOIDOMYCOSIS	ICD-10 B41

1. Clinical features—Paracoccidioidomycosis is a systemic granulomatous mycosis that can affect any organ in the human body. It typically presents as a chronic, progressive disease in men from tropical and subtropical Central and South America. There are 2 general clinical forms of the disease that have been described: (a) acute/subacute (juvenile) form and (b) chronic (adult) form.

The juvenile form is characterized by systemic symptoms, including weakness, malaise, fever, and weight loss. Lymphadenopathy and hepatosplenomegaly occur; skin lesions are also common. It occurs more commonly in children, adolescents, and those with immunocompromising conditions.

In the adult form, most patients present with a primary lung infection, with cough, dyspnea, malaise, and fever. Approximately one-third of patients develop chronic pulmonary sequelae (e.g., pulmonary fibrosis, emphysema). Mucous membrane involvement is common, including laryngeal, pharyngeal, and/or nasal lesions. Cutaneous lesions are less common and result from hematogenous dissemination from the lungs.

2. Risk groups—Occurs primarily in adult men, especially those working in agriculture. Immunocompromised individuals may be at risk for severe disease.

3. Causative agents—*Paracoccidioides brasiliensis*, a thermally dimorphic fungus geographically restricted to areas of South and Central America. Four different phylogenetic lineages (S1, PS2, PS3, and PS4) have been recognized. *Paracoccidioides lutzii* was described as a new species in 2014 and is also able to produce active disease.

4. Diagnosis—Direct microscopy and histopathology allow prompt diagnosis of this disease. In tissue, presence of granuloma is an important clue to diagnosis. Another important clue is the visualization of yeast cell surrounded by multiple budding daughter blastoconidia (pilot's wheel). In culture, *Paracoccidioides* spp. show slow mycelial (> 20 days at 22°C–24°C) and yeast growth (~10 days at 36°C–37°C [96.8°F–98.6°F]). Serology for antibody to *Paracoccidioides* spp. is available in some areas. Quantitative tests for antibody detection are useful for treatment follow-up.

5. Occurrence—Endemic in tropical and subtropical regions of Latin America from Mexico to Argentina. Approximately 80% of cases are thought to occur in Brazil, with considerably fewer cases reported from Colombia, Venezuela, Belize, Nicaragua, the Guianas, Ecuador, and Argentina. Highest incidence is in adults aged 30 to 50 years. Although the juvenile form appears to affect both sexes equally, the adult form affects men 6 to 15 times more frequently than women, likely secondary to the ability of *Paracoccidioides* to bind estrogen (which disallows transformation to the yeast phase needed for tissue invasion).

6. Reservoirs—The habitat of *P. brasiliensis* remains unknown; however, cases within endemic regions appear to be restricted to tobacco- or coffee-growing areas with the following characteristics: acidic soil, moderate temperatures (12°C–30°C [53.6°F–86°F]), and annual rainfall between 100 and 400 cm. Infection has been documented in some animals, including dogs and armadillos; however, animal-to-human transmission is not known to occur.

7. Incubation period—Highly variable; can occur months to years after exposure.

8. Transmission—Likely via inhalation of conidia that reside in soil in endemic areas. There is no known animal-to-person or person-to-person transmission.

9. Treatment—Itraconazole is considered first-line therapy for para-coccidioidomycosis. Reports of other extended azoles (voriconazole and posaconazole) suggest they can also be used successfully. Amphotericin B is usually reserved for severely disseminated or critically ill patients but should be followed up with therapy with an oral agent as amphotericin alone is not curative. An imidazole, ketoconazole, is effective; however, it has a less favorable side effect profile.

Sulfonamide antibiotics are another option—they are cheaper but less effective than azole antifungals with higher relapse rates. Sulfadiazine requires 3 to 5 years of treatment and trimethoprim-sulfamethoxazole requires a median time of therapy of 2 years (as compared with 12 months for itraconazole).

Preferred therapy	Mild-to-moderate cases:
	• Itraconazole 200 mg PO once daily for 12 months
	Severe cases:
	• Liposomal AMB 3–5 mg/kg/day IV (preferred) until clinical improvement; followed by itraconazole (see Mild-to-moderate cases)
Alternative therapy options	• Sulfamethoxazole + trimethoprim 160–240 mg + 800–1200 mg PO/IV every 12 hours for 12–24 months based on disease severity
	• Voriconazole 400 mg PO/IV twice daily for 3 days, THEN 200 mg twice daily for 6–9 months
	• Ketoconazole 200–400 mg PO daily for 9–12 months

Note: AMB = amphotericin B; IV = intravenous(ly); PO = oral(ly).

10. Prevention—Not applicable.

11. Special considerations—None.

[D. Caceres, S. Tsay]

PARAGONIMIASIS

DISEASE	ICD-10 CODE
PARAGONIMIASIS	ICD-10 B66.4

1. Clinical features—Paragonimiasis, also known as lung fluke or lung distomiasis, is a trematode infection primarily involving the lungs and pleura. Most patients present with chronic respiratory symptoms, including cough, hemoptysis, and/or pleuritic chest pain.[1,2] Eosinophilia is common and chest X-ray findings include diffuse and/or segmental infiltrates, nodules, cavities, cysts, and/or pleural effusions. The disease is frequently mistaken for pulmonary tuberculosis. Early and extrapulmonary infections can present with a wide array of symptoms. Migratory subcutaneous nodules are the most common extrapulmonary symptom. Central nervous system infections are less common but may have devastating effects. Patients with cerebral infection can present with headache, mental confusion, behavioral and visual changes, seizures, focal motor signs, and cerebral hemorrhage.

2. Risk groups—Those ingesting raw or undercooked freshwater snails, crabs, or crayfish. Children may be at increased risk in endemic areas. Consumption of raw wild boar meat has been reported as a risk factor in Japan. Wild boars act as paratenic hosts where juvenile parasites migrate through tissue without developing into adults.

3. Causative agents—There are more than 50 species of *Paragonimus* reported, some of these are now grouped in complexes. Only 9 species and/ or complexes can infect humans: *Paragonimus westermani*, *Paragonimus skrjabini*, *Paragonimus heterotremus*, and *Paragonimus siamensis* are endemic in Asia; *Paragonimus africanus* and *Paragonimus uterobilateralis* in Africa; *Paragonimus mexicanus* (*Paragonimus peruvianus*) and *Paragonimus caliensis* (previously considered part of *P. mexicanus*)[3] in Latin America; and *Paragonimus kellicotti* in North America. Adult parasites are typically reddish brown in color, plump, and coffee bean-shaped (7-16 mm × 4-8 mm). Eggs are operculated and variable in size (80-120 × 45-70 μm). Species discrimination is done best by molecular methods.

4. Diagnosis—Blood, sputum, and bronchio-alveolar lavage (BAL) specimens with eosinophilia can suggest the diagnosis. Definitive diagnosis is made by demonstration of eggs in the sputum (sensitivity 28%-38%), BAL, and/or in stools. Eggs may be found as orange-brown flecks, in which masses of eggs are seen microscopically. The Ziehl-Nielsen stain used to diagnose tuberculosis is superior to the direct wet mount to detect *Paragonimus* eggs but slides need to be examined at lower magnification.[4,5] Ova are rarely found in pleural fluid but fluid findings may be compatible with empyema. The enzyme-linked immunosorbent assay (ELISA) is highly sensitive (99%) and specific (99%) for *P. westermani*. Other species-specific ELISA tests have been reported with similar performance.[6] CDC performs a highly sensitive (96%) and specific (99%) immunoblot assay for *P. westermani*. Although some cross-reactivity exists, ELISA and immunoblot tests for *P. westermani* may fail to detect antibodies in patients infected with other *Paragonimus* spp. ELISA and immunoblotting tests are particularly helpful in early stages of infection when eggs are not yet excreted by immature parasites. Antibodies against *Paragonimus* can be detected as early as 2 to 3 weeks after infection.

5. Occurrence—Paragonimiasis has been reported in Asia, Africa, and the Americas. It is estimated that 293.8 million people worldwide are at risk of infection and more than 23 million are infected. China has the highest burden (95% of world's cases), followed by India, Korea, the Philippines, eastern Nigeria, southeastern Cameroon, and South America (mostly in Ecuador and Peru).[7,8] The world's burden of paragonimiasis is estimated at 190,000 disability-adjusted life years. However, recent reports suggest that these calculations greatly underestimated the impact of the infection.[9]

6. Reservoirs—Dogs, pigs, cats, and wild carnivores are definitive hosts and act as reservoirs. Humans are accidental hosts. Wild boars act as paratenic hosts in Japan.

7. Incubation period—Immature flukes released in the intestine can migrate through different organs, presenting with nonspecific acute symptoms 2 to 3 weeks after infection. Clinical symptoms can last up to 12 weeks depending on the organs involved and the number of infecting parasites. After mating in the pleural space, flukes finish their migration to the lungs and start producing eggs. Mature flukes cause chronic pulmonary symptoms, which can take as long as 27 months to appear. Most patients with light infections have no symptoms and some may present after being asymptomatic for many years.

8. Transmission—Paragonimiasis is transmitted through consumption of raw or partially cooked freshwater crabs or crayfish containing infective metacercariae. Metacercariae excyst in the duodenum, penetrate the intestinal wall, migrate through the tissues, become encapsulated (usually in the lungs), and develop into egg-producing adults in about 5 to 6 weeks. Eggs, either when expectorated in sputum or passed in the feces, gain access to freshwater and develop an embryo in 2 to 4 weeks. This embryo hatches as a free-swimming miracidium that penetrates suitable freshwater snails (first intermediate host) and undergoes asexual reproduction (3–5 months). Cercariae emerge from the snails and encyst, forming metacercariae in freshwater crabs and crayfish (second intermediate hosts) in 6 to 8 weeks. Ingestion of raw crustaceans with alcohol, brine, or vinegar is common in endemic areas and perpetuates transmission. The consumption of undercooked meat from infected mammalian hosts (e.g., wild boars) may also transmit the infection.[10] Tourists sampling local foods may get infected. Eggs may be excreted by the definitive mammalian hosts for up to 20 years but the duration of infection in snail and crustacean hosts is not well defined. Contaminated cooking utensils, such as knives or cutting boards, have been implicated in transmission.[11] Paragonimiasis is not transmitted from person to person.

9. Treatment—All cases should be treated in order to avoid complications associated with pleuropulmonary and extrapulmonary disease.[12]

Drug	Praziquantel
Dose	75 mg/kg in 3 equally divided doses
Route	PO
Alternative drug	Triclabendazole 10 mg/kg PO every 24 hours[13]
Duration	2–3 days (95% cure rate)[14]
Special considerations and comments	• Pregnancy: category B.[15] • Lactation: found in breast milk. Recommended not to breastfeed during treatment and for 72 hours after last ingestion.[16] • Allergy to praziquantel or any of the contents: desensitization is an option or alternative therapies are recommended.[17] • Use with caution: concomitant GERD medications, neurocysticercosis, and abnormal liver function.[18]

Note: GERD = gastroesophageal reflux disease; PO = oral(ly).

10. Prevention—Education of the population in endemic areas regarding paragonimiasis transmission, diagnosis, and treatment is effective in decreasing the incidence of the disease.[19] Education on safe food-handling and preparation is key to decreasing transmission. CDC recommends cooking or boiling crayfish to reach an internal temperature of 63°C (145°F).[20]

11. Special considerations—None.

References

1. Chai JY. Paragonimiasis. *Handb Clin Neurol.* 2013;114:283–296.
2. Lane MA, Barsanti MC, Santos CA, Yeung M, Lubner SJ, Weil GJ. Human paragonimiasis in North America following ingestion of raw crayfish. *Clin Infect Dis.* 2009;49(6):e55–61.
3. Lenis C, Galiano A, Vélez I, Vélez ID, Muskus C, Marcilla A. Morphological and molecular characterization of Paragonimus caliensis Little, 1968 (Trematoda: Paragonimidae) from Medellin and Pichinde, Colombia. *Acta Trop.* 2018;183:95–102.
4. Ratsavong K, Quet F, Nzabintwali F, et al. Usefulness and limits of Ziehl-Neelsen staining to detect paragonimiasis in highly endemic tuberculosis areas. *Parasite Epidemiol Control.* 2017;2(1):1–7.
5. Slesak G, Inthalad S, Basy P, et al. Ziehl-Neelsen staining technique can diagnose paragonimiasis. *PLoS Negl Trop Dis.* 2011;5(5):e1048.
6. Pothong K, Komalamisra C, Kalambaheti T, Watthanakulpanich D, Yoshino TP, Dekumyoy P. ELISA based on a recombinant Paragonimus heterotremus protein for serodiagnosis of human paragonimiasis in Thailand. *Parasit Vectors.* 2018;11(1):322.
7. Keiser J, Utzinger J. Emerging foodborne trematodiasis. *Emerg Infect Dis.* 2005;11(10):1507–1514.
8. Furst T, Keiser J, Utzinger J. Global burden of human food-borne trematodiasis: a systematic review and meta-analysis. *Lancet Infect Dis.* 2012;12(3):210–221.

9. Feng Y, Fürst T, Liu L, Yang G-J, et al. Estimation of disability weight for paragonimiasis: a systematic analysis. *Infect Dis Poverty*. 2018;7(1):110.

10. Blair D. Paragonimiasis. In: Toledo R, Fried B, eds. *Digenetic Trematodes*. Vol 766. New York, NY: Sprinter-Verlag; 2014:115-152.

11. Choo J-D, Suh B-S, Lee H-S, Lee J-S, Song C-J, Shin D-W, Lee Y-H, et al. Chronic cerebral paragonimiasis combined with aneurysmal subarachnoid hemorrhage. *Am J Trop Med Hyg*. 2003;69(5):466-469.

12. Diaz JH. Paragonimiasis acquired in the United States: native and nonnative species. *Clin Microbiol Rev*. 2013;26(3):493-504.

13. Keiser J, Engels D, Büscher G, Utzinger J. Triclabendazole for the treatment of fascioliasis and paragonimiasis. *Expert Opin Investig Drugs*. 2005;14(12):1513-1526.

14. Chai J-Y. Praziquantel treatment in trematode and cestode infections: an update. *Infect Chemother*. 2013;45(1):32-43.

15. Olveda RM, Acosta LP, Tallo V, et al. Efficacy and safety of praziquantel for the treatment of human schistosomiasis during pregnancy: a phase 2, randomised, double-blind, placebo-controlled trial. *Lancet Infect Dis*. 2016;16(2):199-208.

16. Bayer HealthCare Pharmaceuticals. Biltricide tablets (praziquantel). 2010. Available at: https://www.accessdata.fda.gov/drugsatfda_docs/label/2010/018714s012lbl.pdf. Accessed May 28, 2020.

17. Kyung SY, Cho YK, Kim YJ, et al. A paragonimiasis patient with allergic reaction to praziquantel and resistance to triclabendazole: successful treatment after desensitization to praziquantel. *Korean J Parasitol*. 2011;49(1):73-77.

18. Hong ST. Albendazole and praziquantel: review and safety monitoring in Korea. *Infect Chemother*. 2018;50(1):1-10.

19. Narain K, Devi KR, Bhattacharya S, et al. Declining prevalence of pulmonary paragonimiasis following treatment & community education in a remote tribal population of Arunachal Pradesh, India. *Indian J Med Res*. 2015;141(5):648-652.

20. CDC. Parasites. Available from: https://www.cdc.gov/parasites/paragonimus/index.html. Accessed May 28, 2020.

[M. M. Cabada, C. M. Webb, M. Tanabe]

PEDICULOSIS AND PHTHIRIASIS
(lice)

DISEASE	ICD-10 CODE
PEDICULOSIS AND PHTHIRIASIS	ICD-10 B85

1. Clinical features—Infestation by head lice occurs on hair, eyebrows, and eyelashes; infestation by body lice is of the clothing, especially along the seams of inner surfaces. Pubic lice usually infest the pubic area and, more rarely, facial hair (including eyelashes in heavy infestations), axillae, and body surfaces. Infestation may result in severe itching and excoriation of the scalp or body. Secondary bacterial infection may lead to regional lymphadenitis (especially cervical).

2. Risk groups—Transmission of head lice is not related to cleanliness of the person who acquires an infestation. Transmission usually occurs by direct contact with the hair of any infected person, often among children during play, during sharing of combs, brushes, hats, and helmets, or at slumber parties. Persons at risk for body lice generally have close person-to-person contact in conditions of crowding and poor hygiene. Pubic lice infestation is usually acquired during sexual contact with an infested partner.

3. Causative agents—The ectoparasites *Pediculus capitis* (head louse), *Pediculus corporis* (body louse), and *Phthirus pubis* (pubic louse); adult lice, nymphs, and nits (egg cases) infest people. Lice are host-specific; those that infest nonhuman hosts (e.g., pets) do not infest humans, although they may be present transiently. Both sexes feed on blood. The body louse is the species involved in outbreaks of epidemic typhus caused by *Rickettsia prowazekii*, trench fever caused by *Bartonella quintana*, and epidemic relapsing fever caused by *Borrelia recurrentis*.

4. Diagnosis—A head lice infestation is best diagnosed by finding a live nymph or adult louse in the hair or scalp. However, they are small, move quickly, and can be difficult to see. Use of a fine-toothed louse comb may help in identifying live lice. If they are not found, then finding nits (eggs) on hair shafts (within 0.6 cm [1/4 inch] of the base of the shaft) suggests—but does not confirm—a lice infestation. If no nymphs or adults are seen and the only nits seen are more than 0.6 cm from the base of hair shafts, then the infestation is probably old, is no longer active, and does not need to be treated.

An infestation with body lice is usually diagnosed by finding eggs and crawling lice in the seams of clothing. Sometimes a body louse can be seen crawling or feeding on the skin. Pubic lice infestation is diagnosed by finding excoriations, red flat lesions, or nits on hair in the pubic region or, less commonly, elsewhere on the body.

5. Occurrence—Worldwide. Outbreaks of head lice are common among children in schools and institutions everywhere. Body lice are prevalent among populations with poor personal hygiene, especially in cold climates where heavy clothing is worn and bathing is infrequent, or when people cannot change clothes (e.g., in the case of refugees). The frequency of pubic lice has greatly decreased, attributed to recent changes in pubic hair grooming.

6. Reservoirs—Humans.

7. Incubation period—Life cycle of 3 stages: eggs, nymphs, and adults. The most suitable temperature range for egg production and hatching is 29°C to 32°C (84.2°F–89.6°F). Eggs of human lice do not hatch at temperatures below 22°C (71.6°F). Under optimal conditions, lice eggs hatch in

7 to 10 days. The nymphal stages last about 9 to 12 days for head and body lice and 13 to 17 days for pubic lice. The egg-to-egg cycle averages about 3 weeks. The life cycle of the adult louse is about 1 month.

8. Transmission—For head and body lice, by direct contact with infested persons and objects used by them; for body lice, also by contact with the personal belongings of infested persons, especially shared clothing and headgear. Pubic lice are most frequently transmitted through sexual contact. Because lice leave a febrile host, fever and overcrowding increase transfer from person to person. The period of communicability lasts as long as lice or eggs remain viable on the infested person or on fomites. The adult's life span on the host is approximately 1 month. Nits remain viable on clothing for 1 month. Body lice can survive for up to a week off the host without feeding; head lice and pubic lice only about 2 days. Nymphs can survive 24 hours without feeding. Under suitable environmental conditions, head and pubic lice eggs can remain viable away from the host for up to 7 to 10 days; body lice eggs remain viable for up to a month.

9. Treatment—

Drug	Insecticides (pyrethrins, permethrin 1%, malathion 0.5%)
Dose	Pyrethrins/permethrin:
	• Apply to scalp (head lice) or pubic/perianal/trunk/axillae (pubic lice) for 10 minutes then rinse; repeat in 7–10 days.
	Malathion:
	• Apply to scalp (head lice) or pubic/perianal/trunk/axillae (pubic lice) for 8–10 hours then rinse; repeat in 7–10 days.
	Permethrin 5% cream to entire body skin (body lice)
Route	Topical
Alternative drug	Ivermectin (200–400 μg/kg); usual dose 12 mg PO (4 tablets)
Duration	May repeat in 7–10 days
Special considerations and comments	• Manual removal is an option and is recommended in infants. • Malathion is malodorous. • Avoid ivermectin in pregnancy or children < 15 kg. • Pubic lice: treat sexual contacts < 30 days.

Note: PO = oral(ly).

10. Prevention—

1) Educate the public about diagnosis, treatment, and prevention, including the value of destroying eggs and lice through early detection, safe and thorough treatment of the hair, laundering clothing

and bedding in hot water (55°C [131°F] for 20 minutes), and dry cleaning and/or the use of dryers set on a hot cycle.

2) For head lice, avoid head contact with an infested person and avoid contact with items that have been in contact with hair from an infested person (e.g., hats, scarves, combs, brushes, pillowcases, towels). For body and pubic lice, avoid direct physical contact with infested individuals and their belongings, especially clothing and bedding.

3) Perform direct inspection of body and clothing for evidence of body lice when indicated. Evidence does not support the efficacy and cost-effectiveness of regular screening of children in classroom or schoolwide settings for head lice and nits.

11. Special considerations—

1) School and return to school: children with head lice need not be dismissed early and may return to school after first topical treatment.

2) Epidemic measures: mass treatment with the treatments recommended in Treatment in this chapter, using insecticides clearly known to be effective against prevalent strains of lice. In typhus epidemics, individuals may protect themselves by wearing silk or plastic clothing tightly fastened around wrists, ankles, and neck and by impregnating their clothes with repellents or permethrin.

3) Disaster implications: infectious diseases for which body and head lice are vectors are particularly prone to occur at times of social upheaval, displacement, and prolonged encampment (see Epidemic Louse-Borne Typhus Fever in "Typhus").

[J. Klausner]

PERTUSSIS
(whooping cough)

DISEASE	ICD-10 CODE
PERTUSSIS	ICD-10 A37.0, A37.9
PARAPERTUSSIS	ICD-10 A37.1

1. Clinical features—An acute bacterial infection of the respiratory tract classically characterized by paroxysmal cough and inspiratory whoop. The initial (catarrhal) stage consists of an insidious onset of upper respiratory infection with an irritating cough. Over the course of 1 to 2 weeks, paroxysms develop (paroxysmal phase) and increase in frequency and intensity before gradually improving after 1 to 2 months. Paroxysms are characterized by repeated violent coughing; each series of paroxysms has many coughs without intervening inhalation, which may be followed by a characteristic high-pitched inspiratory whoop. Paroxysms frequently end with the expulsion of clear, tenacious mucus often followed by vomiting. Between paroxysms, infected persons may appear well. Infants younger than 6 months may have cough without the typical whoop or may present with apnea.

In many industrialized countries with long-standing infant immunization and high coverage, an increasing number of cases are reported in adolescents and adults. Many such cases occur in previously immunized persons and suggest waning immunity following immunization. In those with partial immunity, symptoms vary from a mild, atypical respiratory illness to the full whooping syndrome.

Complications include pulmonary hypertension, pneumonia, atelectasis, seizures, encephalopathy, weight loss, hernias, and death. Pulmonary complications are the most common cause of death; fatal encephalopathy, probably hypoxic, and inanition from repeated vomiting occasionally occur. The number of fatalities in vaccinated populations is low. Most cases of severe disease and deaths occur in infants younger than 6 months, often in those too young to have completed primary immunization. Case-fatality rates are less than 1 per 1,000 in industrialized countries; in developing countries they are estimated at 3.7% for children younger than 1 year and 1% for children aged 1 to 4 years. Pertussis remains among the most lethal diseases of unimmunized infants and young children, especially in those with underlying malnutrition and simultaneous enteric or respiratory infections. Parapertussis is a similar but occasional and milder disease.

2. Risk groups—Susceptibility of nonimmunized individuals is universal and pertussis can be severe in immuno-naive individuals of any age. The highest incidence of pertussis, as well as the highest risk for severe or fatal pertussis, is in infants but infection also occurs in adolescents and adults. Incidence, morbidity, and mortality are higher in females than in males for unknown reasons. Secondary attack rates of up to 90% have been observed in nonimmune household contacts. Disease confers immunity but not lifelong. Maternal antibodies are actively transported across the placenta; this observation has formed part of the rationale in certain countries to vaccinate pregnant women to reduce severe and fatal pertussis in young infants.

3. Causative agents—*Bordetella pertussis*, the bacillus of pertussis sensu stricto; *Bordetella parapertussis* causes parapertussis. Bordetellae are Gram-negative aerobic bacteria; *B. pertussis* and *B. parapertussis* are similar species but the latter lacks the expression of the gene coding for pertussis toxin. *Bordetella holmesii* has also been reported to cause a pertussis-like syndrome.

4. Diagnosis—Based on clinical suspicion in the presence of typical signs and symptoms of pertussis. Confirmation requires demonstration of the causal organism from nasopharyngeal specimens obtained during the catarrhal and early paroxysmal stages. Culture is performed on Bordet-Gengou or Regan-Lowe culture media, both supplemented with 15% defibrinated sheep or horse blood; this is considered the gold standard of laboratory confirmation. While it is the most specific diagnosis, culture has limited sensitivity (60%). Polymerase chain reaction (PCR) can be highly sensitive and can be performed on the same biologic samples as cultures. Patient specimens collected by aspirating or swabbing for culture or PCR should be taken from the posterior oral pharynx and not the anterior oral pharynx. PCR sensitivity is also optimized if the specimen is collected during the first 3 weeks of cough. After 4 weeks of cough or after 5 days of antibiotic therapy, PCR will not likely be helpful. Direct fluorescent antibody staining of nasopharyngeal secretions is not recommended because of the occurrence of false-positive and -negative results. Indirect diagnosis is possible by determining a rise in specific immunoglobulin class G (IgG) antibodies directed against the pertussis toxin (anti-PT IgG) in an acute serum of the infected individual collected at the beginning of cough and in a convalescent serum collected 1 month later. In many industrialized countries, single-point anti-PT antibody tests are readily available and useful for diagnosis late in the course of illness when culture and PCR may be negative. Single-point serology results should be interpreted with caution as they do not differentiate between antibodies due to vaccination and those due to infection. Differentiation among *B. parapertussis*, *B. pertussis*, and *B. holmesii* is based on phenotypic, genetic, biochemical, and immunologic differences.

5. Occurrence—An endemic disease common in children everywhere, regardless of ethnicity, climate, or geographic location. Outbreaks occur typically every 3 to 4 years. In communities with active immunization programs and where good nutrition and medical care are available, pertussis still remains endemic, though at greatly reduced rates. Pertussis resurges when immunization rates fall and drops again when immunization programs are reestablished, as seen in Japan, Sweden, and the UK in the 1970s and 1980s. In 2015, WHO reported 142,512 pertussis cases globally and estimated that there were 89,000 deaths, despite an estimated worldwide vaccination coverage of around 86%. Recent modeling suggests annual deaths to be much higher: more than 160,000 deaths globally.

The actual rates of disease are unknown because reporting is incomplete and laboratory confirmation differs from country to country. Since 2004, notable increases in incidence have occurred in Australia, the USA, and some European countries.

6. Reservoirs—Humans are believed to be the only host for pertussis. *B. parapertussis* can also be isolated from ovines.

7. Incubation period—Average 9 to 10 days (range, 6-20 days).

8. Transmission—Through direct contact with discharges from respiratory mucous membranes of infected persons by the airborne route, probably via large droplets. Indirect spread through the air or contaminated objects may occur rarely. Pertussis is highly communicable in the early catarrhal stage and at the beginning of the paroxysmal cough stage (first 2 weeks). Thereafter, communicability gradually decreases and becomes negligible by about 3 weeks despite persisting spasmodic cough with whoop. Patients are considered no longer contagious after 5 days of treatment with erythromycin, clarithromycin, or azithromycin. In vaccinated populations, infants are most often exposed to pertussis in the home by a parent, older sibling, or other caregiver.

9. Treatment—

Drug	Azithromycin[a]
Dose	Infants < 6 months: • 10 mg/kg/day as a single daily dose (≤ 500 mg/day)
	Infants and children ≥ 6 months: • Day 1: 10 mg/kg (≤ 500 mg) • Days 2–5: 5 mg/kg/day (≤ 250 mg) as a single daily dose
	Adults: • Day 1: 500 mg • Days 2–5: 250 mg/day as a single daily dose
Route	PO
Alternative drug	• Erythromycin 40–50 mg/kg PO divided into 4 daily doses for 14 days (≤ 2 g/day) • Clarithromycin 14 mg/kg PO divided into 2 daily doses for 7 days (≤ 1 g/day) • TMP/SMX 8/40 mg/kg PO divided into 2 daily doses for 14 days (≤ 320/600 mg/day)
Duration	• 5 days for azithromycin • 14 days for erythromycin and TMP/SMX • 7 days for clarithromycin

(Continued)

(Continued)

Special considerations and comments	• The earlier the treatment, the better, whether based on strong clinical suspicion, especially in patients at high risk for severe disease, or based on the results of diagnostic testing.
	• As a general rule, CDC recommends that for patients aged > 1 year treatment should start within 3 weeks of cough onset; for children aged < 1 year and for pregnant women (especially close to delivery) treatment should start within 6 weeks of cough onset.
	• Antibiotics should also be administered to close contacts within 3 weeks of exposure. The recommended antimicrobial agents for treatment or chemoprophylaxis of pertussis are azithromycin, clarithromycin, and erythromycin. Clinicians can also use TMP/SMX.
	• Choice of drugs may depend upon drug availability, costs, likelihood of adverse events and drug interactions, and ease of adherence to the regimen prescribed.
	• For infants aged < 1 month, azithromycin is preferred for postexposure prophylaxis and treatment because azithromycin has not been associated with infantile hypertrophic pyloric stenosis, whereas erythromycin has been associated with this condition.
	• Avoid azithromycin in patients with cardiac electrical conduction defects, especially with prolonged QT intervals.
	• In developing countries the only drugs available may be erythromycin or TMP/SMX. They require more doses and longer duration of administration, highlighting the importance of close follow-up and monitoring of compliance in order to help stop transmission in outbreaks.

Note: PO = oral(ly); TMP/SMX = trimethoprim-sulfamethoxazole.
[a]As recommended by CDC.

10. Prevention—

1) Educate the public, particularly parents of infants, about the dangers of whooping cough and the advantages of initiating immunization on time (between 6 weeks and 3 months after birth, depending on the country) and of adhering to the immunization schedule. This is important because of the widespread past and present negative publicity given to adverse immunization reactions associated with pertussis vaccination.

2) Pertussis is generally recalcitrant to routine control measures and immunization is the best means to control pertussis. Active primary immunization against *B. pertussis* infection is by administering 3 doses of either killed whole-cell pertussis (wP) or acellular pertussis (aP) vaccines. The latter contains 1 to 5 different components of *B. pertussis*. These are usually given in combination with diphtheria and tetanus toxoids adsorbed on aluminum salts

(diphtheria/tetanus and whole-cell pertussis vaccine [DTwP] or diphtheria/tetanus and acellular pertussis vaccine [DTaP]). Both aP and wP vaccines are very safe; local and transient systemic reactions are less commonly associated with aP vaccines than with wP vaccines. Similar high efficacy (80%) is observed with the best aP and wP vaccines, although efficacy can differ among available vaccine products. Protection is greater against severe disease and wanes over time; many industrialized and middle-income countries therefore recommend a fourth dose during the second year of life, a fifth dose before school entry, and a reduced dose booster for adolescents and/or adults. Pertussis vaccination does not protect against parapertussis.

Many industrialized and middle-income countries have completely replaced wP vaccines with aP vaccines, largely because of parents' concerns about the comparative increased occurrence of local reactions of wP. Though wP vaccines have a higher occurrence of local and systemic reactions such as fever, price considerations affect the wider implementation of aP vaccines. In most developing countries, however, as per WHO's recommendations, wP vaccines continue to be used in developing countries because they provide longer duration of protection, are less expensive, and effectively reduce the burden of pertussis.

Schedules vary but in all countries the goal should be to reach at least 90% coverage with a primary series of 3 doses of DTwP/DTaP in infants in all areas. In countries where immunization programs have considerably reduced pertussis incidence, a fourth dose is recommended. The optimal timing of a fourth dose and the need and timing for a fifth dose or adolescent/adult booster doses should be based on the local epidemiology. Vaccines containing wP are not recommended after the seventh birthday since local reactions may be increased in older children and adults. Formulations of acellular pertussis vaccine for use in adolescents and adults have been licensed and are available in several countries.

DTwP/DTaP can be given simultaneously with oral poliovirus vaccine and at different sites from inactivated poliovirus vaccine (IPV); *Haemophilus influenzae* type b (Hib) vaccine; hepatitis B (HB) vaccine; pneumococcal and meningococcal conjugate vaccine; and vaccines for measles, mumps, rubella. Combination vaccines with Hib, IPV, and HB are available and are widely used in Europe and North America.

Minor adverse reactions such as local redness and swelling, fever, and agitation often occur after immunization with wP vaccine (1 in 2-10 cases). Prolonged crying and febrile seizures are less common (1 in 1000 cases); hypotonic-hyporesponsive episodes are rare (1 in 2,000 cases). Although febrile seizures and hypotonic-hyporesponsive episodes may follow DTwP and are disturbing to parents and physicians alike, there is no scientific evidence that these reactions have any permanent consequences. Recent detailed reviews of all available studies conclude that there is no demonstrable causal relationship between DTwP and chronic nervous system dysfunction in children. The only true contraindication to immunization with DTwP/DTaP is an anaphylactic reaction to a previous dose or to any constituent of the vaccine. In young infants with suspected evolving and progressive neurologic disease, immunization may be delayed to permit diagnosis and avoid possible confusion about the cause of symptoms.

11. Special considerations—

1) Reporting: case report to local health authority of suspected and confirmed cases is required in most countries; early reporting may permit better outbreak control. The clinical case definition for pertussis is a coughing illness that lasts at least 2 weeks and presents with at least 1 of the following symptoms: paroxysms (fits) of coughing, inspiratory whooping, post-tussive vomiting (vomiting immediately after coughing), or apnea (with or without cyanosis). For further information, see: https://wwwn.cdc.gov/nndss/conditions/pertussis/case-definition/2020.

2) Epidemic measures: a search for unrecognized and unreported cases may be indicated to protect preschool children from exposure and to ensure adequate preventive measures for exposed children younger than 7 years. Accelerated immunization with the first dose as early as 6 weeks old and the second and third doses at 4-week intervals may be indicated; it is more important to make sure that immunization is completed for those whose schedule is incomplete and that the vaccines are given on time according to the national schedule.

3) Disaster implications: pertussis is a potential problem if introduced into crowded refugee camps containing nonimmunized children.

4) Ensure completion of primary immunization of infants and young children before they travel to other countries if possible; review need for a booster dose.

[J. Andrus]

❖

PINTA
(carate)

DISEASE	ICD-10 CODE
PINTA	ICD-10 A67

1. Clinical features—Pinta is a chronic nonvenereal infection limited to the skin without systemic manifestations. This infection is characterized by early and late stages, as seen in other pathogenic treponemal diseases.

The typical initial lesion, occurring 1 to 8 weeks after exposure, consists of 1 or more scaly erythematous papules or small plaques that usually appear on an exposed part of the body—often the legs, dorsum of the foot, forearms, or back of the hands. Over time, the papules or plaques increase in size to form larger patches. Lesions do not ulcerate but can display a pale central area. The primary stage is often pruritic and can be accompanied by regional lymphadenopathy. The primary lesions may resolve spontaneously without treatment or may persist for many years.

During the secondary stage, which occurs after 3 to 12 months, smaller scaly papules disseminate over a wider area of the body. These treponemal-rich lesions (pintids) may vary in size from less than 0.5 cm to several centimeters. Over time, the lesions coalesce into macules or plaques, tending to change in color from an initial copper red to brown, slate blue-gray, or black. Different forms and colorations may occur simultaneously in different pintids or within a single pintid. This secondary stage may last 2 to 4 years, during which some lesions will heal and others persist or enlarge, sometimes leading to extensive hypopigmentation.

The late (tertiary) stage is characterized by patches or plaques of altered (dyschromic) skin pigmentation of variable size and is accompanied by skin atrophy and hyperkeratosis. The extent of skin pigmentation can vary, resulting in a mottled appearance of the skin. Lesions may change color (brown, gray, slate blue, or black) or lack any color, often coexisting at different stages of evolution and most commonly involving the face and extremities (e.g., wrists, elbows, and ankles).

The differential diagnosis includes syphilis, the late scars of yaws, psoriasis, vitiligo, tinea versicolor, pityriasis alba, melasma, discoid lupus erythematosus, leprosy, and other pigmentary disorders.

2. Risk groups—Pinta usually occurs in children and young adults living in endemic areas (hot, humid areas of Mexico, Central America, and South America). Children are at risk for developing pinta, although peak incidence is in 15- to 30-year-olds. The incidence is similar in males and females.

3. Causative agents—*Treponema carateum*, a species of spirochete bacteria in the genus *Treponema*. The organism multiplies very slowly in humans and has not been cultured.

4. Diagnosis—Based on clinical and epidemiologic findings along with direct microscopic examination (confirmed) and/or serologic tests (presumptive infection) (see "Yaws"). Spirochetes are demonstrable in primary, secondary, and dyschromic (but not achromic) lesions through dark-field microscopic examination. The treponemes that cause pinta, yaws, endemic syphilis (bejel), and syphilis have almost identical morphology on dark field. There are no published data on the use of molecular methods for direct detection of *T. carateum*. Treponemal and nontreponemal serologic tests usually become reactive before or during the secondary lesions and thereafter behave as in venereal syphilis. Rapid treponemal diagnostic tests are increasingly available and do not require laboratory support (see "Yaws"). Other diseases in the differential might be ruled out by histologic examination of the skin lesions.

5. Occurrence—Pinta is increasingly rare and today is found only among isolated rural populations living in crowded conditions in the American tropics. It is predominantly a disease of older children and young adults. Surveys carried out during the mid-1990s by the Pan American Health Organization in targeted Amazonian populations in Brazil, Peru, and Venezuela found few cases. Isolated foci may still exist in Central America and Cuba.

6. Reservoirs—Humans.

7. Incubation period—Usually 2 to 3 weeks.

8. Transmission—Transmissibility is low. The exact mechanism of transmission is unknown but is presumed to be through repeated direct lesion-to-skin contact with an infected person. Treponemes are abundant in initial and early dyschromic skin lesions and can persist even in later disease with the exception of late hypopigmented lesions. Various biting and sucking arthropods, especially blackflies, are suspected (but not proven) biologic vectors. Pinta is not highly contagious and several years of intimate contact may be necessary for transmission. Vertical transmission from mother to fetus during pregnancy is not known to occur; however, the disease could be transmitted from mother to infant through close contact.

9. Treatment—

Preferred therapy	Benzathine penicillin 1.2 MU (adults) or 600,000 units (infants > 10 kg and children < 15 years) IM as a single dose
Alternative therapy options	• Azithromycin 30 mg/kg PO (≤ 2 g) as a single dose • Doxycycline 100 mg PO BID for 7 days for patients allergic to penicillin and azithromycin
Special considerations and comments	Early pinta lesions heal within several months after administration of penicillin but treatment cannot reverse the skin changes of late treatment.

Note: BID = twice daily; IM = intramuscular(ly); MU = million units; PO = oral(ly).

10. Prevention—Those applicable to other nonvenereal treponematoses apply to pinta; see "Yaws."

11. Special considerations—

1) Reporting: pinta should be reported to the local health authority.
2) For disaster implications and international measures, see "Yaws."

[M. Kamb, A. Pillay]

PLAGUE
(pestis)

DISEASE	ICD-10 CODE
PLAGUE	ICD-10 A20

1. Clinical features—Plague has 3 principal presentations: bubonic, septicemic, and pneumonic. Initial signs and symptoms for all phases may be nonspecific, with fever, chills, malaise, myalgia, nausea, prostration, and headache. All forms can be complicated by bacteremia with spread to other organs, disseminated intravascular coagulation, and endotoxic shock. Bubonic plague is characterized by swollen lymph nodes (buboes) in the region of a fleabite or other percutaneous exposure. Fleabites on the legs typically result in buboes in the inguinal area, whereas axillary buboes are often associated with handling or butchering infected animals, though they may also arise through fleabites to the arms. Cervical buboes are rare in industrialized countries but are relatively common in many developing countries where people sleep on dirt floors of flea-infested huts. Regardless of the location, buboes are inflamed and tender and may suppurate. The septicemic form of plague can occur subsequent to bubonic plague (secondary septicemic plague) or without prior lymphadenopathy (primary septicemic plague) and involves bloodstream dissemination to diverse parts of the body, including in some instances the meninges. Septicemic plague is characterized by sudden onset of fever and endotoxemia without prior lymphadenopathy or other localizing symptoms, although some patients experience abdominal pain and other gastrointestinal symptoms. Septicemic plague accounts for approximately 5% to 15% of cases in most series. Pneumonic plague is of special significance because of the potential for person-to-person transmission. Pneumonic plague arises either through hematogenous spread in a patient with untreated bubonic, septicemic plague (secondary pneumonic plague), or inhalation of respiratory droplets from another person or an animal with pneumonic or pharyngeal infection (primary pneumonic plague). Pneumonic transmission can lead to localized outbreaks of primary pneumonic or pharyngeal plague in close contacts. Though naturally acquired plague usually presents as bubonic plague, intentional aerosol dissemination for the purposes of terrorism or warfare would be expected to manifest primarily as pneumonic plague.

Untreated bubonic plague has a case-fatality rate of approximately 50% to 60%. Untreated primary septicemic plague and pneumonic plague are almost invariably fatal. Modern therapy markedly reduces fatalities from bubonic plague; pneumonic and septicemic plague also respond if recognized and treated early (i.e., ≤ 2 days). Plague is a medical and a public health emergency. Further information on this and other plague-related topics or updates can be found at: http://www.cdc.gov/plague.

2. Risk groups—All humans should be considered susceptible to plague. Immunity after recovery is relative; it may not protect against a future large inoculum. Those who live in areas with poor rodent sanitation practices and hunters, trappers, trekkers, veterinary staff, and farmers operating during or following an epizootic are at increased risk of exposure.

3. Causative agents—*Yersinia pestis*, the plague bacillus.

4. Diagnosis—Visualization of characteristic bipolar-staining, safety pin ovoid, Gram-negative organisms in direct microscopic examination of material aspirated from a bubo, sputum, or cerebrospinal fluid (CSF) is suggestive, but not conclusive, evidence of plague infection. Examination by fluorescent antibody test, antigen capture by enzyme-linked immunosorbent assay (ELISA) or dipstick formats, or polymerase chain reaction are more specific and particularly useful in some instances. In the USA, cases are considered confirmed following isolation of *Y. pestis* by culture of bubo aspirates, blood, CSF, or sputum samples or by demonstration of a 4-fold or greater rise or fall in antibody titer. Automated biochemical identification systems occasionally misidentify the organism as a different species (e.g., *Pseudomonas luteola*). A passive hemagglutination test using *Y. pestis* fraction-1 antigen or ELISA are used for serodiagnosis. WHO and others have proposed the use of dipstick (horizontal flow) assays designed to detect *Y. pestis* antigen in clinical samples as a means of rapid diagnosis; however, these tests are not widely available and may not be reliable on all specimen types (e.g., sputum). Medical personnel should be aware of areas where the disease is endemic and should entertain the diagnosis of plague early on; unfortunately, plague is often misdiagnosed, especially in travelers who develop illness after returning from an endemic area, and delays in diagnosis can result in fatalities.

5. Occurrence—While rat-associated plague has been controlled or eliminated from most urban areas of the world, foci of plague persist among wild rodent populations in rural areas on most continents, causing sporadic cases and occasional outbreaks among humans. In the Americas, plague foci are found in northeastern Brazil, the Andean region near the border of Ecuador and Peru, and the western half of the USA. Active and historic foci are also found in scattered locations in East, Central, and southern Africa, the interior of Algeria, and perhaps other African countries bordering the Mediterranean Sea. In Asia, foci of endemic disease occur from northeastern China westward to the Caspian Sea, including boundary areas with Mongolia and Russia. Worldwide a total of 3,248 cases of human plague were reported to WHO from 2010 to 2015, including 584 fatalities. Madagascar accounted for nearly 75% of these cases, with far smaller numbers reported from the Democratic Republic of Congo, Tanzania, Uganda, Peru, Bolivia, the USA, China, Kyrgyzstan, Mongolia, and Russia. It should be noted that routine notification of cases to WHO was discontinued after 2007 and that cases and outbreaks occasionally appear in areas that have been free of the disease for many decades. In 2017, an unprecedented outbreak of pneumonic plague occurred in the capital of Madagascar. The true number of infections was likely much smaller than the approximately 1,800 suspected cases reported; however, the social and economic impact was substantial. In the USA, an average of 7 cases (range, 1–16) are reported annually, usually as sporadic cases or small common source clusters following exposure to wild rodent fleas or bodily fluids from infected rabbits, wild carnivores, or domestic cats or dogs. Average mortality in the USA is approximately 15% and up to 10% of patients have pulmonary involvement. Person-to-person transmission is rare, however. The last confirmed case of person-to-person transmission in the USA occurred in 1924, although a possible instance was also reported in 2014.

6. Reservoirs—Wild rodents are the natural vertebrate hosts of plague and play a key role in maintaining natural plague cycles by serving as sources of infection (amplifying hosts) for the flea vectors of the disease. Some of these species can survive for weeks to months in the burrows of their hosts and appear to represent a significant reservoir of infection. Certain other mammals, including lagomorphs (rabbits and hares), wild carnivores, and domestic cats, may also become infected and act as sources of infection to people. In many developing countries, commensal rats play epidemiologically important roles by moving infected fleas into human dwellings from wild lands or agricultural fields.

7. Incubation period—From 1 to 7 days; for primary plague pneumonia, incubation period is short, lasting 1 to 4 days.

8. Transmission—Two main patterns of transmission for naturally acquired human plague can be distinguished:

1) Human intrusion into the zoonotic (sylvatic) cycle during or following an epizootic. Cases typically result from being bitten by infectious wild rodent fleas. Some of these flea species may remain infective for months under suitable conditions of temperature and humidity. Human cases have also been linked to handling infected animals and domestic pets, particularly house cats and dogs, which can carry *Y. pestis*-infected wild rodent fleas into homes. Cats, and less commonly dogs, may occasionally transmit infection through bites, scratches, or respiratory droplets to owners and veterinary personnel.

2) Infection in commensal rodents (e.g., *Rattus rattus*, *Rattus norvegicus*) and their fleas leads to an entry of the bacteria into human habitat. In that case, the disease is a manifestation of poverty and insufficient conditions of hygiene. Person-to-person transmission by *Pulex irritans* fleas may be important in the South American Andes and a few other places around the world where plague occurs; this flea is abundant in homes or on domestic animals. Risk of exposure concerns the community as a whole in Africa, India, and South America. On a worldwide basis, the most frequent source of exposure for human cases is the bites of infected rat fleas, especially the Oriental rat flea (*Xenopsylla cheopis*). In some countries, wild rodent hosts of plague live in close proximity to humans, as is the case for certain ground squirrels infested with *Oropsylla montana*, the primary vector of plague to humans in North America.

Other important sources of human infection include the handling of infected animals, especially rodents and rabbits but also wild carnivores and domestic cats; rarely, airborne droplets from human patients or household cats with plague pharyngitis or pneumonia; and careless manipulation of laboratory cultures. Human cases acquired by inhalation (primary pneumonic plague) have been reported in the past couple of decades in developing countries. Bubonic plague is not usually transmitted directly unless there is contact with pus from suppurating buboes. Pneumonic plague may be highly communicable under appropriate climatic conditions; overcrowding and cool temperatures facilitate transmission.

In the case of deliberate use, plague bacilli would possibly be transmitted as an aerosol.

9. Treatment—For seriously ill patients, begin parenteral therapy as soon as plague is suspected. Duration of treatment is 10 to 14 days or until 2 days after fever subsides. Oral therapy may be substituted once the patient improves. The regimens listed in the treatment table are guidelines only and may need to be adjusted depending on a patient's age, medical history, underlying health conditions, or allergies. Most recommended antibiotics for plague have relative contraindications for use in children and pregnant women; however, use is justified in life-threatening situations.

Antibiotic	Adult Dose	Route	Notes
Streptomycin	1 g BID	IM	Not widely available in many countries.
Gentamicin	• 5 mg/kg once daily OR • 2 mg/kg loading dose, THEN 1.7 mg/kg every 8 hours	IM/IV	• Not approved by FDA but considered an effective alternative to streptomycin. • Because of poor abscess penetration, consider alternative or dual therapy for patients with bubonic disease.
Levofloxacin	500 mg once daily	IV/PO	Bactericidal. Approved by FDA based on animal studies but limited clinical experience treating human plague. A higher dose (750 mg) may be used if clinically indicated.
Ciprofloxacin	• 400 mg every 8–12 hours OR • 500–750 mg BID	IV/PO	Bactericidal. Approved by FDA based on animal studies but limited clinical experience treating human plague.
Doxycycline	• 100 mg BID OR • 200 mg once daily	IV/PO	Bacteriostatic but effective in a randomized trial when compared with gentamicin.
Chloramphenicol	25 mg/kg every 6 hours	IV	Not widely available in the USA.

Note: BID = twice daily; IM = intramuscular(ly); IV = intravenous(ly); PO = oral(ly).

10. Prevention—The basic objective is to reduce the likelihood of people being bitten by infectious fleas, having direct contact with infective tissues and exudates, or being exposed to patients with pneumonic plague.

1) Educate the public in enzootic areas on the modes of human and domestic animal exposure; on rat-proofing buildings and preventing access to food and shelter by peridomestic or wild rodents through appropriate storage and disposal of food, garbage, and refuse; and on the importance of avoiding fleabites by use of insecticides and repellents. In sylvatic or rural plague areas, the public should be advised to use insect repellents when walking or working in suspect areas and be warned not to camp near rodent burrows and not to handle rodents. Dead or sick animals should be reported to health authorities or other appropriate persons. Dogs and cats in such areas should be protected periodically with

appropriate insecticides to reduce the risk that infectious fleas will be transported into human environs and should not be allowed to roam freely in plague-affected areas. Any animal carcasses brought home by these animals should be disposed of safely.

2) Consider monitoring rodent populations to determine whether epizootics are in progress or conditions indicate that one is likely. The effectiveness of rodent sanitation measures in homes and public areas should also be evaluated. Although flea control is the primary means of controlling plague, rat suppression by poisoning may be used to augment basic environmental sanitation measures; rat control should always be preceded by measures to control fleas (see later). Areas of plague activity can be identified by surveillance of natural foci by testing of fleas collected from rodents and their burrows or nests, by bacteriologic testing of sick or dead wild rodents, and by serologic analyses of samples from wild carnivores and outdoor-ranging dogs and cats. Regular testing should take place to ensure the effectiveness of insecticides on target flea populations.

3) Control rats on ships, on docks, and in warehouses by rat-proofing or periodic fumigation, combined when necessary with destruction of rats and their fleas in vessels and in cargoes, especially containerized cargoes, before shipment and on arrival from locations endemic for plague.

4) Wear gloves when hunting and handling wildlife. Veterinarians and their staff should wear gloves and masks when examining sick cats.

5) Plague vaccine is unavailable in most countries and should not be relied upon as the sole preventive measure; immunized persons should take other appropriate prevention precautions as indicated in this chapter. Live attenuated vaccines are used in some countries but can produce adverse reactions and their efficacy has not been proven. Different vaccination strategies have been used in the past involving both a killed and a live attenuated vaccine but these strategies have only conferred protection against bubonic plague and not against primary pneumonic plague. Currently, the next generation of plague vaccines is being researched; in some cases, vaccines are in clinical trials.

11. Special considerations—

1) Reporting: report any suspected case to the local health authority. In many developed countries, because of the rarity of naturally acquired primary plague pneumonia, even a single case should initiate prompt investigation. In the unlikely circumstance that a natural source of infection cannot be identified, public health and law enforcement authorities might be reasonably suspicious of deliberate use. For more information, see later.

Any event of potential international concern is subject to a notification to WHO under the International Health Regulations. Plague cases are to be reported to WHO only if the assessment done by the country shows that the public health impact can be considered as serious with at least 1 of the following characteristics: unusual or unexpected event, risk of international spread, and significant risk of international travel or trade restriction. Thus, the occurrence of a pneumonic plague case in a well-known focus should not be systematically notified. Conversely, the appearance of a bubonic case in a nonendemic region is typically an event to be notified.

2) Epidemic measures:

- Investigate all suspected plague deaths with autopsy and laboratory examinations when indicated. Develop and carry out case finding. Establish the best possible facilities for diagnosis and treatment. Alert existing medical facilities to report cases immediately and to use full diagnostic and therapeutic services.

- Attempt to prevent or mitigate public hysteria by prompt and accurate informational and educational releases through the news media, information leaflets, websites, and social media channels.

- Institute intensive flea control in affected areas and during epidemics. Apply flea control measures in expanding circles from known outbreak sites. Flea control should precede antirodent measures; the latter should not be executed until the efficacy of the flea control measures has been demonstrated.

- To control fleas, apply insecticidal dusts to rodent runs, harborages, nests, and burrows in and around known or suspected plague areas. All insecticides used for such control should be safe for human residents, labeled for flea control, and known to be effective against local fleas. If nonburrowing rodents are involved, insecticide bait stations can be used. If urban rats are involved, disinsect houses and other structures with insecticidal dusts; dust the bodies and clothing of all residents in the immediate vicinity. After appropriate flea control measures have been taken, rat populations can be suppressed by environmental modifications intended to reduce rodent food and harborage and applications of appropriate rodent poisons or traps can be considered.

- Implement tracing of contacts for cases of pneumonic plague and medical surveillance/chemoprophylaxis for high-risk populations.

- Protect field workers against fleas, dust clothing with insecticide powder, and use insect repellents daily. Antibiotic prophylaxis should be provided for those with documented close exposure.

3) Disaster implications: plague could become a significant problem in or near endemic areas when there are social upheavals, crowding, and unhygienic conditions.

4) International measures:

- Notify WHO if necessary (see earlier).
- Measures applicable to ships, aircraft, and land transport arriving from plague areas are specified in the IHR.
- All ships should be free of rodents or periodically deratted.
- Rat-proof buildings at seaports and airports, apply appropriate insecticides, and eliminate rats with effective rodenticides.
- WHO Collaborating Centres provide support as required. Further information can be found at: http://apps.who.int/whocc.

5) Measures in the case of deliberate use: *Y. pestis* is distributed worldwide; techniques for mass production and aerosol dissemination are thought to exist. The fatality rate for primary pneumonic plague is high and there is a real potential for secondary spread, particularly in those circumstances where patients are treated in home environments without modern medical care. For these reasons, the risk of a biologic attack with plague is considered to be a serious public health concern. In some countries, a few sporadic cases may be missed or not attributed to a deliberate act, particularly in those with natural foci. Any suspect case of pneumonic plague should be reported immediately to the local health department. The sudden appearance of many patients presenting with fever, cough, a fulminant course, and high case-fatality rate should provide a suspect alert for plague; if cough is primarily accompanied by hemoptysis, this presentation favors the tentative diagnosis of pneumonic plague. For a suspected or confirmed outbreak of pneumonic plague, follow the treatment and containment measures outlined in this chapter. Depending on the extent of dissemination, mass prophylaxis of potentially exposed populations may be considered.

[P. Mead]

PNEUMONIA

DISEASE	ICD-10 CODE
PNEUMOCOCCAL PNEUMONIA	ICD-10 J13
MYCOPLASMA PNEUMONIA	ICD-10 J15.7
PNEUMOCYSTIS PNEUMONIA	ICD-10 B59
PNEUMONIA DUE TO *CHLAMYDIA TRACHOMATIS*	ICD-10 P23.1
PNEUMONIA DUE TO *CHLAMYDIA PNEUMONIAE*	ICD-10 J16.0
OTHER PNEUMONIAS	ICD-10 J12, J15, J16.8, J18

There are a number of pathogens known to cause pneumonia. This chapter will focus on the most common variants and special cases regarding treatment. However, it should be noted that there are many other forms of pneumonia, some of which are included in other chapters.

Among the known viruses, pneumonitis can be caused by adenoviruses, respiratory syncytial virus, parainfluenza viruses, human bocavirus, and probably others as yet unidentified. Because these agents cause upper respiratory disease more often than pneumonia, they are presented in "Common Cold and Other Acute Viral Respiratory Diseases." Measles, influenza, and chickenpox can cause pneumonia. Pulmonary infection with *Chlamydia psittaci* is presented in "Psittacosis." Pneumonia is also caused by infection with *Coxiella burnetii* (see "Q Fever") and *Legionella* (see "Legionellosis"). Pneumonia can be associated with the invasive phase of nematode infections, such as ascariasis, and with mycoses, such as aspergillosis, histoplasmosis, and coccidioidomycosis.

Various pathogenic bacteria commonly found in the mouth, nose, and throat, such as *Haemophilus influenzae* (see "Meningitis"), *Staphylococcus aureus*, *Klebsiella pneumoniae*, *Streptococcus pyogenes* (group A hemolytic streptococci), *Neisseria meningitidis*, *Bacteroides* spp., *Moraxella catarrhalis*, and anaerobic cocci, can cause pneumonia either as a primary pathogen or as a complication of chronic pulmonary disease after aspiration of gastric contents or in patients with tracheostomy. With increased use of invasive and immunosuppressive therapies, pneumonias caused by enteric Gram-negative bacilli have become more common, especially those caused by *Escherichia coli*, *Pseudomonas aeruginosa*, and *Proteus* spp. Management depends on the organism involved and is beyond the scope of this book.

I. PNEUMOCOCCAL PNEUMONIA

1. Clinical features—Clinical manifestations may include sudden onset, high fever, rigors, pleuritic chest pain, dyspnea, tachypnea, and cough productive of rusty sputum. Onset may be less abrupt, especially among the elderly; fever, shortness of breath, or altered mental status may provide the first evidence of pneumonia. In infants and young children, fever, vomiting, and convulsions may be the initial manifestations. Laboratory findings include leukocytosis (neutrophilia) and elevated C-reactive protein. Typical chest X-ray findings show lobar or segmental consolidation; consolidation may be bronchopneumonic, especially in children and the elderly. Pneumococcal pneumonia is an important cause of death in infants and the elderly.

Infection can be complicated by empyema, acute respiratory distress syndrome, septic shock, and purpura fulminans. The case-fatality rate varies widely from 5% to 35%, depending on the setting (e.g., outpatients vs. inpatients) and the population (e.g., healthy adults vs. persons with alcoholism). In developing countries, case-fatality rates among children are often higher than 10% and as high as 60% among infants younger than 6 months. Pneumococcal pneumonia among previously healthy individuals with other respiratory infections (e.g., influenza) is well described.

2. Risk groups—Susceptibility is increased among certain populations, including infants, the elderly, and persons with underlying illnesses such as anatomic or functional asplenia, sickle cell disease, cardiovascular disease, diabetes mellitus, cirrhosis, Hodgkin's disease, lymphoma, multiple myeloma, chronic renal failure, nephrotic syndrome, human immunodeficiency virus (HIV) infection, and recent organ transplantation. Malnutrition and low birth weight are important risk factors for infection among infants and young children in developing countries. Susceptibility to infection is also increased by processes affecting the integrity of the lower respiratory tract, including influenza, pulmonary edema, aspiration following alcoholic intoxication or other causes, chronic lung disease, or exposure to irritants (e.g., cigarettes, cooking fire smoke). Previously healthy persons can also develop pneumococcal pneumonia.

3. Causative agents—*Streptococcus pneumoniae* (pneumococcus), a Gram-positive, lancet-shaped, encapsulated diplococcus that often asymptomatically colonizes the human nasopharynx. Children are colonized with *S. pneumoniae* more often than adults. There are about 90 serotypes of pneumococcus, most of which cause pneumonia, while invasive disease is associated with fewer serotypes (1, 5, 6B, 7, 14, 19A, 19F, 23F).

4. Diagnosis—A microbiologic diagnosis of pneumococcal pneumonia can guide antibiotic therapy. A Gram stain of sputum showing many Gram-positive diplococci together with polymorphonuclear leukocytes suggests pneumococcal pneumonia; however, Gram stain and culture of respiratory secretions are often not performed, largely because of technical aspects of obtaining good quality specimens and the difficulty of distinguishing infection from respiratory tract colonization. Definitive diagnosis of pneumococcal pneumonia is established by isolation of pneumococci from blood or, less commonly, pleural fluid. Among adults, the diagnosis can also be established by identification of pneumococcal polysaccharide in urine. For children, urine antigen testing is not useful because nasopharyngeal colonization can cause excretion of pneumococcal antigen in urine. Most pediatric cases are diagnosed by isolation of pneumococci from blood. Patients suspected of having pneumococcal pneumonia should be treated promptly, preferably after collection of appropriate diagnostic specimens according to established guidelines. If pneumococcus is isolated, susceptibility testing should be performed and antimicrobial therapy tailored to susceptibility results. The later treatment table gives recommendations for community-acquired pneumonia. If pneumococcus is proven to be the etiology and it is susceptible to penicillin, that should be the antibiotic of choice in the nonallergic patient.

5. Occurrence—*S. pneumoniae* (pneumococcus) is the most common bacterial etiology of community-acquired pneumonia among all ages. Pneumococcal pneumonia is an endemic disease among the elderly and those with underlying medical conditions. Infection is more frequent among malnourished populations and lower socioeconomic groups, especially in developing countries. It occurs in all climates and seasons, peaking in winter in temperate zones. Certain serotypes may cause epidemics, especially among institutionalized populations, the homeless, and those in developing countries. Incidence is high in certain geographic areas (e.g., Papua New Guinea) and in certain ethnic groups, such as Alaska Natives and Australian Aboriginals. In Europe and North America, estimates of the rate of pneumococcal pneumonia vary widely from approximately 30 cases per 100,000 to nearly 100 per 100,000 adults each year, depending on the population studied and the diagnostic tests used. An increased incidence often accompanies epidemics of influenza.

6. Reservoirs—Humans. Pneumococci are commonly found in the upper respiratory tract of healthy people worldwide.

7. Incubation period—Not well determined; may be as short as 1 to 3 days. Infection is thought to be preceded by asymptomatic colonization.

8. Transmission—By droplet spread. Person-to-person transmission is common, but illness among casual contacts and attendants is infrequent. Most transmission results in colonization rather than infection. The disease remains communicable presumably until discharges of mouth and nose no longer contain infectious numbers of pneumococci, which usually occurs within 24 hours of initiation of effective antibiotic therapy.

9. Treatment—Depends on severity.

Community-Acquired Pneumonia

	Outpatient	Inpatient
Drug	β-lactam antibiotics (e.g., amoxicillin)	CTX PLUS azithromycin or doxycycline
Dose	1 g every 8 hours (for children, 90 mg/kg/day divided every 12 hours)	1 g CTX daily PLUS 500 mg once daily or 100 mg BID
Route	PO	IV
Alternative drug	Doxycycline 100 mg PO BID	Not applicable
Duration	≥ 5 days (after 5 days, continue until afebrile for 48–72 hours)	7 days
Special considerations and comments	• Penicillins, doxycycline, and azithromycin are most useful if risk of drug resistance is low. • Consider levofloxacin 750 mg PO daily if resistant strains are common.	• Depending on clinical situation, consider covering for additional pathogens such MRSA. • De-escalate therapy when a pathogen is identified that can be treated with more narrow spectrum agent.

Note: BID = twice daily; CTX = ceftriaxone; IV = intravenous(ly); MRSA = methicillin-resistant *Staphylococcus aureus*; PO = oral(ly).

10. Prevention—

1) Avoid crowding in living quarters whenever practical, particularly in institutions. Prevent malnutrition and encourage physical activity. Bedridden patients should lie in an upright position at a 30° to 45° incline.

2) Protein-polysaccharide conjugate vaccines including 10 or 13 of the commonest serotypes are included in routine infant immunization schedules in many countries. Pneumococcal conjugate vaccines have been shown to be highly effective at preventing invasive pneumococcal disease and pneumococcal pneumonia, with important reductions in disease incidence demonstrated in the target age population (direct effects) and those too old or too young to receive the vaccine (indirect, or herd, effects). It should be noted that the evidence for this is mostly from developed countries; encouraging information about the effectiveness of these vaccines in developing countries is just becoming available.

WHO considers it a priority to include pneumococcal conjugate vaccines in all national immunization programs and recommends that decisions about which conjugate vaccine to introduce should be left to individual country-level policymakers.

3) A 23-valent pneumococcal polysaccharide vaccine (PPV23) is available for persons older than 2 years. In some countries it is recommended for high-risk persons (individuals ≥ 65 years and those with anatomic or functional asplenia, sickle cell disease, HIV infection, and a variety of chronic systemic illnesses, including heart and lung disease, cirrhosis of the liver, renal insufficiency, and diabetes mellitus). In resource-poor settings, WHO recommends placing greater emphasis on the introduction of a conjugate vaccine for children, given their proven efficacy and their demonstrated indirect benefits for adults. PPV23 is not effective in children younger than 2 years and has no impact on pneumococcal carriage. For most eligible patients, PPV23 vaccine needs to be given only once; however, reimmunization is generally safe and vaccine should be offered to eligible patients whose immunization status cannot be determined. Reimmunization is recommended once for persons older than 2 years who are at highest risk for serious pneumococcal infection and those likely to have a rapid decline in pneumococcal antibody levels, provided that 5 years or more have elapsed since receipt of the first dose of vaccine.

4) Pneumococcal resistance is widely prevalent worldwide; it is estimated that between 25% and 30% of all cases involve a strain resistant to at least 1 drug. This number is actually improving with pneumococcal vaccination. 7 serotypes (6A, 6B, 9V, 14, 19A, 19F, 23F), which once accounted for the majority of resistance, are now represented in the PCV13 vaccine. Underuse of PCV13 and PPV23 (when appropriate) is a factor when considering local resistance patterns. Antimicrobial stewardship can curb the development of resistance in pneumococci.

11. Special considerations—See earlier.

II. MYCOPLASMA PNEUMONIA

1. Clinical features—Predominantly a febrile lower respiratory tract infection causing about 2%-11% (depending on population and testing methodology) of pneumonias. Clinical disease due to *Mycoplasma pneumoniae* varies from mild afebrile pharyngitis to febrile illness of the upper or lower respiratory tract. Onset is gradual with headache, malaise, cough (often paroxysmal), sore throat, and sometimes chest discomfort that may be pleuritic. Sputum, scant at first, may increase later. Early patchy infiltration of the lungs is often more extensive on X-ray than clinical findings suggest. In severe cases, the pneumonia may progress from one lobe to another and become bilateral. Leukocytosis occurs after the first week in approximately one-third of cases. Duration varies from a few days to a month or more. Complications such as central nervous system involvement (e.g., encephalitis, acute disseminated encephalomyelitis) and Stevens-Johnson syndrome are infrequent; fatalities are rare. Differentiation is required from atypical pneumonia due to many other agents: other bacteria, adenoviruses, influenza, respiratory syncytial virus, parainfluenza, measles, Q fever, psittacosis, certain mycoses, severe acute respiratory syndrome or other coronavirus infections, and tuberculosis.

2. Risk groups—Primarily school-aged children and young adults, although the disease can occur at any age.

3. Causative agents—*M. pneumoniae* belongs to the mycoplasmas (Mollicutes). Because mycoplasmas lack cell walls, cell wall synthesis inhibitors such as the penicillins and cephalosporins are not effective in treatment. Along with *S. pneumoniae* and *H. influenzae*, *M. pneumoniae* is 1 of the most common agents of community-acquired pneumonia.

4. Diagnosis—Although serology-based tests are commercially available and widely used, many have proven to be unreliable because of inherent difficulties in interpretation. A single positive immunoglobulin class G (IgG) antibody is of little use because of the high seroprevalence in most populations. A 4-fold rise in antibody titers between acute and convalescent sera collected 3 to 6 weeks apart may provide some diagnostic utility. Molecular diagnostics, most notably quantitative real-time polymerase chain reaction (qPCR) assays, have become a more common and reliable method for rapid diagnosis of *M. pneumoniae*. Respiratory specimens such as nasopharyngeal samples and sputum are acceptable specimen types for qPCR testing. These tests are commercially available in some specialty public health laboratories but their main drawback is the lack of standardization between laboratories. Some specialized laboratories can also perform culture using special media. However, because of the low recovery rate and lengthy incubation time required, culturing is not routinely attempted for clinical diagnosis.

5. Occurrence—Worldwide; sporadic, endemic, and occasionally epidemic, especially in institutions and military populations. Outbreaks often occur in schools and households. Attack rates vary from 5 to more than 50 per 1,000 persons per year in military populations and 1 to 3 per 1,000 persons per year in civilians. Epidemics occur more often in late summer and fall; endemic disease is not seasonal but there can be variation from year to year and among different geographic areas. Males and females of all ages are equally affected. Infection is most frequent among school-aged children and young adults.

6. Reservoirs—Humans.

7. Incubation period—6 to 32 days.

8. Transmission—Probably by droplet inhalation and direct contact with an infected person (including those with subclinical infections). Secondary cases of pneumonia among contacts, family members, and attendants are frequent. The period of communicability is probably less than 20 days. Treatment reduces carriage but does not reliably eradicate the organism from the respiratory tract, where it may persist for weeks. Duration of immunity is uncertain. Second attacks of pneumonia may occur. Protection against repeat infection has been correlated with humoral antibodies that persist up to 1 year.

9. Treatment—See also earlier table in this chapter on empiric treatment of community-acquired pneumonia.

Drug	Azithromycin
Dose	500 mg once daily for 3 days OR 500 mg as a single dose, THEN 250 mg daily for 4 days (for children, 10 mg/kg once, THEN 5 mg/kg/day for 4 days)
Route	PO/IV
Alternative drug	• Doxycycline 100 mg once daily (different than pneumococcal dosing) • Erythromycin 250–500 mg (base) every 6–12 hours • Levofloxacin 500 mg once daily
Duration	At least 5 days; depending on patient response for nonazithromycin regimens.
Special considerations and comments	Macrolide resistance in some areas, especially Asia between 5% and 15%.

Note: IV = intravenous(ly); PO = oral(ly).

10. Prevention—Avoid crowded living and sleeping quarters whenever possible, especially in institutions, barracks, and ships.

11. Special considerations—

1) Reporting: obligatory report of epidemics in some countries.
2) Epidemic measures: no reliably effective measures for control are available, although antimicrobial prophylaxis has been used in some institutional outbreak settings.

III. PNEUMOCYSTIS PNEUMONIA (interstitial plasma cell pneumonia, [PCP])

1. Clinical features—An acute-to-subacute, often fatal, pulmonary disease, especially in persons with immunosuppression and in malnourished, premature infants. Clinically, patients present with dyspnea on exertion; hypoxemia; dry, nonproductive cough; and fever. Signs of respiratory distress may be present but auscultatory signs are usually minimal or absent. Chest X-rays typically show bilateral diffuse interstitial infiltrates.

2. Risk groups—Susceptibility is enhanced by prematurity, chronic debilitating illness, and disease or treatments that impair cell-mediated immune function. Infection with HIV is a predominant risk factor.

3. Causative agents—*Pneumocystis jirovecii* (previously known as *Pneumocystis carinii* and classified as a protozoon). Currently, it is considered a fungus, based on nucleic acid and biochemical analysis.

4. Diagnosis—Established through demonstration of the causative agent in material from induced sputum, bronchoalveolar lavage, or transbronchial or open lung biopsy. Staining with methenamine silver or Giemsa can identify the organism. There are no commercially available routine culture methods or serologic tests at present, though several exist in research laboratories. PCR is available and has good sensitivity. Serum β-D-glucan is usually elevated and can be an adjunct in diagnosis. In patients with acquired immunodeficiency syndrome, the diagnosis is often made presumptively, based on clinical presentation. Patients with leukemia and certain other malignancies, as well as those who are on immunosuppressive therapy for bone marrow or solid organ transplants, are also at risk.

5. Occurrence—Worldwide; may be endemic and epidemic in debilitated, malnourished, or immunosuppressed infants. Before the routine use of prophylactic medication and antiretroviral therapy it affected approximately 60% of patients with HIV infection in the USA, Europe, and Australia. It is a common cause of pneumonia in HIV-infected young infants in developing countries with high HIV prevalence, particularly in sub-Saharan Africa. Patients with leukemia and certain other malignancies, as well as those who are on immunosuppressive therapy for bone marrow or solid organ transplants, are also at risk.

6. Reservoirs—Humans. Organisms have been demonstrated in rodents, cattle, dogs, and other animals but the ubiquitous presence of the organism and its subclinical persistence in humans render these potential animal sources of little public health significance.

7. Incubation period—Unknown. Many adults have subclinical colonization with low numbers of organisms. Analysis of data from institutional outbreaks and animal studies indicates that the onset of disease often occurs 1 to 2 months after establishment of the immunosuppressed state.

8. Transmission—The mode of transmission in people is not known. Airborne animal-to-animal transmission has occurred in rats. In 1 study in the USA, approximately 75% of healthy individuals were reported to have humoral antibody to *P. jirovecii* by 4 years old, suggesting that subclinical colonization is common. Pneumonitis in the compromised host is thought to result either from a reactivation of latent infection or from a newly acquired infection.

9. Treatment—

Drug	TMP/SMX
Dose	15–20 mg/kg/day based on TMP component divided TID or QID
Route	PO/IV
Alternative drug	• Desensitization to TMP/SMX may be considered in patients who are allergic • Atovaquone (mild disease) • Clindamycin + primaquine • Pentamidine (IV)
Duration	21 days

Special considerations and comments	• Steroids should be considered in moderate-to-severe disease (especially in HIV-uninfected patients) when hypoxemia is present or Po_2 < 70 mm Hg or alveolar gradient > 35 mm Hg.
	• Proposed regimen for 21-day course:
	  ○ Prednisone 40 mg BID for 5 days
	  ○ Prednisone 40 mg once daily for 5 days
	  ○ Prednisone 20 mg once daily for 11 days
	• Methylprednisolone can be substituted at 75% dosing.
	• G6PD testing should be done prior to using primaquine.
	• Pentamidine can cause hypotension and other severe adverse effects.

Note: BID = twice daily; HIV = human immunodeficiency virus; IV = intravenous(ly); PO = oral(ly); Po_2 = partial pressure of oxygen; QID = 4 times daily; TID = thrice daily; TMP/SMX = trimethoprim-sulfamethoxazole.

10. Prevention—Among immunosuppressed patients—especially those with HIV infection, those treated for leukemia, and those with certain organ transplants—prophylaxis with either oral trimethoprim-sulfamethoxazole (preferred), atovaquone, dapsone, or the combination of dapsone, pyrimethamine, and leucovorin is effective in preventing endogenous reactivation for the period during which the patient receives treatment.

11. Special considerations—

1) Reporting: when cases occur in people with evidence of HIV infection, case report may be required in some countries.
2) Epidemic measures: knowledge of the source and mode of transmission is so incomplete that there are no generally accepted measures.

IV. CHLAMYDIAL PNEUMONIAS (see also "Psittacosis")

A. PNEUMONIA DUE TO *CHLAMYDIA TRACHOMATIS* (neonatal eosinophilic pneumonia, congenital pneumonia due to *Chlamydia*)

1. Clinical features—A subacute chlamydial pulmonary disease typically occurring between 4 and 11 weeks old among infants whose mothers have chlamydial infection of the genitourinary tract. Clinically, the disease is characterized by insidious onset, cough (characteristically staccato in nature), lack of fever, and patchy infiltrates on chest X-ray with hyperinflation, eosinophilia, and elevated immunoglobulin class M (IgM) and IgG. About half the patients show prodromal rhinitis and conjunctivitis. Duration of illness is commonly 1 to 3 weeks but may extend as long as 2 months. The illness is usually moderate but can progress to severe pneumonia. One study suggests that infants with chlamydial pneumonia are at increased risk of chronic cough and abnormal lung function.

2. Risk groups—Infants of mothers with chlamydial infection. Maternal antibody does not protect the infant from infection.

3. Causative agents—*Chlamydia trachomatis* of immunotypes D to K.

4. Diagnosis—A wide variety of diagnostic tests are available, including direct fluorescent antibody tests, enzyme immunoassays, and nucleic acid amplification tests (NAATs). If NAATs are available, nasopharyngeal specimens should be submitted.

5. Occurrence—Probably coincides with the worldwide distribution of genital chlamydial infection. The disease has been recognized in many countries and epidemics do not seem to occur.

6. Reservoirs—Humans. Experimental infection with *C. trachomatis* has been induced in nonhuman primates and mice; animal infections are not known to occur in nature.

7. Incubation period—Pneumonia may occur in infants from 1 to 18 weeks old (most commonly between 4 and 11 weeks). Nasopharyngeal infection is usually not recognized before 2 weeks old.

8. Transmission—From the infected cervix to an infant during birth, with resultant nasopharyngeal infection (and often chlamydial conjunctivitis). Respiratory transmission does not seem to occur.

9. Treatment—

Drug	Azithromycin
Dose	20 mg/kg/day
Route	PO/IV
Alternative drug	Erythromycin 50 mg/kg/day divided every 6 hours for 10–14 days
Duration	3 days
Special considerations and comments	Erythromycin is more highly correlated with the development of pyloric stenosis than azithromycin.

Note: IV = intravenous(ly); PO = oral(ly).

10. Prevention—See Chlamydial Conjunctivitis in "Conjunctivitis and Keratitis."

11. Special considerations—None.

B. PNEUMONIA DUE TO *CHLAMYDIA* (*CHLAMYDO-PHILA*) *PNEUMONIAE*

1. Clinical features—An acute respiratory disease with cough, frequently a sore throat and hoarseness, and fever at the onset; sputum is scanty and chest pain is rare. Inflammatory signs are sometimes subtle. Pulmonary rales and wheezing are usually present. The clinical picture is similar to pneumonia caused by *Mycoplasma*. Radiographic abnormalities include bilateral infiltrates, occasionally with pleural effusions. Illness is usually mild, but recovery is slow with cough persisting for 2 to 6 weeks. Death is rare.

2. Risk groups—Susceptibility is thought to be universal.

3. Causative agents—*Chlamydia pneumoniae* is the species name for the human-specific organism with distinct morphologic and serologic differences from *C. psittaci* and *C. trachomatis.*

4. Diagnosis—Historically, laboratory diagnosis has been primarily serologic. Microimmunofluorescence testing of paired sera collected 4 to 8 weeks apart is commercially available but requires a fluorescent microscope and there are specificity problems owing to cross-reaction with chlamydial antigens of other species. More recently, real-time PCR assays have been employed to provide rapid, specific, and sensitive detection of deoxyribonucleic acid from nasopharyngeal/oropharyngeal sputum or other respiratory tract specimens. The organism can be isolated from throat swab specimens in special cell lines but this is not routinely performed due to cost, length of time to result, and low recovery rates.

5. Occurrence—Presumably worldwide. Age distribution has 2 peaks: 1 among children between 5 and 15 years old and 1 in persons 60 years and older. Antibodies are rare in children younger than 5 years; seroprevalence increases among teenagers and young adults to a plateau of about 50% by age 20 to 30 years, which persists into old age. No seasonality has been noted. Outbreaks in communities, households, day care centers, and schools are often reported.

6. Reservoirs—Presumably humans.

7. Incubation period—Unknown; may be 3 to 4 weeks.

8. Transmission—The mode of transmission has not been defined, although droplet transmission is most likely. The period of communicability also has not been defined but is presumably long; some military outbreaks have lasted as long as 8 months.

9. Treatment—See also earlier table in this chapter on empiric therapy of community-acquired pneumonia.

Drug	Azithromycin
Dose	• 500 mg once daily for 3 days OR • 500 mg once daily for 3 days, THEN 250 mg once daily for 4 days
Route	PO
Alternative drug	• Doxycycline 100 mg BID for 10–14 days • Erythromycin 1 g/day divided every 6 or 12 hours for 5 days

Note: BID = twice daily; PO = oral(ly).

10. Prevention—

  1) Avoid crowding in living and sleeping quarters.
  2) Apply personal hygiene measures: cover mouth when coughing and sneezing and wash hands frequently.

11. Special considerations—

  1) Reporting: report epidemics to local health authority.
  2) Epidemic measures: case-finding and appropriate treatment.

[M. Maguire, S. Eppes]

POLIOMYELITIS
(polioviral fever, infantile paralysis)

DISEASE	ICD-10 CODE
POLIOMYELITIS	ICD-10 A80

1. Clinical features—A viral infection recognized by acute onset of flaccid paralysis. Infection occurs in the gastrointestinal tract with spread to regional lymph nodes and, in a minority of cases, to the central nervous system (CNS). Flaccid paralysis occurs in fewer than 1% of infections (ranging from 1 paralytic case per 200 infections by type 1 poliovirus to 1 in more than 1,000 infections by type 2 or 3 poliovirus); the rate of paralysis among infected nonimmune adults is higher than that among nonimmunized infants and young children and more severe. Approximately 90% of infections are inapparent or result in nonspecific fever. Aseptic meningitis occurs in about 1% of infections. Fever, malaise, headache, nausea, and vomiting are recognized in 10% of infections. If disease progresses to major illness, severe muscle pain and stiffness of the neck and back with flaccid paralysis may occur. Paralysis is usually asymmetric with fever present at onset; maximum extent is usually reached within 3 to 4 days. The site of paralysis depends on the location of nerve cell destruction in the spinal cord or brain stem; legs are affected more often than arms. Paralysis of the respiration and/or swallowing muscles can be life-threatening. Some improvement in paralysis may occur during convalescence but paralysis still present after 60 days is likely to be permanent. Infrequently, recurrence of muscle weakness following recovery may occur many years after the original infection has resolved (postpolio syndrome); this is not believed to be related to persistence of the virus itself.

With progress made towards global eradication, poliomyelitis (polio) must now be distinguished from other paralytic conditions by isolation of virus from stools. Other enteroviruses, echoviruses, and coxsackieviruses have been reported to cause an illness simulating paralytic polio. Polio-like illness can occur in a small minority of persons infected with West Nile virus and Japanese encephalitis virus. The most frequent cause of acute flaccid paralysis (AFP) that must be distinguished from polio is Guillain-Barré syndrome (GBS). Paralysis in GBS is typically symmetrical and may progress for periods as long as 10 days. Fever, headache, nausea, vomiting, and pleocytosis characteristic of polio are usually absent in GBS; high protein and low cell counts in cerebrospinal fluid (CSF) and sensory changes are seen in the majority of GBS cases. Acute motor axonal neuropathy (Chinese paralytic syndrome) is an important cause of AFP in northern China and is probably present elsewhere; it is seasonally epidemic and closely resembles polio. Fever and CSF pleocytosis are usually absent but paralysis may persist for several months. Other causes of AFP include transverse myelitis, traumatic neuritis, infectious and toxic neuropathies, tick paralysis, myasthenia gravis, porphyria, botulism, insecticide poisoning, polymyositis, trichinosis, and periodic paralysis. Differential diagnosis of acute nonparalytic polio includes other forms of acute nonbacterial meningitis, purulent meningitis, brain abscess, tuberculous meningitis, leptospirosis, lymphocytic choriomeningitis, infectious mononucleosis, the encephalitides, neurosyphilis, and toxic encephalopathies.

2. Risk groups—Groups that refuse immunization or others unimmunized or underimmunized; minority populations, migrants, and other unregistered children; nomads, refugees, and the urban poor are at high risk as well as those in areas in geographic proximity to endemic countries and those that are inaccessible because of security issues. Intramuscular injections, trauma, or surgery during the incubation period or prodromal illness may provoke paralysis in the affected extremity. Tonsillectomy increases the risk of bulbar involvement. Excessive muscular activity in the prodromal period may predispose to paralysis. Infants born to immune mothers have transient passive immunity.

3. Causative agents—Poliovirus (genus *Enterovirus*) types 1, 2, and 3; all types can cause paralysis. Wild poliovirus type 1 is isolated from paralytic cases most often and type 3 less so. Wild poliovirus type 2 has not been detected since October 1999 (and it was certified as eradicated in 2015). Wild poliovirus type 3 has not been detected since November 2012. Type 1 most frequently causes epidemics. Paralytic polio cases have also been reported as a result of outbreaks caused by circulating vaccine-derived polioviruses (cVDPVs) types 1, 2, and 3. Paralytic polio also occurs in association with vaccination (vaccine-associated paralytic polio [VAPP]) in vaccine recipients or their healthy contacts at a rate of approximately 1 in every 2.5 million doses administered or 1 in 800,000 first vaccinations. The risk of VAPP is 3,000-fold higher among persons with congenital hypogammaglobulinemia than among immunocompetent people.

4. Diagnosis—Definitive laboratory diagnosis requires isolation of the poliovirus from stool samples, CSF, or oropharyngeal secretions. To increase the probability of isolating poliovirus, at least 2 stool specimens should be collected 24 hours apart as early in the disease as possible, ideally within 14 days of paralysis onset; uncommonly poliovirus can be isolated up to 60 days after onset. Real-time reverse transcription polymerase chain reaction is now used to rapidly differentiate wild from vaccine-derived virus strains. Isolates of wild or vaccine-derived poliovirus should be immediately characterized through genetic sequencing to identify sources of transmission and, in the case of vaccine-derived virus, to differentiate between cVDPV strains and strains excreted by immunodeficient individuals.

Rises in antibody levels (> 4-fold) are less helpful in the diagnosis of wild polio infection; type-specific neutralizing antibodies may already be present when paralysis develops and significant titer rises may therefore not be demonstrable in paired sera. Antibody response following immunization mimics the response after infection with wild-type viruses; the widespread use of live polio vaccines makes interpretation of antibody levels difficult, except to rule out polio in cases where no antibody has developed in immuno-competent children. Poliovirus is demonstrable as early as 36 hours after exposure to infection in throat secretions and 72 hours after exposure to infection in feces in both clinical and inapparent cases.

5. Occurrence—Historically, polio occurred worldwide sporadically and as epidemics with an increase during the late summer and fall in temperate countries. In tropical countries, a less pronounced seasonal peak occurred in the hot and rainy season. With improved immunization and the global initiative to eradicate polio, wild polioviruses at the time of writing were endemic in only 3 countries that have not succeeded in interrupting trans-mission (Afghanistan, Nigeria, Pakistan). Polio remains primarily a disease of infants and young children. In the 3 countries that have not yet succeeded in interrupting transmission, 80% to 90% of cases are in children younger than 3 years and virtually all cases are in those younger than 5 years.

Although wild poliovirus transmission has ceased in most countries, importation remains a threat. A large outbreak of polio occurred in 1992–1993 in the Netherlands among members of a religious group that refuse immunization; virus was also found among members of a related religious group in Canada, although no cases occurred. Since 2000, imported wild poliovirus has caused outbreaks and paralytic cases in more than 30 countries, primarily in Africa, Asia, and the Middle East. In recent years, outbreaks following wild poliovirus importations into polio-free countries have often affected adults owing to the increasing susceptibility of older populations in areas with gaps in routine immunization coverage. With the exception of rare imported cases, the few cases of polio in industrialized countries were caused by vaccine virus strains. About half of VAPP cases occurred among adult contacts of vaccinees. Between 2000 and 2012, polio outbreaks due to cVDPVs were reported from 20 countries, all of which continue to use oral poliovirus vaccine (OPV) for routine immunization. These outbreaks have been associated with areas of low OPV coverage and the cases were clinically indistinguishable from polio caused by wild poliovirus.

6. Reservoirs—Humans, most frequently people with inapparent infections, especially children. No long-term carriers of wild-type poliovirus have been detected. Chronic carriage of vaccine-derived poliovirus has been reported, all from industrialized countries or emerging economies and all associated with primary immunodeficiency syndromes.

7. Incubation period—Commonly 7 to 14 days for paralytic cases; reported range of 3 to possibly 35 days.

8. Transmission—Primarily person-to-person spread, principally through the fecal-oral route; virus is detectable more easily and for a longer period in feces than in throat secretions. Where sanitation levels are high, pharyngeal spread may be relatively more important. In rare instances, milk, foodstuffs, and other materials contaminated with feces have been implicated as vehicles. No reliable evidence of spread by insects. Transmission is possible as long as the virus is excreted. Virus typically persists in the throat for approximately 1 week and in feces for 3 to 6 weeks. Cases are most infectious during the days before and after onset of symptoms. Type-specific immunity, apparently of lifelong duration, follows both clinically recognizable and inapparent infections. Second attacks of polio are rare and result from infection with a poliovirus of a different type.

9. Treatment—There is no specific treatment for polio. Depending on the site of paralysis, specific interventions and modalities may be helpful (e.g., walking aids). Physical therapy and occupational therapy may be helpful to attain maximum function after paralytic polio and may prevent some deformities as late manifestations of the illness. Respiratory complications may require expertise from pulmonary specialists, especially as the patient's ventilation needs increase.

10. Prevention—

1) Educate the public on the advantages of immunization in early childhood.
2) Trivalent OPV was withdrawn globally in April 2016 to ensure cessation of the use of type 2 live attenuated vaccine. Bivalent (types 1 and 3) live attenuated OPV and injectable inactivated poliovirus vaccine (IPV) are commercially available for routine immunization. Since 2005 monovalent OPV types 1 and 3 have been developed and licensed for use in mass campaigns but are not currently in general use; since 2009 bivalent OPV has been used for supplementary immunization, for provision of higher, type-specific seroconversion rates.

   OPV simulates natural infection by inducing both circulating antibody and resistance to infection of the pharynx and intestine (mucosal immunity); it also immunizes some susceptible contacts through secondary spread. In developing countries, lower rates of seroconversion and reduced vaccine efficacy for OPV have been reported; this can be overcome by administration of numerous extra doses in immunization programs and/or supplemental campaigns. Breastfeeding does not cause a significant reduction in the protection provided by OPV. WHO recommends the use of OPV for immunization programs in low/middle-income countries because of the capacity to induce mucosal immunity, low cost, ease of administration, and superior capacity to provide population immunity through secondary spread. IPV, like OPV, provides excellent individual protection by inducing circulating antibodies that block the spread of virus to the CNS and also protect against pharyngeal infection; however, it does not induce intestinal immunity comparable to OPV (though IPV may substantially boost intestinal immunity in children who have previously been vaccinated with OPV). Many high-income countries have switched to IPV alone for routine immunization because wild-type polioviruses have been eliminated in those settings, ongoing global eradication efforts have reduced the risk of importations, and the risk of paralysis from OPV in these countries is considered greater than that from wild poliovirus.

A few individuals with underlying primary immunodeficiency disorders who chronically excreted an OPV-derived poliovirus have been identified in industrialized countries and emerging market economies; the significance of these chronic excreters for polio eradication is under review. More troublesome are outbreaks of polio caused by cVDPVs. These are capable of spreading through populations and infecting nonvaccinated or incompletely vaccinated individuals. The extent of this problem has become clearer in recent years, with at least 4 such outbreaks being detected each year since 2008, arising primarily in areas of low OPV coverage.

3) Recommendations for routine and supplementary childhood immunization: in developing countries, WHO recommends 4 doses of OPV at 6, 10, and 14 weeks old, with an additional dose at birth and/or at the measles contact (usually 9 months of age), depending on the endemicity and/or risk of polio in the country. In endemic countries and countries at high risk of importations or cVDPV emergence, WHO recommends annual national supplemental immunization campaigns to administer 2 or more doses of OPV at least 1 month apart to all children younger than 5 years regardless of prior immunization status. These campaigns should be conducted during the cool, dry season to achieve maximum effect. On the attainment of a high level of control in an endemic country, targeted house-to-house mop-up immunization campaigns in infected and high-risk areas are recommended to interrupt the final chains of transmission. Where polio is still endemic or at high risk of importation and spread, WHO recommends the use of OPV for all infants, including those who may be infected with human immunodeficiency virus in whom study has shown OPV to be safe. Diarrhea is not a contraindication to

OPV. In industrialized countries, contraindications to OPV frequently include congenital immunodeficiency (B-lymphocyte deficiency, thymic dysplasia), current immunosuppressive treatment, disease states associated with immunosuppression (e.g., lymphoma, leukemia, and generalized malignancy), and the presence of immunodeficient individuals in the households of potential vaccine recipients. IPV should be used in such people but this is no longer an issue in most industrialized countries as they have now shifted to IPV.

With progress towards eradication, the risk profile of paralytic polio is changing, particularly in middle- and high-income countries, and many have either replaced OPV with IPV for routine immunization or introduced mixed OPV/IPV immunization schedules. Following withdrawal of type 2 OPV, nearly all countries have added at least 1 full dose or 2 fractional doses of IPV in routine immunizations and low/middle-income countries that have continued to use OPV have shifted from trivalent OPV to bivalent OPV in both the routine schedule and supplementary immunization.

4) Immunization of adults: routine immunization for adults is not considered necessary. Primary immunization is advised for previously nonimmunized adults traveling to endemic countries and countries at high risk of importations, members of communities or population groups in which poliovirus disease is present, laboratory workers handling specimens containing poliovirus, and health care workers who may be exposed to patients excreting wild-type polioviruses. In most industrialized countries, IPV is recommended for adult primary immunization. Those having previously completed a course of immunization and currently at increased risk of exposure are often given an additional dose of IPV. A single, lifetime booster is recommended for previously immunized adults traveling to polio-infected areas. Travelers from polio-infected areas are recommended to have an additional dose of OPV at least 6 weeks before each international journey to reduce the risk of transient virus carriage and international spread. In case of urgent travel, a minimum of 1 dose of OPV should be given ideally 4 weeks before departure. Some polio-free countries have established special immunization requirements for travelers from polio-endemic and reinfected countries (e.g., receipt of an additional dose on arrival); travelers should check immunization requirements prior to departure. All travelers are advised to carry their written vaccination record in the event that evidence of polio vaccination is requested for entry

into countries being visited, preferably using the International Health Regulations (IHR) international certificate of vaccination or prophylaxis. The certificate is available at: http://www.who.int/ihr/IVC200_06_26.pdf.

11. Special considerations—

1) Reporting: polio is a disease under surveillance by WHO and targeted for eradication. Since 2007, countries party to the IHR are required to inform WHO immediately of individual cases of paralytic polio due to wild poliovirus and to report details and extent of virus transmission. Countries should also report wild poliovirus isolated from other sources (e.g., environmental sampling) and polio cases due to cVDPV. In countries undertaking polio eradication and/or certification, each case of AFP, including GBS, in children younger than 15 years must be reported and fully investigated as well as each case of suspected polio in people of any age. Nonparalytic infections should also be reported to the local health authority.

2) Epidemic measures: in any country that has previously interrupted transmission of wild poliovirus, a single case of polio must now be considered a public health emergency, requiring an extensive supplementary immunization response over a large geographic area. Responses should be initiated within 4 weeks of confirmation of the index case and should consist of a minimum of 5 mass immunization rounds, covering a minimum of 2 million to 5 million children and achieving at least 95% coverage in each administrative area. cVDPVs require a similar intensity of response; type 2 cVDPV requires an authorized release of monovalent type 2 OPV by WHO.

3) Disaster implications: overcrowding of nonimmune groups and collapse of the sanitary infrastructure pose an epidemic threat.

4) International measures: cases must be reported to WHO under the IHR (see earlier). Planning of a large-scale immunization response must begin immediately, be completed within 72 hours, and, if appropriate, be coordinated with bordering countries. Primary isolation of the virus is best accomplished in a designated Global Polio Eradication Laboratory. Once a wild poliovirus is isolated, molecular epidemiology can help trace the source and timing. At-risk countries should submit weekly reports on cases of polio, AFP cases, and AFP surveillance performance to their respective WHO offices until the world has been certified polio-free.

International travelers visiting polio-infected areas should be adequately immunized. For further information, see the WHO publication *International Travel and Health* (see: https://www.who.int/ith/en).

WHO Collaborating Centres provide support as required. More information can be found at: http://www.who.int/collaborating-centres/database/en. Further information can be found at: http://www.polioeradication.org.

[O. A. Khan]

PRION DISEASES
(transmissible spongiform encephalopathies)

DISEASE	ICD-10 CODE
CREUTZFELDT-JAKOB DISEASE	ICD-10 A81.0
VARIANT CREUTZFELDT-JAKOB DISEASE	ICD-10-CM A81.01
GERSTMANN-STRÄUSSLER-SCHEINKER SYNDROME	ICD-10-CM A81.09
FATAL FAMILIAL INSOMNIA	ICD-10-CM A81.09

A group of brain diseases characterized by a clinical and neuropathologic picture of progressive neurodegeneration resulting from tissue deposition of prions, which are abnormally folded forms of a host-encoded cellular protein (the prion protein). Prions are believed to be the causative agents and their deposition in neurons is the hallmark of prion disease pathology and pathogenesis. Human prion diseases comprise

1) Creutzfeldt-Jakob disease (CJD), occurring in 3 different forms: sporadic CJD (~85% of cases), familial CJD (10%–15% of cases), and iatrogenic CJD (< 1% of cases)
2) Variant CJD (vCJD), which has been causally linked with bovine spongiform encephalopathy (BSE), a prion disease of cattle
3) Gerstmann-Sträussler-Scheinker syndrome (GSS)
4) Fatal familial insomnia (FFI)

The most common prion disease in humans, sporadic CJD, is not thought to be exogenously acquired and occurs sporadically. Other prion diseases not thought to be exogenously acquired include familial CJD, GSS, and FFI; these diseases are associated with mutations of the prion protein gene and are inherited within families. Other prion diseases in humans (Kuru, vCJD, iatrogenic CJD) are thought to be acquired exogenously. Incubation periods are generally long (many years) and there is no demonstrable inflammatory or immune response. Even those diseases thought not to be acquired exogenously and some that are genetically associated may be transmissible to others in certain settings (e.g., iatrogenic CJD, vCJD).

1. Clinical features—Signs and symptoms of CJD are limited to central nervous system (CNS) dysfunction. It typically presents as a subacute illness in the middle-aged and elderly (median age at death, 68 years) as a rapidly progressive encephalopathy with confusion, dementia, and other neurologic signs such as cerebellar dysfunction and myoclonus. However, clinical heterogeneity and atypical presentations have been reported. Patients have no fever and routine blood tests and cerebrospinal fluid (CSF) cell count are normal. Typical periodic high-voltage complexes are present in the electroencephalogram (EEG) in about 70% of cases and the CSF 14-3-3 and tau proteins are elevated in the majority of patients. Brain magnetic resonance imaging (MRI) shows signal hyperintensity in the caudate/putamen in many cases, especially on fluid-attenuated inversion recovery (FLAIR) sequences. High signal may be seen in some cerebral cortical regions.

vCJD, first identified in 1996, has a longer clinical course (median 14 months vs. 4 months for sporadic CJD) and usually presents with psychiatric or behavioral disturbances, followed by signs of neurologic dysfunction, usually delayed by several months after the onset of illness. The typical EEG changes of sporadic CJD are seen only rarely in vCJD. MRI scan in vCJD shows high signal in the pulvinar area of the posterior thalamus in more than 90% of cases, especially on FLAIR sequences. The CSF 14-3-3 may be elevated but in only about 45% of cases. All tested confirmed cases of vCJD to date have been homozygous for methionine (MM) at the polymorphic codon 129 of the prion protein gene. It remains unclear whether or not vCJD will occur in non-MM individuals who may be infected at present.

The clinical picture for genetic prion diseases is highly variable; traditionally, they have been classified as familial CJD, GSS, and FFI. GSS is used to describe a heterogeneous group of inherited prion diseases that are characterized by long illness duration and the presence of amyloid plaques, primarily in the cerebellum. FFI predominantly involves the thalamus, resulting in an illness characterized by intractable insomnia and autonomic nervous system dysfunction. CJD must be differentiated from other forms of dementia (especially Alzheimer's disease), other infections (including encephalitis and vasculitis), and toxic, endocrine, autoimmune, and metabolic encephalopathies.

2. Risk groups—The following persons have been regarded as at risk for developing a prion disease: recipients of human dura mater graft, human cadaver–derived pituitary hormones (especially human cadaver–derived growth hormone), and corneal transplants; persons undergoing neurosurgery; and members of families with heritable CJD.

Mutations of the prion protein gene are associated with genetic or familial forms of human prion diseases. In human prion diseases, the polymorphic codon 129 of the prion protein gene, which codes for either methionine or valine, influences susceptibility and phenotypic expression of the disease.

3. Causative agents—CJD and other related diseases are believed to be caused by prions, which are abnormally folded versions of the self-replicating, host-encoded prion protein. The normal cellular prion protein is a structural component of cell membranes of neurons and other mammalian cells. Genetic prion diseases are associated with 1 of several mutations in the prion protein gene located on chromosome 20 that encodes for the normal prion protein. The pattern of inheritance is variable but up to 40% of patients may have no family history of a prion disease. Many prion diseases are transmissible in the laboratory to other species, including wild and transgenic mice and nonhuman primates.

4. Diagnosis—All forms of CJD are diagnosed based on clinical features and EEG, CSF 14-3-3, and MRI findings. In vCJD, immunohistochemical or Western blot testing of tonsil biopsy can be very helpful but is probably best reserved for those cases with atypical features and/or without the MRI pulvinar sign. Real-time quaking-induced conversion (RT-QuIC) is a new test that detects a minute amount of prions in the CSF. RT-QuIC is used as an antemortem diagnostic tool in a majority of suspected cases. A definite diagnosis of all prion diseases depends on brain tissue testing and is usually undertaken at postmortem examination. Genetic testing on a simple blood sample is of importance in the diagnosis of suspect genetic prion disease. Brain biopsy can provide antemortem diagnosis but this is an invasive procedure and is arguably best reserved for those patients in whom an alternative diagnosis is otherwise not possible.

5. Occurrence—Sporadic CJD has been reported worldwide with an annual mortality rate of 1 to 2 per million population. The highest age-specific average mortality rate (5 cases/million) occurs in the 65- to 79-year age group. Genetic prion disease foci have been reported in familial clusters in many countries, including Chile, France, Israel, Slovakia, and the USA. vCJD typically affects a younger age group than sporadic CJD (median age at death, 28 vs. 68 years). As of mid-2018, more than 230 cases of vCJD had been identified worldwide, including 178 patients in the UK and 27 in France. Although the incidence of vCJD cases has virtually disappeared because of human dietary protection measures and changes in animal feeding and slaughtering practices, concerns about iatrogenic transmission by blood, surgery, and dentistry still remain. Five instances of blood-borne vCJD transmission have been reported in the UK.

6. Reservoirs—Humans are the only species affected by the CJD prions in nature, with the exception of vCJD, which represents zoonotic spread of BSE from its reservoir, thought to be in cattle. Subclinical infection with the BSE prion appears to be present in human populations (especially in the UK, where the estimated prevalence ranges between 1 in 1,250 and 1 in 3,500).

The magnitude of the risk from such infections is unknown but they may represent a potential reservoir of infection for secondary human-to-human spread by blood transfusion, organ transplantation, or surgery.

7. Incubation period—The concept of incubation period from the time of an external source exposure may not be applicable to sporadic and genetic prion diseases. For acquired forms of human prion diseases (e.g., iatrogenic CJD and vCJD), incubation periods could range from 15 months to more than 30 years. The route of exposure influences the incubation period: a mean of 12 years (range, 1.3-30 years) with direct CNS exposure (dura mater grafts) and a mean of 17 years (range, 5-42 years) with peripheral exposure (human pituitary hormones given by injection). The incubation period for 3 patients with vCJD infected by blood transfusion ranged from 6.6 to 8.5 years. The estimated mean incubation period for vCJD from consuming BSE-contaminated cattle products is between 10 and 20 years.

8. Transmission—There is no firm evidence that sporadic CJD is an exogenously acquired disease. De novo spontaneous generation of the self-replicating, abnormally folded protein has been hypothesized as a source of the disease. Some case-control studies have suggested that surgery may be a risk factor for some sporadic CJD patients. Iatrogenic transmission of CJD has occurred following the use of contaminated cadaver-derived human pituitary hormone, dura mater and corneal grafts, EEG depth electrodes, and neurosurgical instruments. In all these cases, it is presumed that infection from a case, or cases, of sporadic CJD was inadvertently transmitted to another person in the course of medical/surgical treatment. The mechanism of transmission of BSE from cattle to humans has not been established but the favored hypothesis is that humans are infected through dietary consumption of the BSE agent. Three cases of vCJD have resulted from red cell transfusion and a fourth patient heterozygous at codon 129 was positive for the vCJD agent but died of another condition. This agent was also found in a spleen sample of a fifth patient, who received fractionated plasma products partly sourced from a donor who went on to develop vCJD. To date, blood products have not been shown to be a risk factor for other forms of prion diseases in humans. The highest levels of prion infectivity are associated with CNS tissues. In sporadic CJD, infectivity may be present in non-CNS tissues but at much lower levels and probably essentially during the period of clinical illness. In vCJD, infection is present in lymphoid tissues and blood during the incubation period and during clinical illness. The level of infectivity in the CNS rises late in the incubation period and high levels of infectivity occur in the CNS throughout symptomatic illness.

9. Treatment—Prion diseases are uniformly fatal. No agent-specific treatment exists. Clinical management of patients is focused on supportive treatment to ameliorate some symptoms, on monitoring and treating secondary infections, and on maintaining hydration and caloric intake.

10. Prevention—

1) Avoid organ or tissue transplants from infected patients and reuse of potentially contaminated surgical instruments. WHO guidelines to minimize the risk of transmission of CJD and sterilization protocols for CJD-contaminated surgical instruments are available at: http://www.who.int/csr/resources/publications/bse/WHO_CDS_CSR_APH_2000_3/en.

2) Avoid iatrogenic exposures:

   - Specific precautions should be taken in the management of persons with confirmed or suspected prion disease.
   - When determining the risk of iatrogenic transmission, infectivity of a given tissue should be considered together with the route of exposure. Infectivity is found most often, and in the highest concentration, in the CNS. Precautions have been proposed when performing certain interventions in patients with prion disease (dental, diagnostic, surgical procedures) and when handling instruments or cleaning and decontaminating instruments, work surfaces, and waste.
   - Blood transfusion has resulted in the transmission of vCJD. This has not been demonstrated for other forms of prion disease.

3) Avoid exposures to BSE-causing agents in food of bovine origin because BSE is a risk to animal and public health; it is transmissible to humans and food is considered the most likely source of exposure. Bovines, bovine products, and bovine byproducts potentially carrying the BSE agent have been traded worldwide, giving this risk a global dimension with possible repercussions for public health, animal health, and trade. At this time, the 2 key methods used to protect public health are minimizing or eliminating BSE in livestock populations and excluding from human food bovine tissues with the likely potential to contain the BSE agent if an animal were infected. For further information, see the *Joint WHO/FAO/OIE Technical Consultation on BSE: Public Health, Animal Health and Trade*, which is available at: http://whqlibdoc.who.int/publications/2001/9290445556.pdf.

11. Special considerations—

1) Reporting: many countries have made CJD (including vCJD) a notifiable disease. The World Organisation for Animal Health (Office International des Epizooties; OIE) lists BSE as a reportable disease for international trade in livestock and livestock products.

2) International measures for the prevention of vCJD: to avoid human exposures to the BSE agent in food of bovine origin, no part or product of any animal that has shown signs of a prion disease should enter the human food chain. Countries should not permit tissues that are likely to contain the BSE agent to enter any (human or animal) food chain.

- Managing BSE in cattle:

  - All countries should determine the BSE risk status of their cattle population through the outcome of an annual risk assessment, identifying all potential factors for BSE introduction, recycling, and amplification. A BSE surveillance system fitting the estimated level of risk should be put into place.

  - Whenever a risk of BSE is identified, countries can consider taking immediate steps to define the specified risk materials; tissues that have been shown to contain infectivity should be removed and destroyed. If the BSE risk is considered higher, other tissues that under certain conditions may carry infectivity can be added to the specified risk materials list for removal and destruction. Additional precautions may be taken, such as prohibiting cattle over a certain age from entering food or feed chains. WHO, FAO, and OIE continuously review this approach, specifically in relation to public health issues.

  - Countries should monitor the effective application of the regulatory measures that have been decided upon, in particular the effectiveness of their ban (if in place) on feeding ruminant tissues to ruminants.

  - International trade in food products may disseminate tissues containing BSE; control transborder passage of cattle and bovine meat from areas where cattle are infected with BSE. WHO, FAO, and OIE continue to work together to mitigate the risk of dissemination of BSE agents.

- Prevention of blood-borne transmission: as a precautionary measure to reduce the risk of transmission of vCJD through blood or blood products, some countries—including Canada, the USA, and some continental European countries—have requested that blood centers exclude potential blood donors who have resided for a specified period in the UK.

[E. Belay]

❖

PSITTACOSIS

(*Chlamydia* [or *Chlamydophila*] *psittaci* infection, ornithosis, parrot fever, avian chlamydiosis)

DISEASE	ICD-10 CODE
PSITTACOSIS	ICD-10 A70

1. Clinical features—A disease with systemic presentations and respiratory symptoms. Acute onset of fever, chills, headache, and myalgia are typical clinical features. Cough is initially absent or nonproductive; when present, sputum is mucopurulent and scant. Respiratory symptoms are often mild when compared with pneumonia and are demonstrable by chest X-ray. Pleuritic chest pain and splenomegaly occur infrequently; pulse may be slow in relation to temperature. Respiratory failure, hepatitis, endocarditis, and encephalitis are occasional complications; relapses may occur. Although usually mild or moderate, human disease can be severe, especially in untreated elderly persons.

2. Risk groups—Susceptibility is general and postinfection immunity is incomplete and transitory. Older adults may be more severely affected.

3. Causative agents—the bacterium *Chlamydophila* (formerly *Chlamydia*) *psittaci*.

4. Diagnosis—May be suspected in patients presenting with symptoms, a history of exposure to birds, and appropriate laboratory tests (serology). Owing to a lack of specific laboratory testing, there is a possibility that reported cases of psittacosis may have been caused by the recently described *Chlamydophila pneumoniae* rather than *C. psittaci*. Isolation of the infectious agent from sputum, blood, or postmortem tissues, cultured in mice, eggs, or cell culture and under safe laboratory conditions only, confirms the diagnosis. Recovery of the infectious agent from human specimens may be difficult, especially if the patient has received broad-spectrum antibiotics.

5. Occurrence—Worldwide. It is primarily an infection of birds. Outbreaks occasionally occur in households, pet shops, aviaries, avian exhibits, and pigeon lofts. Most human cases are sporadic; many infections are probably not diagnosed.

6. Reservoirs—Birds are the primary reservoir—mainly birds of the parrot family (psittacine birds, including parakeets and parrots); less often poultry, pigeons, and canaries. Apparently healthy birds can be carriers and shed the infectious agent, particularly when subjected to stress through crowding and shipping. Birds may shed the bacteria intermittently, and sometimes continuously, for weeks or months.

7. Incubation period—From 1 to 4 weeks.

8. Transmission—By inhaling the agent from desiccated droppings, secretions, and dust from feathers of infected birds. Imported psittacine birds are the most frequent source of exposure, followed by turkey and duck farms; processing and rendering plants have also been sources of occupational disease. Geese and pigeons are occasionally responsible for human disease. Rarely, person-to-person transmission may occur during acute illness with paroxysmal coughing.

9. Treatment—

Preferred therapy	Doxycycline 100 mg PO BID for $\geq$ 14 days to prevent relapse
Alternative therapy options	• Tetracycline 500 mg PO QID for $\geq$ 14 days OR • Chloramphenicol (no longer available in the USA) OR • Azithromycin 250–500 mg PO daily for 7 days
Special considerations and comments	• Use erythromycin in children and pregnant women (> 8 years: 2 g/day in divided doses; 2–8 years: 30 mg/kg/day in divided doses). • Macrolides and fluoroquinolones have in vitro activity against *Chlamydophila psittaci*; however, limited clinical data are available and macrolide and quinolone failures have been observed.

Note: BID = twice daily; PO = oral(ly); QID = 4 times daily.

10. Prevention—

1) Educate the public to the danger of exposure to infected pet birds. Medical personnel responsible for occupational health in animal processing plants should be aware that febrile respiratory illness with headache or myalgia among employees exposed to birds may be psittacosis.

2) Regulate the importation, raising, and trafficking of birds of the parrot family.

3) Prevent or eliminate avian infections through quarantine of infected farms (or premises with infected birds) until the buildings have been disinfected and diseased birds destroyed or adequately treated with tetracycline.

4) Psittacine birds offered for sale should be raised under psittacosis-free conditions and handled in such a manner as to prevent infection. Tetracyclines can be effective in controlling disease in psittacines and other companion birds if properly administered to ensure adequate intake for at least 30, and preferably 45, days.

5) Conduct surveillance at pet shops and aviaries where psittacosis has occurred or where birds epidemiologically linked to cases

were obtained and at farms or animal processing plants to which human psittacosis was traced. Infected birds must be treated or destroyed and the area where they were housed must be thoroughly cleaned and disinfected with a phenolic compound.

11. Special considerations—

1) Reporting: obligatory case report to health authorities in many countries.

2) Epidemic measures: cases are usually sporadic or confined to families but outbreaks related to infected aviaries or bird suppliers may be extensive. Report outbreaks of avian psittacosis to agricultural and public health authorities. In poultry flocks, large doses of tetracycline can suppress, but not eliminate, infection and thus may complicate investigations.

3) International measures: compliance with national regulations to control importation of psittacine birds.

[H. Badaruddin]

Q FEVER
(query fever)

DISEASE	ICD-10 CODE
Q FEVER	ICD-10 A78

1. Clinical features—Acute Q fever is a febrile disease characterized by chills, headache, malaise, myalgia, and sweats. There is considerable variation in severity and duration; infections may be unapparent or present as a fever of unknown origin. A pneumonitis may be found on radiographic evaluation, although radiographic patterns are nonspecific and do not allow for differentiation from other etiologies. The most common laboratory abnormalities are increased liver enzyme levels. Acute and chronic granulomatous hepatitis, which can be confused with tuberculous hepatitis, has been reported. Chronic Q fever is rare, manifests primarily as culture-negative endocarditis or vascular infection, and occurs primarily in patients with preexisting risk factors such as valvular or vascular defects. Other rare clinical syndromes, including neurologic syndromes, have been described. The case-fatality rate for hospitalized acute cases can be as high as 1%. Q fever endocarditis is fatal if untreated, whereas with treatment the

10-year mortality rate is 19%. A post–Q fever fatigue syndrome has been described.

2. Risk groups—Veterinarians; sheep, goat, and cattle farmers; researchers who work with ruminants; and abattoir workers are at risk for *Coxiella burnetii* infection. Persons with valvular heart disease, vascular defects, or arterial aneurysms; pregnant women; and persons who are immunosuppressed are at risk for chronic Q fever.

3. Causative agents—*C. burnetii*. The organism can be found in biologic excreta of infected animals such as urine, feces, and milk, with the highest numbers of bacteria shed in birth products (e.g., placenta, amniotic fluid). The bacterium is highly resistant to many disinfectants and environmental conditions.

4. Diagnosis—Serologic diagnosis is facilitated by use of 2 antigenic preparations: phase I, which is the virulent form of the agent, and phase II, which is a laboratory-generated attenuated form with truncated lipopolysaccharide. For acute Q fever, a demonstration of a 4-fold rise in immunoglobulin class G (IgG) antibody against phase II antigen between acute and convalescent serum taken 3 to 6 weeks apart is the standard for confirmed diagnosis. A single high serum phase II IgG titer may be considered evidence of probable acute infection in a clinically compatible patient. Laboratory diagnosis by polymerase chain reaction (PCR) of blood or serum can also be used in the first 2 weeks after symptom onset and prior to antibiotic administration. Diagnosis of chronic Q fever requires an identified nidus of infection and laboratory confirmation with PCR or anti-phase I IgG antibody titer greater than or equal to 1:1024. Bacteria may be identified in tissues (e.g., liver biopsy or heart valve) by PCR or immuno-histochemistry. Culture is rarely done owing to strict biosafety and biosecurity requirements. Anti-*C. burnetii* antibodies may be detectable for 10 to 15 years as long as sensitive methods such as immunofluorescence are used for detection.

5. Occurrence—Reported from all continents. *C. burnetii* is endemic in areas where reservoir animals are present. Outbreaks have occurred among workers in stockyards, in meatpacking and rendering plants, in laboratories, and in medical and veterinary centers that use sheep (especially pregnant ewes) in research. An epidemic occurred in the Netherlands from 2007 through 2010 that was linked to infected goat farms. Individual cases may occur where no animal contact can be demonstrated. The lack of animal contact should not preclude a clinical suspicion of diagnosis as infection via airborne transmission can occur miles from the animal reservoir.

6. Reservoirs—Sheep, cattle, and goats are the primary reservoirs for *C. burnetii*. However, infection has been confirmed in multiple vertebrate species, including cats, dogs, wild mammals, birds, and ticks. Transovarial and transstadial transmission are common in ticks that participate in wildlife cycles in rodents, larger animals, and birds. Infected animals are often asymptomatic but shed massive numbers of organisms in placental tissues and birth fluids at parturition. Abortions may occur in infected pregnant sheep and goats, particularly in naive populations where the agent has recently been introduced.

7. Incubation period—Dose-dependent; typically 2 to 3 weeks for acute disease; range 3 to 30 days. Chronic Q fever can present months to years after the initial infection.

8. Transmission—Occurs most commonly through airborne dissemination of *Coxiella* in dust or aerosols from premises contaminated by placental tissues, birth fluids, and excreta of infected animals. Airborne particles containing organisms may be carried downwind for a distance of 1 kilometer or more. Contamination also occurs through direct contact with contaminated materials, such as wool, straw, and laundry. Raw(unpasteurized) milk from infected cattle or goats contains viable organisms and may be responsible for human transmission. Direct transmission by blood or marrow transfusion has been rarely reported. Sporadic cases of nosocomial transmission have been reported in infected women during autopsies and obstetric procedures.

9. Treatment—

Acute Q Fever

	Adults	Children	Pregnant women
Drug	Doxycycline	Doxycycline	TMP/SMX
Dose	100 mg BID	2.2 mg/kg/dose BID	160 mg/800 mg BID
Route	PO	PO	PO
Alternative drug	TMP/SMX 160 mg/ 800 mg BID	• TMP/SMX 1:5 ratio • TMP 4–20 mg/kg/ day divided into 2 doses (≤ 320 mg/day)	Not applicable
Duration	14 days	14 days	≤ 32 weeks of gestation
Special considerations and comments	Not applicable	Drug choice is based on the age of the child, the severity of disease, and the presence of risk factors for chronic Q.[a]	TMP/SMX should be discontinued for the final 8 weeks of pregnancy because of the risk for hyperbilirubinemia.

Note: BID = twice daily; PO = oral(ly); TMP/SMX = trimethoprim-sulfamethoxazole.
[a]For further treatment information, see https://www.cdc.gov/mmwr/preview/mmwrhtml/rr6203a1.htm.

Chronic Q Fever

Drug	Doxycycline AND hydroxychloroquine
Dose	• Doxycycline 100 mg BID AND • Hydroxychloroquine 200 mg TID
Route	PO
Alternative drug	• Doxycycline PLUS • Moxifloxacin OR ciprofloxacin
Duration	• ≥ 18 months for native valve infection and ≥ 24 months for prosthetic valve infection. • For noncardiac organ disease, duration of treatment is dependent on serologic response.
Special considerations and comments	Extended treatment is required to prevent recurrence of chronic Q fever. Outcomes are better with doxycycline and hydroxychloroquine; only use alternative if absolutely necessary.

Note: BID = twice daily; TID = thrice daily.

10. **Prevention—**

   1) Educate persons in high-risk occupations on sources of infection and the necessity for adequate disinfection and disposal of animal birth products; restrict access to sheds, barns, and laboratories with potentially infected animals; and stress the value of pasteurization of milk.

   2) Immunization with vaccines prepared from formalin-inactivated *C. burnetii* is useful in protecting laboratory workers and is strongly recommended for those working with live *C. burnetii*. It should also be considered for abattoir workers and others in hazardous occupations, including those carrying out medical research with pregnant sheep. The only commercially available Q fever vaccine for humans is produced and licensed in Australia (Q-Vax). This vaccine should not be given to individuals with evidence of preexisting immunity to *C. burnetii* owing to the likelihood of adverse skin reactions at the injection site. A Q fever vaccine for cattle and goats (Coxevac) is available in some European countries.

   3) Research workers using live *C. burnetii* and/or pregnant sheep or goats should be identified and enrolled in a health education and surveillance program. This should include a baseline serum evaluation, followed by yearly evaluations. Persons at risk for chronic infection should be advised of the risk of serious illness that may result from Q fever. Laboratory clothes must be appropriately

bagged and washed to prevent infection of laundry personnel. Animal-holding facilities should be away from populated areas and measures should be implemented to prevent airflow to other occupied areas. No casual visitors should be permitted.

11. Special considerations—

1) Reporting: Q fever is a notifiable disease in many countries.
2) Epidemic measures: control measures involve elimination of sources of infection, observation of exposed people, and administration of doxycycline to symptomatic persons. The 2007–2010 Netherlands epidemic resolved after widespread culling of infected goats and repopulation with vaccinated goats nationwide. Detection is particularly important in pregnant women, immunosuppressed persons, and patients with cardiac valve and vascular lesions.
3) Deliberate use: because of its low infectious dose, aerosol transmission, environmental stability, and previous testing as a bioweapon, *C. burnetii* is regulated as a select agent by the US Federal Select Agent Program. The agent is listed as a category B bioterrorism agent by CDC.

[C. C. Cherry, G. J. Kersh]

RABIES
(hydrophobia)

DISEASE	ICD-10 CODE
RABIES, UNSPECIFIED	ICD-10 A82.9
CONTACT WITH AND (SUSPECTED) EXPOSURE TO RABIES	ICD-10 Z20.3

1. Clinical features—An acute viral zoonotic disease that causes a progressive viral encephalomyelitis that is nearly always fatal. Onset is generally heralded by a sense of apprehension, headache, fever, malaise, and sensory changes (paresthesias) at the site of an animal bite. Excitability and aerophobia and/or hydrophobia, often with spasms of swallowing muscles, are frequent symptoms. Delirium with occasional convulsions follows. Such classic symptoms of furious rabies are noted in two-thirds of cases, whereas the remaining present as paralysis of limbs and respiratory muscles with sparing of consciousness. Phobic spasms may be absent in the paralytic form. Coma and death ensue within 1 to 2 weeks, mainly owing to cardiac failure.

2. Risk groups—Persons exposed to rabid animals, particularly veterinarians and veterinary technicians, animal control staff, wildlife researchers, cavers, staff of quarantine kennels, rehabilitators, laboratory and field personnel working with rabies virus or other lyssaviruses, and long-term travelers to rabies-endemic areas. All mammals are susceptible to varying degrees; the degree of susceptibility may be influenced by the virus species and variant as well as by certain host parameters (e.g., age, health, nutrition).

3. Causative agents—Lyssaviruses, such as the classical rabies virus, are in the family Rhabdoviridae in the genus *Lyssavirus*. Genus *Lyssavirus* currently contains 14 species and is divided into 3 phylogroups. Only 1 of the species, classical rabies virus, is currently present in the Americas. Classical rabies virus is the most important for public health as it causes 99.9% of all human rabies cases worldwide. Lyssaviruses in Africa (Mokola and Duvenhage) and Eurasia (European bat lyssaviruses 1 and 2) and the Australian bat lyssavirus, which was first identified in 1996 in several species of flying foxes in Australia, have been associated with human deaths from rabies. All members of the genus are antigenically related, but use of monoclonal antibodies and nucleotide sequencing demonstrates differences according to animal species and/or geographic origin. Rabies caused by other lyssaviruses may be diagnosed by the standard direct fluorescent antibody test on brain tissue or by suggested antemortem tests. Several other lyssaviruses (e.g., Aravan virus, Irkut virus, Khujand virus, Lagos bat virus, West Caucasian bat virus, Shimoni bat virus, Bokeloh bat lyssavirus, Ikoma lyssavirus, Lleida bat lyssavirus) have been characterized as etiologic agents of rabies in mammals but have not so far been identified in human infections.

4. Diagnosis—Rabies can present in atypical forms and medical personnel unfamiliar with the disease may misdiagnose it. Confirmatory diagnosis is made through specific postmortem fluorescent antibody (FA) staining of brain tissue or virus isolation in mouse or cell cultures. Antemortem diagnosis can be made by specific FA staining of viral antigens in frozen skin sections taken from the back of the neck at the hairline, detection of viral antibodies in serum and cerebrospinal fluid, and specific amplification of viral nucleic acids in saliva or skin biopsies by reverse transcription polymerase chain reaction. Serologic diagnosis is based on neutralization tests in cell culture or in mice. Viral shedding in body secretions is intermittent; therefore, the absence of virus or nucleic acids in those secretions does not exclude rabies as a diagnosis. A combination of tests for detection of rabies-specific antibodies, antigens, and nucleic acids is needed for conclusive antemortem diagnosis.

5. Occurrence—Worldwide; more than 10 million human exposures and approximately 55,000 rabies deaths are estimated to occur each year, almost all in developing countries, particularly in Asia (31,000 deaths) and

Africa (24,000 deaths). The disease is underreported worldwide, owing in part to misdiagnosis. Most human deaths follow dog bites for which adequate postexposure prophylaxis (PEP) was not, or could not be, provided. In Latin America, a regional dog rabies control program coordinated by the Pan American Health Organization since 1983 has led to a reduction of almost 95% in the number of human deaths, with only 9 cases reported in 2012, 46% of which followed contact with hematophagous bats. During the past 12 years, although reductions in the numbers of human cases have been reported in several Asian countries (particularly Thailand), increases have occurred in China—where, since 1996, the number of notified human rabies deaths has continuously increased, reaching on average 3,000 to 4,000 in recent years. In Western, Central, and Eastern Europe, including Russia, fewer than 50 human rabies deaths are reported annually. In the USA between 2000 and 2012, 30 of 40 human rabies cases were acquired domestically and almost all were bat-associated infections.

Given the global distribution of bat rabies, few areas are truly free of autochthonous rabies in the animal population. Some sites include insular locations in the western Pacific and parts of the Caribbean. By 2000, many Western European countries had successfully eliminated fox rabies by oral immunization via the distribution of vaccine-laden baits. In Canada and the USA, oral immunization of free-ranging wild terrestrial carnivores has likewise helped to control rabies over large areas.

6. Reservoirs—All mammals are susceptible. Reservoirs and important vectors include wild and domestic Canidae, such as dogs, foxes, coyotes, wolves, and jackals, and also skunks, raccoons, raccoon dogs, mongooses, and other common carnivores, such as cats in North America. In developing countries, dogs remain the principal reservoir. Infected populations of vampire, frugivorous, and insectivorous bats occur in Mexico and Central and South America, and infected insectivorous bats are present throughout Canada, the USA, and Eurasia. In Africa, Asia, and Australia, infected frugivorous and insectivorous bat species are involved in transmission. Many other mammals, such as rabbits, squirrels, chipmunks, rats, mice, and opossums, are very rarely infected.

7. Incubation period—Highly variable but usually 3 to 8 weeks; very rarely as short as a few days or as long as several years. The length of the incubation period depends in part on wound severity, wound location in relation to nerve supply, and relative distance from the brain; the amount, species, and variant of virus; the degree of protection provided by clothing; and other factors.

8. Transmission—Dogs are the main transmitter of rabies to humans in most developing countries, whereas in many developed countries rabies is a disease of wild carnivores with sporadic spillover infection to domestic animals. The most common form of exposure is virus-laden saliva from a rabid animal introduced though a bite or scratch (and very rarely into a pre-existing fresh break in the skin or through intact mucous membranes). Person-to-person transmission is theoretically possible but is rare and not well documented. Several cases of rabies transmission by transplant of cornea, solid organs, and blood vessels from persons dying of undiagnosed central nervous system disease have been reported from Asia, Europe, and North America. Airborne spread has been suggested in a cave where heavy infestations of bats were roosting and demonstrated in laboratory settings, but this is thought to occur very rarely. Transmission from infected vampire bats feeding on domestic animals is common in Latin America. Rabid insectivorous or frugivorous bats can transmit rabies to terrestrial animals, wild or domestic. Defined periods of communicability before onset of clinical signs of animal hosts are only known with reliability in domestic dogs, cats, and ferrets and are usually for 3 to 10 days before onset of clinical signs (rarely 0.4 days) and throughout the course of the disease. Longer periods of excretion before onset of clinical signs (14 days) have been observed with certain canine rabies virus variants in experimental infections, but these are the exception. Excretion in other animals is highly variable. For example, in one study, bats shed virus for 12 to 16 days before evidence of illness, whereas, in another, skunks shed virus for at least 8 days before onset of clinical signs. In general, a 10-day communicability period with intermittent shedding preceding clinical onset for dogs, cats, and ferrets, and 14 days for other mammals (including humans), has been assumed in risk assessments in the majority of countries.

9. Treatment—

Previously vaccinated	<ul><li>Wound cleansing: immediate thorough cleansing of all wounds with soap and water. If available, a virucidal agent such as povidine-iodine solution should be used to irrigate the wounds.</li><li>HRIG: do not administer.</li><li>Vaccine: HDCV or PCECV 1.0 mL IM (deltoid area), on days 0 and 3.</li></ul>
Not previously vaccinated	<ul><li>Wound cleansing: immediate thorough cleansing of all wounds with soap and water. If available, a virucidal agent such as povidine-iodine solution should be used to irrigate the wounds.</li><li>-HRIG: 20 IU/kg. If feasible, the full dose should be infiltrated around and into the wound(s), and any remaining volume should be administered at an anatomic site (IM) distant from vaccine administration. HRIG should not be administered in the same syringe as vaccine because HRIG might partially suppress active production of rabies virus antibody; no more than the recommended dose should be administered.</li><li>Vaccine: HDCV or PCECV 1.0 mL IM (deltoid area) on days 0, 3, 7, and 14.</li></ul>

(Continued)

(Continued)

Special considerations and comments	• For younger children, the outer aspect of the thigh may be used. • For persons with immunosuppression, rabies PEP should be administered using all 5 doses of vaccine on days 0, 3, 7, 14, and 28.

Note: HDCV = human diploid cell vaccine; HRIG = human rabies immunoglobulin; IM = intramuscular(ly); IU = international units; PCECV = purified chick embryo cell vaccine; PEP = postexposure prophylaxis.

10. Prevention—Many preventive measures are possible at the level of the primary animal host(s) and transmitter(s) of rabies to humans. Such measures are part of a comprehensive rabies control program.

1) Register, license, and vaccinate all owned dogs, cats, ferrets, and other pets, when feasible, in enzootic countries; manage population of ownerless animals and strays. Educate pet owners and the public on the importance of local community responsibilities. Pets should be leashed in congested areas when not confined on the owner's premises; strange-acting or sick animals of any species—domestic or wild—should be avoided and not handled; animals that have bitten a person or another animal should be reported to relevant authorities, such as the police or local health departments; if possible, such animals should be confined and observed as a preventive measure or euthanized and tested in a laboratory. Wildlife should be appreciated in nature and not be kept as pets. Where animal population reduction is impractical, animal contraception and repetitive vaccination campaigns may prove effective.

2) Maintain active surveillance for animal rabies. Laboratory capacity should be developed to perform FA diagnosis on all wild mammals involved in human or domestic animal exposures and on all domestic animals clinically suspected of having rabies.

3) Detain and observe for 10 days any healthy-appearing dog, cat, or ferret known to have bitten a person (stray or ownerless dogs, cats, or ferrets may be euthanized and examined for rabies by fluorescent microscopy); animals showing suspicious clinical signs of rabies should be euthanized and tested for rabies. If the biting animal was infective at the time of the bite, it usually develops signs of rabies within 4 to 10 days, such as change in behavior, excitability, or paralysis, followed by acute death. All wild mammals that have bitten a person should be euthanized and the brain examined for evidence of rabies.

4) In a timely manner, submit to a qualified laboratory the intact head of suspect animals, packed in ice (not frozen), for rabies diagnosis.

5) Euthanize unvaccinated domestic animals bitten by known rabid animals; if detention is elected, hold the animal in a secure facility for at least 6 months under veterinary supervision, and vaccinate against rabies at least 30 days before release. If previously vaccinated, booster immediately with rabies vaccine and detain for at least 45 days.

6) Immunize wild carnivore reservoirs and free-ranging domestic dogs, using vaccine-laden baits containing attenuated or recombinant rabies viral vectors, as utilized in Europe and North America.

7) Cooperate with wildlife conservation authorities in programs to reduce the carrying capacity of wildlife hosts of sylvatic rabies with vaccine-laden baits and to reduce exposures to domestic animals and human populations—such as in circumscribed enzootic areas near campsites and in areas of dense human habitation.

8) Vaccinate individuals at high risk of exposure (see Risk Groups in this chapter). Such persons should receive preexposure immunization, using potent and safe cell-culture vaccines. Vaccine can be administered in doses of 1.0 or 0.5 mL intramuscularly on days 0, 7, and 21 or 28. Results with intradermal (ID) immunization (using WHO-recommended schedules) for human diploid cell vaccine (HDCV), purified chick embryo cell vaccine (PCECV), and purified Vero cell vaccines have been equivalent to what is expected from the intramuscular (IM) schedule. Antibody response to ID immunization has, however, been less than ideal in some groups receiving chloroquine for antimalarial chemoprophylaxis and may be the same in persons receiving antimalarials structurally related to chloroquine (e.g., mefloquine, hydroxychloroquine). HDCV was the original gold standard for modern human rabies prophylaxis, but other less expensive cell-culture vaccines fulfilling basic WHO requirements for the ID route, such as purified Vero cell and chick embryo cell vaccines, are widely and successfully used in many canine rabies–endemic countries.

If a risk of exposure continues, single booster doses are given, preferably after serologic testing every 6 months to 2 years, depending upon the defined level of exposure, as long as the risk remains. Cell-culture vaccines are considered to be safe and well-tolerated, although reported reaction rates to primary immunization have varied with the monitoring system. Following IM immunization with HDCV, mild and self-limited local reactions, such as pain at the site of injection, redness, and swelling, occur in 21% to 74% of cases. Mild systemic reactions, such as fever, headache, dizziness, and gastrointestinal symptoms, occur in 5% to 40% of cases, and systemic hypersensitivity following booster injections occurs in 6% of vaccinated individuals but is less common following primary immunization. When further purification steps are added, systemic hypersensitivity reactions become very rare. With chick embryo and Vero cell–based vaccines, the rates of local and mild systemic reactions are similar to those with HDCV, but no systemic hypersensitivity reactions have been reported. Compared with IM vaccination, the ID application is at least as safe and well tolerated.

Prevention of rabies after animal bites (PEP) consists of first aid, passive immunization, and vaccination as follows:

1) First aid: clean and flush the wound immediately with soap or detergent and water, then apply either 70% ethanol, tincture of aqueous solution of iodine or povidone-iodine, or Dakin's solution (household bleach: 3 tablespoons of bleach plus one-half teaspoon baking soda in 1 L boiled water). The wound should not be sutured unless unavoidable. Sutures, if required, should be placed after local infiltration of immunoglobulin (see point 2); they should be loose and should not interfere with free bleeding and drainage.

2) Passive immunization: infiltrate the wound with human (HRIG) or equine (ERIG) rabies immunoglobulin as soon as possible after exposure to neutralize the virus. HRIG should be used in a single dose of 20 international units (IU)/kg and ERIG in a single dose of 40 IU/kg. All, or as much as possible, of the rabies immunoglobulin (RIG) should be infiltrated into and around the bite wound; the remainder, if any, should be given intramuscularly. Where serum of animal origin (ERIG) is used, an ID or subcutaneous test dose preceding administration may detect potential allergic sensitivity, but the utility of this testing for predictive risk has been questionable.

- In previously vaccinated persons, RIG and ERIG are not required or recommended as part of PEP.
- No significant adverse reactions have been attributed to HRIG; however, immunoglobulin from a nonhuman source produces serum sickness in 5% to 40% of recipients. Newer, commercially produced purified animal globulins, in particular purified equine globulin, have only a 1% to 6% risk of serum sickness reactions. The commonly used skin test for

ERIG does not predict serum sickness. Serious anaphylaxis is extremely rare with purified ERIG products (2 in 150,000 cases in one series). The risk of contracting fatal rabies outweighs the risks for allergic reactions.

- Animal studies suggest that passive immunization with HRIG and ERIG, combined with vaccination, is effective after exposure to the majority of known lyssavirus species (phylogroup I). However, currently available rabies biologics do not provide adequate protection against phylogroup II (Mokola virus, Lagos and Shimoni bat viruses) and putative group III lyssaviruses (West Caucasian bat virus and Ikoma lyssavirus). Regardless, although PEP may not always be effective for the management of some bat lyssavirus infections, it should always be used in all the geographic location.

3) Vaccination: WHO-approved cell-culture vaccines should be applied according to the WHO and CDC (Advisory Committee on Immunization Practices)–approved modified Essen regimen in 4 IM doses of 0.5 or 1.0 mL on days 0, 3, 7, and 14 in the deltoid region or for small children in lateral thigh muscles. This is to start as soon as possible after exposure. In Europe, Asia, Africa, and South and Central America, 2 additional WHO-approved regimens are widely used and found to be safe and effective; these are referred to as the Essen regimen, comprising 5 IM doses of vaccine on days 0, 3, 7, 14, and 28, and the 2-1-1 or Zagreb regimen, which consists of 2 full IM doses at 2 sites on day 0 and 1 injection each on days 7 and 21, thus saving 1 vaccine dose and 1 clinic visit.

- Reduced-dose vaccination, WHO-approved, multisite ID postexposure schedules have been approved by local authorities in several rabies-endemic countries of Asia and Africa where the cost of vaccine is a significant deterrent to proper PEP. WHO recommends 2 ID multisite regimens with cell-culture vaccines known to be safe and immunogenic: (a) the 2-site Thai Red Cross regimen (2-2-0-2) and (b) the 8-site Oxford regimen (8-0-4-0-1-1). If properly applied using potent modern vaccines, these schedules result in an antibody response equivalent to that seen with the 3 WHO-approved IM regimens.
- In terms of passive prophylaxis, animal studies suggest that vaccination should be provided as a part of PEP after exposure to any lyssaviruses regardless of the geographic location.

- It has been well documented that subjects with severe immunodeficiency will not respond well to rabies vaccination, and some may not develop neutralizing antibody. Careful wound cleansing and the use of immunoglobulin is thus of great importance in such patients, with the vaccination mandatory and administered via the usual full 5-dose regimen.
- A serum specimen should be collected at the time of the last dose of vaccine and tested for rabies antibodies. If sensitization reactions appear in the course of immunization, consult the health department or infectious disease consultants for guidance. If the immunodeficient person has had a previous full course of preexposure or postexposure rabies immunization with an approved vaccine, only 2 doses of vaccine need to be given—one immediately and one 3 days later.

4) The combination of local wound treatment, passive immunization with RIG, and active vaccination is recommended for all severe exposures (category III; see later) and provides reliable, adequate protection. Pregnancy and infancy are never contraindications to PEP. Persons presenting even months after the bite must be dealt with in the same way as recent exposures. Factors to be considered in the initiation of PEP are the nature of the contact; rabies endemicity at the site of encounter or origin of the animal; the animal species involved; vaccination/clinical status of the animal and of the exposed person; availability of the animal for observation; and laboratory results of the animal for rabies, if available.

11. Special considerations—

1) Reporting: obligatory case report to the local health authority is required in most countries.

2) Epidemic (epizootic) measures: applicable only to animals; a sporadic disease in humans.

- Establish control area under authority of laws, regulations, and ordinances in cooperation with appropriate human, agricultural, and wildlife conservation authorities.
- Immunize dogs and cats through officially sponsored, intensified mass programs that provide immunizations at temporary and emergency stations. For protection of other domestic animals, use approved vaccines appropriate for each animal species.
- In urban areas of industrialized countries, ensure strict enforcement of regulations, entailing collection, detention,

and euthanasia of ownerless and stray dogs and of nonimmu-nized dogs found off owners' premises; control of the dog population by castration, spaying, or drugs, as well as thorough policies for proper waste management, have been effective in breaking transmission cycles.

- Mass immunization of wildlife with baits containing vaccine has contained red fox rabies in Western Europe and southern Canada and coyote, gray fox, and raccoon rabies in the USA.

3) Disaster implications: a potential problem exists if the disease is freshly introduced or enzootic in an area where there are many stray dogs or wild reservoir animals. Similarly, in disaster areas—for example after earthquakes, hurricanes, or tsunamis—stray animals may be present after human evacuations with subsequent bites to animal control or humane society personnel taking part in future rescue attempts.

4) International measures:

- Strict compliance by common carriers and travelers with national laws and regulation (http://www.who.int/ith/en). Immunization of animals, certificates of health and origin, and microchip identification of animals may be required.
- WHO Collaborating Centres and other international organiz-ations and institutions are prepared to collaborate with national services on request. See WHO technical reports.[1,2] Further information on WHO Collaborating Centres can be found at: http://www.who.int/collaboratingcentres/database/en.

POSTEXPOSURE PROPHYLAXIS GUIDE (Tables 1 and 2)

Table 1. WHO Recommendations for PEP Rabies Management

Category of Exposure	Type of Exposure/Contact With a Domestic or Wild Animal[a] Suspected or Confirmed to be Rabid or With an Animal Unavailable for Testing	WHO-Recommended PEP
Category I (no exposure)	Touching or feeding of animal; licks on intact skin. Contact of intact skin with secretions or excretions of a rabid animal or human case.	None, if reliable case history is available.

(Continued)

Table 1. WHO Recommendations for PEP Rabies Management (Continued)

Category of Exposure	Type of Exposure/Contact With a Domestic or Wild Animal[a] Suspected or Confirmed to be Rabid or With an Animal Unavailable for Testing	WHO-Recommended PEP
Category II	Nibbling of uncovered skin. Minor scratches or abrasions without bleeding.	Administer vaccine immediately.[b] Stop prophylaxis if animal remains healthy throughout an observation period of 10 days[c] or is proven to be negative for rabies by a reliable laboratory, using appropriate diagnostic techniques.
Category III	Single or multiple transdermal bites[d] or scratches; contamination of mucous membranes with saliva (licks); licks on broken skin. Exposure to bats.[e]	• Administer rabies vaccine immediately and rabies immunoglobulin, preferably as soon as possible after initiation of PEP. Rabies immunoglobulin can be injected up to 7 days after administration of first vaccine dose. • Stop prophylaxis if animal remains healthy throughout an observation of 10 days or is proven to be negative for rabies by a reliable laboratory using appropriate diagnostic techniques.

Source: Based on WHO.[1,2]

Note: PEP = postexposure prophylaxis.

[a] Exposure to most small mammals, such as insectivores (e.g., shrews), rodents (e.g., mice, rats, squirrels), and lagomorphs (e.g., rabbits and hares), seldom, if ever, requires specific rabies prophylaxis.

[b] The placing of an apparently healthy dog or cat in or from a low-risk area under careful supervision may warrant delaying prophylaxis.

[c] This observation period applies only to dogs, cats, and ferrets. Except for threatened or endangered species, other domestic and wild animals suspected of being rabid should be euthanized and their tissues examined for the presence of rabies antigen by appropriate laboratory techniques.

[d] Bites are category III exposures, especially on the head, neck, face, hands, and genitals because of the rich innervation of these areas.

[e] PEP should be considered when contact between a human and a bat has occurred, unless the exposed person can rule out a bite or scratch or exposure of a mucous membrane.

Table 2. US Recommendations for Postexposure Management

Vaccination Status	Regimen[a]
Not previously vaccinated	• Wound cleansing: all PEP to begin with immediate and thorough cleansing of all wounds with soap and water. If available, a virucidal agent such as a povidone-iodine solution should be used to irrigate the wounds. • HRIG: administer 20 IU/kg. If anatomically feasible, the full dose should be infiltrated around the wound(s); any remaining volume should be administered IM at an anatomic site distant from that of the vaccine administration (such as the deltoid or the anterior-lateral aspect of the thigh). HRIG should not be administered in the same syringe or location as the vaccine. Because HRIG may partially suppress active production of antibody, no more than the recommended dose should be given. • Vaccine: HDCV or PCECV 1.0 mL IM (deltoid area[b]) on days 0, 3, 7, and 14 in immunocompetent individuals and on days 0, 3, 7, 14, and 28 in immunosuppressed individuals.[c]
Previously vaccinated[d]	• Wound cleansing: all PEP to begin with immediate and thorough cleansing of all wounds with soap and water. If available, a virucidal agent such as a povidone-iodine solution should be used to irrigate wounds. • HRIG: HRIG should not be administered. • Vaccine: HDCV or PCECV 1.0 mL IM (deltoid area[b]) on days 0 and 3.[c]

Source: Based on Rupprecht et al.[3] and Manning et al.[4]

Note: HDCV = human diploid cell vaccine; HRIG = human rabies immunoglobulin; IM = intramuscular(ly); IU = international units; PCECV = purified chick embryo cell vaccine; PEP = postexposure prophylaxis.

[a]Regimens are applicable for all age groups, including children.

[b]The deltoid area is the only acceptable site of vaccination for adults and older children. For younger children, the outer aspect of the thigh may be used. Never administer vaccine in the gluteal area.

[c]Day 0 is the day the first dose of vaccine is administered.

[d]History of preexposure vaccination with HDCV, RVA (rabies vaccine, adsorbed), or PCECV; prior PEP with HDCV, RVA, or PCECV; or previous vaccination with any other type of rabies vaccine and a documented history of antibody response to the prior vaccination.

In addition to PEP as described, consult regional, provincial, local, state, or national health officials if questions arise about the need for rabies prophylaxis.

References

1. WHO. *WHO Expert Consultation on Rabies. Second report.* WHO Technical Report Series 982. 2013. Available at: https://apps.who.int/iris/handle/10665/85346. Accessed November 21, 2019.

2. WHO.. *WHO Expert Committee on Specifications for Pharmaceutical Preparations. Fiftieth Report*. WHO Technical Report Series 996. Annex 8. 2016. Available at: http://apps.who.int/medicinedocs/documents/s22397en/s22397en.pdf. Accessed November 21, 2019.

3. Rupprecht CE, Briggs D, Brown CM, et al. Use of a reduced (4-dose) vaccine schedule for postexposure prophylaxis to prevent human rabies: recommendations of the Advisory Committee on Immunization Practices. *MMWR Recomm Rep*. 2010;59(RR-2):1–9.

4. Manning SE, Rupprecht CE, Fishbein D, et al. Human rabies prevention—United States, 2008: recommendations of the Advisory Committee on Immunization Practices. *MMWR Recomm Rep*. 2008;57(RR-3):1–28.

[I. Chuang]

RAT-BITE FEVER
(streptobacillary fever, Haverhill fever, epidemic arthritic erythema, spirillary fever, sodoku)

DISEASE	ICD-10 CODE
STREPTOBACILLOSIS	ICD-10 A25.1
SPIRILLOSIS	ICD-10 A25.0

1. Clinical features—The term "rat-bite fever" refers to 2 rare zoonotic bacterial infections—streptobacillosis and spirillosis—which have similar clinical features. In streptobacillosis, a rapid onset of headache, fever, vomiting, and muscle or joint pain is followed within 2 to 4 days by a maculopapular rash often focused on the extremities. The rash can also be petechial, purpuric, or pustular. Polyarthritis is a common development in cases of streptobacillosis. There is usually a history of a rodent bite, which heals normally within the previous 10 days. In untreated cases of streptobacillosis, bacterial endocarditis, pericarditis, parotitis, tenosynovitis, and focal abscesses of soft tissues or the brain can occur. Symptoms typically resolve within 2 weeks without treatment but relapses can occur. For some it can take a year for symptoms to resolve. Streptobacillosis has an approximate case-fatality rate of 7% to 10%.

Spirillosis is characterized by fever, a rash with reddish or purplish plaques, and the presence of an indurated or ulcerated lesion at the site of the bite; regional lymphadenopathy may occur. Arthritic symptoms are rare in this disease. Otherwise, spirillosis has complications similar to those seen in streptobacillosis. In untreated patients, the case-fatality rate is approximately 10%.

2. Risk groups—Persons who come in direct or indirect contact with rats, mice, and other reported animal reservoirs. These persons include people living in poverty, laboratory technicians, and pet store workers. It is important to note that children account for more than 50% of new cases. This may be an underestimate as rat-bite fever is not a reportable disease.

3. Causative agents—*Streptobacillus moniliformis* causes streptobacillosis. This rod-shaped organism is Gram-negative and nonmotile. *S. moniliformis* is a fastidious, slow-growing organism; thus, cultures should be maintained for at least 7 to 10 days following inoculation. *Spirillum minus* causes spirillosis. This spiral-shaped organism is Gram-negative and uses bipolar flagella for mobility. *S. minus* has not been successfully cultured on laboratory media (similar to other spirochetes).

4. Diagnosis—Laboratory methods are essential for differentiation from other bacterial infections. However, owing to the risk of morbidity and mortality, empiric therapy should not await laboratory confirmation. Microbiologic confirmation of streptobacillosis is done through the isolation of *S. moniliformis* by inoculating matter from the primary lesions, blood, joint fluid, lymph node, or pus into the appropriate bacteriologic medium enriched with 20% serum or ascitic fluid for optimal growth. Culture of *S. moniliformis* may be enhanced by using heart infusion agar plates with 5% rabbit or sheep blood with addition of sterile rabbit or horse serum spread on the agar and dried. Anaerobic blood cultures should be used to optimize yield from blood. To confirm *S. minus* in the laboratory animal, inoculation and direct visualization via Giemsa stain, Wright stain, or dark-field microscopy are used. Additionally, 16S ribosomal ribonucleic acid can be used for diagnosis if that laboratory capability is available.

5. Occurrence—Rat-bite fever is a rare disease that can be found globally. Streptobacillosis occurs more commonly in North and South America and Europe, while spirillosis is more common in Asia and Africa. In the parts of Asia where rat-bite fever is due to *S. minus*, the disease is called sodoku, meaning rat poison.

6. Reservoirs—Infected rats; seldom in other rodents, including mice, gerbils, and guinea pigs; ferrets, weasels, cats, and dogs, which may become infected when consuming infected rodents.

7. Incubation period—For streptobacillosis, usually from 3 to 10 days; can range from 2 days to 3 weeks. For spirillosis, usually between 7 and 21 days with a range of 1 day to 6 weeks.

8. Transmission—*S. moniliformis* and *S. minus* are commensal organisms of rats and can be found in the upper respiratory and conjunctival secretions and urine of an infected animal. Transmission most frequently occurs through biting or scratching but sporadic cases may occur without history of a bite. Infection has occurred through indirect contact such as living or working in rat-infested buildings where exposure to rat saliva, urine, or droppings on surfaces may transpire. Infection can occur through the consumption of contaminated food and drink; an outbreak associated with contaminated milk occurred in 1926 in Haverhill, Massachusetts, giving rise to the moniker of Haverhill fever. No direct person-to-person transmission has been reported.

9. Treatment—

Drug	Penicillin G
Dose	• Adults: 1.2 million IU/day divided every 4 hours • Children: 100,000 IU/kg/day divided every 4 hours
Route	IV and PO
Alternative drug	Erythromycin, doxycycline, tetracycline, chloramphenicol, clindamycin, and cephalosporins
Duration	• Adults: 7 days IV • Children: 7 days IV; some experts recommend another 7 days PO
Special considerations and comments	• Once bitten, clean and disinfect wound as soon as possible and cover with a clean dressing. • Higher penicillin doses should be used for endocarditis. • Prompt treatment may reduce clinical course and subsequent complications.

Note: IU = international units; IV = intravenous(ly); PO = oral(ly).

10. Prevention—Avoid direct contact with rodents by rat-proofing dwellings and reducing reservoir populations. Prevent contamination of food and water sources by rodents. For pet owners and laboratory animal technicians, take proper safety precautions by utilizing appropriate restraining techniques, protective equipment, and hygiene practices such as washing hands when handling rodents. Penicillin (or amoxicillin/clavulanate) may be used as prophylaxis following a rodent bite.

11. Special considerations—

1) Reporting: report of an epidemic to the local health authority is obligatory in most countries; no case report required, although encouraged.
2) Epidemic measures: a cluster of cases requires search for a common source, possibly contaminated food and water.

Bibliography

CDC. Rat-bite fever (RBF). 2019. Available at: https://www.cdc.gov/rat-bite-fever/index.html. Accessed November 26, 2019.

Gupta M, Bhansali RK, Nagalli S, Oliver TI. *Rat-bite Fever (Streptobacillus moniliformis, Sodoku, Spirillum Minor)*—StatPearls Publishing. Available at: https://www.ncbi.nlm.nih.gov/books/NBK448197. Accessed November 26, 2019.

The Center for Food Security and Public Health, Iowa State University. Rat bite fever. 2013. Available at: http://www.cfsph.iastate.edu/FastFacts/pdfs/rat_bite_fever_F.pdf. Accessed November 26, 2019.

[C. Harrison, S. Eppes]

RELAPSING FEVER
(borrelia recurrentis, louse-borne relapsing fever)

DISEASE	ICD-10 CODE
RELAPSING FEVER	ICD-10 A68

1. Clinical features—A systemic louse-borne epidemic or tickborne sporadic spirochetal disease in which periods of fever lasting 2 to 7 days alternate with afebrile periods of 4 to 14 days; the number of relapses varies from 1 to 10 or more. Total duration of louse-borne relapsing fever (LBRF) averages 13 to 16 days; usually longer for tickborne relapsing fever (TBRF). Other nonspecific signs and symptoms include headache, myalgia, arthralgia, shaking chills, and gastrointestinal pain or illness. Patients with LBRF are more likely to have jaundice, central nervous system involvement, petechial rashes, blood-tinged sputum, and epistaxis. In contrast, acute respiratory distress syndrome has been reported more frequently in TBRF. Predisposing factors (poor nutrition and thiamine or vitamin B deficiency) may lead to more severe disease and neurologic involvement. The overall case-fatality rate in untreated cases is between 2% and 10%.

2. Risk groups—Various risk groups in endemic regions. For LBRF, those living in crowded conditions with poor sanitary resources and practice, particularly those sharing clothing and bedding with infected individuals. For TBRF, persons disturbing or inhabiting environments (caves and abandoned human dwellings) where infected ticks and reservoirs are present. Most argasid ticks are indiscriminate feeders and will prey upon humans when their usual blood-meal host is purposely displaced by human intervention or unwittingly displaced by human activity. The developing human fetus is particularly vulnerable to often fatal infection as spirochetes are able to cross the placental barrier and establish a persistent fetal infection while the mother may clear the infection.

3. Causative agents—Helical and motile spirochetes of the genus *Borrelia*. *Borrelia recurrentis* is the sole agent of human-specific LBRF and is spread from person to person by the human body louse. *Borrelia duttoni* also appears to be a human-specific pathogen but is one of more than 10 species that cause TBRF; all TBRF species are transmitted by soft-bodied (argasid) ticks. Both LBRF and TBRF spirochetes demonstrate antigenic variation in parallel with successive relapses. In North America, most human cases are caused by *Borrelia hermsii* transmitted by the soft-bodied tick *Ornithodoros hermsi*. The classical agent of relapsing fever in Europe is *Borrelia hispanica*, also tickborne.

4. Diagnosis—The spiral-shaped bacteria range in length from 7 to 30 μm and in width from 0.2 to 0.5 μm and stain poorly with Gram stain reagents. They are best detected in peripheral blood (febrile periods most sensitive) and visualized in wet mounts by dark-field microscopy (where corkscrew motility assists detection) or in Giemsa- or Wright-based stained smears with bright-field microscopy. Detection of spirochetes during afebrile and late-stage febrile periods is generally insensitive. Weanling mice and specialized liquid culture media (Barbour-Stoenner-Kelly) may serve as amplifying environments to increase the sensitivity of subsequent microscopic detection.

5. Occurrence—Relapsing fever has been reported from all parts of the world except Australia and New Zealand. Louse-borne relapsing fever occurs in limited areas in Asia, eastern Africa (Burundi, Ethiopia, and Sudan), highlands of Central Africa, and South America. Tickborne disease is endemic throughout tropical Africa with other foci in India, Iran, Portugal, Saudi Arabia, Spain, northern Africa, Central Asia, and North and South America. Sporadic human cases and occasional outbreaks of tickborne disease occur in portions of Europe, western Canada, and the USA. In parts of the world, such as Senegal and Tanzania for TBRF and Ethiopia for LBRF, these diseases are among the top 10 bacterial causes of mortality and hospital admissions.

6. Reservoirs—For the singular agent of LBRF (*B. recurrentis*) and 1 species (*B. duttoni*) of TBRF, humans are the reservoir. For other species of TBRF, wild rodents are the primary reservoir. The long life span (years) of argasid (soft) tick vectors of TBRF and transovarial transmission of spirochetes from adult females to eggs may enable ticks themselves to serve as reservoirs during periods of mammalian blood-host absence. With the exception of *B. recurrentis* and *B. duttoni*, humans are incidental and dead-end hosts.

7. Incubation period—LBRF, usually 8 days (range, 5–15 days); TBRF about 7 days (range, 2–18 days).

8. Transmission—The epidemic form (LBRF) is spread by lice, whereas the endemic or sporadic forms are spread by argasid ticks. Repeated infections may occur. There is no direct person-to-person transmission (exception—transplacental transmission in infected pregnant women). LBRF is acquired by crushing an infected louse, *Pediculus humanus*; this results in contamination of the bite wound or an abrasion of the skin. Lice become infective 4 to 5 days after ingestion of blood from an infected person and remain so for life (20–30 days). In tickborne disease, people are infected by the bite of an argasid tick, principally *Ornithodoros moubata* and *Ornithodoros hispanica* in Africa, *Ornithodoros rudis* and *Ornithodoros talaje* in Central and South America, *Ornithodoros tholozani* in the Near East and Middle East, and *O. hermsi* and *Ornithodoros turicata* in the USA. Most argasid ticks are rapid (30 minutes) and nocturnal feeding ticks and bites are often not recognized. Infected ticks can live and remain infective for several years without feeding; they may pass the infection transovarially to their progeny.

9. Treatment—CDC has not developed specific guidelines for relapsing fever. However, expert guidance is noted in the treatment table.

Drug	Tetracycline (for adults)
Dose	500 mg every 6 hours for 10 days
Route	PO
Alternative drug	Erythromycin 500 mg (or 12.5 mg/kg) every 6 hours for 10 days
Duration	10 days for both regimens
Special considerations and comments	Observe patients during the first 4 hours of initiating antimicrobial therapy for the Jarisch-Herxheimer reaction and for respiratory distress syndrome.

Note: PO = oral(ly).

10. Prevention—

1) Control lice using measures prescribed for louse-borne typhus (see Epidemic Louse-Borne Typhus Fever in "Typhus").
2) Control ticks by measures prescribed for spotted fever (see "Rickettsioses"). Soft-tick–infested human habitations may present a major problem and eradication of the ticks may be difficult. Closing crevasses in wall structures and installing rodent proofing to prevent future colonization by rodents and their soft ticks are the mainstay of prevention and control. Spraying with approved acaricides, such as diazinon, chlorpyrifos, propoxur, pyrethrum, or permethrin, may be tried.
3) Use personal protective measures, including repellents and permethrin, on clothing and bedding for people with exposure in

endemic foci. Dimethyl phthalate (5%) and 10% carbolic soap are effective.

4) Antibiotic chemoprophylaxis with tetracyclines may be taken after exposure (arthropod bites) when the risk of acquiring the infection is high.

11. Special considerations—

1) Reporting: report to local health authority of LBRF required as a disease under surveillance by WHO; TBRF—reporting required in some areas.

2) Epidemic measures: for LBRF, when case reporting has been properly done and cases are localized, dust or spray contacts and their clothing with 1% permethrin and apply permethrin spray at 0.03 to 0.3 kg/hectare (2.47 acres) to the immediate environment of all reported cases. Provide facilities for washing clothes and for bathing to affected populations; establish active surveillance, especially in refugee camps. Where infection is known to be widespread, apply permethrin systematically to all people in the community. For TBRF, apply permethrin or other acaricides to target areas where vector ticks are thought to be present; for sustained control, an application cycle of 1 month is recommended during the transmission season. Since animals (horses, camels, cows, sheep, pigs, and dogs) can also play a role in TBRF, persons entering tick-infested areas (hunters, soldiers, vacationers, and others) should be educated regarding the disease.

3) Disaster implications: a serious potential hazard among louse-infested populations. Epidemics are common in wars, famines, and other situations with increased prevalence of pediculosis (e.g., overcrowded, malnourished populations with poor personal hygiene), especially with important population movements and in refugee camps.

4) International measures: prompt notification by governments to WHO and adjacent countries of an outbreak of LBRF in any areas of their territories with further information on the source and type of the disease and the number of cases and deaths.

5) Further information can be found at:
https://www.cdc.gov/relapsing-fever/clinicians/index.html.

[O. A. Khan]

RICKETTSIOSES
(spotted fever group)

DISEASE	CAUSATIVE AGENT	ICD-10 CODE
ROCKY MOUNTAIN SPOTTED FEVER	*Rickettsia rickettsii*	ICD-10 A77.0
MEDITERRANEAN SPOTTED FEVER (BOUTONNEUSE FEVER)	*Rickettsia conorii* and closely related organisms	ICD-10 A77.1
AFRICAN TICK-BITE FEVER	*Rickettsia africae*	ICD-10 A77.8 (other tickborne spotted fevers [specified])
QUEENSLAND TICK TYPHUS	*Rickettsia australis*	ICD-10 A77.3
NORTH ASIAN TICK TYPHUS	*Rickettsia sibirica*	ICD-10 A77.2
TICKBORNE LYMPHADENOPATHY (TIBOLA)	*Rickettsia slovaca*	ICD-10 A77.8
FLINDERS ISLAND SPOTTED FEVER	*Rickettsia honei*	ICD-10 A77.8
AUSTRALIAN SPOTTED FEVER	*Rickettsia marmionii*	ICD-10 A77.8
FAR EASTERN SPOTTED FEVER	*Rickettsia heilongjiangensis*	ICD-10 A77.8
JAPANESE SPOTTED FEVER	*Rickettsia japonica*	ICD-10 A77.8
RICKETTSIA PARKERI RICKETTSIOSIS	*Rickettsia parkeri*	ICD-10 A77.8
RICKETTSIALPOX	*Rickettsia akari*	ICD-10 A79.1

I. TICKBORNE SPOTTED FEVERS
ROCKY MOUNTAIN SPOTTED FEVER (RMSF, fiebre maculosa)
MEDITERRANEAN SPOTTED FEVER (Mediterranean tick fever, boutonneuse fever, Marseilles fever, Kenya tick typhus, Indian tick typhus, Israeli tick typhus, Astrakhan fever)
AFRICAN TICK-BITE FEVER
NORTH ASIAN TICK FEVER (Siberian tick typhus)
TICKBORNE LYMPHADENOPATHY (TIBOLA, *Dermacentor*-borne necrosis erythema and lymphadenopathy [DEBONEL])
FLINDERS ISLAND SPOTTED FEVER (Thai tick typhus)
AUSTRALIAN SPOTTED FEVER
FAR EASTERN SPOTTED FEVER
JAPANESE SPOTTED FEVER
RICKETTSIA PARKERI RICKETTSIOSIS

1. Clinical features—Spotted fever group rickettsial infections are a closely related group of primarily tickborne bacterial infections causing clinically similar diseases characterized by fever, rash, and vasculitis. Although clinical presentations and severity vary by species, some spotted fever infections can be associated with multiorgan involvement such as respiratory failure, hepatosplenomegaly, heart failure, renal failure, dysfunctional bleeding or coagulopathy, and neurologic complications.

1) Rocky Mountain spotted fever (RMSF) ranges greatly in severity and can be mild if treated early or rapidly fatal in some patients if appropriate treatment is not initiated before day 5 of symptoms. It is characterized by the sudden onset of moderate-to-high fever, significant malaise, muscle and joint pain, severe headache, chills, and conjunctival injection. A maculopapular rash typically appears on the extremities between the second and fourth day of illness; however, rash can develop later in the course of the illness and approximately 10% of individuals will never develop a rash. The rash includes the palms and soles in about 30% of those affected and spreads centrally to the trunk. Around days 5 to 7 of illness, the rash can evolve into a petechial exanthema, which is reflective of vascular damage and can be accompanied by end-organ dysfunction. Every effort should be made to treat the disease before these manifestations develop. The case-fatality rate for untreated cases can range from 20% to 25%; in some regions during outbreaks, fatality rates have been reported as high as 80%. Prompt recognition and treatment are most effective at preventing fatal outcome; the median time from onset of symptoms to death is 8 days in fatal cases. Delayed treatment with antibiotics is the single most important risk factor associated with severe disease and death. Factors such as absence, delayed appearance, or failure to recognize rash, along with illness occurrence outside either the typical season or geographic distribution, make diagnosis more difficult and can lead to delayed treatment and severe outcomes, including death. Approximately half of all patients will report a tick bite; tick bites are typically painless and often go unrecognized by patients. The most common laboratory abnormalities in patients with RMSF are low platelets, low sodium, and elevated liver enzymes. In the early stages of RMSF, the disease may be confused with a variety of febrile illnesses, including, but not limited to, ehrlichiosis, meningococcemia (see "Meningitis"), enteroviral infection, dengue, pyelonephritis, and pneumonia.

2) Mediterranean spotted fever (MSF) can range in severity and is characterized by abrupt onset of fever; there may be a primary lesion or eschar at the site of the tick bite. This eschar (tache noire), often evident at the onset of fever, is a small ulcer 2 to 5 mm in diameter with a black center and red areola; regional lymph nodes

are often enlarged. A generalized maculopapular erythematous rash occurs on about the fourth to fifth day. With appropriate antibiotic therapy, fever typically resolves within 48 hours. The case-fatality rate varies by region.

3) African tick-bite fever is similar to MSF but typically presents with a milder course. Fatalities are rarely reported. Abrupt onset of fever, nausea, headache, and myalgia are common and may be accompanied by 1 or more inoculation eschars. Regional draining lymphangitis and aphthous stomatitis may occur. Rash is present in only half the cases and may be maculopapular or vesicular. Complications are rare and symptoms typically resolve within 10 days but resolve more quickly with appropriate antibiotics.

4) Queensland tick typhus is clinically similar to MSF; the rash may be vesicular.

5) North Asian tick typhus is clinically similar to MSF; rash and lymph-adenitis are common.

6) Tickborne lymphadenopathy is a mild rickettsiosis; main symptoms include an eschar, often found on the head; regional lympha-denopathy; low-grade fever; and, in some cases, alopecia at the eschar site.

7) Flinders Island spotted fever is a mild disease with maculopapular rash; eschar and adenopathy are rare.

8) Australian spotted fever manifests with eschar, maculopapular or vesicular rash, and adenopathy; fatalities have been reported.

9) Far Eastern spotted fever is characterized by eschar, faint macular or maculopapular rash, lymphadenopathy, and lymphangitis; con-junctival papulae may be present.

10) Japanese spotted fever similarly involves eschar, macular or mac-ulopapular rash (which may become petechial), and lymphaden-opathy; fatalities have been described.

11) *Rickettsia parkeri* rickettsiosis is a mild febrile illness with eschar and maculopapular or vesicular rash.

2. Risk groups—Anyone engaging in activities placing them in contact with tick environments—including, but not limited to, camping, gardening, hiking, or close contact with animals that are in similar environments—are susceptible. Risk factors for severe or fatal outcome include extremes of age, alcoholism, glucose-6-phosphate dehydrogenase deficiency, and immuno-compromised status; however, fatal outcome can occur in previously healthy people of all ages in severe diseases such as RMSF. Patients with a history of alcoholism may be at increased risk for delayed diagnosis and treatment because abnormal laboratory values may be attributed to alcohol abuse and not appreciated as indicative of an acute rickettsial illness.

3. Causative agents—See earlier table.

4. Diagnosis—Samples from symptomatic patients at the acute stage of illness, including tissue biopsies (eschar and rash), eschar swab sampling, whole blood, and less commonly serum, may be tested by polymerase chain reaction (PCR) for confirmation of disease by the detection of *Rickettsia*-specific nucleic acid sequences. Samples must be collected before or within 48 hours of doxycycline treatment. Because of the low level of bacteria circulating in blood, a negative result does not rule out an active infection, while a positive result is confirmatory. Indirect immunofluorescence assay (IFA) is the reference standard for serologic diagnostic confirmation. Serologic diagnosis is confirmed by a 4-fold or greater rise in specific antibody (immunoglobulin class G) titer between acute and convalescent sera. The acute sample should be taken in the first week of illness and the convalescent sample should be taken 2 to 4 weeks later (for *Rickettsia africae*, the convalescent sample should be collected 4–6 weeks after the acute sampling, owing to a longer latency period). IFA tests become positive generally in the second to third week of illness. Therefore, an acute titer taken in the first week of illness should be used as a baseline for comparison with the convalescent sample; a negative acute result does not rule out active infection—nor does a positive acute result confirm the diagnosis. Confirmatory diagnosis cannot be made with a single serology result. Immunohistochemistry and culture can also be used to confirm diagnosis. Older Weil-Felix tests using Proteus OX-19 and Proteus OX-2 antigens are less sensitive and less specific and are not recommended.

5. Occurrence—

1) RMSF: throughout the USA. Recently, there has been an increasing number of cases reported from the southwestern USA. Cases have also been documented in Argentina, Brazil, Canada, Colombia, Mexico, and Central America. In most of the USA, infections occur from April through September; in the southwest, cases have been reported year-round.

2) MSF: widely distributed throughout the African continent, India, and in parts of Europe and the Middle East adjacent to the Mediterranean and the Black and Caspian seas. Temperate areas report disease during warmer months when ticks are more prevalent; in tropical regions, disease is reported year-round. Tache noir lesions are seen with less frequency in areas such as the Negev, Israel, and Astrakhan, Russia.

3) African tick-bite fever: sub-Saharan Africa, including Botswana, South Africa, Swaziland, and Zimbabwe, and the West Indies, including the Lesser Antilles. Outbreaks of disease may occur when groups

of travelers (such as people on safari in Africa) are bitten by ticks. Cases are occasionally imported into the USA and Europe.

4) Queensland tick typhus: Queensland, New South Wales, Tasmania, and coastal areas of eastern Victoria, Australia.

5) North Asian tick fever: North China, Mongolia, and Asiatic areas of Russia.

6) Tickborne lymphadenopathy: Europe and Asia.

7) Flinders Island spotted fever: Australia, Thailand, Flinders Island, and Tasmania.

8) Australian spotted fever: Australia.

9) Far Eastern spotted fever: Far East of Russia, northern China.

10) Japanese spotted fever: Japan.

11) *R. parkeri* rickettsiosis: coastal regions of southeastern USA; southern South America, including Argentina, Uruguay, and parts of Brazil.

6. Reservoirs—Maintained in nature among a variety of tick species by transovarial and transstadial passage. Organisms from both RMSF and MSF can be transmitted to dogs, rodents, and other animals; animal infections may be subclinical but persistent infections in rodents and disease in dogs have been observed. Dogs are useful sentinels for spotted fever group rickettsiae. Clustering of cases of RMSF in humans and dogs may occur. Rodents and reptiles are the reservoir for Australian spotted fever and Japanese spotted fever; rodents and lagomorphs for Far Eastern spotted fever. The reservoir for Flinders Island spotted fever is not well determined; however, reptiles, migratory birds, and rodents are suspected.

7. Incubation period—Incubation periods for all spotted fever group rickettsial infections range from 2 to 21 days.

8. Transmission—Most spotted fever infections are transmitted by ixodid (hard) ticks, which are widely distributed throughout the world; tick species differ markedly according to geographic area. Primary route of transmission is via tick exposure; however, diagnosis should not depend on the recollection of a tick bite as they are often painless and can go unrecognized. The diseases are not directly transmitted from person to person; however, household clusters may occur because of the possible proximity to the infected tick population. Common vectors are as follows:

1) RMSF: *Dermacentor variabilis* (American dog tick), *Dermacentor andersoni* (Rocky Mountain wood tick), *Rhipicephalus sanguineus* (brown dog tick), and *Amblyomma cajennense* (Cayenne tick)

2) MSF: *Rhipicephalus sanguineus* (brown dog tick)

3) African tickbite fever: *Amblyomma hebraeum* (African bont tick) and *Amblyomma variegatum* (tropical bont tick)

4) Queensland tick typhus: *Ixodes holocyclus* (paralysis tick)
5) North Asian tick fever: *Dermacentor* and *Haemaphysalis* ticks
6) Tickborne lymphadenopathy: *Dermacentor marginatus* (ornate sheep tick)
7) Flinders Island spotted fever: *Aponomma hydrosauri* (southern reptile tick), *Ixodes tasmani* (common marsupial tick), and *Ixodes granulatus*
8) Australian spotted fever: *I. holocyclus* (Australian paralysis tick) and *Haemaphysalis novaeguineae*
9) Far Eastern spotted fever: *Dermacentor silvarum, Haemaphysalis concinna* (relict tick), and *Haemaphysalis japonica douglasii*
10) Japanese spotted fever: *Haemaphysalis flava, Haemaphysalis longicornis* (bush tick), *Dermacentor taiwanensis,* and *Ixodes ovatus*
11) *R. parkeri* Rickettsiosis: *A. maculatum* and *Amblyomma triste*

9. Treatment—

Drug	Doxycycline
Dose	• 100 mg BID for adults and children ≥ 45 kg • 2.2 mg/kg BID for children < 45 kg
Route	PO or IV
Alternative drug	• Alternative therapies have been associated with increased risk of death and severe outcome. • Chloramphenicol is the only acceptable alternative treatment.
Duration	• 5–7 days or ≥ 3 days after defervescence or signs of clinical improvement. • Short courses (≤ 10 days have not been shown to cause enamel hypoplasia or tooth discoloration in children < 8 years)
Special considerations and comments	All efforts should be made to begin treatment before day 5 of symptoms, especially for RMSF.

Note: BID = twice daily; IV = intravenous(ly); PO = oral(ly); RMSF = Rocky Mountain spotted fever.

10. Prevention—

1) See also Prevention in "Lyme Disease." Utilize repellants prior to exposure and search for and remove attached or crawling ticks immediately after exposure to tick-infested habitats.
2) Minimize tick populations near residences by removing ticks from dogs and using collars or other treatment with an anti-tick claim.

3) Vaccines are not available. Antibiotic prophylaxis following a tick bite is not recommended and may delay or confound presentation, making it more difficult to correctly diagnose.

11. Special considerations—Reporting: case reporting is obligatory for many of the spotted fever rickettsioses diseases in certain countries. WHO Collaborating Centres provide support as required. More information can be found at: http://www.who.int/collaboratingcentres/database/en.

II. RICKETTSIALPOX (vesicular rickettsiosis)

1. Clinical features—an acute febrile illness in which an initial skin lesion at the site of a mite bite, often associated with lymphadenopathy, is followed by fever. A disseminated vesicular skin rash appears, which generally does not involve the palms and soles and lasts only a few days. It may be confused with chickenpox. Death is uncommon. Acute hepatitis is one of the more common indicators that can follow infection but precede rash.

2. Risk groups—Individuals residing in urban settings with rodents are more likely to be exposed.

3. Causative agents—*Rickettsia akari.*

4. Diagnosis—Serology, PCR, or immunostains of biopsied tissues as described in Diagnosis under Tickborne Spotted Fevers in this chapter.

5. Occurrence—Urban areas of the eastern USA; most cases have been described in New York City. *R. akari* has also been reported in Russia and neighboring countries, Africa, and Korea.

6. Reservoirs—Mice (*Mus musculus*) in urban sites in the USA. Commensal rats are reported to be the reservoir in Russia and *Apodemus* in Korea.

7. Incubation period—6 to 15 days.

8. Transmission—Rickettsialpox is acquired from *Liponyssoides sanguineus,* the house mouse mite, through either a bite or similar contamination of broken skin with the feces of infected mites. The disease is not directly transmitted from person to person; however, household clusters may occur because of the possible proximity to the infected mite population.

9. Treatment—

Drug	Doxycyline
Dose	• 100 mg BID for adults and children ≥ 45 kg • 2.2 mg/kg BID for children < 45 kg
Route	PO (IV rarely needed)

(Continued)

(Continued)

Alternative drug	Chloramphenicol
Duration	5–7 days or ≥ 48 hours after improvement in symptoms; can resolve without treatment.
Special considerations and comments	None

Note: BID = twice daily; IV = intravenous(ly); PO = oral(ly).

10. Prevention—Includes rodent elimination and mite control.

11. Special considerations—None.

[P. Armstrong, C. Kato]

RIFT VALLEY FEVER

DISEASE	ICD-10 CODE
RIFT VALLEY FEVER	ICD-10 A92.4

1. Clinical features—Rift Valley fever (RVF) is a viral zoonosis that primarily affects animals but also has the capacity to infect humans. RVF virus (RVFV) infection can be unapparent or characterized by a brief, self-limiting febrile illness with a sudden onset of fever, myalgia, chills, dizziness, and headache, lasting for 3 to 4 days. General symptoms also include abdominal pains, severe joint and muscle pains (particularly in the back and extremities), weakness, sweating, and constipation. Recovery is usually without sequelae.

In a small proportion of cases (1%), the clinical syndrome progresses to a severe disease of 3 forms: ocular (0.5%–2% of patients), meningoencephalitis (< 1% of patients), or hemorrhagic with liver failure (< 1% of patients).

In the ocular form of the disease, mild general symptoms are accompanied by retinal lesions. Visual defects tend to occur 1 to 3 weeks after onset of initial symptoms and include photophobia, reduced vision, blind spots, uveitis, retinitis, and retinal hemorrhage. Ocular complications are most frequently reported in all forms of RVF disease, occurring in up to 10% of infected patients, even those with less severe disease. Deaths among patients who present with the ocular form of the disease only are uncommon.

The onset of the meningoencephalitis form occurs 1 to 4 weeks after the first general symptoms appear. The meningoencephalitis form of RVF is characterized by neurocognitive symptoms, including severe headaches, hallucinations, loss of memory, confusion, vertigo, convulsions, and lethargy. Neurologic complications may appear after more than 60 days after initial infection. The meningoencephalitis form is rarely fatal; however, residual neurologic defect is common and may be severe.

Symptoms for the hemorrhagic form of RVF begin 2 to 4 days after onset of illness. General symptoms are accompanied by evidence of liver impairment, including jaundice. Shortly after, hemorrhagic symptoms begin to appear, including vomiting blood; bleeding from the nose, gums, or venipuncture sites; passing blood in stools; and purpuric rashes and ecchymoses. The case-fatality ratio for patients with the severe hemorrhagic form of the disease is approximately 50%. Death occurs 3 to 6 days after symptom onset.

The appearance of shock, multiorgan failure, and disseminated intravascular coagulation indicates a poor prognosis. Laboratory findings may include elevated liver enzyme levels, thrombocytopenia, leukopenia, anemia, and elevated blood urea nitrogen and creatinine. Variable neurologic sequelae are observed in survivors of RVF meningoencephalitis. In about 1% to 5% of all RVF patients, unilateral or bilateral retinal hemorrhages occur, resulting in transitory or permanent scotoma visual field defects. The overall case-fatality rate is low (1%–5%) but can reach up to 50% in hospitalized patients.

2. Risk groups—Humans become infected from contact with blood, organs, and tissues of infected animals; inhalation of airborne droplets from animals; the bite of an infected mosquito; or mechanical transmission via blood-feeding flies. Farmers, herders, owners of livestock, abattoir workers, and veterinary personnel are at risk of RVFV infection. Numerous laboratory infections were described before the systematic use of personnel protective equipment.

3. Causative agents—RVFV is a single-stranded enveloped RNA virus and a member of the genus *Phlebovirus*, family Phenuiviridae.

4. Diagnosis—During the acute phase of the disease (4–5 days post onset), the virus can be detected from blood or serum by conventional or real-time polymerase chain reaction, virus isolation, or antigen detection enzyme-linked immunosorbent assay (ELISA). Serologic diagnosis (immunoglobulin class M [IgM], immunoglobulin class G) is confirmed by ELISA. RVFV-specific neutralizing antibodies persist for years. Antibodies appear a few days after onset of symptoms and the virus is very rapidly cleared. In fatal cases, the virus can be detected in tissues (liver) by molecular techniques, virus isolation, or immunohistochemistry.

5. Occurrence—An RVF-compatible disease in lambs and humans was first reported in East Africa in the 1910s and RVFV was first isolated in 1930 in the Rift Valley region of Kenya. Since then, it has been reported in most sub-Saharan African countries, Egypt, and Madagascar, and in the past 10 years in the Arabian Peninsula (Yemen and Saudi Arabia), marking the first reported occurrences of the disease outside the African continent (see Table 1 in this chapter). Furthermore, in 2016, a Chinese man acquired RVFV after he traveled to Angola and returned home to China, marking the first documented instance of a human RVFV infection in East Asia. This raises concerns that RVFV could extend to other parts of Asia, Europe, and the Middle East. Large livestock and human outbreaks have recurred in East Africa, Egypt, Sudan, Mauritania, Senegal, South Africa, Namibia, Niger, and Madagascar.

The largest human RVF outbreak in recent memory occurred in Niger in 2016. In August of 2016, health officials in the Tahoua region reported cases of acute febrile illness and hemorrhagic symptoms in humans and ruminants. From August 2016 through December 2016, 348 suspected or probable cases of RVF were reported by the WHO Niger Country Office (17 of which were laboratory-confirmed); there were 33 deaths.

Table 1. Rift Valley Fever Outbreaks Since Initial Recognition of the Virus in 1931

Year	Location	Human cases
1930–1931	Rift Valley, Kenya	Not determined
1950–1951	South Africa	Not determined
1974–1975	South Africa	110 confirmed or probable cases; 7 deaths
1977–1979	Egypt	200,000 confirmed or probable cases; 600 deaths
1978	Zimbabwe	3 deaths
1987	Mauritania	220 deaths
1997–1998	East Africa	89,000 confirmed or probable cases; 478 deaths
1998	Mauritania	400 confirmed or probable cases; 6 deaths
2000–2001	Saudi Arabia	886 confirmed or probable cases; 123 deaths
2000–2001	Yemen	1,328 confirmed or probable cases; 166 deaths
2003	Egypt	148 confirmed or probable cases; 27 deaths
2006–2007	Kenya	684 confirmed or probable cases; 155 deaths
2006–2007	Somalia	114 confirmed or probable cases; 51 deaths
2006–2007	Tanzania	309 confirmed or probable cases; 142 deaths
2007–2008	Sudan	747 confirmed or probable cases; 230 deaths
2008–2009	Madagascar	418 confirmed or probable cases; 17 deaths
2010	Mauritania	63 confirmed or probable cases; 13 deaths

(Continued)

Table 1. Rift Valley Fever Outbreaks Since Initial Recognition of the Virus in 1931 (Continued)

Year	Location	Human cases
2010–2011	South Africa	302 confirmed or probable cases; 25 deaths
2012	Mauritania	41 confirmed or probable cases; 18 deaths
2016	China	1 confirmed or probable case
2016	Niger	348 confirmed or probable cases; 33 deaths
2018	South Sudan	20 confirmed or probable cases; 4 deaths
2018	Gambia	1 probable case; 1 death

6. **Reservoirs**—RVFV is a predominantly epizootic virus and is maintained in nature in *Aedes* spp. mosquitoes and in wildlife reservoirs such as rodents, wild ruminants, or bats. Domestic ruminants serve as the main amplifying hosts. Virus has been isolated from male and female mosquitoes, suggesting transovarial transmission. Hatching of infected *Aedes* eggs follows abnormally high rainfall and flooding, and infected mosquitoes feed on susceptible wildlife species or livestock, resulting in abortion storms and virus amplification. Horizontal transmission to other mosquito species (i.e., *Culex*, *Anopheles*, and *Mansonia*) is facilitated by the high viremia observed in domestic ruminants. RVFV has also been isolated in ticks, flies, and midges.

7. **Incubation period**—Usually 2 to 6 days.

8. **Transmission**—RVFV is transmitted through bites of infected mosquitoes, by mechanical transmission via blood-feeding flies, or by direct contact with the blood, body fluids, or abortion products of infected domestic ruminants (e.g., sheep, goats, cattle, camels). The virus infects humans through inoculation—for example, via a wound from an infected knife, through contact with broken skin, or through inhalation of aerosols produced during the slaughter of infected animals. The aerosol mode of transmission has also led to infection in laboratory workers. Ingestion of unpasteurized dairy and undercooked meat has also been reported as a route of transmission. Direct human-to-human transmission has not been reported, but accidental laboratory infections with RVFVs have been frequently described. While nosocomial transmission has not yet been described, it is theoretically possible; therefore, personal protective measures are recommended to prevent exposure to infected blood or bodily fluids.

A few cases of vertical transmission have been independently reported, in Sudan in 2008, when a pregnant Sudanese mother delivered a baby boy with a skin rash and enlarged liver. Both mother and infant tested positive for RVFV-specific IgM, indicating vertical transmission; however, the clinical significance of RVFV vertical transmission and the effects of infection on both mother and infant are not yet understood. Research exploring the mechanisms of vertical transmission is underway in preclinical studies with pregnant rodents, which may set the stage for future vaccine trials.

9. Treatment—There are currently no licensed therapeutics for RVFV and no therapeutic candidates have proceeded to clinical trials in humans. For hospitalized patients with RVFV, supportive care and careful monitoring of hydration and fluid volume are recommended. Oral or intravenous fluid replacement is highly suggested.

10. Prevention—

1) Vaccination: there are currently no licensed RVF vaccines available for use in humans. An inactivated vaccine has been developed for human use in experimental contexts to protect veterinary and laboratory personnel at high risk of exposure to RVF; however, it is not licensed or commercially available for widespread use.

2) Contact and droplet precautions are recommended for management of RVF patients. Personal protective equipment and high-containment laboratories are recommended for RVFV manipulations.

3) Application of insect repellents on clothes in endemic areas; see "Arboviral Encephalitides" for preventive measures against mosquitoes.

4) Handling potentially infected animals or their tissues should be done with protective equipment, using contact and droplet precautions.

5) RVFV infections of humans are most effectively prevented by preventing animal infections through vaccination of livestock. Several vaccines using various strategies for use in livestock have been developed; however, there are no fully licensed RVFV vaccines approved for veterinary use outside endemic areas.

11. Special considerations—

1) Reporting: individual cases should be reported to the local health authority and confirmed cases could be notifiable to national authorities in some countries. Security authorities in some countries also require notification of RVFV isolation. RVFV is listed as an agent that must be assessed in terms of potential to cause public health emergencies of international concern under the International Health Regulations. Suspicion or confirmation of RVF in humans or animals should also be reported to the Food and Agriculture Organization of the United Nations, the World Organisation for Animal Health, and applicable WHO regional bodies.

2) Epidemic measures: limit contact with potentially infected animals. Use of insecticide-treated bed nets and insect repellent is recommended to prevent mosquito transmission of RVFV (see "Arboviral Encephalitides").

3) Human infection as a result of laboratory work is the biggest risk for transmission of RVFV to humans. RVFV is therefore classified as a risk group 3 agent and biosafety level 3 laboratory containment is necessary to work with the virus in the laboratory.

[A. Parikh, M. Amare, I.-M. Vilcins, C. Storme, P. Scott, K. Modjarrad]

ROTAVIRUS INFECTION
(sporadic viral gastroenteritis, severe viral gastroenteritis of infants and children)

DISEASE	ICD-10 CODE
ROTAVIRUS INFECTION	ICD-10 A08.0

1. Clinical features—A sporadic, seasonal, often severe gastroenteritis of infants and young children, characterized by vomiting, fever, and watery diarrhea. Rotavirus infection is occasionally associated with severe dehydration and death in young children. Secondary symptomatic cases among adult family contacts can occur, although subclinical infections are more common. Rotavirus is a major cause of nosocomial diarrhea of children younger than 5 years. Although rotavirus diarrhea is generally more severe than acute diarrhea owing to other agents, illness caused by rotavirus is not distinguishable from that caused by other enteric viruses for any individual patient.

2. Risk groups—Susceptibility is greatest in those aged between 6 and 24 months. By 3 years, most children have acquired rotavirus antibodies. Diarrhea is relatively uncommon in infected infants younger than 3 months. Immunocompromised individuals are at particular risk for prolonged rotavirus antigen excretion and intermittent rotavirus diarrhea. Ninety percent of pediatric deaths from rotavirus occur in low-income countries.

3. Causative agents—The 70-nm rotavirus belongs to the Reoviridae family. Group A is most common in humans, group B is uncommon in infants but has caused large epidemics in adults in China, and group C appears to be uncommon in humans. Groups A, B, C, D, E, and F occur in animals. There are 6 major serotypes of group A human rotavirus, based on antigenic differences. The main target of rotavirus is mature intestinal enterocytes mostly concentrated at the tips of intestinal villi. The major neutralization antigen is the VP7 outer capsid surface protein; another outer capsid protein, VP4, is associated with virulence and also plays a role in virus neutralization.

4. Diagnosis—Commercially available enzyme-linked immunosorbent assay (ELISA) kits have long been the standard method for diagnosis and the most commonly used worldwide, with sensitivity and specificity at 90% to 95%. Electron microscopy, latex agglutination, and other immunologic techniques, some of which are commercially available, can also identify rotavirus in stool specimens or rectal swabs but are not commonly used. False-positive ELISA reactions are common in newborns; thus, positive reactions in newborns require confirmation by an alternative test. Polymerase chain reaction (PCR)–based assays are helpful in determining genotypes of the virus but are less widely available than ELISA tests. PCR-based enteric pathogen panels are increasingly available and include rotavirus testing.

5. Occurrence—Historically rotavirus has been associated with about one-third to one-half of hospitalized cases of diarrheal illness in infants and children younger than 5 years. The introduction of rotavirus vaccine has reduced rotavirus-associated hospitalizations by 67% worldwide. Neonatal rotaviral infections are frequent in certain settings but are usually asymptomatic. Essentially, all children are infected by rotavirus in their first 2 to 3 years of life, with peak incidence of clinical disease in the 6- to 24-month age group. Rotavirus is more frequently associated with severe diarrhea than other enteric pathogens; in developing countries, it is responsible for an estimated 200,000 to 250,000 diarrheal deaths each year. Although not consistent in all settings, in temperate climates rotavirus diarrhea often occurs in seasonal peaks during cooler months, while in tropical climates diarrhea usually occurs throughout the year with a moderate peak in the cooler dry months. Rotavirus infection of adults is usually mild and is a cause of travelers' diarrhea, diarrhea in the immunocompromised (including those with human immunodeficiency virus infection), diarrhea in parents of children with rotavirus infection, and diarrhea in the elderly (sometimes in outbreaks in geriatric units).

6. Reservoirs—Probably humans. The animal viruses do not typically produce disease in humans.

7. Incubation period—Approximately 24 to 72 hours.

8. Transmission—Probably fecal-oral with possible contact with contaminated hands, environmental surfaces, and sometimes contaminated food and water reservoirs. The virus is communicable during the acute stage and later while viral shedding continues. Rotavirus is not usually detectable after about the eighth day of infection, although excretion of virus can last up to

20 days (in immunocompromised hosts viral shedding may last 30 days or more). Symptoms last for an average of 4 to 6 days.

9. Treatment—Focused on acute management of dehydration. Oral and intravenous rehydration is the main treatment for dehydration from rotavirus or other acute gastroenteritis etiology. In mild-to-moderate dehydration in children and adults, oral rehydration therapy is the preferred treatment. If there is concern for intestinal ileus or inaudible bowel sounds on examination, oral rehydration should be avoided. Intravenous rehydration is reserved for severe dehydration. Children who appear ill and lethargic, are drinking poorly, or have vital signs near or at criteria for hypovolemic shock should be started on intravenous rehydration. Using fluid-deficient calculations will estimate the amount of fluid needed to rehydrate.

Drug	There is no medication that is used to treat rotavirus. Symptoms of dehydration are managed with fluid resuscitation and electrolytes. If malnutrition is suspected, ensuring protein caloric intake is adequate.
Dose	Not applicable
Route	PO or IV fluids
Alternative drug	There is some evidence that the introduction of probiotics (e.g., *Lactobacillus rhamnosus*, *Lactobacillus plantarum*, several strains of *bifidobacteria* and *Enterococcus faecium* [the SF68 strain], and yeast such as *Saccharomyces boulardii*) may help to reduce pro-inflammatory cytokines caused by rotavirus infection.
Duration	Typically, 1–5 days of fluid and electrolyte management is indicated for rotavirus.
Special considerations and comments	Breastfeeding should continue throughout acute rotavirus infection for breastfed infants.

Note: IV = intravenous(ly); PO = oral(ly).

10. Prevention—

1) WHO has prequalified 4 oral live attenuated rotavirus vaccines: Rotarix, RotaTeq, Rotavac, and RotaSiil. Rotarix and RotaTeq are the 2 vaccines marketed worldwide and most commonly used. Rotarix is dosed at 2 months and 4 months. RotaTeq is dosed at 2 months, 4 months, and 6 months. Clinical trials in both developed and developing countries have demonstrated their safety and efficacy (80%–90%) in preventing rotavirus-associated severe gastroenteritis. Data from many countries in the developed world that have implemented routine rotavirus vaccination show

marked declines in the incidence of severe diarrhea, including declines in diarrhea mortality.

2) The effectiveness of other preventive measures is undetermined. Hygienic measures applicable to diseases transmitted via the fecal-oral route may not be effective in preventing transmission. The virus survives for long periods on hard surfaces, in water, and on hands. It is relatively resistant to some commonly used disinfectants but is inactivated by chlorine.

3) Prevent exposure of infants and young children to individuals with acute gastroenteritis in family and institutional (day care or hospital) settings by maintaining a high level of sanitary practices.

4) Exclusively breastfed infants are partially protected against rotavirus infection during the period of breastfeeding; however, immunity typically decreases in those aged around 4 months. Mothers should continue to breastfeed even during acute rotavirus infection to provide adequate hydration to infected infants.

11. Special considerations—

1) Reporting: obligatory report of epidemics in some countries; no individual case report required.

2) Rotavirus is a potential problem with dislocated populations and dense populations.

[M. Molnar, S. Eppes]

RUBELLA
(German measles)

DISEASE	ICD-10 CODE
RUBELLA	ICD-10 B06

1. Clinical features—Rubella is usually a mild febrile viral disease with a diffuse punctate and maculopapular rash. Clinically similar to other febrile rash illnesses (e.g., measles, dengue, parvovirus B19, human herpesvirus 6, coxsackievirus, echovirus, adenovirus, scarlet fever). Children usually present few or no constitutional symptoms, but adults may experience a 1- to 5-day prodrome of low-grade fever, headache, malaise, mild coryza, and conjunctivitis. Postauricular, occipital, and posterior cervical lymphadenopathy is the most characteristic clinical feature and precedes the rash by

5 to 10 days. Thrombocytopenia can occur but hemorrhagic manifestations are rare. Arthralgia and, less commonly, arthritis complicate a substantial proportion of infections, particularly among adult females. Encephalitis is seen in 1 out of 6,000 cases and occurs with a higher frequency in adults. Up to 50% of rubella infections are either without rash or subclinical.

Rubella is important because it can produce a constellation of anomalies in the developing fetus, called congenital rubella syndrome (CRS). CRS may occur in up to 90% of infants born to women who are infected with rubella during the first 10 weeks of pregnancy. Fetuses infected early are at greatest risk of intrauterine death, spontaneous abortion, and CRS. Clinical manifestations of CRS include single or combined defects or symptoms such as hearing impairment, cataracts, microphthalmia, congenital glaucoma, microcephaly, meningoencephalitis, developmental delay, congenital heart defects (e.g., patent ductus arteriosus, atrial or ventricular septal defects), purpura, hepatosplenomegaly, jaundice, and radiolucent bone disease. Moderate and severe CRS is usually recognizable at birth; mild CRS with only slight cardiac involvement or hearing impairment may not be detected for months or even years after birth. Insulin-dependent diabetes mellitus is recognized as a frequent late manifestation of CRS. Congenital malformations and fetal death can also occur following inapparent maternal rubella. Defects are rare when maternal infection occurs after the twentieth week of gestation.

2. Risk groups—Immunity is usually permanent after natural infection and thought to be long-term, probably lifelong, after immunization; infants born to immune mothers are ordinarily protected for 6 to 9 months, depending on the amount of maternal antibodies acquired transplacentally.

3. Causative agents—Rubella virus (family Togaviridae, genus *Rubivirus*).

4. Diagnosis—Laboratory diagnosis of rubella is required since clinical diagnosis is often inaccurate. Laboratory confirmation is usually based on a positive rubella-specific immunoglobulin class M (IgM) enzyme-linked immunosorbent assay (ELISA) test on a blood specimen obtained within 28 days after the rash onset. An epidemiologically confirmed rubella case is a patient with suspected rubella with an epidemiologic link to a laboratory-confirmed case.

Other methods for rubella diagnosis include paired serum specimens that show seroconversion or at least a 4-fold rise in rubella-specific immunoglobulin class G (IgG) antibody titer, positive rubella reverse transcription polymerase chain reaction (RT-PCR) test, and virus isolation; RT-PCR and virus isolation may be only available in higher-level reference laboratories.

Laboratory confirmation of CRS in an infant is based on a positive rubella-specific IgM ELISA test on a blood specimen, the persistence of a rubella-specific IgG antibody titer in a blood specimen beyond the time expected from passive transfer of maternal IgG antibody, isolation of the virus from a throat swab or urine specimen, or detection of rubella virus by PCR. Almost all infants with CRS have a positive rubella IgM test from 0 to 3 months old and more than 30% of infants remain positive from 4 to 9 months old. Rubella virus has been isolated from throat and urine specimens of infants with CRS and from cataract surgery aspirates in children aged up to 3 years.

5. Occurrence—In the absence of generalized immunization, rubella has occurred worldwide at endemic levels with epidemics every 5 to 9 years. Large rubella epidemics have resulted in very high levels of morbidity. For example, the US epidemic in 1964–1965 led to an estimated 12.5 million cases of rubella, more than 20,000 cases of CRS, and 11,000 fetal deaths; the incidence of CRS during endemic periods was 0.1 to 0.2 per 1,000 live births and 1 to 4 per 1,000 live births during epidemics. In countries where the rubella vaccine has not been introduced, rubella remains endemic. In 2010, an estimated 103,000 CRS cases occurred worldwide. Since 2009, surveillance data have provided evidence that the interruption of rubella virus transmission among countries has occurred in the WHO Region of the Americas and rubella is now only endemic in the rest of the world.

As of 2013, 135 countries/territories (70% of the world total) have introduced rubella vaccine in their national immunization programs, with the highest percentage in the WHO Region of the Americas (100% of countries) and Europe (100%), followed by the Western Pacific Region (81%), the Eastern Mediterranean Region (64%), the South-East Asia Region (45%), and the African Region (13%). In many countries, sustained high levels of rubella immunization have drastically reduced or eliminated rubella and CRS.

6. Reservoirs—Humans.

7. Incubation period—From 14 to 17 days, with a range of 14 to 21 days.

8. Transmission—Through contact with nasopharyngeal secretions of infected people. Infection is by droplet spread or direct contact with patients. Infants with CRS shed large quantities of virus in their pharyngeal secretions and urine and serve as a source of infection to their contacts. The disease is highly communicable. The period of communicability is about 1 week before and at least 4 days after onset of rash. Infants with CRS may shed virus for up to 1 year after birth.

9. Treatment—There are no specific medications for treating rubella. Antipyretics such as acetaminophen, dosed age-appropriately, may be helpful in cases of febrile illness.

10. Prevention—Rubella control is needed primarily to prevent fetal death and/or CRS in the offspring of women who acquire the disease during pregnancy.

1) Educate the general public on modes of transmission and stress the need for rubella immunization. Health care providers must be aware of the risks caused by rubella in pregnancy.

2) A single dose of live attenuated rubella virus vaccine elicits a significant and long-lasting antibody response in about 95% to 100% of susceptible individuals aged 9 months or older. Rubella vaccines are cold-chain dependent and should be protected from light. Several rubella vaccines are available as a single antigen—measles and rubella (MR); measles, mumps, and rubella (MMR); or measles, mumps, rubella, and varicella vaccines. Most of the currently licensed vaccines are based on the live attenuated RA27/3 strain of rubella virus; other live attenuated rubella virus strains are used in China and Japan.

3) WHO recommends use of the vaccine in all countries where control or elimination of rubella and CRS are considered a public health priority. The primary purpose of rubella vaccination is to prevent the occurrence of congenital rubella infection, including CRS. This can be achieved using combined vaccines (MR or MMR), and current efforts in global measles control should be used as an opportunity to pursue control of rubella. Two general approaches are recommended to prevent the occurrence of CRS: (a) prevention of CRS only through immunization of adolescent girls or women of childbearing age and (b) elimination of rubella as well as CRS.

For countries undertaking the elimination of both rubella and CRS, the preferred approach is to begin with MR vaccine or MMR vaccine in a campaign targeting a wide range of ages that is followed immediately by the introduction of MR or MMR vaccine into the routine childhood vaccination program. The first dose of a rubella-containing vaccine should be delivered with MCV1 (first dose of measles-containing vaccine at either 9 months or 12 months old), depending on the level of measles virus transmission. All subsequent follow-up campaigns should use MR vaccine or MMR vaccine. In addition, countries should make efforts to reach women of childbearing age by immunizing adolescent girls or women of childbearing age, or both, through routine services. If countries conduct any supplementary immunization activities targeting immunity gaps in adults, the supplementary immunization activity should include both males and females.

Depending on the burden of disease and the available resources, countries may choose to accelerate their progress towards elimination by conducting campaigns targeting a wide range of ages of both adult males and females. The precise target population depends on the country's susceptibility profile, cultural acceptability, and operational feasibility. Following well-designed and well-implemented programs, rubella and CRS have disappeared from many countries. Two regions—the Americas and Europe—have adopted a goal of rubella elimination.

Inadequately implemented childhood vaccination programs may run the risk of increasing the number of susceptibles among women—and the possibility of increased numbers of cases of CRS—but the risk decreases as immunized child cohorts become adults. To avoid the potential of an increased risk of CRS, countries should achieve and maintain immunization coverage of 80% or greater with at least 1 dose of a rubella-containing vaccine delivered through routine services with MCV1 or regular supplemental immunization activities, or both.

Following the introduction of large-scale rubella vaccination, coverage should be measured periodically by age and locality. In addition, surveillance is needed for rubella and CRS. If resources permit, longitudinal serologic surveillance can be used to monitor the impact of the immunization program, especially through assessing rubella IgG antibody in serum samples from women attending antenatal clinics.

Rubella vaccine should be avoided in pregnancy because of the theoretical—but never demonstrated—teratogenic risk. To date, CRS has not occurred in almost 3,000 susceptible pregnant women who were unknowingly pregnant and received RA27/3 rubella vaccine in early pregnancy. If pregnancy is being planned, however, an interval of 1 month should be observed after rubella immunization. Receipt of rubella vaccine during pregnancy is not an indication for abortion. Rubella vaccine should not be given to anyone with an immunodeficiency or who receives immunosuppressive therapy. Asymptomatic persons infected with human immunodeficiency virus can, however, be safely immunized.

4) In cases of infection with wild rubella virus early in pregnancy, culturally appropriate counseling should be provided. Abortion may be considered in those countries where this is an option.

5) Intramuscular immunoglobulin (IG) given within 72 hours of rubella exposure may lessen clinical disease, viral shedding, and the rate of viremia in exposed susceptible persons. IG may be considered for a susceptible pregnant woman exposed to the disease who would not be in a position to consider abortion. The absence of clinical signs in a pregnant woman who has

received IG does not guarantee that fetal infection has been prevented. Infants with congenital rubella have been born to mothers who were given IG shortly after exposure.

11. Special considerations—

1) Reporting: in countries where rubella elimination is a goal, all cases of rubella and of CRS should be reported. In many countries, reporting is obligatory. Early reporting of suspected cases permits early establishment of control measures.

2) For surveillance purposes, the WHO-recommended case definition of a suspected rubella case is any person with fever, non-vesicular (maculopapular) rash, and adenopathy (cervical, suboccipital, or postauricular).

3) Epidemic measures: prompt reporting of all confirmed and suspected cases; the country's established goal for rubella control/elimination will dictate the level of investigation required. During an outbreak, a limited number (5–10) of suspect cases (definition discussed earlier) should be investigated with laboratory tests to confirm that disease is due to rubella. However, during an outbreak, all rash illnesses in pregnancy should be investigated. The medical community and general public should be informed about rubella epidemics in order to identify and protect susceptible pregnant women. Active surveillance for infants with CRS should be carried out until 9 months after the last reported rubella case.

[O. A. Khan, E. Healy]

SALMONELLOSIS

DISEASE	ICD-10 CODE
SALMONELLOSIS	ICD-10 A02

This chapter is about illness caused by nontyphoidal *Salmonella* organisms. Illness caused by *Salmonella* serotypes Typhi and the paratyphoidal serotypes is described in "Typhoid Fever and Paratyphoid Fever."

1. Clinical features—Illness typically begins as a mild-to-moderate diarrhea with abdominal cramps, initially accompanied by nausea, vomiting, headache, and chills. Typical illness lasts about 7 days. Severe enterocolitis may be dysenteric (with blood in the stools) or cholera-like (with profuse watery diarrhea). Bacteremia occurs in approximately 5% of cases and is more likely to be the primary presentation in immunocompromised persons or patients in resource-poor settings. In some patients, bacterial seeding may lead to focal, suppurative infection. The most frequent extraintestinal infections are osteomyelitis, meningitis, endocarditis, endarteritis, septic arthritis, skin and soft-tissue infections, genital or intra-abdominal abscess, and urinary tract infection. Although mortality is less than 1% in well-resourced settings, the case-fatality rate from invasive disease globally is estimated to be approximately 20%. Following acute illness, some patients develop reactive arthritis or irritable bowel syndrome or have diarrhea associated with persistent infection.

2. Risk groups—Risk of infection can be increased by eating contaminated foods, animal contact, and travel. Stomach acid and healthy bowel flora provide some protection. Risk of infection increases with use of proton pump inhibitors, following gastrointestinal surgery, among infants fed with formula milk, and with antibiotic use. Bacteremia is more likely to occur in infants and adults aged 65 years or over and immunocompromised patients, such as those with human immunodeficiency virus, lymphoproliferative disorders, sickle cell disease, and transplants. Endovascular infections, abscesses, and focal bone and joint infections are more likely if there is localized inflammation or prosthetic material. Atherosclerotic plaques increase the risk of endovascular infection, osteomyelitis is more likely to occur in patients with hemoglobinopathies, and most cases of meningitis occur in infants.

3. Causative agents—Nontyphoidal *Salmonella* bacteria. *Salmonella* is a predominantly motile, Gram-negative bacterium found in the intestinal tract of mammals, birds, amphibians, and reptiles and ubiquitously in the environment. More than 2,500 *Salmonella* serotypes have been identified but just 10 serotypes account for approximately 80% of the reported salmonellosis cases. The prevalence of serotypes varies by geographic region. Nearly all *Salmonella* isolated from ill persons are serotypes of *Salmonella enterica* subsp. I; this includes serotypes Typhimurium and Enteritidis, which are the most commonly reported serotypes in countries with surveillance data. In sub-Saharan Africa, invasive disease has been associated with serotype Typhimurium multilocus sequence type ST313. Infections with resistant strains usually have poorer outcomes, including hospitalization and invasive disease.

4. Diagnosis—*Salmonella* may be isolated from stools, blood, urine, and other tissues or fluids. Serologic tests are not useful for diagnosis. Bacteremic patients should be investigated for extraintestinal infection, including by repeat blood cultures and, when indicated, imaging and culture of suspected sites. Culture-independent diagnostic tests are faster than culture, are increasingly available, and can have excellent sensitivity and specificity. However, isolation of organisms from clinical samples remains necessary for antimicrobial susceptibility testing, serotyping, and strain characterization. Detailed subtyping (including determination of serotype, subtype, and predicted resistance profile, and the search for closely related strains that might indicate an outbreak) is being increasingly performed using whole-genome sequencing.

5. Occurrence—Worldwide, salmonellosis is a leading cause of diarrheal illness, causing an estimated 153 million cases each year. In the USA, an estimated 374 salmonellosis cases (including those who do not seek medical care) per 100,000 population occur each year, with a 0.4% mortality rate among confirmed cases. Risk of infection is highest among children younger than 5 years, especially infants, and among adults aged 70 years and older. The serotypes most commonly reported among invasive disease cases in the USA are Choleraesuis, Enteritidis, Dublin, Heidelberg, Schwarzengrund, and Typhimurium. Approximately 6% of salmonellosis cases in the USA are part of an outbreak; cases that appear to be sporadic may actually be part of larger, unrecognized outbreaks. *Salmonella* can cause outbreaks in settings where food, restrooms, or living quarters are shared, such as in restaurants, nursing homes, schools, and hospitals, as well as in dispersed settings when people eat food that has been distributed widely.

6. Reservoirs—Serotypes causing human infections are mainly found in warm-blooded animals, including food animals (e.g., chickens, swine, cattle, turkeys), pets (dogs, cats, guinea pigs, hedgehogs), and other animals that may transfer *Salmonella* between animal reservoirs (e.g., rodents, wild birds). Other subspecies of *S. enterica* are predominantly found in cold-blooded animals, including reptiles (e.g., turtles, iguanas, snakes) and amphibians (e.g., frogs, toads), and in the environment. Human reservoirs may be important in some resource-poor settings; asymptomatic carriage may occur in household members of cases. *Salmonella* can survive in dry environments or in water for years, depending on the type of environment and temperature.

7. Incubation period—Typically about 6 to 96 hours. Incubation periods as long as 10 days can occur. Longer incubation periods of up to 16 days have been documented but are uncommon. Incubation period is likely dependent on the ingested dose.

8. Transmission—

1) Foodborne salmonellosis, which occurs by ingestion of contaminated food, is estimated to account for more than 80% of cases. Risk is increased by inadequate cooking, eating food raw, and eating outside the home. In the USA, approximately 90% of foodborne infections have been attributed to—based on outbreak-based

models—fresh produce, eggs, poultry, pork, and beef; less frequent sources include fish and seafood. Widespread outbreaks have been linked to ingestion of eggs, poultry, ground beef, tomatoes, leafy greens, and melons from single suppliers that distribute products over a wide geographic area; outbreaks have also occurred from commercially processed foods including frozen pot pies, peanut butter, dry snack foods, and cereals.

2) Transmission may occur via direct or indirect contact with animal reservoirs, including farm animals and pets. Colonized animals typically appear healthy and clean but their bodies (hide, fur, feathers, and scales) and their environments (e.g., water in a turtle tank) can be contaminated. Large outbreaks have resulted from contact with high-risk animals, including live poultry in backyard flocks, reptiles, and amphibians. Rodents used to feed reptiles and raw pet food have caused outbreaks.

3) Person-to-person fecal-oral transmission occurs. Patients with diarrhea and those in diapers (e.g., infants and incontinent adults) likely pose the greatest risk of transmission. Approximately 1% of infected adults and 5% of children younger than 5 years may shed the organism for up to 1 year after infection, depending on the serotype. Transmission from asymptomatic carriers may be important in some settings with high incidence; reported transmission in child care settings in the USA is uncommon.

4) Many environments (e.g., a field, a water system contaminated with human or animal feces) can transmit infection. Hospital-acquired infection may occur through contaminated equipment and environments.

9. Treatment—

Preferred therapy	• Provide supportive care with fluids and nutrition and ensure adequate contact precautions are taken to prevent transmission. If dehydration occurs, use appropriate IV fluids or oral rehydration solution. • Antibiotics are not recommended for mild-to-moderate diarrheal illness because they do not shorten the overall duration of the illness but do increase the risk of side effects and prolonged carriage. Antibiotics are indicated if invasive disease suspected (e.g., blood in the stools, profuse diarrhea, prolonged fever) or elevated risk of invasive disease (patients aged < 3 months or ≥ 50 years; those who are immunocompromised or who have hemoglobinopathies, vascular grafts, or prosthetic joints).
	When antibiotics are indicated: • Children: ceftriaxone 100 mg/kg/dose IV in 1–2 divided doses OR azithromycin PO 10 mg/kg/dose once daily (3–7 days for severe diarrheal illness; ≥ 7 days for bacteremia) • Adults: ciprofloxacin 500–750 mg PO BID (3–7 days for severe diarrheal illness; ≥ 7 days for bacteremia) OR levofloxacin 500 mg PO once daily (3–7 days for severe diarrheal illness; ≥ 7 days for bacteremia) OR ceftriaxone 1–2 g IV daily (3–7 days for severe diarrheal illness; ≥ 7 days for bacteremia)[a]

(Continued)

(Continued)

Alternative therapy options	When antibiotics are indicated:
	• Children: ciprofloxacin 10–15 mg/kg/dose (≤ 750 mg/dose) PO BID (3–7 days for severe diarrheal illness; ≥ 7 days for bacteremia)[a,b]
	• Adults: azithromycin 500 mg PO daily (3–7 days for severe diarrheal illness; ≥ 7 days for bacteremia)
Special considerations and comments	• For patients with diarrheal illness, obtain blood cultures before first dose and obtain stool culture. If bacteremia is present, repeat blood cultures and exclude extraintestinal infection before changing to oral therapy. Bacteremia should be treated for ≥ 7–14 days while excluding focal extraintestinal infection.
	• If available, local antibiogram should be checked to guide choice of antibiotic agent. Consider changing to TMP/SMX or ampicillin if the isolate is susceptible.
	• For patients with diarrheal illness, obtain blood cultures before first dose and obtain stool culture.
	• For patients with bacteremia, repeat blood cultures and exclude extraintestinal infection.
	• Treatment of focal extraintestinal infection depends on the site. Localized collections or abscesses, infected prostheses, and endovascular infections usually require surgery in addition to a prolonged course of antibiotics; consult appropriate specialists and more detailed recommendations.
	• If HIV infection with a low CD4+ count or high viral load, see guidelines (https://aidsinfo.nih.gov/guidelines) for the treatment of opportunistic infections. For pregnant women, ceftriaxone (for bacteremia) and azithromycin (for diarrhea) are generally considered safe; caution is advised for ciprofloxacin.
	• Carriage of *Salmonella* is typically for several weeks following infection; therefore, handwashing precautions should be taken to prevent transmission. Some jurisdictions and situations require stool culture to confirm eradication of *Salmonella*. However, routine follow-up cultures are not recommended after uncomplicated *Salmonella* diarrheal illness in immunocompetent patients, particularly if symptoms have resolved. Antibiotic treatment is also not indicated for patients incidentally found to have continued *Salmonella* isolation from the stools following an episode of diarrhea.

Note: BID = twice daily; CD4+ = cluster of differentiation 4; HIV = human immunodeficiency virus; IV = intravenous(ly); PO = oral(ly); TMP/SMX = trimethoprim-sulfamethoxazole.
[a]Do not give ciprofloxacin or levofloxacin if the infection was acquired in Asia or another region where a high percentage of isolates are not susceptible to quinolones.
[b]Ciprofloxacin is not routinely recommended in children but may be considered if the benefits outweigh the risks.

10. Prevention—Because of the ubiquity of *Salmonella,* infection prevention measures must be multifaceted and should include consumers, health care providers, veterinarians, food handlers, regulatory agencies, public health officials, and industry. Key prevention elements for patients include the following:

1) Food safety

- Educate patients about safe food preparation:

   o Wash hands before, during, and after food preparation.
   o Thoroughly cook all foods of animal origin, particularly poultry, meat, and egg products.
   o Thoroughly rinse produce when it is to be eaten raw.

- o Use pasteurized eggs in recipes that result in consumption of raw or undercooked eggs (e.g., hollandaise sauce, Caesar salad dressing, eggnog, homemade ice cream).
- o Refrigerate prepared foods at a safe temperature (between 0°C and 4°C [32°F-40°F]).
- o Refrigerate cooked foods within 2 hours.
- o Use a food thermometer to ensure that poultry and meat reach a safe minimum internal temperature.
- o Avoid recontamination in the kitchen after cooking is completed by washing hands, cutting boards (one for raw meat, one for other foods when possible), counters, knives, and other utensils thoroughly after they contact uncooked foods.
- o Keep uncooked meats separate from produce, cooked foods, and ready-to-eat foods.
- o Protect prepared foods against rodent and insect contamination.

- Educate patients that eating the following foods increases the risk of infection:

  - o Raw or undercooked eggs (e.g., eggs over easy or sunny-side up) and dirty or cracked eggs
  - o Raw milk, raw milk yogurt, and unpasteurized soft cheese
  - o Ciders and juices that are not pasteurized (e.g., raw apple cider)
  - o Raw or undercooked meat and poultry
  - o Raw sprouts of any kind, e.g., alfalfa, clover, radish, and mung beans. (These should be avoided by children, older adults, pregnant women, and persons with weakened immune systems.)

2) Prevention in the household

- Educate known carriers about the need for careful handwashing after defecation and before handling food and discourage them from handling food for others as long as they shed organisms.
- Educate patients about the risk of healthy pets and other animals carrying or transmitting *Salmonella*, particularly to young children.
- Keep high-risk animals (live poultry, reptiles, and amphibians) out of child care facilities that have children younger than 5 years and out of nursing homes and other facilities with high-risk persons. Because small turtles are particularly

hazardous to young children, their distribution has been banned in the USA since 1975.

- Wash hands thoroughly after handling animals and pet foods and after cleaning animal enclosures, especially before handling food, drinks, or other items that will be touched by babies (e.g., bottles).
- Avoid giving pets raw foods of animal origin because such foods can contain pathogens that are shed in pets' feces and transmitted to people.

3) Community: salmonellosis is a nationally notifiable disease; patients may be contacted by their local public health department about possible sources of infection.

11. Special considerations—

1) Reporting: case report obligatory.

2) In situations where large numbers of people must be fed in an area with poor sanitation, WHO Collaborating Centres may provide support. See http://www.who.int/gfn/en for more information.

3) Other references include:

- http://www.who.int/news-room/fact-sheets/detail/salmonella-(non-typhoidal)
- https://www.cdc.gov/salmonella/index.html
- https://wwwnc.cdc.gov/travel/yellowbook/2018/infectious-diseases-related-to-travel/salmonellosis-nontyphoidal

Bibliography

Crump JA, Sjölund-Karlsson M, Gordon MA, Parry CM. Epidemiology, clinical presentation, laboratory diagnosis, antimicrobial resistance, and antimicrobial management of invasive *Salmonella* infections. *Clin Microbiol Rev*. 2015;28(4):901–937.

Kirk MD, Pires SM, Black RE, et al. World Health Organization estimates of the global and regional disease burden of 22 foodborne bacterial, protozoal, and viral diseases, 2010: a data synthesis. *PLoS Med*. 2015;12(12):e1001921.

Shane AL, Mody RK, Crump JA, et al. 2017 Infectious Diseases Society of America clinical practice guidelines for the diagnosis and management of infectious diarrhea. *Clin Infect Dis*. 2017;65(12):e45–e80.

[J. M. Healy, I. D. Plumb, B. B. Bruce]

SARS, MERS, COVID-19, AND OTHER CORONAVIRUS INFECTIONS

DISEASE	ICD-10 CODE
SEVERE ACUTE RESPIRATORY SYNDROME (SARS)	ICD-10 U04.9 (provisional)
MIDDLE EAST RESPIRATORY SYNDROME (MERS)	
CORONAVIRUS DISEASE 2019 (COVID-19)	ICD-10 U07.1, U07.2
Common cold (see "Common Cold and Other Acute Viral Respiratory Diseases")	

I. SEVERE ACUTE RESPIRATORY SYNDROME (SARS)

1. Clinical features—Early signs and symptoms of severe acute respiratory syndrome (SARS) are nonspecific and consistent with influenza-like illness, with a spectrum of disease ranging from milder or atypical presentations to severe respiratory illness. SARS should be considered in the differential diagnosis in an individual presenting with fever above 38°C (100.4°F) and with symptoms of lower respiratory tract illness (e.g., cough, dyspnea, shortness of breath), with radiologic evidence of lung infiltrates consistent with pneumonia or adult respiratory distress syndrome (ARDS), or with autopsy findings consistent with pneumonia or ARDS without an identifiable cause and with no alternative diagnosis that can fully explain the illness. Cases can become severe quickly, progressing to respiratory distress coinciding with peak viremia that occurs during the second week of illness (e.g., 10 days), with about 20% to 30% requiring intensive care.

2. Risk groups—The primary risk factor is contact with a person infected with the SARS coronavirus (SARS-CoV) or the SARS-CoV itself secondary to a laboratory breach in infection control. Health workers are at great risk of infection, especially before the diagnosis of SARS is suspected and when involved in aerosol-generating procedures such as intubation or nebulization.

3. Causative agents—SARS is caused by the SARS-CoV. CoVs are enveloped, single-stranded, positive-sense ribonucleic acid (RNA) viruses that infect mammals and birds. In humans, CoVs are mainly associated with upper respiratory tract infections but can cause severe disease. Bats are most likely the natural reservoirs for SARS-CoV. Other animals, such as the masked palm civet, probably serve as intermediate hosts between bats and humans.

4. Diagnosis—SARS is diagnosed by exclusion of more usual causes of severe respiratory disease. It is unlikely that sporadic cases of SARS will be detected unless a patient with pneumonia gives a history of 1 or more of the following:

1) Exposure to an animal host
2) SARS-CoV–related laboratory work
3) Travel to southern China or another area with increased likelihood of animal-to-human transmission of SARS-CoV–like viruses from wildlife or other animal reservoirs

Diagnosis requires both a compatible clinical illness and definitive laboratory tests for SARS-CoV infection. As there has been no documented human-to-human transmission of SARS-CoV worldwide since 2004, the number of qualified laboratories that test for SARS-CoV is limited. WHO recommends that testing for SARS-CoV only be undertaken when there is compelling clinical and/or epidemiologic evidence that SARS may be the cause of an individual case or cluster of acute respiratory illness.

A variety of diagnostic tests are available. Their reliability depends on the type of clinical specimens collected and the timing of collection relative to symptom onset. Respiratory samples and stool samples should be routinely collected for nucleic acid detection by reverse transcription polymerase chain reaction (RT-PCR) or virus isolation during the first and second weeks of illness, as these specimens are most likely to yield virus. Sensitivity of newer RT-PCR assays has improved, with approximately 80% SARS-CoV RNA detected in stored respiratory specimens that had been collected within the first few days of symptom onset. When upper respiratory tract specimens are negative, lower respiratory specimens may be useful. Persons infected with CoVs often shed virus in stools for days to weeks. In stools, RT-PCR assays can detect SARS-CoV RNA for more than 4 weeks after illness onset. A confirmed positive PCR test for the global surveillance of SARS requires at least 2 different clinical specimens (e.g., nasopharyngeal and stool), the same type of specimen collected on 2 or more days during illness (e.g., 2 or more nasopharyngeal aspirates), 2 different assays, or repeat PCR using a new extract from the original clinical sample on each occasion of testing. Serologic testing is also available, and acute- and convalescent-phase sera should also be collected if possible.

All positive test results should be independently verified by a WHO International SARS Reference and Verification Network laboratory. WHO has published guidance on the clinical and laboratory diagnosis of SARS, as follows:

1) http://www.who.int/csr/resources/publications/WHO_CDS_CSR_ARO_2004_1/en/index.html
2) http://www.who.int/csr/sars/guidelines/en/SARSLabmeeting.pdf
3) http://www.who.int/csr/resources/publications/en/SARSReferenceLab.pdf

5. Occurrence—SARS is thought to have first appeared in human populations in November 2002. The 2002–2003 epidemic was characterized by outbreaks worldwide, including in Canada, Singapore, Vietnam, and

China (originating in Guangdong Province and spreading to major cities in other areas, including Beijing, Taipei, and Hong Kong). The disease spread internationally along major airline routes and resulted in 8,096 reported SARS cases in 29 countries with 774 deaths (9.6%). The last reported cases of SARS were in a cluster linked to a laboratory worker in China who was thought to have been infected in April 2004 at a laboratory where the virus was being studied.

It remains very difficult to predict when or whether SARS will reemerge in epidemic form. China has implemented strict market and food safety and other measures to prevent the transmission of SARS-like CoVs from animal hosts to humans. However, clustering of SARS-like illness in persons exposed to potential animal hosts—among health care workers or others exposed to a health care facility—remains an important sentinel event that may indicate the reemergence of SARS.

6. Reservoirs—The Himalayan masked palm civet (*Paguma larvata*) is considered the main source of animal-to-human transmission of SARS-CoV. Cave-dwelling Chinese horseshoe bats (of the genus *Rhinolophus*) are a reservoir of SARS-like CoVs that are closely related to those responsible for the SARS epidemic but display greater genetic variation than SARS-CoV isolated from humans or civets. Initial studies in Guangdong Province, China, showed similar CoVs in civets and in a small number of other wildlife species sold in wet markets.

7. Incubation period—From 2 to 10 days (mean of 5-6 days), with isolated reports of longer incubation periods.

8. Transmission—SARS-CoV–like viruses are thought to have been introduced into the human population from wildlife hosts in 2002. SARS is usually transmitted from person to person by direct contact and respiratory droplets and in some situations by fomites. Caring for, or living with, an infected person or having direct contact with respiratory secretions, body fluids, and excretions from someone infected with SARS-CoV are high-risk exposures in the absence of appropriate levels of infection control. In one recorded instance, it is thought the virus was transmitted by an environmental vehicle, possibly aerosolized sewerage or transport of sewerage by mechanical vectors. Nosocomial transmission of SARS-CoV was common early in the 2002-2003 outbreak but subsequently declined as a result of early diagnosis and strengthening infection control practices. Transmission studies have suggested that each SARS patient infected an average of 3 additional persons. During the 2002-2003 outbreak, several SARS patients were recognized as superspreaders because of the high number of persons secondarily infected (average, 36 patients). The superspreading phenomenon was associated with several factors, including a large number of close contacts, delayed diagnosis, more severe illness, and poor infection control practices.

The period of communicability is not yet completely understood. Epidemiologic and virologic studies and clinical follow-up during the epidemic indicated that transmission does not occur before onset of clinical signs and symptoms and that the maximum period of communicability is usually less than 21 days.

9. Treatment—Supportive at this point.

10. Prevention—Health services should develop clinical algorithms to assist clinicians in assessing patients with acute febrile respiratory infection for their risk of SARS, based on the national and global risk assessment of SARS reemergence. *WHO Guidelines for the Global Surveillance of SARS* (https://www.who.int/csr/resources/publications/WHO_CDS_CSR_ARO_2004_1/en) and *WHO SARS Risk Assessment and Preparedness Framework* (http://www.who.int/csr/resources/publications/WHO_CDS_CSR_ARO_2004_2/en) provide detailed guidance on SARS alert and triage of acute respiratory illness in the current epidemiologic situation.

1) Identify all suspect and probable cases using the WHO case definitions for SARS.

2) Health care workers involved in the triage process should wear a face mask (N/R/P 95/99/100 or filtering facepiece 2/3 or equivalent national manufacturing standard) with eye protection, wear gloves, and wash hands before and after contact with any patient, especially after activities likely to cause contamination and after removing gloves. Triage and waiting areas need to be adequately ventilated.

3) Soiled gloves, stethoscopes, and other equipment must be treated with care as they have the potential to spread infection. Broad-spectrum disinfectants of proven antiviral activity, such as fresh bleach solutions, must be widely available at appropriate concentrations and must be used according to manufacturers' instructions.

11. Special considerations—

1) Reporting: SARS is a notifiable disease under the International Health Regulations (IHR).

2) Should SARS reemerge, WHO will provide regular information updates and evidence-based travel recommendations to limit the international spread of infection in accordance with the IHR. A global response, facilitating exchange of information among scientists, clinicians, and public health experts, has been shown to be effective in providing information and real-time evidence-based policies and strategies.

3) The laboratory-associated outbreaks of SARS highlight the importance of strict adherence to biosafety procedures and practices

for laboratory work with SARS-CoV. WHO strongly recommends biosafety level 3 (BSL-3) for working with live SARS-CoV material.

4) During an epidemic, establish a multisectoral national SARS advisory group to oversee control measures. Traditional public health measures, including active case finding, case isolation, strict adherence to infection control in health care settings, contact tracing, fever monitoring, and enhanced surveillance, have been successful in controlling the spread of SARS. Ensure adequate triage facilities and clearly indicate to the general public where they are located and how they can be accessed.

5) Risk communication and community education should be an integral part of epidemic control measures. Establish telephone hotlines or other means of dealing with enquiries from the general public, health professionals, and the media. Ensure that all stakeholders have access to these resources.

II. MIDDLE EAST RESPIRATORY SYNDROME (MERS) CORONAVIRUS (CoV)

1. Clinical features—Since its emergence in 2012, signs and symptoms of Middle East respiratory syndrome CoV (MERS-CoV) infections in the majority of primary human cases have been reported as severe respiratory disease, as judged by admission to intensive care, mechanical ventilation, use of extracorporeal membrane oxygenation and vasopressors, and death; however, recently, milder clinical presentations and even some asymptomatic cases have been reported. Secondary human cases have had a spectrum of disease ranging from milder influenza-like illness to severe respiratory illness. There have also been cases with atypical presentation, such as immunosuppressed individuals presenting with gastric involvement. Coinfections with other respiratory viruses (in particular influenza A [H1N1], herpes simplex virus, rhinovirus, parainfluenza virus, influenza B) have been reported.

2. Risk groups—A variety of comorbidities have been associated with either MERS-CoV severe disease or death in sporadic cases, with diabetes, immunosuppression, and heart disease being the most commonly reported comorbidity conditions. The main risk factor for infection is contact with a person infected with MERS-CoV. Health care workers involved in aerosol-generating procedures, such as intubation or nebulization, are at greatest risk of infection, especially before the diagnosis of MERS-CoV is suspected and when infection control may not have been adequately instigated.

3. Causative agents—MERS-CoV. CoVs are enveloped, single-stranded, positive-sense RNA viruses that infect a wide range of mammals and birds. In humans, CoVs are mainly associated with seasonal upper respiratory tract infections similar to the common cold but can cause severe disease.

4. Diagnosis—All cases to date have had a direct or indirect link to the Middle East, and so relevant travel history should be obtained in any individual presenting with a febrile acute respiratory illness.

Both upper and lower respiratory and serum samples should be collected for nucleic acid detection. If available, serologic testing should be considered. Rapid real-time PCR diagnostic assays have been developed for the specific detection and confirmation of MERS-CoV. WHO has published guidance on the clinical and laboratory diagnosis of MERS-CoV and defines laboratory confirmation of a case as a person testing positive in at least 2 different PCR targets on the viral genome or positive for a single PCR target with sequence confirmation from a different genomic site. A number of laboratories have successfully established a PCR screening assay and accept samples from probable cases for confirmation. Within the Middle East, MERS-CoV screening of severe acute respiratory illness cases with no known etiology is encouraged. Only laboratories with adequate biosafety containment should attempt virus culture. Further information can be found at

1) http://www.who.int/csr/disease/coronavirus_infections/ MERS_Lab_recos_16_Sept_2013.pdf
2) http://www.who.int/csr/disease/coronavirus_infections/ InterimRevisedSurveillanceRecommendations_nCoVinfection_ 27Jun13.pdf

5. Occurrence—MERS-CoV was first identified in a fatal case of acute pneumonia with renal failure in a 60-year-old man from Saudi Arabia in June 2012, but phylogenetic analyses of the MERS-CoV full-genome sequences currently available indicate that it likely was introduced into the human population in mid-2011. By June 11, 2014, 699 laboratory-confirmed cases, including at least 209 deaths, had been officially reported to WHO. Sporadic cases have been identified in a number of countries in the Middle East, Europe, North Africa, and North America, all with a direct/ indirect link to the Middle East. Retrospective testing of a cluster of fatal pneumonia cases (with no known etiology), which occurred in Jordan in April 2012, identified this cluster to have been the earliest known human infections with MERS-CoV. Full-genome analyses of viruses to date suggest there have been multiple introductions into the human population rather than a single common source with undetected transmission. The level of undetected circulation in the human population remains unknown. Sporadic human cases of MERS-CoV infections are likely to continue until the source of infection and risk factors for transmission have been definitely established and prevention is possible or until the presumed epizootic ends.

6. Reservoirs—Although the reservoir remains unknown, the search for the source of MERS-CoV infection has uncovered many closely related betacoronaviruses in numerous bat species, including insectivorous bats common in the Middle East (e.g., the Egyptian tomb bat, *Taphozous perforates*). None of the full genomes detected thus far have been sufficiently similar to MERS-CoV to suggest it as the parental strain. Other animals common to the area have also been implicated. Serologic cross-sectional studies in dromedary camels across the Middle Eastern region have demonstrated a high seropositivity rate to MERS-CoV or a virus very antigenically similar to MERS-CoV. Sequence comparisons between the viruses detected in the human and camel samples cannot firmly conclude the direction of transmission or rule out a potential common infection source for both, and studies are ongoing.

7. Incubation period—The incubation period for primary cases with environmental exposure is unknown as the source of infection has not yet been identified. However, from case-contact studies following person-to-person transmission events, the incubation period is estimated to be between 2 and 14 days (median 5-6 days).

8. Transmission—The source of infection for index cases with environmental exposure is still unknown; however, person-to-person transmission is thought to be by direct contact, by fomites, and by respiratory droplets. Transmission has occurred in household, hospital, and work settings. Nosocomial transmission of MERS-CoV has been seen across the Middle East with nonsustained human-to-human transmission, including secondary cases in health care workers who sometimes remain asymptomatic. The period of communicability is not yet understood and studies are ongoing. Further information can be found at: https://www.who.int/emergencies/mers-cov/en.

9. Treatment—Treatment for MERS is supportive. The WHO guidelines *Clinical Management of Severe Acute Respiratory Infections When Novel Coronavirus Is Suspected* (https://www.who.int/csr/disease/coronavirus_infections/case-management-ipc/en/) provide detailed guidance on MERS alert and triage of acute respiratory illness.

10. Prevention—

1) Identify all possible and probable cases using the WHO case definitions for MERS.
2) Apply standard infection control measures, including hand hygiene, and use of personal protective equipment, including eye protection, to avoid direct contact with patients' blood, body fluids, secretions (including respiratory secretions), and nonintact skin.
3) When working within 1 m (3 ft) of the patient, droplet precautions should be taken by placing patients in single rooms when

possible, limiting patient movement, and ensuring that patients wear appropriate personal protective equipment when outside their rooms.

4) Health care workers performing aerosol-generating procedures should use personal protective equipment, including gloves, long-sleeved gowns, eye protection, and particulate respirators (N95 or equivalent). Whenever possible, use adequately ventilated single rooms when performing aerosol-generating procedures.

11. Special considerations—

1) Reporting: MERS is a notifiable disease under the IHR.

2) WHO provides regular information updates and evidence-based travel recommendations during an outbreak to limit the international spread of infection in accordance with the IHR. A global response, facilitating exchange of information among scientists, clinicians, and public health experts, has been an effective means to support the development of evidence-based policies and intervention strategies.

3) WHO strongly recommends BSL-3 for working with live MERS-CoV material.

4) Implementation of infection control in health care settings appears to prevent onward transmission of MERS-CoV to health care workers and patients without spread to the wider community.

5) Establish good communication routes with regular updates to clinicians and other health care workers to keep awareness of MERS-CoV high both inside and outside the affected countries. Establish easily accessible Web tools or other means of dealing with enquiries from health professionals, the general public, and the media.

III. COVID-19

Scientific and epidemiological knowledge of coronavirus disease 2019 (COVID-19) is evolving rapidly as the pandemic unfolds. The following text describes what is known at the time as of May 3, 2020.

In late November or early December 2019, another novel zoonotic coronavirus that causes lethal human disease, SARS-CoV-2, emerged in human populations and came to the attention of medical workers in Wuhan (capital of Hubei Province in China) where a cluster of patients with pneumonia was first noted. The Chinese Center for Disease Control and Prevention (China CDC) linked the source of the outbreak to Wuhan's Huanan Seafood Market, where game meat was also available. It has been hypothesized, based on subsequent analysis of the genetic sequence, that the virus emerged several weeks earlier than first thought. The outbreak spread rapidly within Wuhan, and China CDC instituted public health measures including intensive surveillance, epidemiological investigations, and closure of the market on January 1, 2020.

A novel coronavirus was identified from patients' samples using whole-genome sequencing and was named several weeks later as SARS-CoV-2. The disease caused by SARS-CoV-2 has been abbreviated to COVID-19.

On January 23, 2020, China imposed a strict lockdown of Wuhan and took similar measures in 15 other cities in the subsequent days. The lockdowns slowed the epidemic in China and its international spread. By mid-April China began to ease them. However, WHO declared the outbreak a public health emergency of international concern on January 30, 2020 and announced the extent and evolution of the global outbreak of COVID-19 as reaching a pandemic on March 11, 2020, with cases being reported from around the world and severe epidemics in some countries in Europe that threatened to overwhelm demand on the health systems.

The genetic sequence of SARS-CoV2 has 79.5% similarity to SARS-CoV and 96% similarity, at the whole-genome level, to a bat CoV.[1] While an intermediary animal source is still unknown and not yet proven, pangolins are implicated as a potential source.[2]

Initial studies of the natural history of infection describe common clinical features of COVID-19 as fever (44% on admission, then increased to 89% during hospitalization) and nonproductive cough (67.8%). Diarrhea is uncommon (3.8%). Absence of fever in COVID-19 is more common than in SARS (1%) and MERS (2%). Loss of smell and/or taste sensation has been observed but these symptoms appear transient in most patients. The median incubation period of COVID-19 is 4 days (interquartile range, 2–7 days). Ground-glass opacity (56.4%) is a common finding on chest computerized tomography (CT) upon hospital admission. Neither radiographic nor CT abnormality was found in 157 of 877 patients (17.9%) with nonsevere disease and in 5 of 173 patients (2.9%) with severe disease.

Up to 80% of those infected in China had mild symptoms not requiring hospitalization. Similar to SARS and MERS, children infected with SARS-CoV2 generally have mild disease.[3] Viral kinetic studies have shown that the viral load peaks on days 2–3 of the patient's illness, and this may explain the high transmission potential of SARS-CoV2 in causing community outbreaks, especially among close contacts.[4] Serology response has been demonstrated to start on day 7 of illness while PCR positivity in deep throat saliva could last for more than 3 weeks in one-third of patients. The risk factors associated with more severe disease include comorbid illness such as diabetes, hypertension, cardiac disease, and being older than 65 years. The case-fatality ratio has ranged from less than 1% to 13%–14% depending on the case definition used and, to some extent, the intensive care capacity of hospitals.

As it is a novel virus newly emerged in humans, the world's population is completely immune-naïve to SARS-CoV2 and therefore vulnerable. There has been clear human-to-human transmission in family clusters in China and beyond; transmission from close face-to-face social contact, especially in small enclosed spaces; and transmission from failed infection prevention and control measures in health facilities. In addition, the experience in Wuhan shows that transmission can be massive in a short period of time, with thousands of new patients diagnosed daily. Presymptomatic transmission has been observed 1 or 2 days before onset of symptoms. The role of transmission from asymptomatic persons is not completely understood. The immune response is not fully understood.

The aim of the response has been to flatten the epidemic curve so that transmission is slowed and to interrupt transmission where possible. While all countries have attempted to limit population exposure with personal protection policies such as frequent handwashing and physical distancing, response strategies have varied.

While there is clearly mortality linked to the virus, the most concerning problem is when a health system is overwhelmed in the wake of rapid transmission, which prevents affected patients from receiving the care they need. Furthermore, patients with other urgent medical conditions are at risk of not obtaining their necessary care as hospitals focus on isolation and management of COVID-19 patients. Countries with vulnerable health systems are particularly of concern.

The economic fallout of the COVID-19 pandemic will be severe, as many countries initially locked down industrial sectors, small businesses, and schools with mandatory home isolation in order to slow the arrival in hospital of patients requiring intensive care and ventilation. Although the final destiny of the virus is not yet known, it is feared that it will continue to transmit in human populations well into 2021 and beyond.

References

1. Zhou P, Yang XL, Wang XG, et al. A pneumonia outbreak associated with a new coronavirus of probable bat origin. *Nature*. 2020;579(7798):270–273.
2. Zhang T, Wu Q, Zhang Z. Probable pangolin origin of SARS-CoV-2 associated with the COVID-19 outbreak. *Curr Biol*. 30(7):1346–1351.e2.
3. Ludvigsson JF. Systematic review of COVID-19 in children show milder cases and a better prognosis than adults [published online ahead of print March 23, 2020]. *Acta Paediatr*. doi:10.1111/apa.15270.
4. To KK, Tsang OT, Leung WS, et al. Temporal profiles of viral load in posterior oropharyngeal saliva samples and serum antibody responses during infection by SARS-CoV-2: an observational cohort study. *Lancet Infect Dis*. 2020;20(5):565–574.

[O. A. Khan, D. S. Hui, E. Azhar, A. Zumia]

SCABIES
(sarcoptic itch, sarcoptic acariasis)

DISEASE	ICD-10 CODE
SCABIES	ICD-10 B86

1. Clinical features—A parasitic infestation of the skin caused by a mite whose presence is evident as papules, vesicles, or tiny, superficial, linear burrows containing the mites and their eggs. Itching is intense, especially at night, but complications are limited to lesions infected by bacteria due to scratching. Lesions are prominent around finger webs, anterior surfaces of wrists and elbows, anterior axillary folds, beltlines, and thighs. Nipples, abdomen, and the lower portion of the buttocks are frequently affected in women, as are external genitalia in men. In infants, the head, neck, palms, and soles may be involved; these areas are usually spared in older individuals. In immunosuppressed individuals, infestation may appear as a generalized dermatitis more widely distributed than the burrows with extensive scaling and sometimes vesiculation and crusting (Norwegian or crusted scabies); the usual severe itching may be reduced or absent. When scabies is complicated by β-hemolytic streptococcal infection, there is a risk of acute glomerulonephritis.

2. Risk groups—Household members and sex partners of persons infested with scabies and other persons living in conditions in which close body and skin contact is common. When scabies outbreaks occur, they tend to be in nursing homes, child care centers, extended-care facilities, and prisons. The risk groups for crusted (Norwegian) scabies are immunocompromised, elderly, disabled, or debilitated persons.

3. Causative agents—*Sarcoptes scabiei* subsp. *hominis*, a mite. Other *Sarcoptes* spp. and other animal (e.g., canine) mites, including other variants of *S. scabiei*, can live but not reproduce on humans; such infestations are self-limiting.

4. Diagnosis—Typically done by clinical examination of papules and burrows. Diagnosis can be confirmed by microscopic identification of the mite, eggs, or mite feces (scybala) from lesions. Care should be taken to choose lesions for scraping or biopsy that have not been excoriated by repeated scratching. Prior application of mineral oil facilitates collecting the scrapings and examining them microscopically under a coverslip. Applying ink to the skin and then washing it off will disclose the burrows.

5. Occurrence—Widespread and endemic in many countries. Causes of epidemics are not clear but past epidemics were attributed to poor sanitation and crowding associated with poverty, war, mass movement of people, and economic crises. Recent epidemics have affected people of all socioeconomic levels and standards of personal hygiene.

6. Reservoirs—Humans.

7. Incubation period—In persons without previous exposure, 2 to 6 weeks. Persons who have been previously infested develop symptoms 1 to 4 days after reexposure.

8. Transmission—Transfer of parasites commonly occurs through prolonged direct contact with infested skin or sexual contact. Transfer from undergarments and bedding occurs only if these have been infested immediately beforehand. Mites can burrow beneath the skin surface in about 1 hour. Persons with the crusted scabies are highly contagious because of the large number of mites present in the exfoliating scales. Transmission can occur until mites and eggs are destroyed. Crusted scabies can require multiple treatments to eliminate an infestation.

9. Treatment—

Drug	Permethrin 5% lotion or cream
Dose	8- to 14-hour application, THEN rinse off
Route	Topical[a]
Alternative drug	Ivermectin 200 μg/kg PO once (3-mg tablets; typical dose 4–6 tablets)
Duration	Once
Special considerations and comments	• Topical or PO treatments similar efficacy at 4 weeks (~95% cure) • No benefit of multiple treatments

Note: PO = oral(ly).
[a]After a shower or bath, apply from head (including scalp) to toe, including groin. Avoid mucous membranes.

10. Prevention—Educate the public and medical community on the mode of transmission, early diagnosis, and treatment of infested patients and contacts.

11. Special considerations—A potential nuisance in situations of overcrowding.

Bibliography

Chosidow O. Clinical practices. Scabies. *N Engl J Med.* 2006;354(16):1718-1727.
Rosumeck S, Nast A, Dressler C. Ivermectin and permethrin for treating scabies. *Cochrane Database Syst Rev.* 2018;(4):CD012994.

[J. Klausner]

SCHISTOSOMIASIS
(bilharzia, snail fever, Katayama fever)

DISEASE	ICD-10 CODE
SCHISTOSOMIASIS	ICD-10 B65

1. Clinical features—Chronic blood fluke (trematode) infection characterized by rash or itchy skin that occurs within days of exposure, although many early infections are asymptomatic. Within about 2 to 6 weeks of initial infection, acute schistosomiasis (Katayama fever) can present with systemic symptoms including fever, chills, fatigue, malaise, abdominal pain, diarrhea, dry cough, and/or myalgia. These symptoms are due to the host response to initial deposition of parasite eggs. Chronic symptoms vary by frequency and location and are also due to host immune responses to schistosome eggs traveling either through the bowel wall to the intestinal lumen and then being shed in feces (*Schistosoma mansoni, Schistosoma japonicum*) or through the bladder wall and then being shed in urine (*Schistosoma haematobium*). Eggs that fail to pass out of the body may produce inflammation or scarring (granulomata, fibrosis) in organs where they lodge. Depending on the species, adult worms tend to inhabit different anatomic sites of the venous system. Species residing in the mesenteric venules of the large (more often *S. mansoni*) and small (more often *S. japonicum*) intestine give rise primarily to hepatic and intestinal pathology. Symptoms may include diarrhea, abdominal pain, bloody stools, and/or hepatosplenomegaly; long duration and high-intensity infections can lead to liver fibrosis and portal hypertension. By contrast, *S. haematobium* worms most often inhabit the venous plexus of the bladder and give rise to urinary manifestations. Symptoms may include dysuria, urinary frequency, and/or hematuria at the end of urination; prolonged infections may lead to hydronephrosis or changes to the female genital tract and have been associated with bladder cancer in both sexes. Rarely, neuroschistosomiasis may develop when ectopic eggs lodge in the spinal cord (more common with *S. mansoni* or *S. haematobium*) or brain (more often associated with *S. japonicum*), causing seizures, paralysis, or spinal cord inflammation. Children who are repeatedly infected may develop anemia, malnutrition, growth stunting or wasting, and learning difficulties.

Swimmers itch occurs when the larvae of certain schistosomes of birds and mammals penetrate the human skin and cause dermatitis. These schistosomes do not mature in humans but die in the skin. The rash develops in response to the parasite antigens.

2. Risk groups—Susceptibility is universal. Because infection occurs through skin contact with freshwater inhabited by snails carrying schistosomes, risk is higher in those with greatest exposure to contaminated water containing cercariae (free-swimming larval forms). Any immunity developing as a result of infection is variable and not yet fully understood.

3. Causative agents—*S. mansoni*, *S. haematobium*, and *S. japonicum* are the major species causing human disease. *Schistosoma mekongi* and *Schistosoma intercalatum* are only important in limited areas.

4. Diagnosis—Through demonstration of eggs in the stools by direct smear or using the Kato-Katz technique (*S. mansoni* or *S. japonicum*). *S. haematobium* infection is diagnosed by the examination of a urine sediment or Nuclepore filtration. Serologic testing is useful for diagnosis of traveler infections. Useful immunologic tests include enzyme-linked immunosorbent assay and immunoblot analysis using egg or adult worm antigens; positive results on serologic antibody detection tests could be indicative of prior infection and are not proof of current infection.

5. Occurrence—*S. mansoni* is found in Africa; the Arabian Peninsula; Brazil, Suriname, and Venezuela in South America; and in some Caribbean island nations (Dominican Republic, Guadeloupe, Martinique, Saint Lucia). *S. haematobium* occurs in Africa and the Middle East. *S. japonicum* occurs in southern China, the Philippines, and Central Sulawesi in Indonesia. *S. mekongi* is found in the Mekong River area of Cambodia and Laos. *S. intercalatum* occurs in parts of Central and western Africa. Recently, a focus of transmission has been identified in Corsica. Some of these parasites are hybrids of *S. haematobium* and *Schistosoma bovis*.

6. Reservoirs—Humans are the principal reservoir of *S. haematobium*, *S. intercalatum*, and *S. mansoni*. Humans, dogs, cats, pigs, cattle, water buffalo, and wild rodents are potential hosts of *S. japonicum*; their relative epidemiologic importance varies in different regions. Epidemiologic persistence of the parasite depends on the presence of an appropriate snail as intermediate host (i.e., species of the genera *Biomphalaria* for *S. mansoni*; *Bulinus* for *S. haematobium* and *S. intercalatum*; *Oncomelania* for *S. japonicum*; and *Tricula* for *S. mekongi*).

7. Incubation period—Acute systemic manifestations (Katayama fever) may occur in primary infections 2 to 6 weeks after exposure, immediately preceding and during initial egg deposition.

8. Transmission—Schistosomiasis is not communicable directly from person to person. Transmission is maintained when infected persons defecate or urinate, thereby shedding eggs, into freshwater containing appropriate intermediate snail hosts. The eggs hatch in water and the liberated larvae (miracidia) penetrate into suitable freshwater snail intermediate hosts. After several weeks of amplification through asexual reproduction, the cercariae (free-swimming larval forms) emerge from the snail; infected snails continue to release cercariae for as long as they live. Human infection occurs when cercariae penetrate the skin. In the human host, cercariae become schistosomula following skin penetration; the schistosomula migrate through various tissues before developing into adult worms. Mated female worms release eggs into the circulation and may have a life span of up to 10 years. Adult forms usually remain in mesenteric veins with the exception of those of *S. haematobium*, which usually migrate to the venous plexus of the urinary bladder. Eggs are deposited in venules and escape into the lumen of the bowel or urinary bladder, where they are excreted in feces or urine.

9. Treatment—Infection with all major *Schistosoma* spp. can be safely and effectively treated with praziquantel. Dosing varies depending upon the species.

Drug	Praziquantel
Dose	*Schistosoma mansoni, Schistosoma haematobium, Schistosoma intercalatum*: • 40 mg/kg/day divided into 2 daily doses *Schistosoma japonicum, Schistosoma mekongi*: • 60 mg/kg/day divided into 3 daily doses
Route	PO
Alternative drug	Oxamniquine had been used to treat *S. mansoni* but is no longer commercially available. It is ineffective in other schistosomal infections.
Duration	• A single course is usually curative. • Repeat treatment after 2–4 weeks may increase effectiveness in persons from nonendemic areas who may have a less robust immune response to the parasite.
Special considerations and comments	• For travelers to endemic areas, treatment should occur ≥ 6–8 weeks after last exposure to contaminated freshwater. • If eggs were identified in stools or urine prior to treatment, follow-up examination at 1–2 months is suggested to help confirm successful cure. • Limited safety data exist in children < 4 years or pregnant women but WHO recommends praziquantel treatment of these groups in field settings.

Note: PO = oral(ly).

10. Prevention—

1) In endemic areas, regular mass drug treatments with praziquantel are recommended for populations at risk, including school-aged children, women of childbearing age, and certain groups with occupational water exposure.

2) Avoid swimming or wading in freshwater in countries where schistosomiasis occurs.

3) Ensure adequate sanitation with disposal of feces and urine so that viable eggs will not reach bodies of freshwater containing intermediate snail hosts. Control of animals infected with *S. japonicum* is desirable but difficult.

4) Improve irrigation and agriculture practices. Reduce snail habitats by removing vegetation, draining and filling marshy areas, or lining canals with concrete.

5) Where appropriate, treat snail breeding sites with molluscicides. Cost and environmental impact may limit the utility of these agents.

6) Minimize exposure to contaminated water (e.g., by wearing rubber boots). Application of topical water-resistant preparations containing N,N-diethyl-meta-toluamide may prevent cercarial penetration but total coverage is difficult. Immediate vigorous towel drying of exposed skin has been suggested to reduce cercarial penetration after accidental water contact but is ineffective for all but the briefest of exposures.

7) Provide safe water for drinking, bathing, and washing clothes from sources free of cercariae or treated to kill them. Effective measures for inactivating cercariae include heating bath water to a rolling boil for at least 1 minute; holding water in a storage tank for 48 to 72 hours prior to bathing; and filtering water before drinking it. Water treatment with iodine or chlorine will not guarantee that water is safe and free of all parasites and may not inactivate other pathogens.

8) Advise travelers visiting endemic areas of the risks and inform them about preventive measures. Local tourist information suggesting freshwater bodies are free of schistosomiasis is not reliable.

11. Special considerations—

1) Reporting: reporting requirements vary by country and region.

2) Surveillance case definition: for endemic areas, screening for urinary schistosomiasis is based on the presence of visible hematuria, a positive reagent strip for hematuria, or detection of *S. haematobium* eggs in urine. Screening for intestinal schistosomiasis is based on detection of eggs in stools.

3) Epidemic measures: examine for schistosomiasis and treat all who are infected, especially those with disease and/or moderate-to-heavy intensity of infection; pay particular attention to children. Provide clean water, warn people against contact with water

potentially containing cercariae, and prevent contamination of water with urine and feces. Treat areas that have high snail densities with molluscicides as appropriate.

4) Further information may be found at:

- http://www.who.int/topics/schistosomiasis/en
- http://www.cdc.gov/parasites/schistosomiasis/index.html

[M. Kamb]

SHIGELLOSIS
(bacillary dysentery)

DISEASE	ICD-10 CODE
SHIGELLOSIS	ICD-10 A03

1. Clinical features—An acute bacterial disease involving the distal small intestine and colon, characterized by loose stools accompanied by fever, nausea, and sometimes toxemia, vomiting, cramps, and tenesmus. Stools may contain blood and mucus (dysentery) resulting from mucosal ulcerations and confluent colonic crypt microabscesses caused by the invasive organisms; however, many cases present with nonbloody diarrhea. Convulsions may be an important complication in young children. Bacteremia is uncommon. Severity and case-fatality rate vary with the host (age and preexisting nutritional state) and serotype. *Shigella dysenteriae* type 1 (Shiga bacillus) spreads in epidemics and is often associated with serious disease and complications, including toxic megacolon, intestinal perforation, and hemolytic uremic syndrome; case-fatality rates have been as high as 20% among hospitalized patients even in recent years.

Mild and asymptomatic infections occur. These are usually self-limited, lasting on average 4 to 7 days. Many infections with *Shigella sonnei* result in a short clinical course and an almost negligible case-fatality rate except in immunocompromised hosts. Certain strains of *Shigella flexneri* can cause a reactive postinfectious arthropathy (formerly known as Reiter syndrome), especially in persons who are genetically predisposed by having HLA-B27 antigen.

2. Risk groups—Two-thirds of cases and most of the deaths are in children younger than 10 years. Illness in infants younger than 6 months is unusual and breastfeeding is protective for infants and young children. The elderly, the debilitated, and the malnourished of all ages and those infected with human immunodeficiency virus are particularly susceptible to severe disease and death. Secondary attack rates in households can be as high as 40%. Outbreaks occur in crowded conditions and where contact with fecal material is possible, such as in prisons, institutions for children, child care centers, mental health facilities, and crowded refugee camps, as well as among men who have sex with men (MSM).

3. Causative agents—*Shigella* strains are Gram-negative, facultatively anaerobic, nonmotile rods classified in the family Enterobacteriaceae. *Shigella* strains cause dysentery symptoms by invading and destroying the cells that line the large intestine. These symptoms are mediated by several invasion-related factors including *ipaC* and *ipaH*, which are encoded on a characteristic, large 120- to 140-MDa plasmid. The *ipaH* factor is also chromosomally encoded. The severity of symptoms associated with infection by *S. dysenteriae* type 1 is thought to be related to its production of Shiga toxin type 1. Rarely, nontype 1 strains of *S. dysenteriae* and certain strains of *S. flexneri* also produce Shiga toxin type 1. With the exception of *Shigella boydii* serotype 13, *Shigella* and *Escherichia coli* represent a single genomospecies. *S. boydii* 13 has been determined to be a separate species, *Escherichia albertii*. There are 4 subgroups of *Shigella*, which have traditionally been regarded as separate species:

1) Group A: *S. dysenteriae*
2) Group B: *S. flexneri*
3) Group C: *S. boydii*
4) Group D: *S. sonnei*.

Groups A, B, and C are further divided into 15, 8, and 19 serotypes, respectively, and *S. flexneri* serotypes 1 through 5 are further subdivided into 11 subserotypes designated by numbers and lowercase letters (e.g., *S. flexneri* 2a). *S. sonnei* (group D) consists of a single serotype.

4. Diagnosis—Isolation of *Shigella* from feces or rectal swabs provides bacteriologic diagnosis. Outside the human body, *Shigella* remains viable only for a short period, which is why stool specimens for culture must be processed rapidly after collection. *Shigella* isolates should be tested for antimicrobial susceptibility. Commercial rapid diagnostic tests or antigen detection assays are not available.

5. Occurrence—Shigellosis causes an estimated 125 million illnesses and 14,000 deaths per year. Shigellosis is endemic in both tropical and temperate climates. Reported cases represent only a small proportion of cases, even in developed areas. Mixed infections with other intestinal pathogens also occur.

The geographic distribution of the 4 *Shigella* serogroups is different, as is their pathogenicity. More than 1 serotype is commonly present in a community. In general, *S. flexneri*, *S. boydii*, and *S. dysenteriae* account for most isolates from developing countries. *S. dysenteriae* type 1 is of particular concern in developing countries and complex emergency situations where huge outbreaks can occur. *S. sonnei* is most common in industrialized countries where the disease is generally less severe. Multidrug-resistant *Shigella* (including *S. dysenteriae* type 1) with considerable geographic variations have appeared worldwide in association with the widespread use of antimicrobial agents.

6. Reservoirs—The only significant reservoir is humans, although prolonged outbreaks have occurred in primate colonies.

7. Incubation period—Usually 1 to 3 days, but may range from 12 to 96 hours and up to 1 week for *S. dysenteriae* type 1.

8. Transmission—Mainly by direct or indirect fecal-oral transmission from a symptomatic patient or asymptomatic carrier. The infective dose can be as low as 10 to 100 organisms. Individuals primarily responsible for transmission include those who fail to clean hands and under fingernails thoroughly after defecation. They may spread infection to others directly by physical contact or indirectly by contaminating food, water, or fomites. Transmission via drinking or recreational water may also occur as the result of direct fecal contamination. Flies can transfer organisms from latrines to uncovered food items. Certain sexual practices, particularly among MSM, also increase risk of transmission.

The period of communicability continues during the acute infection and until the infectious agent is no longer present in feces, usually for less than 4 weeks after illness. Very rarely, the asymptomatic carrier state may persist for months or longer; appropriate antimicrobial treatment usually reduces duration of carriage to a few days.

9. Treatment—As with all diarrheal diseases, early rehydration with oral fluids is important. Intravenous rehydration is recommended for patients who are unable to tolerate oral intake or for those who are severely ill. Antimotility agents are not recommended. Unfortunately, shigellae tend to acquire resistance against formerly effective antimicrobials (for further information on treatment failures with ciprofloxacin and azithromycin, see: https://emergency.cdc.gov/han/han00411.asp). It is therefore critical to assess local antimicrobial resistance patterns prior to initiating therapy. If resistance patterns allow, treatment options can include ciprofloxacin, azithromycin, and ceftriaxone. If using ciprofloxacin, a dosing regimen per WHO guidelines of 15 mg/kg orally twice daily for 3 days can be considered in children. Alternatively, ceftriaxone 50 to 100 mg/kg intramuscular injection daily for 5 days. For adults, ciprofloxacin dosing of 500 mg orally twice daily for 5 days is reasonable.

10. Prevention—

1) General measures to improve hygiene are important. An organized effort to promote careful handwashing with soap and water is the single most important control measure to decrease transmission rates in most settings. Provide soap and hand dryers or individual paper towels in public settings if otherwise not available. Prophylactic administration of antibiotics is not recommended.

2) Use of barriers during oral-, digital-, and genital-anal contact, accompanied by washing hands and genitals with soap before and after sexual contact, may help prevent transmission.

3) Studies with experimental serotype-specific live oral vaccines and parenteral polysaccharide conjugate vaccines show protection of short duration (1 year) against infection with the homologous serotype.

4) Closure of child care centers or prolonged exclusion of ill children from child care centers may lead to placement of infected children in other centers with subsequent transmission in the latter; few data exist to assess whether these are effective control measures.

11. Special considerations—

1) Reporting: case report to the local health authority is obligatory in many countries. Any group of cases of acute diarrheal disorder should be reported at once to the local health authority, even without specific identification of the causal agent.

2) Common-source foodborne or waterborne outbreaks require prompt investigation and intervention whatever the infecting species. Institutional outbreaks may require special measures, including separate housing for cases and new admissions, a vigorous program of supervised handwashing, and repeated cultures of patients and attendants. The most difficult outbreaks to control are those that involve groups of young children (not yet or recently toilet-trained) or the intellectually disabled and those without an adequate supply of water.

3) *Shigella* infection, particularly that caused by *S. dysenteriae* type 1, is a potential problem in a disaster situation when personal hygiene and environmental sanitation are deficient (see "Typhoid Fever and Paratyphoid Fever").

Bibliography

Christopher PR, David KV, John SM, Sankarapandian V. Antibiotic therapy for *Shigella* dysentery. *Cochrane Database Syst Rev.* 2010;(8):CD006784.

Williams PCM, Berkley JA. Guidelines for the treatment of dysentery (shigellosis): a systematic review of the evidence. *Paediatr Int Child Health.* 2018;38(suppl 1): S50–S65.

[O. A. Khan]

SMALLPOX AND OTHER POXVIRUS DISEASES

DISEASE	ICD-10 CODE
SMALLPOX	ICD-10 B03
VACCINIA	ICD-10 B08.0
MONKEYPOX	ICD-10 B04
ORF VIRUS DISEASE	ICD-10 B08.0

Smallpox is caused by the variola virus, genus *Orthopoxvirus*. Vaccinia virus and monkeypox virus are both members of the same genus and also cause infection in humans. Vaccinia virus is the live *Orthopoxvirus* immunizing agent that was used to eradicate smallpox and is protective against other *Orthopoxvirus* infections. Human monkeypox is a sporadic zoonotic infection first identified in humans in 1970 from remote, heavily forested villages in Central and West African countries during smallpox eradication. Clinically, the disease closely resembles ordinary or modified smallpox, with the addition of lymphadenopathy. Orf virus, a zoonotic infection belonging to the genus *Parapoxvirus*, is acquired from goats and sheep. It manifests as a proliferative cutaneous disease, generally with a solitary lesion on hands, arms, or face.

I. SMALLPOX

The last naturally acquired case of smallpox occurred in October 1977 in Somalia; global eradication was certified 2 years later (1979) by WHO and by World Health Assembly (WHA) in May 1980. Except for a limited outbreak after a laboratory accident at the University of Birmingham (UK) in 1978, no further cases have been identified. All known smallpox (variola) virus stocks are held under security in 2 WHO Collaborating Centre laboratories: CDC,

Atlanta, Georgia, USA, and the State Research Centre of Virology and Biotechnology, Koltsovo, Novosibirsk Region, Russia. Because of concerns that the world would be unable to respond to and contain an accidental or intentional release of smallpox, WHA has authorized the retention of virus at the laboratories in Russia and the USA. A biosafety inspection program for the 2 laboratories was created and an appointed group of experts determine and oversee the research. Because few health care workers today have ever encountered smallpox or have ever managed cases of the illness, it is important that they become familiar with the clinical and epidemiologic features of smallpox and how it can be distinguished from chickenpox—a herpesvirus—and other rash illnesses. Laboratory confirmation of variola virus from suspect smallpox patients is performed at the 2 WHO Collaborating Centre laboratories, using appropriate biosafety containment practices.

1. Clinical features—Smallpox was a systemic viral disease generally presenting with a characteristic skin eruption. Preceding the appearance of the rash was a prodrome of sudden onset with high fever (40°C [104°F]), malaise, headache, prostration, severe backache, and occasional abdominal pain and vomiting—a clinical picture that resembled influenza. After 2 to 4 days, the fever began to decrease and a deep-seated rash developed in which individual lesions containing infectious virus progressed through successive stages of macules, papules, vesicles, pustules, and then crusted scabs, which fell off 3 to 4 weeks after the appearance of the rash. The lesions first appeared on the face and extremities, including the palms and soles, and subsequently on the trunk—the so-called centrifugal rash distribution. They were well circumscribed and at the same stage of development in a given area.

Two types of smallpox were recognized during the 20th century: variola minor (including a genetically and biologically distinct subgroup described as alastrim), which had a case-fatality rate of less than 1%, and variola major, which had a case-fatality rate among unvaccinated populations of 20% to 50% or higher (30% on average). Fatalities normally occurred between the fifth and seventh day after onset of illness and occasionally as late as the second week. Fewer than 3% of variola major cases experienced a fulminant hemorrhagic course, characterized by a severe prodrome, prostration, and bleeding into the skin and mucous membranes; such hemorrhagic cases were rapidly fatal. In hemorrhagic smallpox the usual vesicular rash did not appear and the disease might have been confused with severe leukemia, meningococcemia, or idiopathic thrombocytopenic purpura. The rash of smallpox could also be significantly modified in previously vaccinated persons to the extent that only a few highly atypical lesions might be seen. In such cases, prodromal illness was not modified but the maturation of lesions was accelerated with crusting by the tenth day.

Smallpox was most frequently confused with chickenpox (varicella), in which skin lesions commonly occur in successive crops with several stages of maturity visible at the same time. The chickenpox rash is more abundant on covered than on exposed parts of the body, is centripetal rather than centrifugal, and is usually intensely itchy. However, the appearance of the rash in the early florid stage of a very severe chickenpox case may generate diagnostic confusion for those unfamiliar with smallpox or monkeypox. The smallpox vesicles are firm (bullet-like) and deep-seated, whereas the chickenpox vesicles are more superficial and easily deroofed.

2. Risk groups—Smallpox research scientists. Susceptibility among the unvaccinated is universal.

3. Causative agents—Variola virus, a species of *Orthopoxvirus*.

4. Diagnosis—Smallpox was indicated by a clear-cut prodromal illness; the more or less simultaneous appearance of all lesions when the fever broke; the similarity of appearance of all lesions in a given area rather than successive crops; and deep-seated lesions with no surrounding inflammatory flare, often involving sebaceous glands and scarring of the pitted lesions. By contrast, chickenpox lesions are superficial, not well circumscribed, and manifest with irregular borders; the vesicle or pustule is surrounded by an inflammatory flare; and chickenpox rash is usually pruritic. Smallpox lesions were virtually never seen at the apex of the axilla and chickenpox lesions are rarely, if ever, seen on the palms and soles of the feet—a distribution characteristic of smallpox in many cases. Outbreaks of variola minor were recognized by low case-fatality rates in the late 19th century. Although the rash was like that in ordinary smallpox, patients generally experienced less severe systemic reactions and hemorrhagic cases were virtually unknown.

Prior to eradication, laboratory confirmation of smallpox used isolation of the virus on chorioallantoic membranes or tissue culture from the scrapings of lesions, from vesicular or pustular fluid, from crusts, and sometimes from blood during the febrile prodrome. Electron microscopy or immunodiffusion technique often permitted a rapid provisional diagnosis—though eradication was made possible on the basis of clinical, not laboratory, diagnosis. It should be remembered that all orthopoxviruses look alike on electron microscopy, so it cannot be used to distinguish smallpox from other orthopoxviruses that infect humans, such as vaccinia or monkeypox. Molecular methods, such as polymerase chain reaction (PCR) or virus isolation, are available for rapid diagnosis of smallpox and other *Orthopoxvirus* infections.

Should smallpox infection be suspected, immediate communication by national authorities to WHO is obligatory under the International Health Regulations (IHR). Advice will be provided on appropriate laboratories to confirm the diagnosis and guidance will be provided on management of the suspected case and follow-up of contacts.

5. Occurrence—Formerly a worldwide disease; no known human cases since 1978.

6. Reservoirs—As epidemiologically described in the 19th and 20th centuries, smallpox was exclusively a human disease with no known animal or environmental reservoir.

7. Incubation period—From 7 to 19 days; commonly 10 to 14 days to onset of illness and 2 to 4 days more to onset of rash.

8. Transmission—Infection usually occurred via the respiratory tract (droplet spread) or skin inoculation. The conjunctivae or the placenta were occasional portals of entry. The period of communicability extended from the time of development of the earliest rash lesions to disappearance of all scabs—about 3 weeks. Risk of transmission appears to have been highest in the first week after appearance of the earliest lesions through droplet spread from the oropharyngeal enanthem and subsequent oropharyngeal excretion of virus.

9. Treatment—Antiviral therapy was not effective and, apart from vaccination, control of smallpox in the preeradication era was based on identification and isolation of cases and supportive treatment. New antivirals are in advanced stages of regulatory assessment but have not yet been approved.

The historic control strategy included vaccination of contacts and those living in the immediate vicinity (ring vaccination), surveillance of contacts (including daily monitoring of temperature), and isolation of those contacts in whom fever developed. This approach would be implemented if an outbreak of the disease were to occur in the present-day setting.

10. Prevention—Prevention and eradication of smallpox were based on vaccination (vaccinia virus). Because of the relatively long period of incubation for smallpox, vaccination within a 4-day period after exposure prevented or attenuated clinical illness. Two newer, more attenuated, vaccines have been developed and have been approved for specified uses by several national regulatory authorities.

11. Special considerations—Reporting: patients with acute, generalized vesicular, or pustular rash illness should be evaluated. For more details on evaluating the risk for smallpox, see: https://www.cdc.gov/smallpox/clinicians/algorithm-protocol.html. If a nonvaricella, smallpox-like/high-risk case is suspected, immediate telephone communication (without waiting for laboratory results) to hospital infection control and applicable local and national health authorities is obligatory. National health authorities should inform WHO immediately. Notification of smallpox is mandatory under the IHR.

Further information can be found at: https://www.cdc.gov/smallpox and http://www.who.int/csr/disease/smallpox.

II. VACCINIA

Vaccinia virus is the live, fully replicative *Orthopoxvirus* immunizing agent that was used to eradicate smallpox. Discovery of vaccinia variants causing human infection in the Indian subcontinent and in South America (Brazil) has led to the consideration that vaccines may have escaped into animal populations; alternatively, these occurrences may be indicative of the origins of vaccinia virus. Vaccinia virus was genetically engineered and biologically derived into candidate and approved vaccines (some are in clinical trials) with low potential for spread to nonimmune contacts.

Vaccination with licensed (fully replicative) vaccinia vaccine is recommended for all laboratory workers at high risk of contracting smallpox infection, such as those who directly handle cultures or animals contaminated or infected with vaccinia or other orthopoxviruses that infect humans. It may also be considered for other health care personnel who are at lower risk of infection, such as doctors and nurses whose contact with these viruses would be limited to contaminated dressings. WHO does not recommend vaccination in the general public because the risk of death (1/1,000,000 doses) or serious side effects is greater than the known risk of infection with smallpox. Vaccination is contraindicated in persons with deficient immune systems, persons with eczema or certain other dermatitis disorders, and pregnant women.

Vaccine immunoglobulin can be obtained for laboratory workers in the USA through the CDC Drug Service (1-404-639-3670) and in other industrialized countries from public health agencies. Vaccination should be repeated unless a major reaction (one that is indurated and erythematous 7 days after vaccination) or take has developed. Booster vaccinations are recommended within 10 years in categories for which vaccine is recommended. WHO maintains a supply of the vaccine seed lot (vaccinia virus strain Lister Elstree) at the WHO Collaborating Centre for Smallpox Vaccine at the National Institute of Public Health and Environmental Protection in Bilthoven, the Netherlands. WHO also maintains a stockpile of vaccine to be used if needed to control a proven outbreak of smallpox.

III. MONKEYPOX

1. Clinical features—Human monkeypox is a sporadic zoonotic infection first identified in humans in 1970 from rural, heavily forested villages in Central and West African countries as smallpox was in the final stages of eradication. Clinically, the disease closely resembles ordinary or modified smallpox but lymphadenopathy is a more prominent feature in many cases and occurs in the early stage of the disease. Pleomorphism and cropping similar to that seen in chickenpox are observed in 20% of patients, depending on strain. The case-fatality rate among children not vaccinated against smallpox ranges from 1% to 14%.

2. Risk groups—Hunters in tropical rainforests of West and Central Africa and their families, laboratory workers, and others exposed either directly or indirectly to rodent populations and nonhuman primates from West and Central Africa.

3. Causative agents—Monkeypox virus is a species of the genus *Orthopoxvirus* with biologic properties and a genome distinct from variola virus. At least 2 genetically distinct clades of monkeypox exist with different human clinical and epidemiologic manifestations. To date, West African clade monkeypox manifests without apparent human-to-human transmission and without human mortality, whereas the Congo Basin clade is associated with human-to-human transmission and case-fatality rates historically reported at an average of approximately 10% in unvaccinated persons.

4. Diagnosis—Identification of the characteristic lesion; ascertainment of a history of direct or indirect contact with animals of West and Central African origin; through demonstration of poxvirions in the lesion by means of electron microscopy; by growth of the virus primate cell cultures; or through positive molecular (e.g., PCR), virus isolation, or serologic tests. The CDC smallpox Web page (https://emergency.cdc.gov/agent/smallpox) provides guidance for a clinical algorithm designed to aid in distinguishing *Orthopoxvirus* infections from other disseminated rash illnesses, such as chickenpox.

5. Occurrence—Between 1970 and 1994, more than 400 cases of human monkeypox were reported from West and Central Africa; the Democratic Republic of the Congo (DRC; formerly Zaire) accounted for about 95% of reported cases during a 5-year surveillance period from 1981 to 1986. However, poor public health infrastructure and other factors complicate accurate case reporting. In the late 1990s, a prolonged outbreak of human monkeypox was recognized in DRC; it has been postulated that lack of vaccination and an epizootic event(s) allowed virus transmission to humans. In 2003, a prolonged and efficient chain of human-to-human transmission was described in a hospital setting in the Republic of Congo. The 2003 introduction of monkeypox in the USA related to importation and sale of exotic animals from West Africa as pets resulted in infection of North American prairie dogs for sale in pet shops and at least 50 probable and confirmed human cases, mainly among prairie dog owners and animal handlers. Outbreaks of monkeypox are regularly reported in DRC and have been reported sporadically in the Republic of Congo in 2010 and again in 2017. Most recently a large monkeypox outbreak was reported in Nigeria. The disease affects all age groups; children younger than 16 years have historically constituted the greatest proportion of cases.

6. Reservoirs—The natural history of the disease is unclear; humans, primates, and squirrels appear to be involved in the enzootic cycle. Ecologic studies in the 1980s point to squirrels (*Funisciurus* and *Heliosciurus*), abundant among the oil palms surrounding the villages at the study sites, as a significant local reservoir host. Monkeypox has been demonstrated in terrestrial giant pouched Gambian rats (*Cricetomys* spp.) and dormice (*Graphiurus* spp.) The virus was isolated in a rope squirrel (*Funisciurus anerythrus*) in the Équateur province of DRC in 1985 and in a dead sooty mangabey found in Taï National Park, Côte d'Ivoire, in 2012. Maintenance of an animal reservoir and animal contact appear to be required to sustain the disease among humans.

7. Incubation period—7 to 17 days; usually around 12 days.

8. Transmission—In the 1980s about 75% of reported cases of human monkeypox were attributable to contact with affected animals; in one outbreak in the DRC in 1996–1997, it appeared that a larger number of cases were attributable to person-to-person contact. Unaccustomed conditions of crowding at the start of that event due to civil disruption may have contributed to this unusual pattern. The longest chain of person-to-person transmission was 7 reported serial cases but serial transmission usually did not extend beyond secondary cases. Epidemiologic data suggest a secondary attack rate of about 8%. In a 2013 outbreak in the DRC, the proportion of household contacts infected with monkeypox ranged from 50% to 100%, suggesting an increased risk for human-to-human transmission. Most cases have occurred either singly or in clusters in small remote villages, usually in tropical rainforest where the population has multiple contacts with several types of wild animals.

9. Treatment—Patients should be managed symptomatically and, if hospitalized, placed under strict infection control measures with sterilization of any implements used in patient management and safe disposal of bandages by boiling, autoclaving, or incineration; physical contact with others should be avoided until lesions have completely resolved.

10. Prevention—Vaccination with vaccinia is believed to be protective. However, the protection provided by childhood smallpox vaccination is waning in the general populations at risk since the cessation of smallpox vaccination in the 1980s. Currently, because of adverse event profiles and anticipated clinical and epidemiologic risk-benefit ratios, cross-protective prophylactic vaccination with smallpox vaccine (fully replicative vaccinia) is not routinely recommended by WHO.

Human infection may be controllable to some extent by education to limit contact with infected cases and potentially infected animals. However, in areas where the disease is endemic in the zoonotic reservoirs and the population relies on hunting as an important food source, sporadic infections continue to occur.

The 2003 outbreak in the USA clearly demonstrates potential for monkeypox to be a public health threat outside enzootic areas and there is evidence that infection has also emerged in nature outside of historic known enzootic areas. It is not fully understood whether this represents a real extension of enzootic areas or is the result of ascertainment of human infection. Full evaluation of the ecology, epidemiology, and virology associated with monkeypox outbreaks in endemic areas will enable understanding of prevention and control measures.

11. Special considerations—No information is available on the efficacy of postexposure vaccination with vaccinia virus; however, postexposure vaccination may potentially prevent monkeypox disease or reduce severity if given within 3 days of exposure. Smallpox (vaccinia) vaccination was used as an outbreak response intervention in the USA outbreak in 2003. A WHO technical advisory committee on variola virus research met in 2016 and recommended that progress of monkeypox research be accelerated, particularly in diagnostics and therapeutics. A prospective cohort study evaluating the immunogenicity and safety of Imvamune, a live attenuated smallpox vaccine in health care personnel is currently being conducted in Tshuapa province in the DRC.

IV. ORF VIRUS DISEASE (contagious pustular dermatitis, human orf, ecthyma contagiosum)

1. Clinical features—A proliferative cutaneous viral disease in which the lesion, usually solitary and located on hands, arms, or face, is a red-to-violet vesiculonodule, maculopapule, or pustule, progressing to a weeping nodule with central umbilication. There may be several lesions, each up to 3 cm in diameter and lasting 3 to 6 weeks. With secondary bacterial infection, lesions may become pustular. Regional adenitis occurs in a few cases. A maculopapular rash may occur on the trunk. Erythema multiforme and erythema multiforme bullosum are rare complications. Disseminated disease and serious ocular damage have been reported but are uncommon. The disease has been confused with cutaneous anthrax and malignancy.

2. Risk groups—Susceptibility is probably universal; recovery produces variable levels of immunity. A common infection among shepherds, veterinarians, and abattoir workers in areas producing sheep and goats and an important occupational disease in New Zealand.

3. Causative agents—Orf virus, a deoxyribonucleic acid virus belonging to the genus *Parapoxvirus* of poxviruses (family Poxviridae). The agent is closely related to other parapoxviruses that can be transmitted to humans as occupational diseases, such as milker's nodule virus of dairy cattle and bovine papular stomatitis virus of beef cattle. Contagious ecthyma parapoxvirus of domesticated camels may infect people on rare occasions.

4. Diagnosis—Identification of the characteristic lesion and ascertainment of a history of contact with sheep, goats, or wild ungulates, in particular their young; through electron microscopy demonstration of ovoid parapoxvirions in the lesion or by growth of the virus in ovine, bovine, or primate cell cultures; or through positive molecular (e.g., PCR) or serologic tests.

5. Occurrence—Probably worldwide among farm workers.

6. Reservoirs—Probably in various ungulates (sheep, goats, reindeer, musk oxen). The virus is very resistant to physical factors, except ultraviolet light, and may persist for months in soil and on animal skin and hair.

7. Incubation period—Generally 3 to 6 days.

8. Transmission—Through contact with infected sheep and goats and, occasionally, wild ungulates (deer, reindeer). Direct contact with the mucous membranes of infected animals, with lesions on udders of nursing dams, or through intermediate passive transfer from apparently normal animals contaminated by contact, knives, shears, trucks, and clothing. Human infection may follow production and administration of vaccines to animals. Person-to-person transmission is rare. Human lesions show a decrease in the number of virus particles as the disease progresses.

9. Treatment—Boil, autoclave, or incinerate dressings. There is no specific treatment.

10. Prevention—

1) Good personal hygiene and use of gloves.
2) Washing of hands and exposed areas with soap and water.
3) Domestic and wild ungulates should be considered a potential source of infection. Ensure general cleanliness of animal housing areas. The efficacy and safety of parapoxvirus vaccines in animals has not been fully determined.

11. Special considerations—Reporting: check local reporting requirements. Case report to local health authority is not usually required but may be desirable when a human case occurs in areas not previously known to have the infection.

[A. Rimoin, N. Hoff, R. Doshi]

SPOROTRICHOSIS

DISEASE	ICD-10 CODE
SPOROTRICHOSIS	ICD-10 B42

1. Clinical features—A fungal disease, usually of the skin, often of an extremity. It begins as a single nodule at the site of traumatic inoculation. As this grows, lymphatics draining the area become firm and cord-like and form a series of nodules, which in turn may soften and ulcerate. Osteoarticular, pulmonary, and multifocal infections occur but are relatively rare, except multifocal disseminated infections in patients with human immunodeficiency virus. Fatalities are uncommon.

2. Risk groups—Farmers, gardeners, and horticulturists are occupational groups at risk of infection from environmental reservoirs. Persons handling animals infected with sporotrichosis are also at risk.

3. Causative agents—*Sporothrix schenckii* spp. complex, consisting of *S. schenckii* sensu stricto, *Sporothrix mexicana*, *Sporothrix globosa*, *Sporothrix brasiliensis*, and *Sporothrix luriei*. *Sporothrix pallida* (formerly *Sporothrix albicans*) is also sometimes considered part of this species complex.

4. Diagnosis—Culture of a biopsy, pus, or exudate confirms the diagnosis in skin lesions. Organisms are rarely visualized by direct smear. Biopsied tissue should be examined with fungal stains. Serologic testing is available for detection of antibodies, though these tests have limited sensitivity in cutaneous cases.

5. Occurrence—Reported worldwide but characteristically sporadic and relatively uncommon. One of the largest known outbreaks in humans affected more than 3,000 gold miners in South Africa during the 1930s and 1940s. Outbreaks of cutaneous infection have occurred among children playing in baled hay and adults working with it. A cluster of cutaneous infections was also reported in gardeners who had stuffed topiaries with contaminated sphagnum moss. Contact with infected cats was an exposure risk in a Brazilian outbreak of lymphocutaneous infection in 2003. Cases continue to spread between cats and humans throughout Brazil, with thousands of cases recorded to date.

6. Reservoirs—Soil and plant matter such as moss, wood, and hay.

7. Incubation period—The lymphatic form usually develops 1 week to 3 months after injury.

8. Transmission—Fungus is introduced through skin pricks from thorns or barbs, through handling of sphagnum moss, or through slivers from wood or lumber. Bites or scratches from infected animals can also transmit the infection. Pulmonary sporotrichosis arises through inhalation of conidia. Person-to-person transmission has only rarely been documented.

9. Treatment—In lymphocutaneous infection, itraconazole is the drug of choice but treatment options include terbinafine, supersaturated potassium iodide, or fluconazole. In extracutaneous forms, amphotericin B is often recommended for initial treatment.

Preferred therapy	Lymphocutaneous infection: • Itraconazole 200 mg PO daily for 3–6 months usually and 2–4 weeks after all lesions have resolved
	Osteoarticular infection: • Itraconazole 200 mg PO BID for 12 months
	Pulmonary infection, severe: • AMB lipid formulation 3–5 mg/kg IV daily • AMB deoxycholate 0.7–1 mg/kg IV daily • If response occurs to AMB, change to itraconazole 200 mg PO BID for 12 months
	Pulmonary infection, nonsevere: • Itraconazole 200 mg PO BID for 12 months
	Meningeal or disseminated infection: • AMB lipid formulation 3–5 mg/kg IV daily (disseminated) OR 5 mg/kg IV daily (meningeal) for 4–6 weeks • If response occurs to AMB, change to itraconazole 200 mg PO BID for 12 months
	Pregnant women: • Local hyperthermia for cutaneous infection • If treatment required, liposomal AMB 3–5 mg/kg IV daily OR AMB deoxycholate 0.7–1 mg/kg IV daily • Avoid azoles
	Children: • For cutaneous or lymphocutaneous infection, itraconazole 6–10 mg/kg (≤ 400 mg) PO daily[a] OR, as an alternative, SSKI 1 drop PO TID, increasing as tolerated ≤ 1 drop/kg in divided doses TID (≤ 40–50 drops daily) • For disseminated infection, AMB deoxycholate 0.7 mg/kg IV daily • If response occurs to AMB, change to itraconazole 6–10 mg/kg (≤ 400 mg) PO daily for 12 months

(Continued)

(Continued)

Alternative therapy options	Lymphocutaneous infection: • Itraconazole 200 mg PO BID • Terbinafine 500 mg PO BID • SSKI (associated with many side effects) • Fluconazole 400–800 mg daily if no response to primary or other alternative therapy • Local hyperthermia for patients with fixed cutaneous sporotrichosis who cannot tolerate other regimens
	Osteoarticular infection: • Liposomal AMB 3–5 mg/kg IV daily • AMB lipid complex 5 mg/kg IV daily • AMB deoxycholate 0.7–1 mg/kg IV daily • If response occurs to AMB, change to itraconazole 200 mg PO BID for 12 months
	Meningeal or disseminated infection: • AMB deoxycholate 0.7–1 mg/kg IV daily
Special considerations and comments	• Surgery combined with medical therapy recommended for localized pulmonary disease. • Improvement of immune function (introducing antiretroviral therapy in patients with HIV or reducing immunosuppressive therapy) may be helpful. • Patients with AIDS or other immunosuppressed patients who have disseminated disease should receive itraconazole 200 mg daily to prevent relapse. • Itraconazole levels are recommended for ensuring adequate concentrations in extracutaneous disease after ≥ 2 weeks of therapy. • Dosing and appropriate dosing weights between AMB formulations vary.

Note: AIDS = acquired immunodeficiency syndrome; AMB = amphotericin B; BID = twice daily; HIV = human immunodeficiency virus; IV = intravenous(ly); PO = oral(ly); SSKI = saturated solution of potassium iodide; TID = thrice daily.

[a]Because Infectious Diseases Society of America guidelines do not specify treatment duration for children, assume same as for adults.

10. Prevention—

1) Wear gloves and long sleeves when handling sphagnum moss or other plant material. Use personal protective equipment when handling infected animals. Dispose of or disinfect material known to be contaminated as appropriate.

2) Management of contacts and the immediate environment: search for undiagnosed cases by investigating household or occupational contacts for evidence of infection from a common environmental source. Determine source to limit future exposures.

11. Special considerations—None.

Bibliography

Bennett JE, Dolin R, Blaser MJ. *Mandell, Douglas, and Bennett's Principles and Practice of Infectious Diseases.* 8th ed. Philadelphia, PA: Elsevier; 2014:3271–3277.

Gremião IDF, Miranda LHM, Reis EG, Rodrigues AM, Pereira SA. Zoonotic Epidemic of Sporotrichosis: Cat to Human Transmission. *PLoS Pathog.* 2017;13(1):e1006077.

Kauffman CA, Bustamante B, Chapman SW, Pappas PG. Clinical practice guidelines for the management of sporotrichosis: 2007 update by the Infectious Diseases Society of America. *Clin Infect Dis.* 2007;45(10):1255–1265.

[B. Jackson]

STAPHYLOCOCCAL DISEASES

DISEASE	ICD-10 CODE
BOILS, CARBUNCLES, FURUNCLES, ABSCESSES	ICD-10 L02; B95.6–B95.8
IMPETIGO	ICD-10 L01
CELLULITIS	ICD-10 L03
STAPHYLOCOCCAL SEPSIS	ICD-10 A41.0–A41.2
STAPHYLOCOCCAL PNEUMONIA	ICD-10 J15.2
ARTHRITIS	ICD-10 M00.0
OSTEOMYELITIS	ICD-10 M86
ENDOCARDITIS	ICD-10 I33.0
IMPETIGO NEONATORUM	ICD-10 L00
ABSCESS OF THE BREAST	ICD-10 P39.0
STAPHYLOCOCCAL DISEASE ON HOSPITAL MEDICAL AND SURGICAL WARDS	ICD-10 T81.4
TOXIC SHOCK SYNDROME	ICD-10 A48.3
Staphylococcal food poisoning (see "Foodborne Intoxications")	

The genus *Staphylococcus* contains more than 50 species that are ubiquitous colonizers of skin and mucosa of almost all animals. In the absence of immunosuppression and implanted foreign materials, only a few of these are pathogenic to humans. The most virulent ones include *Staphylococcus aureus* and *Staphylococcus lugdunensis*. *Staphylococcus epidermidis* and *Staphylococcus haemolyticus* are related to device-associated infections and *Staphylococcus saprophyticus* to urinary tract infections but these produce less severe disease. Methicillin resistance mediated by the production of PBP-2a, a penicillin-binding protein encoded by the *mecA* gene, was first described in *S. aureus* (methicillin-resistant *S. aureus* [MRSA]) in 1961. In 2007, livestock-associated *mecC* MRSA (LA-MRSA) was detected in Western Europe. LA-MRSA has also been associated with human disease and studies of archived isolates indicate that it may have been circulating since 1975. MRSA may be health care–associated or community-associated (CA-MRSA).

Virulence of bacterial strains varies greatly. The most important human pathogen is *S. aureus*. Most strains ferment mannitol and are coagulase-positive. However, coagulase-negative strains are increasingly important, especially in bloodstream infections among patients with intravascular catheters, in infections of prosthetic materials, and in other health care–associated infections. Antibiotic resistance of staphylococci has risen over the last 60 years and continues to cause adverse health-economic outcomes.

Clinical manifestations include skin and soft-tissue infections, bacteremia and its complications (including infective endocarditis), bone and joint infections, and meningitis.

Staphylococcal disease has different clinical and epidemiologic patterns in the general community, in newborns, in menstruating women, and among hospitalized patients; each will be presented separately in this chapter. Staphylococcal toxic shock syndrome (TSS) represents a rare but potentially lethal complication of staphylococcal carriage and is presented at the end of the chapter.

I. STAPHYLOCOCCAL DISEASE IN THE COMMUNITY

1. Clinical features—The common bacterial skin lesions are impetigo, folliculitis, furuncles (boils), carbuncles, abscesses, and infected lacerations. The basic lesion of impetigo is described in this chapter (see Clinical Features under Staphylococcal Disease in Hospital Nurseries). A distinctive scalded skin syndrome is associated with certain strains of *S. aureus* that produce an epidermolytic toxin. Other skin lesions are localized and discrete. If lesions extend or are widespread, fever, malaise, headache, and anorexia may develop. Usually, lesions are uncomplicated but seeding into the bloodstream may lead to lung abscess, osteomyelitis, arthritis, endocarditis, or meningitis. In addition to primary skin lesions, staphylococcal conjunctivitis occurs in newborns and the elderly. Staphylococcal pneumonia is a well-recognized complication following influenza infection. Staphylococcal endocarditis and other complications of staphylococcal bacteremia may result from parenteral use of illicit drugs or nosocomially from intravenous catheters and other devices. Embolic skin lesions are frequent complications of endocarditis due to *S. aureus*. Coagulase-negative staphylococci may cause sepsis, meningitis, endocarditis, or female urinary tract infections.

These are increasing in frequency, usually in connection with prosthetic devices or indwelling catheters.

2. Risk groups—Immune mechanisms depend mainly on an intact opsonization/phagocytosis axis involving neutrophils. Susceptibility to infection is therefore greatest among newborns and the chronically ill. Elderly and debilitated people, injecting drug users, and those with diabetes mellitus, cystic fibrosis, chronic renal failure, agammaglobulinemia, disorders of neutrophil function (e.g., chronic granulomatous disease), neoplastic disease, and burns are particularly susceptible. Use of steroids also increases susceptibility.

3. Causative agents—Various coagulase-positive strains of *S. aureus*. Epidemics are caused by relatively few strains. The majority of clinical isolates of *S. aureus*, whether community- or hospital-acquired, are resistant to penicillin G and multiresistant (including methicillin-resistant) strains have become widespread. CA-MRSA is spreading quickly in many parts of the world; however, its prevalence and molecular epidemiology varies considerably from continent to continent. Evidence suggests that biofilm-producing strains of coagulase-negative staphylococci may be more pathogenic but the data are inconclusive. *S. saprophyticus* is a common cause of urinary tract infection in young women.

4. Diagnosis—Confirmed by isolation of the organism on culture. Most strains of staphylococci can be characterized through antibiotic resistance profile, spa typing, multilocus sequence typing, and whole-genome sequencing.

5. Occurrence—Worldwide. Highest incidence is in areas where hygiene conditions are suboptimal and people are crowded together; common among children, especially in warm weather. The disease occurs sporadically and as small epidemics in families, sports teams, and summer camps, with various members developing recurrent illness due to the same staphylococcal strain. Asymptomatic carriers may serve as an unrecognized reservoir. Also a problem in nursing homes and other health care institutions.

6. Reservoirs—Humans; rarely animals. The animal reservoir of CA-MRSA (mostly farm pigs but also horses and companion animals) appears to be increasing with new implications for MRSA control in human medicine.

7. Incubation period—Variable, but colonization usually precedes infection.

8. Transmission—The major site of colonization is the anterior nasal passages; 20% to 30% of the general population are nasal carriers of coagulase-positive staphylococci. Autoinfection is responsible for at least two-thirds of infections. Persons with a draining lesion or purulent discharge are the most common sources of epidemic spread. Transmission is through contact with a person who has a purulent lesion or is an asymptomatic carrier of a pathogenic strain. Some carriers are more effective disseminators of infection than others. Hands are the most important instruments for staphylococcal transmission. The period of communicability continues as long as purulent lesions continue to drain or the carrier state persists. Autoinfection may continue for the period of nasal colonization or duration of active lesions.

9. **Treatment**—Should be tailored according to sensitivity patterns of staphylococci. Some commonly used antimicrobials for *S. aureus* are listed in the treatment table (dose may vary depending on renal function and presence of complications).

Sensitivity Pattern of *Staphylococcus aureus*	Choice of Antimicrobial Agents	Note
MSSA	<ul><li>Nafcillin</li><li>Oxacillin</li><li>Flucloxacillin</li><li>Cefazolin</li></ul>	Vancomycin is less effective than β-lactams for MSSA bacteremia and should be avoided if a β-lactam can be used.
MRSA	<ul><li>Vancomycin</li><li>Daptomycin</li><li>Teicoplanin</li></ul>	None
	Alternative agents:<ul><li>Ceftaroline</li><li>Ceftobiprole</li><li>Telavancin</li><li>Dalbavancin</li><li>Oritavancin</li><li>Linezolid</li><li>Tedizolid</li><li>TMP/SMX</li><li>Clindamycin</li><li>Doxycycline</li><li>Omadacycline</li><li>Eravacycline</li><li>Delafloxacin</li></ul>	<ul><li>Ceftaroline and ceftobiprole are fifth-generation cephalosporins with MRSA activity. Ceftaroline was approved by FDA for ABSSIs and community-acquired bacterial pneumonia. Ceftobiprole is approved in Canada and Europe but not in the USA.</li><li>The following are generally used in nonbacteremic ABSSIs:<ul><li>TMP/SMX</li><li>Clindamycin</li><li>Doxycycline</li></ul></li></ul>

Note: ABSSI = acute bacterial skin and soft-tissue infection; MRSA = methicillin-resistant *Staphylococcus aureus*; MSSA = methicillin-susceptible *S. aureus*; TMP/SMX = trimethoprim-sulfamethoxazole.

Once treatment has been initiated for *S. aureus* bacteremia, blood culture should be repeated approximately 2 days after initiation of treatment to document clearance of bacteremia. Failure to clear bacteremia within 2 to 3 days should prompt further evaluation.

Duration of treatment is 14 days for patients with uncomplicated *S. aureus* bacteremia. Longer durations of treatment and further evaluation and interventions (e.g., drainage of abscess) are warranted for patients with complicated bacteremia. Patients are considered to have uncomplicated bacteremia if infective endocarditis has been ruled out and if they do not have indwelling devices (e.g., pacemakers), are not immunocompromised (e.g., neutropenic), the bacteremia clears within 72 hours, and there is no evidence of metastatic infection.

10. Prevention—Educate the public and health care personnel in personal hygiene, especially hand hygiene and the importance of not sharing bath towels. Treat initial cases in children and families promptly. Staphylococcal decolonization with topical antimicrobials or antiseptics (e.g., mupirocin or chlorhexidine baths) may be a reasonable preventive option in patients with multiple documented recurrences of staphylococcal infection or ongoing transmission in a close cohort of individuals (i.e., household spread).

11. Special considerations—

1) Reporting: outbreaks in schools, summer camps, and other population groups should be reported to the local health authority. In many industrialized countries, any recognized clusters of cases in the community should also be reported.
2) Epidemic measures:

- Search for and treat those with clinical illness, especially those with draining lesions.
- Strict personal hygiene with emphasis on handwashing should be encouraged. Culture for nasal carriers of the epidemic strain and treat locally with mupirocin or, if unsuccessful, oral antimicrobials.
- Investigate unusual or abrupt prevalence increases in community staphylococcal infections for a possible common source (e.g., an unrecognized hospital epidemic).

II. STAPHYLOCOCCAL DISEASE IN HOSPITAL NURSERIES

1. Clinical features—Impetigo or pustulosis of the newborn and other purulent skin manifestations are the staphylococcal diseases most frequently acquired in nurseries. Characteristic skin lesions develop secondary to colonization of the nose, umbilicus, circumcision site, rectum, or conjunctivae. Colonization of these sites with staphylococcal strains is a normal occurrence and does not imply disease. Lesions most commonly occur in diaper and intertriginous areas. They are initially vesicular, rapidly turning seropurulent, surrounded by an erythematous base. Rupture of pustules favors their spread. Complications are unusual, although lymphadenitis, furunculosis, breast abscess, pneumonia, arthritis, osteomyelitis, and others have been reported.

Though uncommon, staphylococcal scalded skin syndrome (Ritter's disease, pemphigus neonatorum) may occur. Clinical manifestations range from diffuse scarlatiniform erythema to generalized bullous desquamation. Like bullous impetigo, it is caused by strains of *S. aureus*, which produce an epidermolytic toxin.

2. Risk groups—Susceptibility of newborns appears to be general. For the duration of colonization with pathogenic strains, infants remain at risk of disease.

3. Causative agents—Strains of *S. aureus*.

4. Diagnosis—See Staphylococcal Disease in the Community in this chapter.

5. Occurrence—Worldwide. Problems occur mainly in hospitals, are promoted by lax aseptic techniques, and are amplified by the emergence and transmission of antibiotic-resistant strains, in particular CA-MRSA.

6. Reservoirs—See Staphylococcal Disease in the Community in this chapter.

7. Incubation period—Commonly 4 to 10 days; disease may not occur until several months after colonization.

8. Transmission—Primarily spread by hands of hospital personnel; rarely, airborne via droplets. The period of communicability is as described in Staphylococcal Disease in the Community in this chapter.

9. Treatment—

1) Localized pustulosis:

- Term neonate without systemic finding: topical treatment (e.g., mupirocin) with close follow-up.
- Term neonate with systemic finding: parenteral treatment with antistaphylococcal agents, depending on local resistance profile.
- Preterm low birth weight neonates: parenteral treatment until bacteremia is excluded.

2) Skin and soft-tissue infections more severe than localized pustulosis: infants should be hospitalized and closely monitored. Parenteral antimicrobials should be administered. Purulent or fluctuant lesions should be drained.

10. Prevention—

1) Use aseptic techniques when necessary and clean hands with alcohol-based hand rubs before contact with each infant in nurseries.

2) Personnel with minor lesions (pustules, boils, abscesses, paronychia, conjunctivitis, severe acne, otitis externa, or infected lacerations) must not be permitted to work in nurseries.

3) Supervision through an active hospital infection control committee, including a regular system for investigating, reporting, and reviewing hospital-acquired infections.

11. Special considerations—

1) Reporting: obligatory reporting of epidemics to local health authority.

2) Control measures in case of outbreaks:

- Two or more concurrent cases of staphylococcal disease related to a nursery or maternity ward is presumptive evidence of an outbreak and warrants investigation.

- Culture all lesions to determine antibiotic resistance pattern and type of epidemic strain. Laboratories should keep clinically important isolates for genotyping to support epidemiologic investigations.

- In nursery outbreaks, start isolation precautions for cases and contacts until all have been discharged. Colonized or infected infants should be grouped (cohorting). Assignments of personnel should be restricted to specific cohorts.

- Before admitting new patients, wash cribs, beds, and other furniture with an approved disinfectant.

- Examine all personnel for draining lesions anywhere on the body. Perform an epidemiologic investigation and, if 1 or more personnel are associated with the disease, culture nasal specimens from them and all others in contact with infants. It may become necessary to exclude and treat all carriers of the epidemic strain until cultures are negative. Treatment of asymptomatic carriers aims to suppress the nasal carrier state, usually through local application of appropriate antibiotic ointments to the nasal vestibule, sometimes with concurrent systemic antibiotics for 5 to 7 days.

- Investigate adequacy of nursing procedures, especially availability of alcohol-based hand rubs. Emphasize strict hand hygiene. Personnel assigned to infected or colonized infants should not work with noncolonized newborns.

III. STAPHYLOCOCCAL DISEASE AMONG HOSPITALIZED PATIENTS

1. Clinical features—Clinical features of staphylococcal infection among hospitalized patients vary depending on the type of infection. Infections among hospitalized patients range from uncomplicated wound infections, including surgical site infections, to more invasive infections such as bacteremia from catheter-related infections, lower respiratory tract infections, and urinary tract infections. Infection with MRSA is a bigger concern among hospitalized patients than infection with methicillin-susceptible *S. aureus* (MSSA).

2. Risk groups—Risk factors for staphylococcal infections among hospitalized patients include presence of invasive devices (prosthetic joints and devices, central lines and indwelling urinary catheters), history of MRSA colonization or infection, recent surgery, and prolonged hospitalization.

3. Causative agents—*S. aureus*, either MSSA or MRSA.

4. Diagnosis—Verification depends on isolation of *S. aureus* associated with a clinical illness compatible with the bacteriologic findings.

5. Occurrence—Worldwide. Staphylococcal infection is a major cause of hospital-acquired infection in the general wards of hospitals. Attack rates may assume epidemic proportions and community spread may occur when hospital-infected patients are discharged. Misuse of antimicrobials has increased the prevalence of antibiotic-resistant staphylococci.

6. Reservoirs—See Staphylococcal Disease in the Community in this chapter.

7. Incubation period—See Staphylococcal Disease in the Community in this chapter.

8. Transmission—See Reservoirs, Incubation Period, and Transmission under Staphylococcal Disease in the Community in this chapter.

9. Treatment—See Staphylococcal Disease in the Community in this chapter.

10. Prevention—

1) Hand hygiene compliance
2) Contact precautions for MRSA carriers
3) Antimicrobial stewardship
4) Surgical prophylaxis with appropriate antibiotics
5) Decolonization, especially for cardiac and bone and joint surgeries

11. Special considerations—

1) Reporting: obligatory report of epidemics; no individual case report.

2) Control measures in case of outbreaks:

- The occurrence of 2 or more cases with epidemiologic association is sufficient to suspect epidemic spread and to initiate investigation.
- See Special Considerations under Staphylococcal Disease in Hospital Nurseries in this chapter.
- Review and enforce strict aseptic techniques.

IV. TOXIC SHOCK SYNDROME

TSS has been reported in staphylococcal scarlet fever since 1927 but gained traction in the 1980s when it was described to be associated with the use of highly absorbent tampons during menses. The commonest *S. aureus* toxin associated with TSS is TSST-1.

The clinical signs and symptoms of TSS develop rapidly (within 48 hours) and usually in otherwise healthy individuals. The clinical manifestations include rapid onset hypotension, dermatologic manifestations including diffuse macular erythrodermic rash and desquamation (1–2 weeks after onset of rash), and multisystem involvement. According to the criteria established by CDC for epidemiologic surveillance, involvement of 3 or more of the following organ systems is required:

1) Gastrointestinal: vomiting or diarrhea at onset of illness.
2) Muscular: severe myalgia or creatine phosphokinase elevation more than 2 times the upper limit of normal.
3) Mucous membranes: vaginal, oropharyngeal, or conjunctival hyperemia.
4) Renal: blood urea nitrogen or serum creatinine more than 2 times the upper limit of normal or pyuria (> 5 leukocytes/high-power field) in the absence of urinary tract infection.
5) Hepatic: bilirubin or transaminases more than 2 times the upper limit of normal.
6) Hematologic: platelets lower than $100,000/\mu L$.
7) Central nervous system: disorientation or alterations in consciousness without focal neurologic signs when fever and hypotension are absent.

Diagnosis of TSS can be done with the aid of the surveillance criteria developed by CDC (see Box 1 later in this chapter).

Treatment of TSS includes good supportive care, treatment of shock, appropriate antibiotic therapy, surgical debridement (if warranted), and removal of offending foreign materials (e.g., tampon). Clindamycin or linezolid may help reduce toxin production.

Box 1. Toxic Shock Syndrome Case Definition

Clinical criteria:

- Fever: temperature $\geq$ 38.9°C ($\geq$ 102.0°F)
- Rash: diffuse macular erythroderma
- Desquamation: 1–2 weeks after onset of rash
- Hypotension: systolic blood pressure $\leq$ 90 mm Hg for adults or < fifth percentile by age for children younger than 16 years
- Multisystem involvement (3 or more of the following organ systems):
  - Gastrointestinal: vomiting or diarrhea at onset of illness
  - Muscular: severe myalgia or creatine phosphokinase level at least twice the upper limit of normal
  - Mucous membrane: vaginal, oropharyngeal, or conjunctival hyperemia
  - Renal: blood urea nitrogen or creatinine at least twice the upper limit of normal for laboratory or urinary sediment with pyuria ($\geq$ 5 leukocytes/high-power field) in the absence of urinary tract infection
  - Hepatic: total bilirubin, alanine aminotransferase enzyme, or aspartate aminotransferase enzyme levels at least twice the upper limit of normal for laboratory
  - Hematologic: platelets < 100,000/mm^3
  - Central nervous system: disorientation or alterations in consciousness without focal neurologic signs when fever and hypotension are absent

Laboratory criteria:

- Negative results on the following tests for alternative pathogens, if obtained:
  - Blood or cerebrospinal fluid cultures (blood culture may be positive for *Staphylococcus aureus*, but only in ~5% of patients)
  - Negative serologies for Rocky Mountain spotted fever, leptospirosis, or measles

Case classification:

- Probable: a case that meets the laboratory criteria and in which 4 of the 5 clinical criteria described earlier are present
- Confirmed: a case that meets the laboratory criteria and in which all 5 of the clinical criteria described earlier are present, including desquamation, unless the patient dies before desquamation occurs

Source: Data from CDC. Toxic Shock Syndrome (Other Than Streptococcal) (TSS) 2011 Case Definition. 2011. Available at: https://wwwn.cdc.gov/nndss/conditions/toxic-shock-syndrome-other-than-streptococcal/case-definition/2011. Accessed January 24, 2019.

[K. Marimuthu, S. Vasoo]

STREPTOCOCCAL DISEASES

DISEASE	ICD-10 CODE
STREPTOCOCCAL SORE THROAT	ICD-10 J02.0
IMPETIGO	ICD-10 L01.0
CELLULITIS	ICD-10 L03.90
ERYSIPELAS	ICD-10 A46
SCARLET FEVER	ICD-10 A38
PUERPERAL FEVER	ICD-10 O85
SEPSIS DUE TO STREPTOCOCCUS, GROUP A	ICD-10 A40.0
STREPTOCOCCAL TOXIC SHOCK SYNDROME	ICD-10 B95.0
NECROTIZING FASCIITIS	ICD-10 M72.6
RHEUMATIC HEART DISEASE	ICD-10 I09.9
OTHER GROUP A STREPTOCOCCAL INFECTIONS	ICD-10 A49.1
GROUP B STREPTOCOCCAL SEPSIS OF THE NEWBORN	ICD-10 P36.0
Streptococcus pneumoniae infections (see "Pneumonia")	

Group A streptococci (GAS) cause a wide spectrum of diseases from superficial infections such as pharyngitis, impetigo, and cellulitis to severe invasive disease, necrotizing fasciitis, and toxic shock syndrome. In addition, the immunologic complications of GAS infections, namely poststreptococcal glomerulonephritis and particularly acute rheumatic fever (ARF) and rheumatic heart disease (RHD), are responsible for significant morbidity and mortality globally (> 500,000 estimated deaths annually), with the highest burden of disease in low-resource settings (see Group A Streptococcal Infections in this chapter). GAS infections affect all age groups, with infants, children, and the elderly overrepresented.

Group B β-hemolytic streptococci, found in the human vagina and gastrointestinal tract, may cause neonatal sepsis and meningitis (see Group B Streptococcal Sepsis of the Newborn in this chapter) as well as stillbirth, preterm labor, and postpartum endometritis. Group B streptococci (GBS) cause skin infections and sepsis in the elderly and immunocompromised.

Streptococci of other groups can also produce infections in humans; these are discussed briefly here but a detailed examination of these organisms is beyond the scope of this chapter. Groups C and G streptococci have produced outbreaks of streptococcal tonsillitis, usually foodborne. Their role in sporadic cases is less well defined but they can both cause invasive diseases similar to group A streptococcal infections; outbreaks of puerperal fever due to these organisms have been reported. Groups C and G streptococci are also commonly implicated in cellulitis. Glomerulonephritis has followed group C infections but has very rarely been reported after group G infections; neither group is proven to cause rheumatic fever. Group D organisms (including enterococci), both hemolytic and nonhemolytic, are involved in bacterial endocarditis and urinary tract infections. Nosocomial spread of vancomycin-resistant enterococci is of increasing concern worldwide.

I. GROUP A STREPTOCOCCAL INFECTIONS (streptococcal sore throat, scarlet fever, impetigo, erysipelas, cellulitis, puerperal fever, invasive group A strep, streptococcal toxic shock syndrome (STSS), necrotizing fasciitis, poststreptococcal glomerulonephritis, rheumatic fever)

1. Clinical features—The most frequently encountered GAS conditions are pharyngitis/tonsillitis and superficial skin infections such as impetigo or pyoderma. Other acute infections include erysipelas, cellulitis, wound infections, otitis media, and invasive infections including puerperal fever, pneumonia/empyema, osteomyelitis, septic arthritis, meningitis, septicemia, and necrotizing fasciitis. Toxin-mediated disease includes scarlet fever and its more severe form—STSS. One or other form of clinical disease often predominates during outbreaks. Postinfectious sequelae including ARF and acute poststreptococcal glomerulonephritis (APSGN) may develop after pharyngeal or skin infection.

1) Streptococcal sore throat: patients with streptococcal sore throat typically exhibit sudden onset of fever, throat pain and difficulty swallowing, exudative tonsillitis, and tender, enlarged anterior cervical lymph nodes. The pharynx, the tonsillar pillars, and soft palate may be injected and edematous with exudate seen; petechiae may be present against a background of diffuse redness. Coincident or subsequent otitis media, peritonsillar abscess, or retropharyngeal collection may occur.

2) Streptococcal skin infections:

- Pyoderma, impetigo: usually superficial and may proceed through vesicular, pustular, and encrusted stages. GAS is the major pathogen implicated in impetigo in tropical climates and coinfection with *Staphylococcus aureus* is common. (See images at: https://www.dermnetnz.org/topics/impetigo.)

- Erysipelas and cellulitis: acute skin infections characterized by fever with a red, tender, edematous spreading lesion of the skin, sometimes accompanied by lymphangitis and/or lymphadenitis.

  In erysipelas the superficial dermis and cutaneous lymphatics are involved, typically producing a distinct area of erythema with a defined, raised border. The central point of origin tends to clear as the periphery extends. Face and legs are common sites. Recurrences are frequent and disease is more common among persons with underlying skin conditions. GAS is the predominant causative pathogen. (See images at: https://www.dermnetnz.org/topics/erysipelas.)

In cellulitis the deep dermis and subcutaneous tissues are involved; the borders of inflammation are less well demarcated than in erysipelas. Cellulitis most commonly involves the lower limbs and is nearly always unilateral. β-Hemolytic streptococci including GAS (and groups C and G streptococci) are the causative agents of nonpurulent cellulitis based on epidemiologic studies comprising a combination of culture, streptococcal serology, and response to treatment with penicillin; however a pathogen is rarely cultured. (See images at: https://www.dermnetnz.org/topics/cellulitis.)

- Perianal cellulitis (due to GAS): occurs among all ages but is primarily a disease of early childhood. It can also result in disease outbreaks.
- Scarlet fever: a form of GAS infection characterized by a skin rash, occurring when the infecting strain produces a pyrogenic exotoxin (erythrogenic toxin). Clinical characteristics include symptoms associated with a streptococcal sore throat (or with a streptococcal skin or puerperal infection) as well as enanthem, strawberry tongue, and exanthem. The rash is usually a fine erythema, commonly punctate, blanching on pressure, often felt (like sandpaper) better than seen, and appearing most often on the trunk and spreading to the limbs and neck with accentuation in the axilla and groin. Typically, there is sparing of the palms, soles, and face with flushing of the cheeks and circumoral pallor. (See images at: https://www.dermnetnz.org/topics/scarlet-fever.) High fever, nausea, and vomiting often accompany severe infections. During convalescence, skin peeling occurs at the tips of fingers and toes and less often over wide areas of the trunk and limbs; peeling is more pronounced where the exanthem was severe. The case-fatality rate in some parts of the world has been as high as 3% but generally deaths due to scarlet fever are rare; severe forms are likely to be STSS (see later).

3) GAS puerperal fever: an acute disease, usually febrile, characterized by abdominal pain with or without purulent vaginal discharge, uterine tenderness, vomiting, diarrhea, and/or hypotension in the peripartum patient. Case-fatality rate is low when adequately

treated: 2% in the USA; up to 10% in resource-limited settings. Puerperal infections may be caused by organisms other than hemolytic streptococci; they are clinically similar but differ bacteriologically and epidemiologically (see "Staphylococcal Diseases").

4) Invasive GAS disease: defined as an infection associated with isolation of GAS from a sterile site (or from a nonsterile site in patients with necrotizing fasciitis or STSS). Clinical syndromes include pneumonia/empyema, osteomyelitis, septic arthritis, meningitis, epiglottitis, quinsy, endocarditis, septicemia, and necrotizing fasciitis (the last 2 are discussed in detail separately in this chapter). Reported mortality rates range from 8% to 16% with higher case-fatality rates in lower income countries ($\leq$ 25%), among the elderly, and in patients with meningitis.

5) STSS: may occur with either invasive or focal infections caused by superantigen toxin-producing strains of GAS. Defined as isolation of GAS from a sterile site (or nonsterile in probable cases) with associated hypotension and 2 or more of the following: fever; renal impairment; thrombocytopenia; disseminated intravascular coagulation; serum transaminase or bilirubin elevation; acute respiratory distress syndrome; a generalized erythematous macular rash; or soft-tissue necrosis (necrotizing fasciitis). Mortality is high: 35% to 50%; rapid diagnosis and aggressive management including supportive care and early use of appropriate antibiotics are critical.

6) Necrotizing fasciitis: can be caused by multiple pathogens but the most common etiology is GAS. It is a rapidly progressive infection involving the deep fascia that destroys muscles, fat, and skin tissue. Patients often present with skin that is erythematous, edematous, and hot to the touch. The pain is described as out of proportion to what is expected by physical examination. Patients often have fever and chills, fatigue, vomiting, and diarrhea. Up to 50% of patients have associated STSS. In the USA the mortality rate is 25% to 30%.

7) APSGN: presents with hematuria, edema, and hypertension with or without oliguria. APSGN may occur following skin or throat infection with particular nephritogenic strains of GAS associated with specific *emm* types. Occurs an average of 10 days following pharyngitis or 3 weeks after skin infection. Although episodes are generally self-limiting, acute complications including hypertensive encephalopathy and heart failure have been reported. Moreover, recurrent episodes of APSGN may contribute to the burden of chronic renal failure in populations where GAS infection is highly prevalent.

8) ARF and RHD: ARF occurs an average of 2 to 3 weeks following an acute GAS infection (predominantly pharyngitis but also impetigo) and presents with carditis, arthritis, Sydenham's chorea, and/or, rarely, skin changes (erythema marginatum, subcutaneous nodules). RHD results from cumulative valvular damage following recurrent episodes of ARF with significant associated morbidity and mortality due to sequelae such as complications of pregnancy, heart failure, and stroke.

2. Risk groups—Patients with physical skin breakdown (e.g., burns, wounds, primary varicella infection), eczema, chronic limb edema, and those with scabies infestation are highly susceptible to streptococcal infections of the affected area. Social deprivation, household overcrowding, homelessness, intravenous drug use, and alcohol abuse are all associated with an increased risk of GAS disease. Persons with acute influenza infection, primary varicella zoster infection, chronic underlying medical conditions (e.g., diabetes, heart disease, malignancy, human immunodeficiency virus [HIV]), children younger than 2 years, peripartum women, and patients older than 65 years are all at increased risk for invasive GAS infections.

Household contacts of patients with invasive GAS infection are also at increased risk of invasive infection (incidence risk ratio of $\leq$ 2,000 times the background population incidence in the 30 days following first exposure to the index case). Most secondary invasive GAS cases in household contacts occur within the first week of exposure.

Susceptibility to streptococcal pharyngitis/tonsillitis and scarlet fever is general, although many people develop either antitoxin or type-specific antibacterial immunity, or both, through unapparent infection. Antibacterial immunity develops against the specific *emm* type of GAS that induced infection, although the development of antibodies is inconsistent and may not be completely protective against future infection.[1] Repeated attacks of pharyngitis/tonsillitis or other disease due to different types of streptococci are not uncommon. However, when a child or adolescent experiences multiple episodes of culture-positive or rapid test–positive acute pharyngitis within a period of months to years, this person is most likely a pharyngeal carrier of GAS who is actually experiencing viral pharyngitis.

Patients who have had 1 attack of rheumatic fever have a significant risk of recurrence of rheumatic fever following GAS infections, often with further cardiac damage.

3. Causative agents—*Streptococcus pyogenes*—or GAS—is a Gram-positive β-hemolytic bacterium. While the critical virulence factor, the M protein, generates type-specific immunity, distinct GAS serotypes are generally identified through sequence typing the 5, end of the *emm* gene (the hypervariable region of the gene encoding the M protein). More than 240 distinct *emm* types that vary by geographic and time distributions have been recognized. Skin infections caused by GAS usually differ in *emm* type from

GAS associated with throat infections. A relatively small number of *emm* types are known to cause the majority of GAS infections in the industrialized world, whereas a much greater range of *emm* types cause disease in developing countries. In STSS, superantigen exotoxins are produced that directly stimulate a large proportion of circulating T cells, leading to massive cytokine release. The most commonly implicated of these toxins is pyrogenic exotoxin A, which is produced by 80% of GAS strains causing STSS.

4. Diagnosis—Either clinical for skin infections or based on the isolation of the organism from affected tissues (e.g., blood, sterile sites, wound and throat swabs) using blood agar or other appropriate media. Colony morphology and the production of clear β-hemolysis on blood agar identify streptococci on cultures; inhibition by special antibiotic discs containing bacitracin (0.02–0.04 units) constitutes tentative identification. Automated platforms including matrix-assisted laser desorption ionization time-of-flight mass spectrometry and rapid molecular technologies, where available, are readily able to identify GAS isolates. Antigen detection tests allow rapid point-of-care identification (most often used in GAS pharyngitis). Point-of-care polymerase chain reaction kits are emerging for rapid diagnosis of GAS pharyngitis. Serologic testing has utility in establishing a diagnosis of ARF or APSGN where elevated serum antibody titers (antistreptolysin O and anti–DNase B) confirm a recent GAS infection; however, high titers may persist for months to years. For APSGN, low serum complement (particularly C3) levels are helpful in establishing a diagnosis. For ARF, electrocardiogram and echocardiography should be performed in suspected cases to diagnose carditis.

For epidemiologic surveillance, specific serotyping based on the M protein has largely been replaced by *emm* sequence typing. Classification into 48 *emm* clusters sharing similar properties has been proposed.

In many industrialized countries, current recommended practice for diagnosis of GAS pharyngitis is to first do a rapid antigen-detection test (high specificity but low sensitivity) or a throat culture; if this is positive, assume the patient has a GAS infection. If the result of a rapid test used in a child or adolescent is negative or equivocal, a throat culture should be done to guide management and prevent superfluous use of antibiotics.

In developing countries, where ARF incidence may be high and laboratory or rapid antigen diagnosis not possible or practical, clinical algorithms or a treat-all approach are used for managing sore throats.

CDC guidance for laboratories is available at: https://www.cdc.gov/groupastrep/lab.html.

5. Occurrence—Streptococcal (GAS) pharyngitis/tonsillitis is common in temperate zones and semitropical areas; it is less frequently recognized in tropical climates. In temperate zones, streptococcal pharyngitis is unusual in those younger than 3 years, peaks in children aged 5 to 15 years, and declines thereafter.

GAS pharyngitis occurs year-round but peaks in late winter and spring.

The highest incidence of streptococcal impetigo occurs in young children (< 5 years) in the latter part of the hot season in tropical climates. An estimated 162 million children in low- and low- to middle-income countries are affected by impetigo at any one time. Geographic and seasonal distribution of erysipelas is similar to that of streptococcal sore throat; erysipelas is most common in infants and those older than 20 years. Occurrence is sporadic, even during epidemics of streptococcal infection. Cellulitis is common in childhood and increases in incidence with increasing age in adulthood. It is estimated that 2 million patients are admitted to the hospital annually in the USA for treatment of cellulitis.

The incidence of scarlet fever declined dramatically in industrialized countries over the course of the 20th century, although recent increase in disease incidence has been reported in the UK and throughout Asia. Similar to GAS pharyngitis, scarlet fever predominantly affects children and follows a similar seasonal pattern.

In industrialized countries, morbidity and mortality due to puerperal fever have declined, although outbreaks may still occur in institutions often related to GAS-colonized health care staff and breaches in infection control practices. In the USA annual incidence is 6 per 100,000 live births but the disease continues at high rates in many developing countries. Worldwide, an estimated 75,000 maternal deaths are caused by puerperal sepsis annually.

In the USA, of the estimated 11,000 to 13,300 annual invasive GAS infections, 1,250 to 1,600 patients die. Active surveillance in the USA and UK has suggested a recent increase in cases of invasive GAS as has been observed in other countries including the UK and Australia. Globally, the incidence of invasive GAS infections ranges from 2.5 to 46 cases per 100,000 population, with the highest reported rates in indigenous populations of the USA and Australia and in low- and middle-income countries, including Kenya and Fiji. It is estimated that 663,000 new cases and 163,000 deaths related to invasive GAS occur annually worldwide. The incidence of invasive GAS infections follows a seasonal pattern similar to that of noninvasive infections in temperate climates with peaks in winter and early spring. Certain *emm* sequence types (1, 3, 12, 28, and 89) account for the majority of invasive GAS cases in the USA, whereas in resource-poor settings a wider variety of *emm* types are implicated.

Outbreaks of APSGN secondary to GAS skin infection and pharyngitis are well recognized; elsewhere cases occur sporadically. A range of nephritogenic *emm* types have been identified in various outbreaks (types 1, 2, 4, 12, 47, 49, and 55). Overall incidence has declined in industrialized countries but recent large outbreaks have been described in indigenous populations in Australia and a significant burden of disease in developing nations persists.

RHD remains a major cause of cardiovascular disease in the developing world and in indigenous populations in developed countries. It is estimated that 33.4 million people worldwide have RHD, with the highest age-related prevalence seen in Oceania, central sub-Saharan Africa, and South Asia (> 1%). Many reported cases have followed infections by specific GAS *emm* types (3, 5, 6, and 18, particularly among highly mucoid strains of *emm* type 18). The highest incidence, during late winter and spring, corresponds to that of pharyngitis. ARF has virtually disappeared from industrialized countries; however, it persists in some marginalized populations therein. Among indigenous populations in Australia and the Pacific, high rates of impetigo accompanied by a great diversity of skin-associated strains and low rates of GAS pharyngitis suggest that ARF can also occur as a complication of impetigo.

6. Reservoirs—Humans.

7. Incubation period—Short, usually 1 to 3 days, for pharyngitis; estimated 7 to 10 days for impetigo.

8. Transmission—GAS is a human-only pathogen. Transmission is through large respiratory droplets or direct contact with patients or carriers; extremely rarely through indirect contact with contaminated objects. Individuals with acute upper respiratory tract (especially nasal) infections are particularly likely to transmit infection. Casual contact rarely leads to infection. In populations where impetigo is prevalent, GAS may be recovered from normal skin for 1 to 2 weeks before skin lesions develop; the same strain may appear in the throat (without clinical evidence of throat infection), usually late in the course of the skin infection.

Anal, vaginal, skin, and pharyngeal carriers have been responsible for nosocomial outbreaks of serious streptococcal infection, particularly following surgical procedures.

Explosive outbreaks of streptococcal sore throat following ingestion of contaminated food occur rarely. Milk and milk products have been associated most frequently with foodborne outbreaks; egg salad and similar preparations have been implicated.

Transmissibility of GAS pharyngitis generally ends within 24 hours of beginning appropriate antibiotic treatment. Patients with untreated streptococcal pharyngitis may carry the organism for weeks or months, usually in decreasing numbers; contagiousness of these patients decreases sharply in 2 to 3 weeks after onset of infection. In untreated, uncomplicated impetigo, the period of communicability extends to 10 to 21 days; in untreated conditions with purulent discharge, it lasts weeks or months.

9. Treatment—

Drug	• Penicillin (penicillin V or benzylpenicillin) • TMP/SMX
Dose	• Pharyngitis: penicillin V 500 mg PO BID (children: 15 mg/kg, ≤ 500 mg) • Cellulitis: penicillin V 500 mg PO QID (children: 12.5 mg/kg, ≤ 500 mg) • Extensive impetigo: TMP/SMX 160 + 800 mg PO BID (children: 4 + 20 mg/kg, ≤ 160 + 800 mg) • Invasive disease, necrotizing fasciitis, STSS: benzylpenicillin 1.8 g IV 4 hourly (child 50 mg/kg ≤ 1.8 g) AND clindamycin 600 mg IV TID (children: 15 mg/kg, ≤ 600 mg)
Route	• Pharyngitis: penicillin V PO • Cellulitis: penicillin V PO • Impetigo: TMP/SMX PO • Invasive disease, necrotizing fasciitis, STSS: benzylpenicillin IV
Alternative drug	• Pharyngitis: cephalexin 500 mg PO BID for 10 days OR clindamycin 300 mg PO TID for 10 days • Cellulitis: cephalexin 500 mg PO QID OR TMP/SMX 160 + 800 mg PO QID • Extensive impetigo: benzathine penicillin 1.2 MU IM (> 20 kg) and 0.6 MU IM (< 20 kg) once. • Invasive disease, necrotizing fasciitis, STSS: vancomycin IV (dose based on body weight and renal function) PLUS clindamycin 600–900 mg IV every 8 hours (children: 10–15 mg/kg)
Duration	• Pharyngitis: 10 days • Skin infection: 3–5 days • Invasive GAS: variable
Special considerations and comments	• Impetigo: for localized disease in low-burden settings, apply mupirocin ointment 2% topically to crusted area TID for 5 days. • Invasive GAS/necrotizing fasciitis: add clindamycin 600 mg TID (children: 15 mg/kg, ≤ 600 mg); early surgery to remove infected tissue/drain abscesses is key. • STSS: add clindamycin 600 mg TID (children: 15 mg/kg, ≤ 600 mg) IVIG 2 g/kg as a single dose

Note: BID = twice daily; GAS = group A streptococci; IM = intramuscular(ly); IV = intravenous(ly); IVIG = intravenous immunoglobulin; MU = million units; PO = oral(ly); QID = 4 times daily; STSS = streptococcal toxic shock syndrome; TID = thrice daily; TMP/SMX = trimethoprim-sulfamethoxazole.

1) Streptococcal pharyngitis:

Preferred therapy	• Penicillin VK 500 mg (> 27 kg) and 250 mg (< 27 kg) PO BID for 10 days • Benzathine penicillin G 1.2 MU IM (> 20 kg) and 0.6 MU IM (< 20 kg) once • Amoxicillin 500 mg PO BID for 10 days (children: 25 mg/kg)
Alternative therapy options	• Cephalexin 500 mg PO BID for 10 days (children: 25 mg/kg) • Clindamycin 300 mg PO TID for 10 days (children: 7 mg/kg) • Clarithromycin 250 mg PO BID for 10 days (children: 7.5 mg/kg) • Azithromycin 500 mg PO on day 1, THEN 250 mg PO daily on days 2-5 (children: 12 mg/kg PO daily for 5 days) • Cephalexin 25–50 mg/kg/day PO in 2 divided doses for 10 days • Cefdinir 7 mg/kg/dose BID for 5–10 days • Cefpodoxime 5 mg/kg/dose every 12 hours for 5–10 days (≤ 100 mg/dose) • Clindamycin 7 mg/kg/dose PO TID for 10 days • Clarithromycin 7.5 mg/kg/dose PO BID for 10 days (≤ 250 mg/dose) • Azithromycin 12 mg/kg/dose PO once daily for 5 days (≤ 500 mg/dose)
Special considerations and comments	• GAS isolates are universally susceptible to penicillin. • While antibiotics may shorten clinical illness somewhat, it is also recognized that patients with streptococcal pharyngitis improve in 3–4 days without antibiotics. Appropriate antibiotic use reduces the frequency of suppurative complications, prevents the development of most cases of acute rheumatic fever, prevents further spread of the organism in the community, and may reduce the risk of acute glomerulonephritis after pharyngeal and skin infection. • Resistance to macrolides is common in some countries; use local data on macrolide resistance rates to guide treatment. • For acute poststreptococcal glomerulonephritis, a course of penicillin should be given (see earlier in the table) if throat or skin infection is present. Management is otherwise largely supportive and directed at managing hypertension, edema, and renal failure.

Note: BID = twice daily; GAS = group A streptococci; IM = intramuscular(ly); MU = million units; PO = oral(ly); TID = thrice daily.

2) GAS skin infection:

Preferred therapy	Cellulitis: • Penicillin VK 500 mg PO QID for 5 days (children: 12.5 mg/kg) • Penicillin G 1 MU IV every 4–6 hours for 5 days (children: 50,000 units/kg) • Cephalexin 500 mg PO QID daily for 5 days (children: 12.5–25 mg/kg) Cefazolin 1–2 g IV every 8 hours for 5 days (children: 25–50 mg/kg)
	Extensive impetigo: • TMP/SMX 160 + 800 mg PO BID for 3 days (children: 4 + 20 mg/kg) • Benzathine penicillin 1.2 MU (≥ 20 kg) and 0.6 MU (< 20 kg) IM onc
Alternative therapy options	• Clindamycin 300 mg PO QID for 5 days • Clindamycin 600 mg IV TID for 5 days • Vancomycin IV (dose based on body weight and renal function) for 5 days
Special considerations and comments	• Most patients with uncomplicated cellulitis can be treated as outpatients with oral antibiotics. Elevation of the effected limb can hasten resolution. Treatment of any underlying skin condition or skin breakdown is important in preventing recurrence. • For impetigo, topical antibiotics including mupirocin ointment 2% TID for 5 days and retapamulin ointment 1% BID for 5 days are recommended for limited disease in nonendemic settings. • In endemic settings, a single dose intramuscular benzathine or oral amoxicillin can be used where GAS infection is confirmed or strongly suspected (based on local epidemiology). • TMP-SMX is recommended in the Sanford guidelines for impetigo and as an alternative for cellulitis, with reports of in vitro resistance most likely related to laboratory methods. There is now extensive in vitro data to support use of TMP-SMX in GAS infection.[2–5]

Note: GAS = group A streptococci; IM = intramuscular(ly); IV = intravenous(ly); MU = million units; PO = oral(ly); QID = 4 times daily; TMP/SMX = trimethoprim-sulfamethoxazole.

3) GAS invasive infection and necrotizing fasciitis:

Preferred therapy	• Penicillin G 4 MU IV every 4 hours PLUS • Clindamycin 600–900 mg IV every 8 hours
Alternative therapy options	• Vancomycin IV (dose based on body weight and renal function) PLUS • Clindamycin 600–900 mg IV TID (children: 10–15 mg/kg)

(Continued)

(Continued)

Special considerations and comments	• Treatment of necrotizing fasciitis involves prompt and extensive surgical debridement of devitalized tissue in combination with IV antibiotics—broad-spectrum empirical therapy (including cover for Gram-negative and anaerobic organisms) is recommended pending culture results. Combined penicillin and clindamycin is used for directed therapy once GAS is confirmed.
	• Treatment of invasive infections overall depends on the site of infection and clinical progress—surgery to remove infected tissue (e.g., drainage of a septic joint, drainage of empyema, debridement of necrotic tissue) in combination with appropriate antibiotic therapy is critical.
	• Clindamycin suppresses the synthesis of bacterial toxins, has a long-lasting effect, and is effective regardless of the inoculum size or stage of growth of GAS.
	• If clindamycin cannot be used, may consider use of linezolid for suppression of bacterial toxins in place of clindamycin.
	• IVIG should be initiated early where available in cases of streptococcal toxic shock. Adjuvant IVIG should also be considered in necrotizing fasciitis and severe cases of invasive GAS disease.
	• Antibiotic therapy should be continued until further debridement is no longer needed, patient has clinically improved, and fever has been absent for at least 48–72 hours.

Note: GAS = group A streptococci; IV = intravenous(ly); IVIG = intravenous immunoglobulin; MU = million units.

4) Treat associated STSS if present. Treatment of STSS includes intravenous antibiotics and hemodynamic support with fluids and inotropes. Directed therapy with a combination of penicillin and clindamycin is recommended. Adjuvant intravenous immunoglobulin should be considered early in the course of illness where available. Supportive care often includes aggressive fluid resuscitation, inotropic support, and, in some patients, renal replacement therapy and/or ventilatory support.

5) Acute rheumatic fever:

Preferred therapy	• Benzathine penicillin 1.2 MU (≥ 20 kg) and 0.6 MU (< 20 kg) IM initially, THEN ongoing secondary prophylaxis 3–4 times weekly.
	• Penicillin VK 250 mg (< 12 years) and 500 mg (≥ 12 years) PO BID for 10 days initially.

(Continued)

(Continued)

Alternative therapy options	Adults:
	• Cephalexin 500 mg PO BID for 10 days • Azithromycin 500 mg PO on day 1, THEN 250 mg PO daily on days 2–5
	Children:
	• Cephalexin 50 mg/kg/day PO in 2–4 divided doses for 10 days • Azithromycin 10 mg/kg PO ($\leq$ 500 mg) on day 1, THEN 5 mg/kg PO daily on days 2–5 ($\leq$ 250 mg)
Special considerations and comments	• The initial therapy of IM benzathine penicillin G or antibiotic for 10 days is to eradicate any GAS persisting in the respiratory tract. • Arthritis can be managed using NSAIDs or aspirin. • Chorea may require steroids or antiepileptic agents. • Heart failure requires urgent management with diuretics and other cardiac medications. • Resistance to macrolides is common in some countries; use local data on macrolide resistance rates to guide treatment. • Secondary prevention is important to prevent streptococcal reinfection and possible recurrence of rheumatic fever among patients with acute rheumatic fever. Administer benzathine penicillin G 1.2 MU IM every 3–4 weeks OR Penicillin VK 250 mg PO BID for $\geq$ 10 years after the most recent episode (or $\leq$ 21 years old). A longer duration is recommended for those with moderate rheumatic heart disease ($\leq$ 35 years old) and for those with severe valve disease or after valve surgery. Lifelong prophylaxis is recommended. Those who do not tolerate penicillin may be given azithromycin (250 mg PO once daily) if necessary.

Note: BID = twice daily; GAS = group A streptococci; IM = intramuscular(ly); MU = million units; NSAID = nonsteroidal anti-inflammatory drug; PO = oral(ly); TID = thrice daily.

10. Prevention—

1) Contact and droplet precautions for patients hospitalized with GAS disease (may be terminated after 24 hours of effective antibiotic therapy).

2) Alert household contacts of patients with invasive GAS regarding the risk of secondary cases; consider antibiotic prophylaxis (see later).

3) Primary prevention of ARF through treatment of symptomatic GAS pharyngitis targeting high-risk individuals (children aged 5–15 years) in endemic settings may limit the incidence of disease.

4) Primordial prevention strategies such as improving housing conditions, reducing overcrowding, and improving access to water and sanitation have the potential to reduce the incidence of all manifestations of GAS infection in low-resource settings.

5) Vaccination: several vaccine candidates are under active investigation but currently no licensed GAS vaccine is available for clinical use (see Special Considerations under Group A Streptococcal Infections in this chapter).

6) Management of contacts and the immediate environment: in cases of invasive GAS, timely education of household or contacts to ensure a heightened awareness of the risk of secondary cases is required and antibiotic prophylaxis should be considered. A warn-and-inform strategy is a pragmatic approach. This includes systematically advising household contacts of their increased risk of becoming unwell with a GAS infection and to seek medical care in case of suggestive symptoms. National recommendations concerning antibiotic prophylaxis for household contacts of patients with invasive GAS vary; the attack rate in household contacts of index invasive GAS cases is comparable to that of meningococcal disease (where prophylaxis is commonly recommended); however, data demonstrating the efficacy of chemoprophylaxis in preventing secondary cases of invasive GAS are lacking. Considering the increased risk in contacts and the relatively brief time period between exposure and disease in secondary cases, either administering antibiotic prophylaxis to all household contacts or targeting high-risk contacts (e.g., mother-baby pairs or elderly couples > 65 years) are reasonable approaches. The optimal prophylactic antibiotic regimen is unclear; options include azithromycin for 3–5 days, cephalexin for 10 days, or clindamycin for 10 days.

In APSGN outbreaks the administration of intramuscular benzathine penicillin G to household contacts of confirmed cases is an effective control strategy.

11. **Special considerations—**

1) Reporting: obligatory report of epidemics in some countries. ARF, APSGN, and/or STSS or other invasive GAS infections are also reportable in some localities.

2) In settings with endemic scabies, mass drug administration for scabies using ivermectin or permethrin can reduce the prevalence of GAS skin disease and potentially the burden of sequelae including APSGN.

3) GAS vaccine: at the time of writing, several vaccine candidates are at varying stages of investigation and development, including some phase I and phase II trials. Candidates include multivalent M-protein vaccines, vaccines containing antigens from conserved portions of the M protein, and some containing other non–M-protein antigens.

4) Useful publications are available at: https://www.cdc.gov/group-astrep/publications.html#prevention-guidelines.

5) WHO Collaborating Centers provide support as required. Further information can be found at: http://www.who.int/collaborating-centres/database/en.

II. GROUP B STREPTOCOCCAL SEPSIS OF THE NEWBORN

1. Clinical features—Human subtypes of GBS (*Streptococcus agalactiae*) remain a major cause of neonatal death and morbidity globally owing to neonatal invasive disease. GBS can also cause neonatal encephalopathy, preterm delivery, stillbirth, and maternal disease, including chorioamnionitis and occasionally puerperal sepsis.

1) Neonatal invasive GBS disease: GBS can produce invasive disease in the newborn in 2 distinct forms. Early onset GBS (EOGBS) disease (0–6 days old) is acquired just prior to or during delivery and presents with sepsis, pneumonia, occasionally meningitis, and, less frequently, osteomyelitis or septic arthritis. Signs of infection are almost always apparent within the first 24 hours of birth and rapid clinical deterioration is characteristic. Late onset GBS (LOGBS) disease (7–89 days old) is acquired either from the mother or from environmental sources (rarely nosocomially) and presents as sepsis and/or meningitis in about 40% of cases. Advances in neonatal care have led to a fall in the case-fatality rate in the USA from 50% to 4%. Globally the case-fatality rate is estimated between 8% and 10%. Neurodevelopmental sequelae are present in 20% of survivors of GBS meningitis.

2) Maternal disease: GBS is an important pathogen in peripartum sepsis, presenting predominantly during or just after labor. Manifestations include chorioamnionitis, pyelonephritis, and invasive disease including bacteremia, puerperal sepsis, and meningitis. Case-fatality rate of invasive maternal GBS disease in developed settings is less than 0.3%. Maternal GBS disease is associated with a significantly increased risk of preterm birth, stillbirth, and EOGBS disease.

2. Risk groups—The main risk factor for EOGBS disease is maternal GBS colonization.

Prematurity and low birth weight, prolonged rupture of membranes for longer than 18 hours prior to delivery, and maternal fever are additional risk factors for EOGBS disease. A history of GBS disease in an older sibling increases the risk of GBS disease in a newborn (see Prevention under Group

B Streptococcal Sepsis of the Newborn in this chapter). Infants born to HIV-positive mothers have an increased risk of LOGBS disease.

3. Causative agents—*S. agalactiae* is a Gram-positive organism that produces β-hemolysis on blood agar and expresses Lancefield group B antigens.

4. Diagnosis—For neonatal GBS disease and maternal infection, diagnosis is based on culture and isolation of GBS from blood, cerebrospinal fluid, or other normally sterile bodily fluid. Maternal screening (see Prevention under Group B Streptococcal Sepsis of the Newborn in this chapter) is recommended at 35 to 37 weeks' gestation by culture from rectovaginal swabs utilizing a selective enrichment broth. Further guidance on sample processing for screening is available at: https://www.cdc.gov/groupbstrep/lab/index.html.

5. Occurrence—Globally, an estimated 18% of pregnant women are colonized with GBS in the lower genital tract and/or the gastrointestinal tract. There is considerable variability between regions with prevalence of colonization. Around 50% of colonized women will transmit the organism to their offspring, of whom 1% to 2% will develop symptomatic EOGBS disease (in the absence of antibiotic prophylaxis; see Prevention under Group B Streptococcal Sepsis of the Newborn in this chapter).

1) Neonatal invasive GBS disease: global incidence is estimated at 0.5 cases per 1,000 live births overall; EOGBS 0.41 and LOGBS 0.26 cases per 1,000 live births. Incidence varies by setting and generally burden of disease is highest in low- and middle-income countries. Incidence of EOGBS disease in the USA has fallen from 1.7 to 0.21 cases per 1,000 live births since the introduction of intrapartum antibiotic prophylaxis and subsequently universal GBS screening (see Prevention under Group B Streptococcal Sepsis of the Newborn in this chapter). Incidence of late onset disease in the USA has remained unchanged during the same time period. Globally an estimated 205,000 cases of EOGBS disease and 114,000 cases of LOGBS disease occur annually, resulting in 90,000 neonatal deaths.

2) Stillbirth and preterm delivery: it is estimated that globally 57,000 stillbirths and up to 3.5 million preterm births are caused by GBS infection annually.

3) Maternal GBS disease: invasive GBS disease is estimated to occur in 0.23 per 1,000 births from data limited to developed settings. An estimated 33,000 cases of invasive maternal GBS infection occur annually worldwide.

6. Reservoirs—Humans; commonly found in the gastrointestinal and female reproductive tracts and in the urinary tract in cases of heavy colonization.

7. Incubation period—From 1 to 6 days after birth (early onset disease).

8. Transmission—Early onset disease is transmitted to infants by ascending infection to the amniotic fluid during or just prior to labor. The mechanism of GBS transmission to infants with late onset disease is not fully understood but the source of colonization is most commonly the infant's mother, either through colonization at birth or from horizontal transmission after birth; breast milk has been implicated in some case reports. In rare nosocomial outbreaks of late onset disease transmission via the hands of health care workers is thought to have been the mode of spread.

9. Treatment—

Drug	Benzylpenicillin
Dose	<ul><li>Neonates 0–7 days: 60 mg/kg BID</li><li>Neonates 8–28 days: 60 mg/kg QID</li><li>Infants, children, and adults > 1 month: 60 mg/kg ($\leq$ 2.4 g) 4–6 hourly (meningitis dose)</li></ul>
Route	IV
Alternative drug	Penicillin-allergic patients:<ul><li>Vancomycin (dose based on body weight and renal function)</li></ul>OR<ul><li>Clindamycin 600 mg IV TID for adults (if confirmed susceptibility)</li></ul>
Duration	<ul><li>Uncomplicated bacteremia: 10 days</li><li>Neonatal meningitis: 2–3 weeks</li></ul>
Special considerations and comments	Initial empiric treatment of neonatal sepsis should include an agent with activity against Gram-negative bacteria (e.g., gentamicin).

Note: BID = twice daily; IV = intravenously; QID = 4 times daily.

Invasive Neonatal Group B Streptococci (GBS) Diseases

Preferred therapy	<ul><li>Meningitis (2–3 weeks): penicillin G 450,000 units/kg/day IV in 3–4 divided doses</li></ul>PLUS<ul><li>Bacteremia (10 days) and soft tissue or other infections: penicillin G 200,000–400,000 units/kg/day in 2 divided doses</li></ul>
Alternative therapy options	<ul><li>Ampicillin 100 mg/kg IV QID</li></ul>

(Continued)

Invasive Neonatal Group B Streptococci (GBS) Diseases (Continued)

Special considerations and comments	<ul><li>Any infant with clinical signs of sepsis should have blood and cerebrospinal fluid sent for bacterial culture and empirical antibiotic therapy should be initiated immediately.</li><li>Well-appearing infants whose mothers have suspected chorioamnionitis should have blood sent for culture and CBC with antibiotics commenced empirically pending results.</li><li>Well-appearing term infants born to GBS-colonized mothers without a history of suspected chorioamnionitis do not require specific investigation or empiric antibiotics but should be observed for 48 hours for signs of sepsis.</li><li>In some instances, where available, the use of a neonatal early onset sepsis calculator can inform the use of empiric antibiotics term neonates (> 35 weeks) gestation.</li><li>Penicillin is the drug of choice for directed therapy for GBS. When used empirically to cover suspected neonatal sepsis, penicillin is often administered together with another agent (e.g., gentamicin) to provide Gram-negative cover for enterobacteriacaea, particularly *Escherichia coli*, pending culture results.</li><li>Nurse patients using standard infection control precautions; strict adherence to hand hygiene is important in preventing potential nosocomial transmission.</li><li>Neurodevelopmental follow-up is recommended for survivors of GBS meningitis, including assessment of hearing and vision.</li></ul>

Note: CBC = complete blood count; IV = intravenously.

Maternal/Adult Disease

Preferred therapy	<ul><li>Meningitis: penicillin G 4 MU IV every 4 hours for 14 days</li><li>Endocarditis: add gentamicin 1 mg/kg IV every 8 hours to penicillin G 4 MU IV every 4 hours, THEN discontinue gentamicin once infection is under control and continue penicillin for 4–6 weeks total.</li><li>Other infections: penicillin G 2 MU IV every 4 hours for 10–14 days</li></ul>
Alternative therapy options	<ul><li>Vancomycin IV (dose based on body weight and renal function)</li><li>Cefazolin 1–2 g IV TID</li><li>Clindamycin 600 mg IV every TID</li></ul>
Special considerations and comments	Penicillin is the drug of choice. Surgical intervention to drain any purulent collection is recommended in the case of puerperal sepsis.

Note: IV = intravenously; MU = million units; TID = thrice daily.

10. Prevention—Intrapartum antibiotic prophylaxis (IAP) is a well-established intervention to prevent EOGBS sepsis and much progress has been made in developing a maternal GBS vaccine in recent years. Two approaches have been used successfully:

1) Screening-based method: screen all pregnant women for vaginal and rectal GBS colonization at 35 to 37 weeks' gestation and offer women with colonization intrapartum antibiotics during labor. Women whose culture results are unknown at the time of delivery should be managed according to the risk-based method.

2) Risk-based method: identify candidates for intrapartum chemo-prophylaxis according to the presence of any of the following intrapartum risk factors for early onset disease:

   - Delivery at less than 37 weeks.
   - Intrapartum temperature greater than or equal to 38°C (100.4°F).
   - Rupture of membranes for 18 hours or longer.

3) In both cases, women with GBS bacteriuria during the current pregnancy or who previously gave birth to an infant with EOGBS disease are candidates for IAP.

4) Intravenous penicillin is the preferred agent for IAP. The preferred agent for penicillin-allergic patients is cefazolin (or clindamycin if history of immediate penicillin allergy and isolate susceptible).

5) Evidence from a large multicenter cohort study for a strong protective effect of the screening-based method relative to the risk-based strategy has led to the current recommendation in the USA, Australia, and many European countries for use of a screening-based approach. However, the cost-effectiveness of the screening-based approach has not been established and a larger proportion of women (up to 30%) receive antibiotics when using this strategy. In the UK, the Netherlands and Scandinavia, the risk-based method is the foundation of IAP policy.

6) CDC GBS prevention guidelines and further resources are available at: https://www.cdc.gov/groupbstrep/guidelines/index.html.

7) Maternal vaccination: at the time of writing there is no licensed vaccine available; however, a number of capsular polysaccharide-protein conjugate vaccine candidates (and 1 based on conserved GBS surface proteins) are currently progressing through phase I, phase II, and proof-of-concept trials. It is estimated that a vaccine with 90% efficacy and 80% coverage globally could prevent 107,000 stillbirths and infant deaths annually.

11. Special considerations—

1) Nosocomial outbreaks have been reported sporadically in the nursery setting. Any unusual cluster of GBS cases in a neonatal unit should prompt an epidemiologic investigation and a review of local infection control practices. Strains implicated in a suspected outbreak can be examined using pulsed-field gel electrophoresis or sequencing to determine relatedness.

2) Useful publications are available at: https://www.cdc.gov/groupbstrep/references.html.

3) A special issue of *Clinical Infectious Diseases* from 2017 summarizing the global burden of GBS disease is available at: https://academic.oup.com/cid/issue/65/suppl_2?browseBy=volume.

4) Useful guidelines can be found at:

- Neonatal sepsis: https://pediatrics.aappublications.org/content/142/6/e20182894
- Infants at risk of GBS disease: https://pediatrics.aappublications.org/content/early/2019/07/04/peds.2019-1881
- Early onset GBS disease: https://www.acog.org/Clinical-Guidance-and-Publications/Committee-Opinions/Committee-on-Obstetric-Practice/Prevention-of-Group-B-Streptococcal-Early-Onset-Disease-in-Newborns

References

1. Campbell PT, Tong SYC, Geard N, et al. Longitudinal analysis of group A *Streptococcus emm* types and emm clusters in a high-prevalence setting: relationship between past and future infections. *J Infect Dis.* 2020;221(9):1429–1437.

2. Bowen AC, Tong SYC, Andrews RM, et al. Short-course oral co-trimoxazole versus intramuscular benzathine benzylpenicillin for impetigo in a highly endemic region: an open-label, randomised, controlled, non-inferiority trial. *Lancet.* 2014;384(9960):2132–2140.

3. Miller LG, Daum RS, Creech CB, et al. Clindamycin versus trimethoprim-sulfamethoxazole for uncomplicated skin infections. *N Engl J Med.* 2015;372:1093–1103.

4. Ralph AP, Holt DC, Islam S, et al. Potential for molecular testing for group A *Streptococcus* to improve diagnosis and management in a high-risk population: a prospective study. *Open Forum Infect Dis.* 2019;6(4):ofz097.

5. Daum RS, Miller LG, Immergluck L, et al. A placebo-controlled trial of antibiotics for smaller skin abscesses. *N Engl J Med.* 2017;376(26):2545–2555.

[D. Yeoh, J. Carapetis, A. Bowen]

STRONGYLOIDIASIS

DISEASE	ICD-10 CODE
STRONGYLOIDIASIS	ICD-10 B78

1. Clinical features—Strongyloidiasis is often an asymptomatic helminthic infection of the gastrointestinal tract that can remain undetected for decades. The symptoms can include rash, diarrhea, and shortness of breath; it can also result in life-threatening disseminated disease usually in immunosuppressed patients, especially those who have been on corticosteroids. Clinical manifestations may include transient pruritic dermatitis when larvae of the parasite penetrate the skin on initial infection; cough, rales, and sometimes demonstrable pneumonitis when larvae pass through the lungs; or abdominal symptoms caused by adult worms in the intestinal mucosa.

Symptoms of chronic infection may be mild or severe, depending on the intensity of infection. Classic symptoms of chronic infection include abdominal pain (usually epigastric, often suggesting peptic ulcer disease), diarrhea, and urticaria; and sometimes also nausea, weight loss, vomiting, weakness, and constipation. A frequent complaint is nonspecific bloating. Intensely pruritic dermatitis (larva currens) radiating from the anus may occur, as can stationary wheals lasting 1 to 2 days. A migrating serpiginous rash may move several centimeters per hour across the trunk. Eosinophilia is usually moderate (10%–25%) in the chronic stage but may be normal or low with dissemination. Some individuals may have eosinophilia without other symptoms.

More severe symptoms are associated with hyperinfection syndrome and a concomitantly greater parasite burden. Intestinal autoinfection, when it becomes unregulated in the immunocompromised host, results in an increasing worm burden (hyperinfection), which may lead to disseminated strongyloidiasis with wasting, pulmonary involvement, and death (up to 80%). In these cases, secondary Gram-negative sepsis is common.

2. Risk groups—Immunosuppressed persons, including those with human T-cell lymphotropic virus 1, those with malnutrition, those on oral or intravenous steroids, and those receiving chemotherapy for malignancies as well as transplant patients, are at increased risk for disseminated or hyperinfection strongyloidiasis. Steroid courses lasting more than 5 days have been linked to hyperinfection and death.

3. Causative agents—*Strongyloides stercoralis* (major pathogen). *Strongyloides fuelleborni* occurs rarely in Africa and has not been reported to cause disseminated disease in humans.

4. Diagnosis—Strongyloidiasis is one of the most difficult parasitic diseases to diagnose. Eosinophilia is sometimes the only clue but it is mild (5%–15%) and nonspecific. Diagnosis involves identifying motile larvae in concentrated stool specimens of freshly passed feces, in duodenal aspirates, or occasionally in sputum. Sputum Gram stain has been shown to be helpful when hyperinfection syndrome is suspected. Stool samples are often insensitive because larvae are excreted intermittently but a clue to diagnosis may be the larval tracks that can be seen on blood agar. Serologic tests based on larval-stage antigens are positive in 80% to 85% of infected patients.

Patients with presenting symptoms as described earlier, immigrants from endemic areas, and those with unexplained eosinophilia (particularly those who are immunocompromised) are appropriate for strongyloidiasis testing.

5. Occurrence—Common in warm, wet regions such as tropical areas. The highest infection rates in the USA are in southeastern states, particularly in the more mountainous areas of Tennessee and Kentucky. Prevalence in endemic areas is not accurately known. *Strongyloides* may be prevalent in residents of institutions where personal hygiene is poor. The parasite is found frequently in the stools of previous prisoners of war even decades after imprisonment. Human infection with *S. fuelleborni* has been reported only in Africa and Papua New Guinea.

6. Reservoirs—Humans are the principal reservoir of *S. stercoralis*, with occasional transmission of dog and cat strains to humans. Nonhuman primates are the reservoir of *S. fuelleborni* in Africa.

7. Incubation period—From 2 to 4 weeks from penetration of the skin by larvae until rhabditiform larvae appear in the feces; the period until symptoms appear is indefinite and variable.

8. Transmission—Parthenogenetic female worms that are capable of reproducing without male worms inhabit the duodenum, where they lay eggs. In the intestine, eggs hatch into rhabditiform larvae; these larvae migrate into the intestinal lumen and ultimately leave the body with the feces. The free-living rhabditiform larvae may either directly molt into infective filariform larvae that are capable of repenetrating the skin of a suitable host or shift to a free-living cycle. In this latter indirect heterogonic cycle, following several molts, adult male and female worms are developed that mate and produce a generation of offspring whose filariform stage will have the ability to reenter parasitic life. A distinctive characteristic of *S. stercoralis* is that a small percentage of the rhabditiform larvae molt within the host's intestine into the filariform stage. These tissue-penetrating infective larvae may penetrate the colonic wall or the perianal skin; they complete an internal cycle, maturing into adult females in the small intestine. This process is known as autoinfection and is perhaps the phenomenon by which *S. stercoralis* can persist indefinitely in infected hosts. Person-to-person transmission may also occur; the period of communicability lasts as long as living worms remain in the intestine—up to 75 years in cases of continuous autoinfection.

9. Treatment—

Drug	Ivermectin
Dose	200 µg/kg daily for 2 days
Route	PO
Alternative drug	Albendazole 400 mg BID for 3–7 days
Special considerations and comments	• Acute and chronic strongyloidiasis: first-line therapy is ivermectin with eradication reaching as high as 97%. Thiabendazole is no longer available in the USA but is in use in many other countries. A newer drug, tribendimidine, remains under investigation in China and shows some promise in the treatment of strongyloidiasis. Optimal treatment for disseminated disease is uncertain given limited data. • Disease treatment can be monitored by trending eosinophilia and serologic titers.

Note: BID = twice daily; PO = oral(ly).

10. Prevention—

1) Dispose of human feces in a safe manner.
2) Pay strict attention to hygienic habits, including use of footwear in endemic areas.
3) Rule out suspected strongyloidiasis through serologic or stool testing before initiating immunosuppressive treatment for any reason.
4) Examine and treat infected dogs, cats, and monkeys in contact with humans.
5) Reduce immunosuppression if concern for disseminated infection.
6) Avoid going barefoot in endemic areas; outhouses should be built far from where children are at play.

11. Special considerations—None.

[J. Berk, A. Siddiqui, S. Berk]

SYPHILIS
(lues)

DISEASE	ICD-10 CODE
SYPHILIS	ICD-10 A50–A52

1. Clinical features—Syphilis is a systemic treponemal infection characterized by progression through clinical stages and variable periods of latency. The primary stage is characterized by an indurated, painless ulcer known as a chancre. About 3 weeks after sexual contact, the primary chancre develops at the site of exposure. Chancres can appear anywhere on the skin or mucous membranes; although they commonly occur on the penis, vulva, mouth, or perianal skin, they might occur internally on the cervix or anus and go unnoticed. Firm, nonfluctuant, painless, regional lymphadenopathy frequently develops with the primary lesion. The chancre involutes in 4 to 6 weeks without treatment.

Within several weeks to months of the primary lesion, and occasionally at the same time as the primary lesion, a secondary skin eruption appears. Symmetric macular-to-papulosquamous skin lesions develop, classically occurring on the trunk, palms, and soles. Mucous patches (glistening, white-to-red patches) can be seen in the mouth or on other mucous membranes and condyloma lata (white, smooth papules or plaques) can be seen in the genital area. The secondary stage can be accompanied by fever, sore throat, malaise, and generalized lymphadenopathy. Secondary manifestations resolve without treatment in weeks to 12 months; all untreated cases will go on to latent infection. In the early years of latency, there might be recurrences of lesions of the skin and mucous membranes. Up to one-third of untreated patients will eventually exhibit signs and symptoms of tertiary syphilis (i.e., inflammatory or gummatous lesions of the cardiovascular system, skin, bone, or other tissue; or tabes dorsalis or general paresis).

Neurosyphilis must be considered in the differential diagnosis of individuals with central nervous system (CNS) symptoms and ocular or otologic complaints. In the primary and secondary stages, treponemal invasion of the CNS and abnormalities in the cerebrospinal fluid (CSF) are common. Patients are most often asymptomatic but some might develop acute syphilitic meningitis with cranial nerve palsies and deafness. CNS disease in the form of meningovascular syphilis can occur with early syphilis or can develop 5 to 12 years after initial infection; paresis or tabes dorsalis can develop 15 to 20 years after initial infection.

Most untreated patients do not go on to develop tertiary syphilis but remain in the latent period for the rest of their lives. Between 5 and 20 years after initial infection some untreated patients develop gummas of the skin, musculoskeletal system, or internal organs; syphilitic endarteritis with aortic and coronary artery disease; or CNS disease described earlier. The widespread use of antimicrobials has decreased the frequency of these tertiary manifestations.

Concurrent human immunodeficiency virus (HIV) infection might change the appearance and behavior of the primary and secondary mucocutaneous lesions and increase the risk of CNS disease in patients with syphilis.

A woman with untreated early (primary, secondary, or early latent) syphilis during pregnancy has a very high risk of transmitting the infection to her fetus. Congenital syphilis can cause stillbirth, prematurity, neonatal death, or a live-born infant with a spectrum of clinical manifestations of congenital syphilis. Although these infants often appear normal at birth, early manifestations of congenital syphilis appear by 2 months old and include failure to thrive, mucocutaneous abnormalities similar to those seen in secondary syphilis, organomegaly, anemia, bony lesions, and CNS abnormalities. Congenital infection might also result in late manifestations that appear by 2 years old. These late manifestations include CNS abnormalities; interstitial keratitis; deafness; and bony or dental abnormalities, such as notched incisors, saddlenose deformities, or saber shins.

2. Risk groups—All people are considered susceptible to syphilis, though only approximately 30% of exposures result in infection. Patients treated for syphilis do not typically develop immunity and therefore remain susceptible to reinfection following treatment. Health care professionals have developed primary lesions on the hands following unprotected clinical examination of infectious lesions.

3. Causative agents—*Treponema pallidum* subsp. *pallidum*, a spirochete.

4. Diagnosis—A presumptive diagnosis of syphilis requires 2 serologic tests, as no direct detection methods are commercially available. Serologic testing usually begins with a nontreponemal test such as the rapid plasma reagin test. If that test is positive, a confirmatory treponemal serologic test, such as the *T. pallidum* particle agglutination test, is performed. When both tests are positive and the patient has never been treated for syphilis, the diagnosis is confirmed. For patients with a history of treatment for syphilis, the treponemal test usually remains positive after treatment. Reinfection is determined by a 4-fold increase in nontreponemal test titer compared with previous titers.

Some clinical laboratories may begin testing with a treponemal test, such as an enzyme immunoassay or a chemiluminescence immunoassay. Patients with a positive treponemal test should be tested with a nontreponemal test to guide management decisions. If the treponemal test is positive and nontreponemal test is negative, this combination of test results may indicate previous treatment for syphilis, untreated or incompletely treated syphilis, or a false-positive test result. In this scenario, persons with a history of previous treatment for syphilis require no further management unless sexual history suggests likelihood of reexposure. For persons without a history of treatment for syphilis and those with concern for recent exposure to syphilis, a second treponemal test should be done (preferably one based on different antigens than the original treponemal test); if positive (or no second test is available), the patient should be treated. Unless history or results of physical examination suggest a recent infection, previously untreated persons should be treated for late latent syphilis.

Patients in the early stage of disease with primary lesions may have negative serologic tests. Smears of lesion exudate can be examined for spirochetes using dark-field microscopy or polymerase chain reaction (PCR) or biopsy of the lesion can be performed for histology with immunofluorescent or other specific staining for spirochetes; however, these techniques may not be available in many laboratories. In cases where confirmatory tissue diagnosis is not available, patients should be treated based on clinical findings. Other infectious causes of genital ulcers should also be considered in the evaluation.

The diagnosis of congenital syphilis can be difficult as maternal and nontreponemal and treponemal immunoglobulin class G antibodies can be transferred through the placenta, complicating interpretation of positive serologic syphilis tests in neonates. Therefore, the diagnosis and decision to treat for congenital syphilis depend on (a) identification of syphilis in the mother; (b) adequacy of maternal treatment; (c) presence of clinical, laboratory, or radiographic evidence of syphilis in the infant; and (d) comparison of maternal (at delivery) and neonatal nontreponemal serologic titers. Infants should be screened by testing the mother's serum. This is because the infant's serum may be nonreactive if the mother's serologic test result is of low titer or if the mother was infected late in pregnancy. If maternal serum is not available, infant serum is preferred to cord blood. All infants born to women who have reactive serologic tests for syphilis should be examined thoroughly for evidence of congenital syphilis. Infants with physical findings consistent with congenital syphilis, a serum quantitative nontreponemal titer that is 4-fold higher than the mother's titer, or a positive dark-field microscopy or PCR of lesions or bodily fluid should be treated for congenital syphilis. In addition, because infected infants can be asymptomatic at birth, asymptomatic infants born to infected mothers who did not initiate adequate treatment at least 4 weeks prior to delivery should also be treated for congenital syphilis.

Patients with syphilis and neurologic abnormalities or evidence of treatment failure may have neurosyphilis and should have CSF testing performed.

5. Occurrence—Syphilis occurs worldwide and is usually more prevalent in urban areas. After a period of decline from the late 1970s to the late 1990s, incidence in developed countries has increased again in recent years, notably in Western Europe and the USA and in particular among men who have sex with men.

6. Reservoirs—Humans.

7. Incubation period—10 days to 3 months; usually 3 weeks.

8. Transmission—Transmission of syphilis occurs when a person comes into direct contact with the primary or secondary lesions of an infected person. These lesions contain infectious spirochetes. Exposure is almost always through sexual contact during oral, vaginal, or anal sex. Because primary lesions might occur internally and secondary lesions may go unnoticed or undiagnosed, transmission might occur without either partner being aware of the disease. Transmission can also occur through blood transfusion if the donor is in the early stages of disease.

Fetal infection is most likely to occur if the mother is in the primary, secondary, or early latent stage but it can occur throughout the latent period. Infants can have infectious mucocutaneous lesions.

9. Treatment—All patients with syphilis should be tested for other sexually transmitted infections (STIs), particularly HIV. Universal precautions should be used when coming into contact with blood, lesion exudates, or other bodily fluids from patients with syphilis. Ideally, all patients should receive parenteral long-acting penicillin. The form and dose of penicillin depend on the stage and clinical manifestations of syphilis in the particular patient. Primary, secondary, and early latent syphilis (those known to be infected < 1 year) are treated with 1 dose of intramuscular benzathine penicillin G; late latent syphilis or those with unknown duration of latency are treated with 3 doses. Patients with CNS disease at any stage require intravenous aqueous crystalline penicillin G or procaine penicillin plus probenecid for 2 weeks.

There are limited data on the effectiveness of nonpenicillin regimens for syphilis. In nonpregnant penicillin-allergic patients, regimens of doxycycline, tetracycline, or ceftriaxone can be tried with close follow-up. Pregnant penicillin-allergic patients should have their allergy verified with testing if possible; if true allergy exists, they should be desensitized and treated with penicillin.

Patients should abstain from sexual contact until their treatment is completed and lesions disappear. To avoid reinfection, patients should not have sex with previous partners until the partners have also been treated.

Treatment failures might occur with any regimen. In patients who develop new clinical signs and symptoms of syphilis or a sustained 4-fold increase in nontreponemal titers, reinfection or treatment failure should be suspected. These patients should be evaluated and retreated. Most patients have a 4-fold decline in nontreponemal titers 6 to 12 months after appropriate therapy. Patients who do not have this expected titer drop should be tested for HIV and evaluation for CNS disease with CSF testing should be considered; however, the ideal management of these patients is unclear. In HIV-infected patients, close follow-up with repeat serologic testing should be considered at 3, 6, 9, 12, and 24 months. Clinicians should examine the CSF of HIV-infected patients who do not respond appropriately to therapy.

Primary, Secondary, and Early Latent Syphilis

Preferred therapy	Adults:
	• Benzathine penicillin G 2.4 MU IM as a single dose
	Infants and children:
	• Benzathine penicillin G 50,000 units/kg IM (≤ 2.4 MU) as a single dose
Alternative therapy options	Nonpregnant adults[a]:
	• Doxycycline 100 mg PO BID for 14 days OR
	• Tetracycline 500 mg PO QID for 14 days OR
	• Ceftriaxone 1–2 g either IM or IV daily for 10–14 days
Special considerations and comments	Azithromycin therapy is not recommended as first-line therapy owing to concerns with resistance.

Note: BID = twice daily; IM = intramuscular(ly); IV = intravenous(ly); MU = million units; PO = oral(ly); QID = 4 times daily.

[a]No proven alternatives to penicillin are available for treatment of syphilis during pregnancy. Pregnant women who have a history of penicillin allergy should be desensitized and treated with penicillin.

Late Latent Syphilis or Latent Syphilis of Unknown Duration

Preferred therapy	Adults:
	• Benzathine penicillin G 7.2 MU total, administered as 3 doses of 2.4 MU IM each at 1-week intervals
	Infants and children:
	• Benzathine penicillin G 50,000 units/kg IM (≤ 2.4 MU) administered as 3 doses at 1-week intervals (total 150,000 units/kg; ≤7.2 MU)
Alternative therapy options	Nonpregnant adults[a]:
	• Doxycycline 100 mg PO BID for 28 days OR
	• Tetracycline 500 mg PO QID for 28 days

Note: BID = twice daily; IM = intramuscular(ly); MU = million units; PO = oral(ly); QID = 4 times daily.

[a]No proven alternatives to penicillin are available for treatment of syphilis during pregnancy. Pregnant women who have a history of penicillin allergy should be desensitized and treated with penicillin.

Tertiary Syphilis With Normal Cerebrospinal Fluid Examination

Preferred therapy	Benzathine penicillin G 7.2 MU total, administered as 3 doses of 2.4 MU IM each at 1-week intervals

Note: IM = intramuscular(ly); MU = million units.

Neurosyphilis and Ocular Syphilis

Preferred therapy	Aqueous crystalline penicillin G 18–24 MU/day, administered as 3–4 MU IV every 4 hours or continuous infusion, for 10–14 days.
Alternative therapy options	• Procaine penicillin G 2.4 MU IM once daily for 10–14 days PLUS • Probenecid 500 mg PO QID for 10–14 days[a]

Note: IM = intramuscular(ly); IV = intravenous(ly); MU = million units; PO = oral(ly); QID = 4 times daily.
[a]If regimen is selected, patient compliance must be ensured.

Congenital Syphilis

Preferred therapy	Infants < 30 days: • Aqueous crystalline penicillin G 100,000–150,000 units/kg/day, administered as 50,000 units/kg/dose IV every 12 hours during the first 7 days of life and every 8 hours thereafter for a total of 10 days OR • Procaine penicillin G 50,000 units/kg/dose IM as a single daily dose for 10 days
	Infants and children ≥ 1 month: • Aqueous crystalline penicillin G 200,000–300,000 units/kg/day IV, administered as 50,000 units/kg/dose every 4–6 hours for 10 days
Special considerations and comments	If > 1 day of antibiotic therapy is missed, it is recommended to restart the entire antibiotic therapy course.

Note: IM = intramuscular(ly); IV = intravenous(ly).

Interviewing patients to identify sexual contacts is a fundamental part of syphilis control. The patient's stage of disease determines which partners should be notified and tested:

1) For primary syphilis, all sexual contacts during the 3 months preceding onset of symptoms.
2) For secondary syphilis, all sexual contacts during the 6 months preceding onset of symptoms.
3) For early latent syphilis, those of the preceding year.

10. Prevention—

1) Patients and their partners must be encouraged to obtain HIV counseling and testing. All infants born to seroreactive mothers should be treated unless it is documented that the mother had adequate penicillin-based treatment at least 4 weeks prior to delivery.

2) Individuals can decrease their number of sex partners, establish mutually monogamous partnerships, and practice the correct and consistent use of condoms to decrease their risk of syphilis.

3) Health care providers should screen all patients with a confirmed or suspected STI, including HIV, for syphilis. High-risk groups according to local epidemiology, such as commercial sex workers and sexually active men who have sex with men, should be screened on a regular basis.

4) Pregnant women should be screened for syphilis at their first prenatal visit; in high-prevalence areas they should be screened again at 28 to 32 weeks' gestation and at delivery.

5) Culturally appropriate prevention interventions should be available at low or no cost, including condoms, community-level education on the prevention of STIs, and health care for early diagnosis and treatment.

6) Through health care providers or public health organizations, patients should be interviewed to identify partners and partners should be notified and treated.

11. Special considerations—

1) Reporting: case report of early infectious syphilis and congenital syphilis is required in most countries; laboratories must report reactive serology and positive dark-field examinations in many areas. Confidentiality of the individual must be ensured.

2) Epidemic measures: intensification of measures outlined under Prevention in this chapter. In protracted epidemics in selected populations (e.g., commercial sex workers) that remain refractory to standard interventions, mass treatment of the at-risk population might be considered.

3) International measures:

- Examine groups of adolescents and adults who emigrate from areas of high prevalence for treponemal infections.
- Adhere to international agreements concerning records, provision of diagnostic and treatment facilities, and contact interviews at seaports for foreign merchant seamen (e.g., Brussels Agreement).
- Provide for rapid international exchange of information about contacts.

4) WHO Collaborating Centres provide support as required. Further information can be found at: http://www.who.int/collaboratingcentres/database/en.

[K. Workowski]

TAPEWORM

DISEASE	ICD-10 CODE
DWARF TAPEWORM	ICD-10 B71.0
RAT TAPEWORM	ICD-10 B71.0
DOG TAPEWORM	ICD-10 B71.1
BROAD OR FISH TAPEWORM	ICD-10 B70.0
TAENIASIS	ICD-10 B68
TAENIA SOLIUM TAENIASIS, INTESTINAL FORM	ICD-10 B68.0
TAENIA SAGINATA TAENIASIS	ICD-10 B68.1
TAENIASIS, UNSPECIFIED	ICD-10 B68.9
CYSTICERCOSIS	ICD-10 B69
Echinococcosis (see "Echinococcosis")	

I. DWARF TAPEWORM (hymenolepiasis due to *Hymenolepis nana*)

1. Clinical features—An intestinal infection with very small tapeworms; usually an infection of children. Light infections are usually asymptomatic. Massive numbers of worms may cause enteritis with or without diarrhea, abdominal pain, and other nonspecific symptoms such as pallor, loss of weight, and weakness.

2. Risk groups—Children are more likely to be infected and susceptible to disease than adults; severe infection occurs in immunodeficient and malnourished children.

3. Causative agents—*Hymenolepis nana* (dwarf tapeworm), the only human tapeworm without an obligatory intermediate host.

4. Diagnosis—Identification of eggs in feces; may require examination of multiple stool samples.

5. Occurrence—Cosmopolitan; more common in warm than cold and in dry than wet climates. Dwarf tapeworm is the most common human tapeworm in children and has been reported in Australia, India, Latin America, Mediterranean countries, the Middle East, and the USA.

6. Reservoirs—Humans and rodents.

7. Incubation period—Onset of symptoms is variable; the development of mature worms requires about 3 weeks from ingestion of eggs.

8. Transmission—Eggs of *H. nana* are infective when passed in feces and both internal and external autoinfection are possible as well as person-to-person transmission. Infection is acquired through ingestion of eggs in contaminated food or water; directly from fecal-contaminated fingers; or through ingestion of insects such as mealworms, larval fleas, and beetles bearing larvae (cysticercoids) that have developed from eggs ingested by the insect. *H. nana* eggs, once ingested by humans, hatch in the intestine, liberating oncospheres that enter mucosal villi and develop into cysticercoids; these rupture into the lumen and grow into adult tapeworms. The infection is communicable for as long as eggs are passed in feces and may persist for years.

9. Treatment—

Drug	Praziquantel
Dose	25 mg/kg
Route	PO
Alternative drug	• Niclosamide: ○ Adults: 2 g/day as a single dose for 7 days ○ Children 11–34 kg: 1 g as a single dose on day 1, THEN 500 mg/day PO for 6 days ○ Children > 34 kg: 1.5 g as a single dose on day 1, THEN 1 g/day PO for 6 days OR • Nitazoxanide: ○ Adults: 500 mg PO BID for 3 days ○ Children 12–47 months: 100 mg PO BID for 3 days ○ Children 4–11 years: 200 mg PO BID for 3 days
Duration	Single dose
Special considerations and comments	• Niclosamide is not available in the USA. • Niclosamide must be given daily for 1 week.

Note: BID = twice daily; PO = oral(ly).

10. Prevention—

1) Educate the public in personal hygiene, especially handwashing and safe disposal of feces.
2) Provide and maintain clean toilet facilities.
3) Protect food and water from contamination with human and rodent feces.
4) Treat those infected to remove sources of infection.
5) Eliminate rodents from home environment.

11. Special considerations—Outbreaks in schools and institutions can best be controlled through treatment of infected persons and special attention to personal and group hygiene.

II. RAT TAPEWORM (hymenolepiasis due to *Hymenolepis diminuta*)

Infection with the rat tapeworm, *Hymenolepis diminuta*, occurs accidentally in humans, usually in young children. Eggs passed in rodent feces are ingested by insects such as flea larvae, grain beetles, and cockroaches, in which cysticercoids develop in the hemocoel. The mature tapeworm develops in rats, mice, or other rodents when the insect is ingested. People are rare accidental hosts, usually having a single or few tapeworms; human infections are rarely symptomatic. Definitive diagnosis is based on finding characteristic eggs in the feces and treatment is as for *H. nana*.

III. DOG TAPEWORM (dipylidiasis)

Toddler-aged children are occasionally infected with the dog tapeworm (*Dipylidium caninum*), a parasite of dogs and cats worldwide. Infected children are usually asymptomatic but parents may be alarmed by motile, seedlike proglottids (tapeworm segments) at the child's anus or on the surface of the stools. Infection is acquired when the child accidentally ingests adult fleas that, in their larval stage, have eaten eggs from proglottids. In 3 to 4 weeks the tapeworm becomes mature. Infection is prevented by keeping dogs and cats free of fleas and worms; treatment is as for *H. nana*.

IV. BROAD OR FISH TAPEWORM (diphyllobothriasis)

1. Clinical features—An intestinal tapeworm infection of long duration. Symptoms are commonly trivial or absent; some patients, however, develop vitamin B12 deficiency anemia (*Diphyllobothrium latum*, now renamed as *Dibothriocephalus latus*). Massive infections may be associated with diarrhea, obstruction of the bile duct or intestine, and toxic symptoms.

2. Risk groups—Those eating raw or undercooked fish that was harvested in geographic areas where transmission occurs. Infection has been acquired by eating raw or undercooked freshwater, saltwater, and anadromous fish (e.g., salmon).

3. Causative agents—*Diphyllobothrium latum* (*Dibothriocephalus latus*) and 14 other primarily zoonotic species, including *Diphyllobothrium nihonkaiense* (*Dibothriocephalus nihonkaiense*), *Diphyllobothrium pacificum* (*Adenocephalus pacificus*), *Dibothriocephalus dendriticum* (*Dibothriocephalus dendriticus*), *Diphyllobothrium ursi* (*Dibothriocephalus ursi*).

4. Diagnosis—Identification of eggs or segments (proglottids) of the worm in feces; may require examination of multiple stool samples.

5. Occurrence—The disease occurs in areas where eating raw or partly cooked fish is popular. Prevalence increases with age. Fish infected with diphyllobothrid larvae may be transported to and consumed in any area of the world.

6. Reservoirs—Primarily humans for *D. latum*; dogs, bears, and other fish-eating mammals and seagulls for the other *Diphyllobothrium* spp.

7. Incubation period—5 to 6 weeks from ingestion of infected fish to passage of eggs in the stools.

8. Transmission—Humans acquire the infection by eating raw or inadequately cooked fish. Eggs in mature segments of the worm are discharged in feces into bodies of freshwater or salt water, where they mature and hatch; ciliated embryos (coracidium) infect the first intermediate host, usually copepods of the genera *Cyclops* and *Diaptomus*, and become procercoid larvae. Depending on the parasite species, freshwater, anadromous, or marine fish are second intermediate hosts when they ingest infected copepods; freshwater fish hosts include trout, pike, turbot, and perch; anadromous and saltwater hosts include Pacific and Atlantic salmon and whitefish. The procercoid larvae transform into plerocercoids in the fish. This stage is infective for people, fish-eating mammals (e.g., foxes, mink, bears, cats, dogs, pigs, walruses, seals), and seagulls.

No direct person-to-person transmission. Humans and other definitive hosts disseminate eggs into the environment as long as worms remain in the intestine, sometimes for many years.

9. Treatment—

Drug	Praziquantel
Dose	5–10 mg/kg
Route	PO
Alternative drug	• Niclosamide: ○ Adults: 2 g PO once ○ Children: 50 mg/kg ($\leq$ 2 g) PO once
Duration	Single dose
Special considerations and comments	Niclosamide is not available for human use in the USA.

Note: PO = oral(ly).

10. Prevention—Cooking fish to an internal temperature of 63°C (145°F); freezing at -35°C (-31°F) or below until solid and storing at that temperature or below for 15 hours or storing at -20°C (-4°F) or below for 24 hours; freezing at -20°C (-4°F) or below for 7 days.

11. Special considerations—Reporting: report indicated if a commercial source is implicated.

V. TAENIASIS AND CYSTICERCOSIS

1. Clinical features—Taeniasis is an intestinal infection with the adult stage of large tapeworms; cysticercosis is a potentially fatal tissue infection with the larval stage of 1 species, *Taenia solium*. Clinical manifestations of infection with the adult worm are mild, if present, and may include abdominal pain, distension, diarrhea, and nausea. Except for the annoyance of having segments of worms emerging from the anus, many infections are asymptomatic.

Cysticercosis may produce serious somatic disease when larvae localize in the eye or central nervous system (CNS). Clinical manifestations of cysticercosis depend on the number, location, and stage (viable, degenerating, or calcified) of the cysticerci and the intensity of the inflammatory response. The most important clinical manifestations occur when cysticerci are located in the brain. Seizures are the most common CNS manifestation; encephalitis, intracranial hypertension, hydrocephalus, chronic meningitis, and cranial nerve abnormalities are less frequent. CNS cysticercosis, or neurocysticercosis, may cause serious disability but with a relatively low case-fatality rate.

2. Risk groups—People who consume undercooked or raw pork or beef in areas with poor sanitation are at risk for adult tapeworm infection. People are at risk for cysticercosis if they live in areas where *T. solium* tapeworm infection is common. The greatest risk for cysticercosis is being a household member of a *T. solium* adult tapeworm carrier.

3. Causative agents—*T. solium*, the pork tapeworm, causes both intestinal infection with the adult worm and extraintestinal infection with the larvae (cysticerci). *Taenia saginata*, the beef tapeworm, only causes intestinal infection with the adult worm in humans. *Taenia asiatica* is a recently classified organism that causes human infections similar to those caused by *T. saginata*.

4. Diagnosis—Infection with an adult tapeworm is diagnosed by identification of proglottids (segments), eggs, or antigens of the worm in the feces; examination of several samples may be necessary to detect eggs. Eggs of *T. solium* and *T. saginata* cannot be differentiated morphologically. Specific diagnosis is based on the morphology of the scolex (head) and/or gravid proglottids. Subcutaneous cysticerci may be visible or palpable; microscopic examination of an excised cysticercus confirms the diagnosis. Cysticercosis in intracerebral and other tissues may be recognized by computerized axial tomography scan or magnetic resonance imaging. Standard radiography is of limited use for detection of calcified cysticerci. Specific serologic tests may support the clinical diagnosis of cysticercosis.

5. Occurrence—Worldwide; particularly frequent wherever beef or pork is eaten raw or insufficiently cooked and where sanitary conditions allow pigs and cattle to have access to human feces. Prevalence is highest in parts of Latin America, Africa, southern and southeastern Asia, and eastern Europe. In Latin America, seroprevalence of cysticercosis in endemic villages has been reported to be 10% to 25%. In some of the *T. solium*-endemic regions this tapeworm is considered responsible for more than 10% of acute case admissions to neurologic wards and one-third of late onset seizures. Transmission of *T. solium* is rare in Canada, the USA, western Europe, and most parts of Asia and the Pacific. Human infections with *T. asiatica* have been reported in several countries in South Asia, Southeast Asia, and East Asia.

6. Reservoirs—Humans are the definitive host of all 3 species of *Taenia*; cattle are the intermediate hosts for *T. saginata* and pigs for *T. solium* and *T. asiatica*.

7. Incubation period—Symptoms of cysticercosis may appear from months to years after infection. For tapeworm infections, eggs appear in the stools 8 to 12 weeks after consumption of infected pork for *T. solium* and 10 to 14 weeks after consumption of infected beef for *T. saginata*.

8. Transmission—Eggs of *T. saginata* passed in the stools of an infected person are infectious only to cattle. The eggs develop into cysticerci in the muscle tissue of the cow. In humans, infection follows ingestion of raw or undercooked beef containing cysticerci; in the intestine, the adult worm develops attached to the jejunal mucosa. Intestinal tapeworm infection due to *T. solium* in humans follows ingestion of raw or undercooked pork infected with cysticerci (measly pork), with subsequent development of the adult worm in the intestine. Human cysticercosis occurs when a person ingests *T. solium* eggs that are passed in the feces of a human tapeworm carrier. This can happen by ingesting contaminated food and possibly water or by putting contaminated fingers in the mouth. Importantly, a human tapeworm carrier can infect himself or herself with tapeworm eggs, resulting in cysticercosis (autoinfection), and can contaminate others in the household.

Ingested eggs hatch in the small intestine and the larvae migrate hematogenously to the subcutaneous tissues, striated muscles, and other tissues and vital organs of the body, where they form cysticerci.

T. asiatica infection is acquired by eating uncooked liver and other viscera of pigs infected with cysticerci of the parasite. In experimental studies this organism produced cysticerci only in the viscera of pigs, cattle, goats, and monkeys. It is unknown if human cysticercosis occurs with this species.

Eggs of both *T. solium* and *T. saginata* are disseminated into the environment as long as the worm remains in the intestine; the tapeworm lives about 3 to 5 years, while eggs may remain viable in the environment for months.

9. Treatment—

Drug	Praziquantel
Dose	5–10 mg/kg
Route	PO

Alternative drug	• Niclosamide:
	  ○ Adults: 2 g PO once
	  ○ Children: 50 mg/kg PO once

Duration	Single dose
Special considerations and comments	The choice of treatment for neurocysticercosis depends on the clinical manifestations and the location, number, size, and stage of cysticerci. Anthelmintic chemotherapy for symptomatic neuro-cysticercosis is almost never a medical emergency. The focus of initial therapy is control of seizures, edema, intracranial hypertension, or hydrocephalus, when 1 of these conditions is present. Under certain circumstances, a ventricular shunt or other neuro-surgical procedure may be indicated. Rarely, neuro-cysticercosis—especially large and/or subarachnoid (racemose) lesions—may present with imminent threat of intracranial herniation, a neurosurgical emergency. Both albendazole and praziquantel are acceptable and can be used in combination; niclo-samide is not recommended for neurocysticercosis.

Note: PO = oral(ly).

10. Prevention—

1) Cysticercosis can be prevented by improving public health education and sanitary measures.
2) Educate the public to prevent fecal contamination of soil, water, and human and animal food; to avoid use of sewage effluents for pasture irrigation; and to cook beef and pork thoroughly.
3) Identification and immediate treatment or institution of enteric precautions for people harboring adult *T. solium* are essential for prevention of human cysticercosis. *T. solium* eggs are infective immediately on leaving the host and may produce severe human illness.
4) Thoroughly cook meat to an internal temperature of 63°C (145°F) and ground meat to at least 71°C (160°F). Freezing pork or beef at a temperature below 25°C (23°F) for more than 4 days kills the cysticerci effectively. Irradiation is very effective at 1 kGy.
5) Inspection of carcasses of cattle and swine will detect only a proportion of those that are infected; these should be condemned, irradiated, or processed into cooked products.
6) Prevent swine and cattle access to latrines and human feces.

11. Special considerations—Reporting: report to local health authority may be required in some locations.

[S. Montgomery]

TETANUS
(lockjaw)

DISEASE	ICD-10 CODE
TETANUS	ICD-10 A35
OBSTETRICAL TETANUS	ICD-10 A34
TETANUS NEONATORUM	ICD-10 A33

1. Clinical features—Tetanus is an acute disease that is caused by an exotoxin produced by the anaerobic bacterium *Clostridium tetani* at the site of an injury. However, history of an injury or an apparent portal of entry may be lacking. Four clinical types of disease are often described: generalized, localized, cephalic, and neonatal. Generalized tetanus is characterized by painful muscular contractions, primarily of the masseter and neck muscles (trismus) and secondarily of trunk muscles. Generalized spasms are frequently induced by sensory stimuli; typical features of the tetanic spasm are extreme hyperextension of the body, in which the head and heels are bent backward and the spine arches forward (opisthotonos), and the facial expression known as risus sardonicus. A common first sign suggestive of tetanus in older children and adults is abdominal rigidity, though rigidity is sometimes confined to the region of injury (localized tetanus). Infected wounds of the head and neck area can lead to cranial nerve dysfunction or cephalic tetanus.

Tetanus neonatorum (neonatal tetanus) is typified by a newborn infant who sucks and cries well for the first few days after birth but who subsequently develops progressive difficulty and then inability to feed because of trismus—generalized stiffness with spasms or convulsions and opisthotonos.

The case-fatality rate of tetanus ranges from 10% to greater than 80% depending on age, the quality of care available, and the length of the incubation period. Case-fatality rates for neonatal tetanus are highest, exceeding 80% among those with short incubation periods. Neurologic sequelae including cognitive delay occur in 5% to more than 20% of those infants who survive. The case-fatality rate is also high in the elderly and varies inversely with the availability of experienced intensive care unit personnel and resources and with the length of the incubation period.

2. Risk groups—Those with greater than usual risk of traumatic and puncture injury, especially workers in contact with soil, sewage, and domestic animals; members of the armed forces; police officers and others with greater than the usual risk of traumatic injury; adults with diabetes mellitus; older adults who are currently at highest risk for tetanus and tetanus-related mortality; and unvaccinated women of reproductive age and their newborns. Most newborn infants with neonatal tetanus are born to nonimmunized mothers delivered by an untrained birth attendant outside a hospital.

3. Causative agents—*C. tetani*, the tetanus bacillus.

4. Diagnosis—Attempts at laboratory confirmation are of little help. A negative culture does not rule out the diagnosis as the organism is rarely recovered from the site of infection and anti-tetanus antibodies are undetectable in most cases.

5. Occurrence—Worldwide. The disease is sporadic and relatively uncommon in most industrialized countries but is more common in agricultural regions and in areas where contact with animal excreta is more likely and immunization is inadequate. Parenteral use of drugs, particularly intramuscular (IM) or subcutaneous injection, can result in individual cases and occasional circumscribed outbreaks. In 2006, an estimated 290,000 people worldwide died of tetanus, most of them in Asia, Africa, and South America. Populations in rural and tropical areas are especially at risk and tetanus neonatorum is common.

Tetanus neonatorum is a serious health problem in many developing countries where maternity care services are limited and immunization against tetanus is inadequate. In the past 10 years the incidence of tetanus neonatorum has declined considerably in many developing countries as a result of improved training of birth attendants, hygienic deliveries, and immunization coverage with tetanus toxoid for women of childbearing age. Despite this decline, WHO estimated in 2011 that tetanus neonatorum still caused about 61,000 deaths, mainly in the developing world.

6. Reservoirs—Spores of *C. tetani* are ubiquitous in the environment and are normal but harmless inhabitants of intestines of horses and other animals. Tetanus spores in soil or fomites contaminated with animal and human feces can contaminate wounds of all types.

7. Incubation period—Usually 3 to 21 days, although it may range from 1 day to several months, depending on the character, extent, and location of the wound. Most cases occur within 14 days. In general, shorter incubation periods are associated with more heavily contaminated wounds, more severe disease, and a worse prognosis.

For tetanus neonatorum, the average incubation period is about 6 days, with a range from 3 to 28 days.

8. Transmission—No direct person-to-person transmission. Tetanus spores are usually introduced into the body through a puncture wound contaminated with soil, street dust, or animal or human feces; through a laceration, burns, and even a trivial or unnoticed wound; or by injected contaminated drugs (e.g., street drugs). Tetanus occasionally follows surgical procedures, such as circumcision and abortions performed under unhygienic conditions. The presence of necrotic tissue and/or foreign bodies favors growth of the anaerobic pathogen. Cases have followed injuries considered too trivial for medical consultation.

Tetanus neonatorum usually occurs through introduction of tetanus spores via the umbilical cord during delivery through the use of an unclean instrument to cut the cord or after delivery by dressing the umbilical stump with substances heavily contaminated with tetanus spores, frequently as part of natal rituals.

Recovery from tetanus may not result in immunity; second attacks can occur and primary immunization is indicated after recovery.

9. Treatment—

Wound management	• All wounds should be cleaned, dirt or foreign material removed, and necrotic material removed or debrided. • Evaluate the immunization status of the patient. • Assess the need for administering TIG.

Symptom management	• Intensive supportive care
	• Toxin neutralization with TIG 500 IU IM single dose
	• Treat muscle spasms: benzodiazepines, neuromuscular blockade if needed
	• Manage autonomic instability
	• Stop toxin production: antibiotics, metronidazole is the antibiotic of choice:
	  o Adults: metronidazole 500 mg IV every 8 hours (infused over 20 minutes) for 7–14 days
	  o Children: metronidazole 7.5 mg/kg IV every 8 hours for 7–14 days
	• Wound therapy as indicated
	• Immunize with Tdap or DTaP as indicated as infection does not produce immunity

Vaccine status unknown or < 5 years since last vaccine	TIG plus DTaP, Tdap, or Td
Vaccine status known and > 5 years since last vaccine	DTaP, Tdap, or Td only

(*Continued*)

(Continued)

Special considerations and comments	• DTaP is recommended for children < 7 years. Tdap is preferred to Td for persons aged ≥ 7 years.
	• Tdap is recommended at > 20 weeks in every pregnancy regardless of previous vaccination status.
	• Immunocompromised persons who have contaminated wounds should receive TIG regardless of their history of tetanus immunizations.

Note: DTaP = combined diphtheria/tetanus and acellular pertussis vaccine; IM = intramuscular(ly); IU = international units; IV = intravenous(ly); Td = combined tetanus and diphtheria vaccine; Tdap = combined tetanus, diphtheria, and acellular pertussis vaccine; TIG = tetanus immunoglobulin.

10. Prevention—

1) Educate the public on the necessity for complete immunization with tetanus toxoid, the hazards of puncture wounds and closed injuries that are particularly liable to be complicated by tetanus, and the potential need after injury for active and/or passive prophylaxis.

2) Universal active immunization with adsorbed tetanus toxoid, which gives durable protection for at least 10 years; after the initial basic series has been completed, single booster doses elicit high levels of immunity.

   • For children younger than 7 years, tetanus toxoid is generally administered together with diphtheria toxoid and pertussis vaccine as a triple (diphtheria/tetanus and whole-cell pertussis vaccine [DTP] or diphtheria/tetanus and acellular pertussis vaccine [DTaP]) antigen or as a double (diphtheria/tetanus vaccine [DT]) antigen when contraindications to pertussis vaccine exist. Immunization should be initiated in infancy with a formulation containing diphtheria toxoid, tetanus toxoid, and either acellular pertussis antigens (DTaP, preferred in many industrialized countries) or whole-cell pertussis antigens (DTP). WHO recommends at least 3 primary IM DTP or DTaP doses starting as early as 6 months old with a minimum interval of 4 weeks between doses and a DTP booster given at 1 to 6 years. Some currently available formulations combine DTP or DTaP with 1 or more of the following: *Haemophilus influenzae* type b vaccine, poliomyelitis vaccine, or hepatitis B vaccine.

   • For persons older than 7 years, tetanus and diphtheria (Td) vaccine is recommended for primary vaccination and boosters. For adolescents and adults, combined tetanus, diphtheria, and acellular pertussis (Tdap) vaccine, where available, can be safely used as a single dose and for boosting as part of wound prophylaxis instead of Td. In countries with inadequate immunization coverage for children, all pregnant women should receive 2 doses of tetanus toxoid in the first pregnancy with an interval of at least 1 month and with the second dose at least 2 weeks prior to childbirth in order to prevent maternal and neonatal tetanus. Booster doses may be necessary to ensure ongoing protection (discussed later).

- Nonadsorbed (plain) tetanus toxoid vaccines, as opposed to alum adjuvant tetanus toxoid preparations, are less immunogenic for primary immunization or booster shots. Minor local reactions following tetanus toxoid injections are relatively frequent but not clinically significant; severe local and systemic reactions are infrequent but do occur, particularly in persons who have received an excessive number of prior doses.

- Active immunity induced by tetanus toxoid persists for at least 10 years after full primary immunization and should be maintained by administering a dose of Td every 10 years thereafter. For added protection against pertussis, a onetime dose of Tdap may be substituted for the next Td dose in a person older than 18 years.

- Tetanus toxoid is recommended for universal use regardless of age; it is especially important for workers in contact with soil, sewage, and domestic animals; members of the armed forces; police officers and others with greater than the usual risk of traumatic injury; adults with diabetes mellitus; older adults who are currently at highest risk for tetanus and tetanus-related mortality; and women of reproductive age and newborns.

- For children and adults who are severely immunocompromised or infected with human immunodeficiency virus, tetanus toxoid is indicated in the same schedule and dose as for immunocompetent persons, even though the immune response may be suboptimal.

- Transient passive immunity follows injection of tetanus immunoglobulin (TIG) or tetanus antitoxin (equine origin). Infants of actively immunized mothers acquire passive immunity that protects them from neonatal tetanus.

3) Prevention of tetanus neonatorum: improving maternity care, with emphasis on clean deliveries and increasing the tetanus toxoid immunization coverage of women of childbearing age (especially pregnant women).

- Nonimmunized pregnant women should receive at least 2 doses of tetanus toxoid, preferably as Td, with the first dose at initial contact or as early as possible during pregnancy and the second dose 4 weeks after the first and preferably at least 2 weeks before delivery. A third dose could be given 6 to 12 months after the second or during the next pregnancy. An additional 2 doses should be given at annual intervals or during subsequent pregnancies. In some industrialized countries, including the USA, Tdap is recommended during pregnancy, preferably after the first trimester. A 5-dose series of tetanus toxoid protects previously unimmunized women throughout the entire childbearing period. Women whose infants have a risk of neonatal tetanus but who themselves have received 3 or 4 doses of DTP/DTaP as children need only receive 2 doses of tetanus toxoid during each of their first 2 pregnancies.

- Increase the proportion of deliveries attended by trained attendants: Important control measures include licensing of midwives; providing professional supervision and education as to methods, equipment, and techniques of asepsis in childbirth; and educating mothers, relatives, and attendants in the practice of strict asepsis of the umbilical stump. The last is especially important in many areas where strips of bamboo are used to sever the umbilical cord or where ashes, cow dung poultices, or other contaminated substances are traditionally applied to the umbilicus. In those areas, any woman of childbearing age visiting a health facility should be screened and offered immunization, no matter what the reason for the visit.

4) Prophylaxis in wound management: tetanus prophylaxis in managing patients with wounds is based on careful assessment of whether the wound is clean or contaminated and the immunization status of the patient. It requires proper use of tetanus toxoid and/or TIG, wound cleaning, and—where required—surgical debridement and the proper use of antibiotics.

- Those who have been completely immunized and who sustain minor and uncontaminated wounds require a booster dose of toxoid only if more than 10 years have elapsed since the last dose was given. For major and/or contaminated wounds, a single booster injection of tetanus toxoid (preferably as Td or Tdap) should be administered promptly on the day of injury if the patient has not received tetanus toxoid within the preceding 5 years.

- Persons who have not completed a full primary series of tetanus toxoid require a dose of toxoid as soon as possible following the wound and may require passive immunization with human TIG if the wound is major and/or if it is contaminated with soil containing animal excreta. DTP/DTaP, DT, or Td, as determined by the age of the patient and previous immunization history, should be used at the time of the wound and ultimately to complete the primary series. Passive immunization with at least 250 international units (IU) of human-derived TIG IM (or 1,500–5,000 IU of antitoxin of animal origin if human TIG is not available), regardless of the patient's age, is indicated for patients with other than clean, minor wounds and a history of none, unknown, or fewer than 3 previous tetanus toxoid doses. When tetanus toxoid is given concurrently with human TIG (or equine antitoxin), separate syringes and separate sites must be used. When antitoxin of animal origin is given, it is essential to avoid anaphylaxis by first injecting 0.02 mL of a 1:100 dilution in physiologic saline intradermally with a syringe containing epinephrine on hand. Pretest with a 1:1,000 dilution if there has been prior animal serum exposure, together with a similar injection of physiologic saline as a negative control. If after 15 to 20 minutes there is a wheal with surrounding erythema at least 3 mm larger than the negative control, it is necessary to desensitize the individual.
- Antibiotics may theoretically prevent the multiplication of *C. tetani* in the wound, and thus reduce production of toxin, but this does not obviate the need for prompt treatment of the wound together with appropriate immunization. Metronidazole is the most appropriate antibiotic in terms of recovery time and case-fatality rate and should be given for 7 to 14 days in large doses; this also allows for a reduction in the amount of muscle relaxants and sedatives required.
- The wound should be debrided widely if possible. Wide debridement of the umbilical stump in neonates is not indicated.

11. Special considerations—

1) Reporting: case report to the local health authority required in most countries.
2) Epidemic measures: in the rare case of an outbreak, search for the source, especially contaminated street drugs or other common-use injections.

3) Disaster implications: social upheaval (military conflicts, riots) and natural disasters (floods, hurricanes, earthquakes) that cause many traumatic injuries in nonimmunized populations may result in an increased need for TIG or tetanus antitoxin and toxoid for injured patients.

4) Up-to-date immunization against tetanus is advised for international travelers.

[I. Chuang]

TOXOPLASMOSIS

DISEASE	ICD-10 CODE
TOXOPLASMOSIS	ICD-10 B58
CONGENITAL TOXOPLASMOSIS	ICD-10 P37.1

1. Clinical features—A systemic coccidian protozoan disease. Infections are frequently asymptomatic or present as acute disease, with lymphadenopathy only, or resemble infectious mononucleosis, with fever, lymphadenopathy, and lymphocytosis persisting for days or weeks. Development of an immune response decreases parasitemia but *Toxoplasma* cysts remaining in the tissues contain viable organisms that can persist, likely for the life of the host. These cysts may reactivate if the immune system becomes compromised. Among immunodeficient individuals, including patients infected with human immunodeficiency virus (HIV), primary or reactivated infection may cause a maculopapular rash, generalized skeletal muscle involvement, cerebritis, chorioretinitis, pneumonia, myocarditis, and/or death. Toxoplasmic encephalitis is the most frequent manifestation of toxoplasmosis among patients with acquired immunodeficiency syndrome (AIDS) and is generally fatal if untreated. Among pregnant women, a primary infection during early pregnancy may lead to fetal infection with death of the fetus or manifestations such as chorioretinitis, brain damage with intracerebral calcification, hydrocephaly, microcephaly, fever, jaundice, rash, hepatosplenomegaly, xanthochromic cerebrospinal fluid, and convulsions evident at birth or shortly thereafter. Later in pregnancy, maternal infection results in milder or subclinical fetal disease with delayed manifestations, such as recurrent or chronic chorioretinitis. Fetal infection can occur even when the mother's infection is asymptomatic. In immunosuppressed pregnant women who are *Toxoplasma*-seropositive, a reactivation of latent infection may result in congenital toxoplasmosis, though this is thought to be a rare event.

2. Risk groups—Risk for infection is primarily from ingestion of oocysts in cat feces or soil contaminated with cat feces and from ingestion of undercooked meat contaminated with tissue cysts. In addition, infection can occur through blood transfusion or organ transplantation from an infected donor. Pregnant women who have not previously been infected with *Toxoplasma gondii* are at risk for acute infection and congenital transmission to the fetus. Patients undergoing cytotoxic or immunosuppressive treatment and HIV-infected patients are at high risk of developing illness from primary or reactivated infection.

3. Causative agents—*T. gondii*, an intracellular coccidian protozoan that belongs to the family Sarcocystidae, in the class Sporozoa, and completes its sexual life cycle phase in cats.

4. Diagnosis—Based on clinical signs and supportive serologic results, demonstration of the agent in body tissues or fluids by biopsy or necropsy, or isolation in animals or cell culture. The presence of specific immunoglobulin class M and/or rising immunoglobulin class G (IgG) titers in sequential sera from newborns is conclusive evidence of congenital infection. The presence of immunoglobulin class A (IgA) is also helpful in determining infection in newborns. Among postnatally infected individuals, rising antibody titers are corroborative of active infection. However, high IgG antibody levels may persist for years with no relation to active disease. Reference laboratories may use the IgG avidity test, differential agglutination test, and IgA-specific and immunoglobulin class E-specific antibody tests to help determine the timing of infection. In addition, polymerase chain reaction assays of bodily fluids have been used to assist with the diagnosis. Physicians caring for pregnant women with suspected acute toxoplasmosis or for newborns suspected of having congenital toxoplasmosis are strongly encouraged to enlist the services of a reference laboratory to confirm the diagnosis and determine the timing of infection.

5. Occurrence—Worldwide in mammals and birds. Infection in humans is common.

6. Reservoirs—The definitive hosts of *T. gondii* are cats (felines), which acquire infection mainly from eating infected mammals (especially rodents) or birds and probably also from oocysts in soil contaminated with cat feces, acquired during licking/grooming. Felines alone harbor parasites in the intestinal tract, where the sexual stage of the protozoan life cycle occurs, resulting in excretion of oocysts in feces for 10 to 20 days, and rarely longer. Infected cats are rarely symptomatic, even during the period of oocyst shedding. Intermediate hosts include sheep, goats, rodents, swine, cattle, chickens, and other birds; all may carry an infective stage encysted in tissue, especially muscle and brain. Tissue cysts remain viable for long periods, perhaps lifelong. Cattle seem to be only minimally affected by natural *Toxoplasma* infection.

7. Incubation period—From 10 to 23 days from ingestion of undercooked meat in one common-source outbreak; 5 to 20 days in another outbreak associated with cats.

8. Transmission—Transplacental infection occurs in humans when a pregnant woman has rapidly dividing cells (tachyzoites) circulating in the bloodstream, usually during primary infection. Children may become infected by ingesting infective oocysts from sandboxes, playgrounds, and yards in which cats have defecated. Infections arise also from eating raw or undercooked infected meat containing tissue cysts (pork, mutton, or wild game; very rarely beef), ingesting infective oocysts on food such as raw vegetables, or ingesting water contaminated with feline feces. Presumed inhalation of sporulated oocysts was associated with one outbreak; another was associated epidemiologically with consumption of raw goat milk. Infection may occur through blood transfusion or organ transplantation from an infected donor. No direct person-to-person transmission occurs except in utero. Oocysts shed by cats sporulate and become infective 1 to 5 days later and may remain infective in water or moist soil for more than a year. Cysts in the flesh of infected animals remain infective throughout the period during which fresh meat is edible and uncooked; freezing meat, however, destroys infectivity.

Susceptibility to infection is general but immunity is readily acquired and most infections are asymptomatic. Duration of immunity is unknown but is assumed to be long-lasting or permanent; antibodies persist for years, probably for life.

9. Treatment—Treatment of acute toxoplasmosis in immunocompetent nonpregnant individuals is rarely indicated as this form of disease is usually self-limited; exceptions are those with severe symptoms that persist, those with ocular toxoplasmosis, and those with potential laboratory-acquired infection.

Treatment is recommended for acutely infected pregnant women, for congenitally infected newborns, and for immunocompromised persons with signs of reactivation. Prophylactic treatment is recommended for immunocompromised persons with serologic evidence of previous infection.

Drug	For immunocompetent patients:
	• Pyrimethamine[a] PLUS sulfadiazine and folinic acid[b]
	For pregnant women[1,c]:
	• Infection acquired at < 18 weeks' gestation and without evidence of fetal infection: spiramycin[d,e] • Infection acquired at ≥ 18 weeks' gestation or with evidence of fetal infection: pyrimethamine[a,f,g] PLUS sulfadiazine and folinic acid[b]
	For congenitally infected infants[1,h]:
	• Pyrimethamine[a] PLUS sulfadiazine and folinic acid[b]
	For immunocompromised patients[2]:
	• For prophylaxis: TMP/SMX • For treatment of toxoplasmic encephalitis: pyrimethamine[a] PLUS sulfadiazine and folinic acid[b]
Dose	For immunocompetent patients:
	• Pyrimethamine loading dose of 100 mg daily for 1 or 2 days, THEN 25–50 mg daily • Sulfadiazine 1 g every 6 hours • Folinic acid 10–20 mg daily
	For pregnant women:
	• Spiramycin 1 g TID (total daily dose 3 g) • Pyrimethamine[g] loading dose of 100 mg daily for 1 or 2 days, THEN 50 mg daily • Sulfadiazine loading dose of 75 mg/kg/dose for 1 day, THEN 100 mg/kg/day divided into 2 doses (≤ 4 g/day) • Folinic acid 10–20 mg/day, continued for 1 week past cessation of pyrimethamine
	For congenitally infected infants[1,h]:
	• Pyrimethamine: ○ Loading dose of 2 mg/kg/day divided into 2 doses/day for 2 days ○ Intensive initial therapy from day 3 to 2–6 months: 1 mg/kg/day ○ After the first 2–6 months of intensive initial therapy: 1 mg/kg/day 3 times/week until 12 months • Sulfadiazine 100 mg/kg/day divided into 2 doses • Folinic acid 10 mg 3 times/week
	For immunocompromised patients[2]:
	• For prophylaxis: TMP/SMX 1 double-strength tablet daily • For treatment of toxoplasmic encephalitis (≤ 60 kg): ○ Pyrimethamine 200 mg loading dose, THEN 50 mg daily ○ Sulfadiazine 1 g every 6 hours ○ Folinic acid 10–25 mg daily (≤ 50 mg daily or BID) • For treatment of toxoplasmic encephalitis (> 60 kg): ○ Pyrimethamine 200 mg loading dose, THEN 75 mg daily ○ Sulfadiazine 1.5 g every 6 hours ○ Folinic acid 10–25 mg daily (≤ 50 mg daily or BID)

(Continued)

(Continued)

Route	• Pyrimethamine: PO • Sulfadiazine: PO • Folinic acid: PO • Spiramycin: PO • TMP/SMX: PO or IV
Alternative drug	• Alternative regimens using atovaquone, or clindamycin, or TMP/SMX are described. • If alternative therapies are desired, consultation with physicians familiar with treating toxoplasmosis is strongly recommended.
Duration	• For immunocompetent patients, treatment may be indicated for 2–4 weeks. • For pregnant women, treatment is indicated until delivery, regardless of the regimen used. • For congenitally infected infants, treatment is usually recommended for 1 year. • For immunocompromised patients, treatment should be administered until significant immunologic improvement is achieved (e.g., from antiretroviral therapy); this may be 4–6 weeks beyond improvement of clinical toxoplasmosis symptoms.
Special considerations and comments	There is no effective treatment that will fully eradicate the encysted stage (bradyzoites) in tissues; available drugs are only active against the tachyzoite stage.

Source: Based on Maldonado and Read[1] and US National Library of Medicine.[2]

Note: BID = twice daily; IV = intravenous(ly); PO = oral(ly); TID = thrice daily; TMP/SMX = trimethoprim-sulfamethoxazole.

[a]Pyrimethamine is a folic acid antagonist and can cause dose-related bone marrow suppression. Patients on pyrimethamine should have blood counts, creatinine, and liver function monitored regularly.

[b]Folinic acid is different from folic acid. Folinic acid protects the bone marrow from the toxic effects of pyrimethamine and should always be given concomitantly with pyrimethamine. Folic acid cannot be substituted for folinic acid. Folic acid will inhibit the action of pyrimethamine and should not be given to patients being treated with pyrimethamine.

[c]Consultation with physicians familiar with treating toxoplasmosis in pregnant women is strongly recommended.

[d]In the USA, spiramycin can be obtained through FDA's Investigational New Drug process by phoning 301-796-1400. Physicians must have a confirmed diagnosis from a reference laboratory.

[e]Amniocentesis with polymerase chain reaction (PCR) of amniotic fluid (AF) is recommended at ≥ 18 weeks' gestation or as soon as possible thereafter to determine if the fetus is infected and fetal ultrasonography to identify abnormalities should be performed. If the AF PCR is positive and/or fetal ultrasonography identifies abnormalities consistent with congenital toxoplasmosis, therapy should be transitioned to pyrimethamine + sulfadiazine + folinic acid combination until delivery.[1]

[f]Amniocentesis with AF PCR is recommended at ≥ 18 weeks' gestation or as soon as possible thereafter to determine if the fetus is infected and fetal ultrasonography should be performed. If the AF PCR is negative and no abnormalities are identified on fetal ultrasonography then consider switching to spiramycin. Alternatively, pyrimethamine + sulfadiazine + folinic acid can be continued until delivery.[1]

[g]Pyrimethamine is potentially teratogenic and should not be used before the 18th week of pregnancy.

[h]Consultations with medical professionals familiar with treating congenitally infected infants is strongly recommended.

10. Prevention—

1) Educate pregnant women and immunocompromised patients about preventive measures.

2) Use irradiated meats or cook them to safe temperatures before eating. Always use a food thermometer to measure the internal temperature of cooked meat (color is not a reliable indicator that meat has been cooked to a temperature high enough to kill harmful pathogens like *Toxoplasma*).

   - For whole cuts of meat (excluding poultry), cook to at least 63°C (145°F).
   - For ground meat (excluding poultry), cook to at least 71°C (160°F).
   - For all poultry (whole cuts and ground), cook to at least 74°C (165°F).

3) Freezing meat at subzero temperatures (-18°C [0°F]) for several days before cooking can greatly reduce chance of infection.

4) Avoid eating raw or undercooked shellfish (e.g., oysters, mussels, and clams).

5) Unless they are known to have antibodies to *T. gondii*, pregnant women should avoid changing cat litter if possible.

   If no one else can perform the task, pregnant women and immunocompromised patients should wear disposable gloves when changing the litter box and wash their hands with soap and water afterwards. They should wear gloves during gardening and wash hands thoroughly afterward.

6) Raw fruits and vegetables should be peeled or thoroughly washed before eating.

7) Wash hands thoroughly before eating and after handling raw meat or after contact with soil possibly contaminated with cat feces. Cutting boards, dishes, counters, and utensils should be washed after contact with raw meat.

8) Cats should be fed dry, canned, or boiled food and discouraged from hunting (i.e., kept as indoor pets only).

9) Dispose of cat feces and litter daily (before oocysts become infective). Feces can be disposed in trash destined for landfills, burned, or deeply buried. Disinfect litter pans by scalding; wear gloves or wash hands thoroughly after handling potentially infective material. Dispose of dried litter without shaking to avoid aerial dispersal of oocysts.

10) Control stray cats and prevent their access to sandboxes and sand piles used by children for play. Keep sandboxes covered when not in use.

11) Avoid drinking untreated water or unpasteurized milk.

12) Toxoplasma-seropositive patients who have cluster of differentiation 4 counts less than 100 cells/μL should be administered prophylaxis against toxoplasmic encephalitis. A double-strength tablet daily dose of trimethoprim-sulfamethoxazole is the preferred regimen.

13) Patients with AIDS who have experienced symptomatic toxoplasmosis must receive prophylactic treatment throughout life with pyrimethamine, sulfadiazine, and folinic acid.

11. Special considerations—

1) Reporting: reportable in certain states in the USA and in some countries to facilitate further epidemiologic understanding of the disease.

2) International measures: the EU zoonosis directive (92/117 EEG) mentions toxoplasmosis under category B (collection of data in member states when available). WHO Collaborating Centres provide support as required. Further information can be found at: http://www.who.int/collaboratingcentres/database/en.

References

1. Maldonado YA, Read JS; Committee on Infectious Diseases. Diagnosis, treatment, and prevention of congenital toxoplasmosis in the United States. *Pediatrics*. 2017; 139(2):e20163860.

2. AIDSinfo. Guidelines for the prevention and treatment of opportunistic infections in HIV-infected adults and adolescents with HIV. July 2017. Available at: https://aidsinfo.nih.gov/guidelines/html/4/adult-and-adolescent-oi-prevention-and-treatment-guidelines/322/toxo. Accessed December 12, 2019.

[A. Straily]

TRACHOMA

DISEASE	ICD-10 CODE
TRACHOMA	ICD-10 A71
Pneumonia due to *Chlamydia trachomatis* (see "Pneumonia")	

1. Clinical features—A chlamydial conjunctivitis that has an insidious or abrupt onset; the infection may persist for a few weeks if untreated and tends to resolve with no consequence; in hyperendemic areas, the characteristic lifetime duration of active disease is the result of frequent reinfections. Conjunctivitis (active disease) is characterized by the presence of lymphoid follicles and diffuse conjunctival inflammation (papillary hypertrophy), particularly on the tarsal conjunctiva lining the upper eyelid. The inflammation can produce superficial vascularization of the cornea (pannus) and scarring of the conjunctiva, which increases with the severity and duration of inflammatory disease. The marked conjunctival scarring causes lid deformities and in-turning of eyelashes (entropion and trichiasis), which later in adult life cause chronic abrasion of the cornea and opacity in some individuals, resulting in visual impairment and blindness. Secondary bacterial infections frequently occur in populations with endemic trachoma and may contribute to the communicability and severity of the disease.

Active trachoma in some developing countries is an endemic early childhood disease. It may be clinically indistinguishable from conjunctivitis caused by other bacteria (including genital strains of *Chlamydia trachomatis*). Differential diagnosis includes molluscum contagiosum nodules of the eyelids, toxic reactions to chronically administered eye drops, and chronic staphylococcal lid-margin infection. An allergic reaction to contact lenses (giant papillary conjunctivitis) may produce a trachoma-like syndrome with tarsal nodules (giant papillae), conjunctival scarring, and corneal pannus.

2. Risk groups—Susceptibility is general; while there is no absolute immunity conferred by infection, the severity of active disease due to reinfection gradually decreases during the childhood years and active trachoma is no longer seen in older children or young adults. In endemic areas, children have active disease more frequently than adults. The severity of disease is often related to living conditions, particularly poor hygiene; exposure to dry winds, dust, and fine sand may also contribute.

3. Causative agents—*C. trachomatis* serovars A, B, Ba, and C; serovars B, Ba, and C have also been isolated from genital chlamydial infections.

4. Diagnosis—Primarily made though clinical observation of the disease-specific signs. Confirmation of the causative organism can be made through polymerase chain reaction, Giemsa-stained smears for the detection of intracellular chlamydial elementary bodies in epithelial cells of conjunctival scrapings, immunofluorescence examination after methanol fixation of the smear, detection of chlamydial antigen by enzyme immunoassay or deoxyribonucleic acid by probe, or isolation of the agent in special cell culture.

5. Occurrence—Worldwide; as an endemic disease, most often of poor rural communities in developing countries. In endemic areas, trachoma presents in childhood then subsides in adolescence, leaving varying degrees of potentially disabling scarring. Blinding trachoma is still widespread in sub-Saharan Africa. Pockets of blinding trachoma also occur in the Middle East, parts of the Indian subcontinent, southeastern Asia and China, Latin America, Australia (among Aboriginal people), and the Pacific islands. The disease occurs among population groups with poor hygiene, poverty, and crowded living conditions, particularly in dry, dusty regions. The late complications of trachoma (trichiasis and corneal opacity) occur in older people who had active trachoma in childhood.

6. Reservoirs—Humans.

7. Incubation period—From 5 to 12 days (based on volunteer studies).

8. Transmission—Through direct contact with infectious ocular or naso-pharyngeal discharges on fingers or indirect contact with contaminated fomites such as towels, clothes, and nasopharyngeal discharges from infected people and materials soiled therewith. Flies, especially *Musca sorbens* in Africa and the Middle East, can contribute to the spread of the disease. In children with active trachoma, *Chlamydia* can be recovered from the nasopharynx and rectum but the trachoma serovars do not appear to have a genital reservoir in endemic communities. The disease is probably communicable as long as active lesions are present in the conjunctivae and adnexal mucous membranes; commun-icability may continue for up to a few years. Concentration of the infectious agent in the tissues is greatly reduced with cicatrization but increases again with reactivation and recurrence of infective discharges. Infectivity ceases within 2 to 3 days of the start of antibiotic therapy, long before clinical improvement.

9. Treatment—

Preferred therapy	• Azithromycin 1 g PO as a single dose OR • Doxycycline 100 mg PO BID for 21 days
Alternative therapy options	• Tetracycline 250 mg PO QID for 14 days OR • Azithromycin 1% drops: instill 1 drop into affected eye(s) QID for 7 days OR • Erythromycin ointment 0.5%: instill approximately 1-cm ribbon into affected eye(s) 2–4 times daily for 3–4 weeks OR • Sulfacetamide ointment 10%: instill approximately 1-cm ribbon 2–4 times daily for 3–4 weeks
Special considerations and comments	Key factors to consider include personal hygiene, examin-ation of close contacts, and insect control.

Note: BID = twice daily; PO = oral(ly); QID = 4 times daily.

10. Prevention—

1) Educate the public on the need for personal hygiene, especially to encourage washing the face and avoiding sharing towels.
2) Improve basic sanitation, including availability and use of soap and water.

3) Provide appropriate community-based (mass) treatment of meso- and hyperendemic populations with oral or topical azithromycin to decrease the reservoir of infection and thereby reduce transmission.

4) Conduct epidemiologic investigations to determine important factors in the occurrence of the disease for specific situations.

5) There is no available vaccine at present.

6) For those with trichiasis, surgery to reposition the eyelashes so that they no longer abrade the cornea.

11. Special considerations—

1) Reporting: case report to local health authority required in some countries of low endemicity.

2) Epidemic measures: in regions of hyperendemic prevalence, mass treatment campaigns have been successful in eliminating the disease as the cause of visual impairment and blindness when associated with education in personal hygiene, especially cleanliness of the face and improvement of environmental hygiene (particularly increases in availability and use of water).

3) The WHO/Alliance for the Global Elimination of Trachoma provides technical and coordination support. WHO Collaborating Centers can also provide support as required. Further information can be found at:

- http://www.who.int/blindness/causes/trachoma/en/index.html
- http://www.who.int/gho/neglected_diseases/en/index.html.

[R. Abel Jr]

TRENCH FEVER
(quintana fever)

DISEASE	ICD-10 CODE
TRENCH FEVER	ICD-10 A79.0

1. Clinical features—Classic trench fever is typically a nonfatal febrile illness with various manifestations and degrees of severity. Onset can be sudden or insidious. Fever may be a single episode lasting 4 to 5 days, relapsing

(3–5 episodes usually lasting 5 days with asymptomatic intervals between episodes), or prolonged (typhoid-like). Other symptoms include headache, malaise, shin pain, and dizziness. Splenomegaly, transient macular rash, and conjunctivitis may also be present. Symptoms may continue to recur many years after the primary infection; persistent bacteremia has been described. Bacteremia associated with bacillary angiomatosis, fever of unknown origin, and occasionally endocarditis can occur in those with human immunodeficiency virus (HIV) (especially in the setting of advanced immunosuppression). *Bartonella quintana* is a cause of culture-negative endocarditis, especially among homeless or alcoholic persons.

2. Risk groups—The disease is usually encountered among the homeless, refugees, and other persons infested with lice.

3. Causative agents—*B. quintana* (formerly *Rochalimaea quintana*).

4. Diagnosis—Laboratory diagnosis is made by culture of the patient's blood on blood or chocolate agar under 5% CO_2. Microcolonies are visible after 8 to 21 days' incubation at 37°C (98.6°F). Serologic testing may be performed using 2 commercially available tests: an indirect immunofluorescence assay and an enzyme-linked immunosorbent assay. Cross-reactivity occurs with other *Bartonella* spp., *Coxiella burnetii*, and *Chlamydia*. Polymerase chain reaction of resected heart valve tissue may aid diagnosis of endocarditis.

5. Occurrence—Epidemics of trench fever occurred in Europe during World Wars I and II among those living in crowded, unhygienic conditions. Since then, *B. quintana* infections have been reported in every inhabited continent. Two forms of infection were documented during the 1990s in France and the USA: (a) an opportunistic febrile infection in patients with HIV infection (sometimes presenting as bacillary angiomatosis; see "Bartonellosis" and "Cat Scratch Disease") and (b) a louse-borne febrile disease in homeless or alcoholic persons, so-called urban trench fever. Endocarditis has been reported in patients with and without typical risk factors for trench fever.

6. Reservoirs—Humans. The intermediate host and vector is the body louse, *Pediculus humanus humanus*. The organism multiplies in the louse intestine for the duration of the insect's life, which is approximately 5 weeks after hatching; however, transovarial transmission does not occur. Cat fleas may also carry the bacteria but their role in transmission is undetermined.

7. Incubation period—Generally 3 to 30 days.

8. Transmission—Humans are infected by inoculation of louse feces through a break in the skin, usually when scratching louse bite sites. Infected lice begin to excrete infectious feces 5 to 12 days after ingesting infective blood; this continues for the remainder of their life span. The disease spreads when lice leave abnormally hot (febrile) or cold (dead) bodies in search of a normothermic host. Organisms may circulate in the host's blood (thus infecting lice) for weeks, months, or years and may recur with or without symptoms. Trench fever is not directly transmitted from person to person.

9. Treatment—

Drug	Doxycycline
Dose	100 mg BID
Route	PO
Alternative drug	No well-established alternative regimen, but macrolides and rifamycins may have efficacy.
Duration	4 weeks for bacteremia; 6 weeks for endocarditis; 3 months for bacillary angiomatosis.
Special considerations and comments	Add gentamycin 3 mg/kg daily (bacteremia) or 1 mg/kg every 8 hours (endocarditis) for the first 2 weeks of treatment.

Note: BID = twice daily; PO = oral(ly).

10. Prevention—Delousing procedures: clothing, bedding, and towels should be boiled or washed in hot water and machine-dried at high heat. The patient's body should be cleaned thoroughly. Insecticide treatment is generally not necessary since body lice reside in clothing and only visit the host's skin to feed; mass treatments of body and clothing with appropriate pediculicides may be necessary in outbreak situations.

11. Special considerations—

1) Reporting: report to local health authority so that an evaluation of louse infestation in the population may be made and appropriate measures taken.
2) Epidemic measures: systematic application of residual insecticide to clothing of all people in affected population.
3) Disaster implications: risk is increased when louse-infested people are forced to live in crowded, unhygienic shelters.

[L. Blanton, D. Walker]

TRICHINELLOSIS
(trichiniasis, trichinosis [obsolete terms])

DISEASE	ICD-10 CODE
TRICHINELLOSIS	ICD-10 B75

1. Clinical features—A roundworm disease in which clinical illness is highly variable and can range from asymptomatic infection to a fatal disease, depending mainly on the number of muscle larvae ingested but also on the *Trichinella* spp. Gastrointestinal (GI) symptoms, such as diarrhea due to the intraintestinal presence of adult worms, characterize the enteral phase of the disease, followed later by the parenteral phase. The latter phase is due to the migration of juvenile larvae and is characterized by the sudden appearance of muscle soreness and pain. Periorbital or facial edema and fever are early characteristic signs. These are sometimes followed by subconjunctival, subungual, and retinal hemorrhages, pain, and photophobia. Thirst, profuse sweating, chills, weakness, prostration, and rapidly increasing eosinophilia may follow shortly after the ocular signs.

Remittent fever is usual, sometimes as high as 40°C (104°F); fever terminates after 1 to 6 weeks, depending on the intensity of infection. Cardiac and neurologic complications, so-called neurotrichinellosis, may appear in the third to sixth week. In the most severe cases, death due to myocardial failure or arrhythmias may occur in either the first to second week or between the fourth and eighth weeks; however, this outcome is now very rare.

2. Risk groups—People who ingest raw or undercooked meat, especially pork and wild animal meat.

3. Causative agents—Nematodes belonging to the genus *Trichinella*. *Trichinella spiralis* has a cosmopolitan distribution and broad host range in primarily temperate areas of the world. Separate taxonomic designations have been accepted for isolates found in carnivorous and omnivorous animals of the Arctic and subarctic (*Trichinella nativa*), Palaearctic (*Trichinella britovi*), and wild animals in temperate North America (*Trichinella murrelli*); in South America (*Trichinella patagoniensis*); in Africa (*Trichinella nelsoni*); in mammals and birds (*Trichinella pseudospiralis*); and in omnivorous and carnivorous animals (*Trichinella papuae*, *Trichinella zimbabwensis*, and T6, T8, and T9 genotypes) in several specific regions of the world.

4. Diagnosis—Serologic tests based on enzyme-linked immunosorbent assay (ELISA) as screening and immunoblot as confirmatory tests (in both cases excretory/secretory antigens must be used to avoid unspecific results), marked eosinophilia, and increased muscle enzyme serum levels may aid in diagnosis. Biopsy of skeletal muscle, taken more than 10 days after infection (most often positive after the fourth or fifth week of infection), frequently provides conclusive evidence of infection by demonstrating the uncalcified parasite cyst.

5. Occurrence—Worldwide, but variable in incidence, depending in part on practices of eating and preparing pork or wild animal meat and the extent to which the disease is recognized and reported. Cases are usually sporadic and outbreaks localized, often resulting from eating sausage and other meat products containing pork or from sharing meat from Arctic mammals. Several outbreaks in the past have been reported in France and Italy through infected horse meat. Ingestion of raw soft-shelled turtles was implicated in Taiwan.

6. Reservoirs—Swine, dogs, cats, horses, rats, and many wild animals, including foxes, wolves, bears, moose, mountain lions, polar bears, wild boars, marine mammals in the Arctic, and hyenas, jackals, lions, and leopards in the tropics. Also found in farmed crocodiles; health risks from consuming raw crocodile meat are unknown.

7. Incubation period—GI symptoms may appear within a few days. Systemic symptoms usually appear about 8 to 15 days after ingestion of infected meat; this varies from 5 to 45 days depending on the number of muscle larvae ingested.

8. Transmission—Only by consumption of raw or insufficiently cooked flesh of animals containing viable encysted larvae, chiefly pork, pork products, and wild game animals such as bear. Occasionally, beef products, such as hamburger that is adulterated intentionally or inadvertently with raw pork, are implicated. In the epithelium of the small intestine, larvae develop into adults. Gravid female worms then produce larvae, which penetrate the lymphatics or venules and are disseminated via the bloodstream throughout the body. The larvae become encapsulated in skeletal muscle (unless nonencapsulating species). Animal hosts remain infective for months and their meat stays infective for appreciable periods unless cooked, frozen, or irradiated to kill the larvae. Infection results in partial immunity.

9. Treatment—

Preferred therapy	Adults:
	• Albendazole 400 mg PO BID administered in 2 doses for 10–15 days
	Children (> 2 years):
	• Albendazole 10 mg/kg/day PO for 10–15 days
Alternative therapy options	Mebendazole 200–400 mg PO TID for 3 days, THEN 400–500 mg PO TID for 10 days

(Continued)

(Continued)

Special considerations and comments	• Albendazole is available in tablets (200 mg) or as a suspension (20 mL bottle at a concentration of 100 mg/5 mL). • Mebendazole is available in tablets (100 mg) or as a suspension (30 mL bottle at a concentration of 100 mg/5 mL). • The whole treatment cycle may be repeated after 5 days (for severe infections). • Albendazole and mebendazole are both pregnancy category C drugs. • Glucocorticosteroids are used by most physicians to treat the signs and symptoms of type I hypersensitivity. They must always be used in combination with anthelmintics and never alone since they could increase the larval burden by delaying the intestinal worm expulsion. • Prednisolone, most commonly used (available in tablets of 1 mg or 5 mg), is administered at a dosage of 30–60 mg/day in multiple doses for 10–14 days.

Note: BID = twice daily; PO = oral(ly); TID = thrice daily.

10. Prevention—

1) Educate the public on the need to cook all fresh pork, pork products, and meat from wild animals at a temperature and for a time sufficient to allow all parts to reach at least 71°C (160°F) or until the meat changes from pink to grey, which allows a sufficient margin of safety. This should be done unless it has been established that these meat products have been processed by heating, curing, freezing, or irradiation adequate to kill the parasite.

2) Grind pork in a separate grinder or clean the grinder thoroughly before and after processing other meats.

3) Adopt regulations to encourage commercial irradiation processing of pork products. Testing carcasses for infection with a digestion technique is useful, as is immunodiagnosis of pigs with an approved ELISA test.

4) Adopt and enforce regulations that allow only certified trichinae-free pork to be used in raw pork products that have a cooked appearance or in products that are traditionally not heated sufficiently in final preparation to kill the larvae.

5) Adopt laws and regulations to require and enforce the cooking of garbage and offal before feeding to swine.

6) Educate hunters to cook the meat of bears, wild boars, walruses, seals, and other wild animals thoroughly.

7) Freezing temperatures maintained throughout the mass of the infected meat are effective in inactivating most *Trichinella* spp. Holding pieces of pork up to 15 cm thick at a temperature of −15°C (5°F) for 20 days or −25°C (−13°F) or lower for 10 days will effectively destroy most types of *Trichinella* cysts. Hold thicker pieces at the lower temperature for at least 20 days. These temperatures will not inactivate the freeze-resistant Arctic strains (*T. nativa*) found in walrus and bear meat and—rarely—in swine.

8) Exposure of pork cuts or carcasses to low-level gamma irradiation effectively sterilizes and, at higher doses, kills encysted larvae.

9) Cooking meat with a microwave oven should be avoided.

11. Special considerations—

1) Reporting: case report required in most countries.

2) Epidemic measures: epidemiologic study to determine the common food involved. Confiscate remainder of suspected food and correct faulty practices. Eliminate infected herds of swine. WHO Collaborating Centres provide support as required. Further information can be found at: http://www.who.int/collaborating-centres/database/en.

Bibliography

Dupouy-Camet J, Bruschi F. Management and diagnosis of human trichinellosis. In: Dupouy-Camet J, Murrell KD, eds. *FAO/WHO/OIE Guidelines for the Surveillance, Management, Prevention and Control of Trichinellosis*. Paris, France: World Organisation for Animal Health (OIE); 2007:37-69.

[F. Bruschi]

TRICHOMONIASIS

DISEASE	ICD-10 CODE
TRICHOMONIASIS	ICD-10 A59

1. Clinical features—Infection affects members of both sexes, preferentially infecting the urethra, vaginal, and vulvar sites in women and the urethra in men. In women, the disease may range from asymptomatic infection ($\leq$ 50% of women) to complaints of vaginal discharge, itching and irritation, and/or pain during urination or sexual intercourse. Signs of infection include vaginal discharge, odor, edema, or erythema. Although men are often asymptomatic, dysuria and discharge can be present. Trichomoniasis is frequently seen concomitantly with other sexually transmitted infections (STIs) and has been recognized to play a critical role in human immunodeficiency virus (HIV) acquisition and transmission. *Trichomonas vaginalis* infection in pregnant women has been associated with adverse pregnancy outcomes, particularly premature rupture of membranes, preterm delivery, and low birth weight.

2. Risk groups—Risk factors associated with trichomoniasis include multiple sex partners, lower socioeconomic status, and history of STIs. While infection primarily occurs during reproductive age, it occurs more commonly in women versus men, in non-Hispanic black women versus other races/ethnicities, and in women who practice vaginal douching.

3. Causative agents—*T. vaginalis*, an anaerobic flagellated protozoan parasite.

4. Diagnosis—The most common method for diagnosing trichomoniasis is microscopic evaluation of genital secretions (wet mount) because of convenience and relatively low cost. However, the sensitivity of wet mount for *T. vaginalis* diagnosis is poor (51%–65%) in vaginal specimens and even less sensitive when used with male urine specimens. Until recently, culture was the gold standard for diagnosis of trichomoniasis. However, a nucleic acid amplification test has demonstrated high sensitivity and specificity and can be used on multiple specimen types, including urinary, urethral, vaginal, and endocervical specimens.

5. Occurrence—Prevalence of *T. vaginalis* in the USA is reported as 3.1% among women of reproductive age (14–49 years) but may be higher in certain subpopulations. Globally, the prevalence of *T. vaginalis* has been estimated at 8.1% for women and 1% for men.

6. Reservoirs—Humans are the only natural host of *T. vaginalis*.

7. Incubation period—The incubation period of this infection is unknown; however, studies suggest an incubation period of 4 to 28 days but asymptomatic infections can last for years.

8. Transmission—The organism is thought to be transmitted almost exclusively by sexual activity. Nonsexual transmission is rare.

9. Treatment—

Preferred therapy	• Metronidazole 2 g PO as a single dose[a] OR • Tinidazole 2 g PO as a single dose
Alternative therapy options	Metronidazole 500 mg PO BID for 7 days

Special considerations and comments	• Alcohol consumption should be avoided during treatment. For metronidazole, avoid alcohol until 24 hours after last dose. For tinidazole, avoid alcohol until 72 hours after last dose.
	 • Persons with *Trichomonas vaginalis* infection should abstain from sex for at least 1 week after their sex partners are treated. Testing for other STIs, including HIV, should be performed.
	 • Owing to the high rate of reinfection among women treated, retesting for *T. vaginalis* is recommended for all sexually active women within 3 months following initial treatment regardless of whether they believe their sex partners were treated.
	 • Treatment failure recommendations:
	  ○ Ensure all partners have been treated.
	  ○ First failure: metronidazole 500 mg PO BID for 7 days.
	  ○ Second failure: metronidazole 500 mg PO BID or tinidazole 2 g PO daily for 7 days.
	  ○ Third failure: tinidazole 2 g PO daily for 7 days.
	  ○ Consultation with an infectious diseases specialist is recommended when managing treatment failures.

Note: BID = twice daily; HIV = human immunodeficiency virus; PO = oral(ly); STI = sexually transmitted infection.

[a]In women with HIV infection, metronidazole 500 mg orally twice a day for 7 days is recommended.

10. Prevention—Symptomatic women (i.e., with vaginal discharge) should be tested for trichomoniasis. Using latex condoms consistently and correctly can reduce the risk of acquiring or transmitting STIs, including trichomoniasis. Concurrent treatment of sexual partners is recommended to prevent reinfection. Retesting for *T. vaginalis* is recommended for sexually active women within 3 months following treatment because of the high rate of reinfection.

11. Special considerations—Routine screening of asymptomatic women with HIV infection is recommended.

[L. Llata]

TRICHURIASIS
(trichocephaliasis, whipworm disease)

DISEASE	ICD-10 CODE
TRICHURIASIS	ICD-10 B79

1. Clinical features—A nematode infection of the large intestine, usually asymptomatic. Heavy infections may cause bloody, mucoid stools and diarrhea; at times they may also cause rectal prolapse, clubbing of fingers, hypoproteinemia, and iron deficiency anemia with growth retardation.

2. Risk groups—Susceptibility is universal. The highest prevalence and intensity of infection are found in school-aged children.

3. Causative agents—*Trichuris trichiura*, or human whipworm, a nematode, soil-transmitted helminth.

4. Diagnosis—Through demonstration of eggs in feces, passage of adult worms, or observation of worms attached to the wall of the lower colon during a sigmoidoscopic examination conducted for other reasons. Eggs must be differentiated from those of *Capillaria* spp. Polymerase chain reaction on deoxyribonucleic acid extracted from feces is increasingly used for surveillance studies.

5. Occurrence—Worldwide, especially in warm, moist regions.

6. Reservoirs—Humans.

7. Incubation period—Indefinite.

8. Transmission—Indirect, particularly through pica (eating of nonfood items; in this context, especially soil contaminated with infective eggs) or ingestion of contaminated vegetables; no person-to-person transmission. Eggs passed in feces require a minimum of 10 to 14 days in warm, moist soil to become infective. Hatching of larvae follows ingestion of infective eggs from contaminated soil, attachment to the mucosa of the cecum and proximal colon, and development into mature worms. Eggs appear in the feces 70 to 90 days after ingestion of embryonated eggs; symptoms may appear much earlier. The female worm can produce between 2,000 and 10,000 eggs per day and has a life span of about 1 year. Untreated carriers can communicate the disease for several years.

9. Treatment—

Drug	Albendazole or mebendazole
Dose	• Albendazole 400 mg once daily for 3 days • Mebendazole 100 mg BID for 3 days or 500 mg single dose • Half-dosage recommended for children < 24 months
Route	PO
Alternative drug	Ivermectin 200 µg/kg once daily for 3 days
Duration	3 days
Special considerations and comments	• Available evidence suggests that these drugs are safe for use among women during the second and third trimesters of pregnancy, among those who are lactating, and among children ≤ 2 years. Although these drugs are generally considered safe, limited data exist on the risk of treatment in pregnant women during the first trimester or in young children < 2 years; thus risk of treatment needs to be balanced with the risk of disease progression in the absence of treatment. If very young children (1–2 years) are treated, they should be given tablets that are crushed and mixed with water; treatment should be supervised by trained personnel. • Mebendazole is available in the USA only through compounding pharmacies.

Note: BID = twice daily; PO = oral(ly).

10. Prevention—

1) Educate all members of the family, particularly children, in the use of toilet facilities and handwashing. Provide adequate facilities for feces disposal.

2) Encourage satisfactory hygienic habits, especially handwashing before food handling and before eating; avoid ingestion of soil by thorough washing of vegetables and other foods contaminated with soil.

3) In endemic areas, WHO recommends a preventive chemotherapy strategy focused on mebendazole or albendazole treatment of high-risk groups (preschool- and school-aged children, including adolescents who are not in school; women of childbearing age) at regular intervals for the control of morbidity due to the soil-transmitted helminths causing ascariasis, trichuriasis, and hookworm disease (https://www.who.int/intestinal_worms/en). See "Ascariasis" for details.

11. Special considerations—Advise school health authorities of unusual frequency in school populations.

[R. S. Bradbury, M. Kamb]

TRYPANOSOMIASIS

DISEASE	ICD-10 CODE
HUMAN AFRICAN TRYPANOSOMIASIS	ICD-10 B56, B56.1
AMERICAN TRYPANOSOMIASIS	ICD-10 B57

I. HUMAN AFRICAN TRYPANOSOMIASIS (HAT, sleeping sickness)

1. Clinical features—A systemic protozoal disease that is generally fatal without treatment. There are 2 parasite species and 2 forms (stages): the East African *Trypanosoma brucei gambiense* has a more chronic course, which may last several years, and the West African *Trypanosoma brucei rhodesiense* has a more acute course, which is lethal within weeks or months. Both species may have either human African trypanosomiasis (HAT) stage. In the early stage, following a painful tsetse fly bite, a chancre, originating as a papule and evolving into a nodule that ulcerates, may be found at the primary bite site and parasites can be found in the chancre (more frequent in rhodesiense infection); there may also be fever, intense headache, painless enlarged lymph nodes (more commonly posterior cervical lymphadenopathy in the gambiense form), local edema (puffy face syndrome), rash, and nonspecific cardiac symptoms. Death in the febrile hematolymphatic HAT stage I phase is often due to myocarditis. In the later meningoencephalitic HAT stage II, after the parasite crosses the blood-brain barrier, neurologic signs are added, such as disturbances of circadian rhythm, sensory disturbances, endocrine dysfunction, disorders of tonus and mobility, abnormal movements, seizures, mental status changes, or psychiatric disorders. Neurologic symptoms correlate with the damaged areas of the central nervous system (CNS). Occasional inapparent or asymptomatic infections have been documented. Spontaneous recovery in patients with the gambiense form without CNS involvement has been described.

2. Risk groups—Susceptibility is general in endemic areas. Children progress to stage II more rapidly.

3. Causative agents—Extracellular hemoflagellate subspecies of *Trypanosoma brucei*: *T. brucei gambiense* and *T. brucei rhodesiense*. There are no morphologic criteria for subspecies differentiation. Clinically, acute cases contracted in eastern and southern Africa have been considered to be due to *T. brucei rhodesiense*, whereas chronic cases infected in western and Central Africa have been considered to be due to *T. brucei gambiense*. It is now possible to differentiate both subspecies by molecular biology methods.

4. Diagnosis—Cannot be based on clinical symptoms. The more rapidly progressive rhodesiense infection is associated with higher parasite counts. Diagnosis relies on finding trypanosomes in blood, lymph, or eventually cerebrospinal fluid (CSF). Parasite concentration techniques are generally required in gambiense and less often in rhodesiense disease; in blood (thick blood films), capillary tube centrifugation or mini-anion exchange centrifugation, and in CSF, single modified centrifugation or double centrifugation may be used. Inoculation into laboratory rats or mice is sometimes useful in rhodesiense disease. The screening test of choice for *T. brucei gambiense* is the card agglutination test for trypanosomiasis (obtain from the Institute of Tropical Medicine [www.itg.be]), a simple 5-minute test based on the agglutination of whole, fixed, and stained trypanosomes in the presence of specific antibodies. The control programs in areas where *T. brucei gambiense* is endemic use it for seroscreening of at-risk populations; there is no seroscreening test available for *T. brucei rhodesiense*. New rapid serologic tests for the *T. brucei gambiense* form have been developed and are under evaluation. All patients must have sampling of the CSF for white blood cells ($> 6/\mu l$) and/or parasites to determine the involvement (late stage) or not (early stage) of the CNS. Molecular diagnostic tests are available using different targets, although these are not recommended for therapeutic decisions because they lack sensitivity to detect low concentrations of parasites.

5. Occurrence—HAT is confined to tropical Africa between 15°N and 20°S latitude, corresponding to the distribution of the tsetse fly. The annual incidence of cases reported to WHO is now fewer than 3,000 cases per year and HAT is a disease targeted for elimination by 2030. WHO reports that 1,447 persons were infected in 2017, with up to 57 million people in 36 countries at risk of contracting the disease. In the past decade 70% of reported cases were from the Democratic Republic of the Congo. The gambiense form of the disease represents 82% of the total cases reported. Sleeping sickness has a focal distribution and occurs at more than 250 foci in the poorest rural areas of some of the least industrialized countries (see atlas at: www.who.int/ trypanosomiasis_african/country/foci_AFRO/en).

Outbreaks can occur when human-fly contact is intensified, when reservoir hosts introduce trypanosome human-infective strains into a tsetse-infested area, or when populations are displaced into endemic areas.

6. Reservoirs—In *T. brucei gambiense* infection, humans are the major reservoir; however, the role of domestic and wild animals is not clear. Wild animals including antelope, cattle, and other domestic animals are the chief reservoirs for *T. brucei rhodesiense*.

7. Incubation period—Symptoms usually appear within 5 days to a few weeks after infection with *T. brucei rhodesiense* but they may not be apparent or may be misdiagnosed for several months with *T. brucei gambiense* infection.

8. Transmission—Through the bite of infective *Glossina*, the tsetse fly. Six species are the main vectors in nature. The riverine species are vectors for *T. brucei gambiense*: *Glossina palpalis*, *Glossina fuscipes*, and *Glossina tachinoides*. The wooded savanna species are vectors of *T. brucei rhodesiense*: *Glossina morsitans*, *Glossina pallidipes*, and *Glossina swynnertoni*. The fly is infected by ingesting blood of a human or animal that carries trypanosomes. The parasite multiplies in the fly for 12 to 30 days, depending on temperature and other factors, until infective forms develop in the salivary glands. Once infected, a tsetse fly remains infective for life (average 3 months but as long as 10 months); infection is not passed from generation to generation in flies. Congenital transmission can occur in humans. Transmission by blood transfusion and needlestick is possible. Direct mechanical transmission by blood on the proboscis of *Glossina* and other biting insects, such as horseflies, or in laboratory accidents is possible. The disease is communicable to the tsetse fly as long as the parasite is present in the blood of the infected person or animal. Parasitemia in humans occurs in waves of varying intensity in untreated cases and occurs at all stages of the disease.

9. Treatment—

Trypanosoma brucei rhodesiense (East African Human African trypanosomiasis)

	Stage I (hemolymphatic)	Stage II (meningoencephalitic)
Drug	Suramin sodium	Melarsoprol
Dose	Adults: • 1 g IV slowly on days 1, 3, 7, 14, 21	Adults: • 2–3.6 mg/kg IV daily for 3 days THEN • After day 7, 3.6 mg/kg/day for 3 days THEN • After 7 more days, give 3.6 mg/kg for 3 days
	Children: • 20 mg/kg IV slowly on days 1, 3, 7, 14, 21	Children: • Same as for adults

(Continued)

Trypanosoma brucei rhodesiense (East African Human African trypanosomiasis) (Continued)

	Stage I (hemolymphatic)	Stage II (meningoencephalitic)
Route	IV	IV
Alternative drug	Pentamidine isethionate is less effective.	None; fexinidazole and oxaborole are in clinical trials.
Duration	Days 1, 3, 7, 14, 21	Three series of 3-day courses (start days 1, 7, 14)
Special considerations and comments	Obtain from CDC Drug Services by contacting parasites@cdc.gov.	• Toxicity of hemorrhagic encephalopathy caused by this arsenical drug; steroids may help. • Obtain from CDC Drug Services by contacting parasites@cdc.gov.

Note: IV = intravenous(ly).

Trypanosoma brucei gambiense (West African Human African trypanosomiasis)

	Stage I (hemolymphatic)	Stage II (meningoencephalitic)
Drug	Pentamidine[a]	Eflornithine
Dose	Adults and children: 4 mg/kg/day	Adults: 400 mg/kg/day in 4 doses
Route	IV or IM	IV
Alternative drug	Suramin	Eflornithine 400 mg/kg/day in 2 doses for 7 days combined with oral nitrofurtimox 15 mg/kg for 10 days is first line per WHO.
Duration	7–10 days	14 days
Special considerations and comments	None	Obtain from CDC Drug Services by contacting parasites@cdc.gov.

Note: CSF = cerebrospinal fluid; IM = intramuscular(ly); IV = intravenous(ly).
[a]As of August 2019, WHO provided interim new guidance: pentamidine to be replaced with fexinidazole, an oral drug dosed by body weight. Doses should be directly preceded by food and medication should be given by direct observed therapy. Candidates for treatment with fexinidazole are ≥ 6 years, > 20 kg, and at either stage I or stage II (CSF for white blood cells $\leq 100/\mu l$). For those > 35 kg, administer 1,800 mg daily for 4 days, THEN drop to 1,200 mg daily for 6 more days. This drug is not approved in the USA and is not currently provided by CDC.

10. Prevention—Selection of appropriate prevention methods must be based on knowledge of the local ecology of vectors and infectious agents. In a given geographic area, priority must be given to 1 or more of the following:

1) Educate the public on personal protective measures against tsetse fly bites—this has limited impact because tsetse flies bite during the day and N,N-diethyl-meta-toluamide is not effective. Bed nets are not useful. Tsetse flies are visually attracted to their reservoirs; wear long clothing in bright colors, but not blue, pretreated with permethrin.

2) Reduce the parasite population by screening and diagnosing exposed populations and treating those infected. This is effective for *T. brucei gambiense*, for which humans are the main reservoir.

3) Reduce the parasite population by diagnosing and treating cattle. This is effective for *T. brucei rhodesiense*, for which cattle are a reservoir.

4) Destroy vector tsetse fly habitats if useful; indiscriminate destruction of vegetation is not recommended.

5) Reduce the tsetse fly population by appropriate use of traps and screens impregnated with insecticide or otherwise; by local use of residual insecticide; or by sequential aerial spraying of insecticide by helicopter or fixed-wing aircraft. Sterile insect technique has been successfully used to eradicate tsetse from Unguja Island in Zanzibar.

6) Check for the disease in case of blood donation from those who have visited or lived in endemic areas in Africa.

11. Special considerations—

1) In some endemic areas, establish records of prevalence and encourage control measures.

2) Epidemic measures: mainly for *T. brucei rhodesiense*; mass surveys, urgent treatment for identified infections, cattle treatment, and tsetse fly control.

3) International measures: the Pan-African Tsetse and Trypanosomiasis Eradication Campaign is an Africa Union program to promote and coordinate antitrypanosomiasis efforts of governments in affected countries. WHO is leading a human African trypanosomiasis surveillance and control program by providing capacity building as well as technical and logistical support (diagnostic reagents and equipment, drugs, training) to countries where the disease is endemic and by carrying out surveillance and control activities as well as improving reporting of the disease. WHO Collaborating Centres provide support as required. Further information can be found at: http://www.who.int/collaboratingcentres/database/en.

4) Further information on trypanosomiasis can be found at: http://www.who.int/trypanosomiasis_african/en and www.cdc.gov/parasites/sleepingsickness.

II. AMERICAN TRYPANOSOMIASIS (Chagas disease)

1. Clinical features—Infection with this parasite is thought to be life-long and the majority of infections are asymptomatic or paucisymptomatic. The acute form of this infection lasts about 2 months with variable fever, lymphadenopathy, malaise, and hepatosplenomegaly. An inflammatory response may be seen at the site of inoculation (chagoma). Unilateral bipalpebral edema (Romaña's sign) occurs in a small percentage of acute cases. Fewer than 1% have life-threatening or fatal manifestations during the acute phase; these include myocarditis and meningoencephalitis. Without treatment most become asymptomatic—the indeterminate phase. In 20% to 30% of indeterminate infections, irreversible chronic manifestations appear later in life. Chronic irreversible sequelae include myocardial damage with cardiac dilatation, arrhythmias, and major conduction abnormalities and intestinal tract involvement with megaesophagus and megacolon. The prevalence of megaviscera and cardiac involvement varies according to region; the cardiac disease is not as common north of Ecuador as in southern areas and megavisceral manifestations occur mainly in central Brazil and in countries of the Southern Cone. In patients with acquired immunodeficiency syndrome (AIDS), acute myocarditis and severe multifocal or diffuse meningoencephalitis with necrosis and hemorrhage occur as relapses of chronic infection. Reactivation of chronic Chagas disease may also occur with non-AIDS immunosuppression and is characterized by skin lesions, panniculitis, blood parasitemia, and, often, acute myocarditis.

Infection with *Trypanosoma rangeli* occurs in foci of endemic Chagas disease; prolonged parasitemia occurs, sometimes coexisting with *Trypanosoma cruzi* flagellates (with which *T. rangeli* shares reservoir hosts)—no clinical manifestations attributable to *T. rangeli* have been noted.

2. Risk groups—All ages are susceptible but the acute disease is usually more severe in younger people. Immunosuppressed people, especially those with AIDS, are at risk of serious infections and complications.

3. Causative agents—*T. cruzi*, a protozoan that occurs in humans as a hemoflagellate (trypomastigote) and as an intracellular parasite (amastigote) without an external flagellum.

4. Diagnosis—In the acute phase (or in reactivation during immuno-suppression) one should look for parasites using a blood smear or a blood concentration technique, such as microhematocrit, buffy coat, or Strout technique. Parasitemia is most intense during febrile episodes early in the course of infection. Polymerase chain reaction (PCR) is the most sensitive assay during the acute phase. In the chronic phase serologic tests should be used, including anti-*T. cruzi* immunoglobulin class G (IgG) antibodies through a conventional or recombinant enzyme-linked immunosorbent assay, indirect hemagglutination assay, indirect immunofluorescence assay, Western blot, and rapid diagnostic tests such as immunochromatography. No single serology is sufficiently sensitive or specific, so it is recommended to use 2 assays with different antigens or techniques. For discordant results radioimmune precipitation assays and trypomastigote excreted-secreted antigen immunoblot are considered reference tests. Special laboratory studies include blood culture, xenodiagnosis (examination of the feces of an uninfected triatomine bug fed with the patient's blood). *T. cruzi* is best differentiated from *T. rangeli* by PCR, though it is distinctive by its shorter length (20 mm vs. 36 mm) and larger kinetoplast. Serologic tests are valuable for individual diagnosis as well as for screening purposes.

5. Occurrence—This infection is mainly confined to the Western Hemisphere, with wide geographic distribution in rural Mexico and Central and South America. However, progress in reduction of vector-borne and blood-borne transmission in endemic countries, together with migration of chronically infected people to nonendemic countries, is changing the epidemiology of the disease. Based on limited data from seroprevalence studies among blood donors and other populations, it is estimated that at least 300,000 people in North America are infected with *T. cruzi*, mainly immigrants from endemic countries.

6. Reservoirs—Humans and more than 150 domestic and wild mammal species, including dogs, cats, pigs, rats, mice, marsupials, edentates, rodents, Chiroptera, carnivores, and primates.

7. Incubation period—About 5 to 14 days after bite of insect vector; 30 to 40 days if infected through blood transfusion; oral (ingestion) may be accelerated, while transplant-related reactivation can be longer.

8. Transmission—Infected vectors—that is, bloodsucking species of Reduviidae (cone-nosed or kissing bugs), especially various species from the genera *Triatoma*, *Rhodnius*, and *Panstrongylus*—have the trypanosomes in their feces. Defecation occurs during feeding; infection of humans and other mammals occurs when the freshly excreted bug feces contaminate conjunctivae, mucous membranes, abrasions, or skin wounds (including the bite wound). The bugs become infected when they feed on a parasitemic animal; the parasites multiply in the bugs' gut. Transmission may also occur by blood transfusion (1.7% per unit of blood; higher [13.3%] if platelet transfusion); there are increasing numbers of infected donors in cities because of migration from rural areas. Organisms may also cross the placenta to cause congenital infection (in 2%–8% of pregnancies for those infected); transmission through breastfeeding seems unlikely, so there is currently no restriction on breastfeeding by chagasic mothers. Transmission through ingestion of food or drink contaminated with triatomine feces has also been reported. Transplantation of organs from chagasic donors presents a growing risk of *T. cruzi* transmission. The countries with the highest seroprevalence were Bolivia, Argentina, El Salvador, and Honduras. Infection is uncommon in returned travelers.

Organisms are regularly present in the blood during the acute period and may persist in very small numbers throughout life in symptomatic and asymptomatic people. The vector becomes infective 10 to 30 days after biting an infected host; gut infection in the bug persists for life (as long as 2 years).

9. Treatment—

Drug	Benznidazole
Dose	• < 12 years: 10 mg/kg/day divided into 2 doses/day • > 12 years: 5–7 mg/kg/day divided into 2 doses/day
Route	PO
Alternative drug	Nifurtimox: • < 10 years: 15–20 mg/kg/day PO for 90 days • 11–16 years: 13.5–15 mg/kg/day PO for 90 days • ≥ 17 years: 8–10 mg/kg/day PO for 90 days
Duration	60 days for benznidazole
Special considerations and comments	• Longer duration used in HIV infection. • Cure in 60%–100% acute and congenital infections. • Recommended for children < 12 years (response rate 60%–85%). • More controversial to treat adults with indeterminate state based on recent results of BENEFIT trial. • Treatment during megaviscera states is not helpful.

Note: HIV = human immunodeficiency virus; PO = oral(ly).

10. Prevention—

1) Educate the public on mode of spread and methods of prevention.

2) In endemic regions, systematically attack vectors infesting poorly constructed houses and houses with thatched roofs using effective insecticides with residual action (spraying, use of insecticidal paints, or fumigant canisters).

3) Construct or repair living areas to eliminate lodging places for insect vectors and shelter for domestic and wild reservoir animals. In certain areas, palm trees close to houses often harbor infested bugs and can be considered a risk factor.

4) Use bed nets (preferably insecticide-impregnated) in houses infested by the vector.

5) Screen blood and organ donors living in or coming from endemic areas to prevent infection by transfusion or transplants as required by law in most countries in the Americas. In the USA, this is voluntary.

6) Screen children of infected mothers. Prenatal serology in pregnant women from endemic regions; if positive, check cord blood of baby and Chagas IgG at 9 months.

11. Special considerations—

1) Reporting: report to local health authority may be required in some endemic areas.

2) Epidemic measures: in areas of high incidence, field survey to determine distribution and density of vectors and animal host; implement measures described in Prevention.

3) Although triatomine vectors are still responsible for most human infections, successful programs based on application of residual insecticides have substantially reduced transmission by this route in the Southern Cone of South America. Uruguay, Chile, and parts of Brazil have been certified free of vector-borne transmission. Further research and implementation efforts are necessary in the Amazonian, Andean, and Central American regions, where transmission occurs through both domiciliated and nondomiciliated vectors. Many Latin American countries have made considerable progress in improving blood safety. Further information can be found at: http://www.who.int/chagas/en.

[N. Aronson]

TUBERCULOSIS AND OTHER MYCOBACTERIAL DISEASES

DISEASE	ICD-10 CODE
TUBERCULOSIS	ICD-10 A15–A19
DISEASES DUE TO OTHER MYCOBACTERIA	ICD-10 A31
Buruli ulcer (see "Buruli Ulcer")	

I. TUBERCULOSIS

1. Clinical features—Tuberculosis (TB) is classically thought to exist in 2 distinct forms: latent TB infection and active TB disease. A more contemporary approach acknowledges that TB exists on a continuum from TB infection to TB disease. Initial TB infection, usually via inhalation of TB bacilli aerosolized by a patient with pulmonary TB, can either be cleared or contained by the immune system. Containment leads to asymptomatic, latent TB infection, which can reactivate and lead to active TB disease. Alternatively, infection can immediately progress to active disease, referred to as primary TB. The transition from asymptomatic infection to symptomatic disease can take much longer than previously thought, giving rise to the concept of incipient (typically subclinical) TB. TB infection generally causes no outward clinical manifestations. It is characterized by microscopic lesions in the lungs that commonly heal, leaving few residual changes other than small pulmonary or tracheobronchial lymph node calcifications called Ghon's complex.

Active TB disease can have pulmonary and/or extrapulmonary manifestations. Pulmonary TB is the more common form in healthy adults. Extrapulmonary TB occurs in 15% to 30% of cases, often in children and people with human immunodeficiency virus (HIV). Any organ or tissue may be affected or the disease can be disseminated and lead to multiorgan involvement. The most common extrapulmonary sites are lymph nodes (33%), pleura (20%), genitourinary tract (5%-10%), bones and joints (5%-10%), meninges (5%), gastrointestinal tract and peritoneum (3.5%), and pericardium (2%-3%).

Cough, fatigue, fever, night sweats, and weight loss are common symptoms associated with active pulmonary TB. The onset is insidious over weeks to months. In most cases, the cough is initially nonproductive, later productive of purulent sputum, and can eventually progress to hemoptysis. Shortness of breath and hypoxia only occur late in the disease. Chest X-ray can show a wide range of findings. In some cases, there are pulmonary infiltrates and/or cavitary lesions in the upper segments of the lungs but other segments and the pleural spaces are frequently affected. Prolonged disease, even if successfully treated, can lead to fibrotic changes with volume loss and subsequent pulmonary hypertension with cor pulmonale.

2. Risk groups—The risk of infection is directly related to the degree of exposure to active pulmonary TB and less so to genetic or other host factors. Airborne transmission of *Mycobacterium tuberculosis* is most efficient in closed spaces with little sunlight. Hence, those in close contact with an infectious individual in a poorly ventilated home or workplace for several hours are most vulnerable. On a population level, the risk is mostly assessed by one's country of origin or residence but can vary significantly by region and socioeconomic status. For example, while the overall risk of TB infection is low in most high-income countries such as the USA, the risk is significantly higher in people who are homeless or incarcerated. Even in high-TB-burden countries, the risk varies between social groups and people of lower sociodemographic status are disproportionally affected.

The risk of progressing to active TB disease once infected is highest in children younger than 5 years, adolescents, young adults, the very old, and the immunocompromised, especially those with untreated HIV infection. Development of active disease is most likely in the first 2 years after infection or in the setting of weakened immunity, such as in the very young, the elderly, and those with immunosuppression. Screening for latent TB infection and treatment to prevent active TB disease therefore focuses on those at high risk of infection, such as contacts of people with infectious pulmonary TB, immigrants from high–TB-burden countries, prisoners, and people who are homeless; or those at high risk of progressing to active disease once infected, such as children younger than 5 years and individuals with some form of immunosuppression, including people living with HIV, patients initiating anti–tumor necrosis factor (anti-TNF) treatment, patients receiving dialysis, patients preparing for organ or hematopoietic stem cell transplantation, patients with diabetes, or patients with silicosis.

3. Causative agents—*M. tuberculosis* complex, which includes *M. tuberculosis, Mycobacterium bovis* (bovine tubercle bacillus, historically an important cause of TB transmitted through unpasteurized milk), and *Mycobacterium africanum* and *Mycobacterium canettii*, which are the causes of a small number of infections in Africa. Occasionally, other members of the *M. tuberculosis* complex, such as *Mycobacterium microti, Mycobacterium caprae, Mycobacterium pinnipedii, Mycobacterium mungi,* and *Mycobacterium orygis* produce disease clinically indistinguishable from TB.

4. Diagnosis—Latent TB infection can be detected by tuberculin skin testing (TST) or blood tests (interferon-gamma release assays [IGRAs]). Two commercially available IGRAs are QuantiFERON-TB Gold Plus and T-SPOT.TB. These tests become positive 2 to 6 weeks after infection. Both TST and IGRAs do not detect *M. tuberculosis* directly but rely on an immune response to TB antigens. While there are differences in test characteristics between TST and IGRAs, the most relevant difference is that TST can be falsely positive in those infected with some nontuberculous mycobacteria and those vaccinated with bacillus Calmette-Guérin (BCG), while IGRAs are specific for *M. tuberculosis* infection.

The diagnosis of active TB disease relies on detection of *M. tuberculosis* from the site of suspected infection. This has traditionally been achieved by microbiologic techniques including microscopic examination of the specimen using specialized staining techniques including the Kinyoun or Ziehl-Neelsen stains for light microscopy or auramine for fluorescence microscopy. Pulmonary TB is usually characterized according to the presence or absence of acid-fast bacilli (AFB) on this staining, which may have implications for infectiousness. At least 2 sputum specimens (1 early morning) should be obtained. Expert microscopy of 2 consecutive sputum specimens can identify the majority (80% or more) of smear-positive TB patients; however, in practice, its sensitivity is generally much lower.

Then the specimen undergoes mycobacterial culture using a solid (e.g., Löwenstein-Jensen or Middlebrook) or liquid (e.g., mycobacteria growth indicator tube) medium. Culture can take up to 6 weeks for growth.

Molecular methods such as the Xpert MTB/RIF have vastly improved the speed and sensitivity of TB diagnosis.

Since 2010, WHO has recommended Xpert for the rapid diagnosis of pulmonary and extrapulmonary TB in adults and children, including in high–HIV-prevalent settings and locations where multidrug-resistant TB (MDR-TB) is potentially present. This method also detects rifampicin resistance as a proxy of MDR-TB.

Persons with presumptive TB disease should have a full diagnostic evaluation, including a chest X-ray. In the absence of bacteriologic confirmation, active disease can be presumed if clinical, histologic, or radiologic evidence is suggestive of TB and other likely diseases can be ruled out. Diagnosis of TB among persons with HIV infection may be complicated by the tendency to yield negative smears. Serologic tests, TST, and IGRAs have no role in diagnosis of active TB, although TST and IGRAs are often used as additional evidence in young children since bacterial confirmation is so difficult to obtain.

All *M. tuberculosis* isolates, especially those from previously treated patients, should be submitted for culture and drug susceptibility testing. Rapid molecular tests such as line-probe assays result in more rapid diagnosis and treatment of drug-resistant TB.

5. Occurrence—Worldwide. It is estimated that 23% of the human population is infected with TB, mostly in low- and middle-income countries. Higher rates of latent TB have been reported in high-income countries in certain at-risk populations within nursing homes, homeless shelters, hospitals, and prisons.

WHO estimated the incidence of TB disease to be 10 million in 2017 but only 6.4 million cases were officially reported. Ninety-four percent of active TB occurred outside of Europe and the Americas, where it remains a dominant cause of morbidity and mortality. Only 8 countries contributed two-thirds of all TB cases: India (27%), China (9%), Indonesia (8%), the Philippines (6%), Pakistan (5%), Nigeria (4%), Bangladesh (4%), and South Africa (3%). People living with HIV continue to be disproportionately affected, representing 9% of all new cases, of which 72% reside in an African country.

TB incidence is increasing among at-risk populations in many high-income countries because of poverty-related living conditions, immigration from high-incidence areas, HIV infection, alcohol and substance use disorder, smoking, and diabetes. Dismantling of well-resourced TB care services has facilitated this. Morbidity and mortality rates are higher among impoverished, disadvantaged, and minority populations, often living in urban areas.

WHO data suggest that globally 3.5% of new TB cases and 18% of cases among previously treated patients are caused by MDR strains, with even higher proportions in countries of the former Soviet Union. Extensively drug-resistant TB (XDR-TB) is defined as MDR-TB plus resistance to any fluoroquinolones and any of the 3 injectable drugs (amikacin, kanamycin, and capreomycin). It has emerged in settings where second-line drug use has been poorly managed. About 8.5% of all MDR-TB cases are estimated to be XDR-TB.

HIV-associated pulmonary TB is common in persons with untreated HIV infection, especially in Africa. The mortality rates are high, as are the rates of transmission to other patients and health care workers. Strict enforcement of infection control, proactive case-finding, intensive contact investigation, and ensuring completion of appropriate treatment regimens are effective in stopping and preventing TB outbreaks.

Human infection with *M. bovis* occurs when bovine TB in cattle is poorly controlled and unpasteurized milk or dairy products are consumed. It is estimated that approximately 2% of active pulmonary TB cases and 9.4% of extrapulmonary TB cases worldwide are caused by *M. bovis*.

6. Reservoirs—Primarily humans; rarely other primates. *M. bovis* is found in cattle and a variety of other wild mammals.

7. Incubation period—For latent TB, it takes 2 to 10 weeks from infection to demonstrable primary lesion or significant TST reaction. IGRAs are usually positive by 10 weeks after exposure but the actual time from infection to IGRA conversion has not been adequately studied. Fewer than 10% of latently infected persons will develop active pulmonary TB disease in their lifetimes; half of those will progress to active pulmonary TB within 18 months after initial infection. Latent TB infection can persist for a lifetime. It is not yet possible to identify those with latent TB who will progress to active pulmonary TB nor the speed with which it will develop, although this is an area of active research. Rapid clinical progression is more common among infants and in the immunosuppressed, such as people living with HIV.

8. Transmission—Persons with active pulmonary TB transmit the tubercle bacilli during coughing, singing, or sneezing. The droplet nuclei are inhaled into the pulmonary alveoli of their contacts. The aerosolized particles containing *M. tuberculosis* are ingested by alveolar macrophages, initiating a new infection. Theoretically, the period of communicability lasts as long as viable tubercle bacilli are discharged in the sputum. Effective antimicrobial chemotherapy usually eliminates communicability (by reducing microbial burden and cough) within 4 to 7 days, although *M. tuberculosis* may still be cultured from sputum. Some untreated or inadequately treated patients with active pulmonary TB can have intermittently AFB-positive sputum and therefore be contagious for years. Studies suggest that persons with smear-negative, culture-positive active pulmonary TB can also be contagious, although to a lesser extent. Younger children with active TB generally are not contagious. The degree of communicability depends on intimacy and duration of exposure, the number of bacilli discharged, virulence of the bacilli, adequacy of ventilation, exposure of bacilli to sun or ultraviolet light, and opportunities for aerosolization through coughing, sneezing, or singing. Health care workers incur additional risk during aerosolizing procedures. The first 18 months after infection constitute the period of greatest risk for the development of active pulmonary TB. Laryngeal TB disease occurs rarely but is also thought to be contagious.

Direct invasion of mycobacteria through mucous membranes or breaks in the skin can occur but is extremely rare. Except for rare situations where there is a draining sinus, extrapulmonary TB (other than laryngeal) is not communicable. Bovine TB (caused by *M. bovis*) results from direct exposure to tuberculous cattle or the ingestion of unpasteurized contaminated milk or dairy products.

9. Treatment—Current national and international guidance recommends that treatment of drug-susceptible pulmonary TB be initiated with 4 drugs—isoniazid, rifampin, pyrazinamide, and ethambutol—administered for 2 months (intensive phase), followed by 2 drugs—isoniazid and rifampin—administered for at least 4 months (continuation phase). Extrapulmonary forms of TB may require longer durations of therapy. Expert consultation should be sought for management of MDR-TB.

Drug	Isoniazid	Rifampin	Pyrazinamide	Ethambutol
Adult dose	5 mg/kg (≤ 300 mg)	10 mg/kg (≤ 600 mg)	20–25 mg/kg (≤ 2,000 mg)	15–20 mg/kg (≤ 1,600 mg)
Route	PO	PO	PO	PO
Frequency and duration	Daily for 6 months	Daily for 6 months	Daily for 2 months	Daily for 2 months
Most common adverse reactions	Mild hepatic enzyme elevation, hepatotoxicity, peripheral neuritis, hypersensitivity.	Orange discoloration of secretions and urine, staining of contact lenses, hepatotoxicity, influenza-like reaction, thrombocytopenia, pruritus, oral contraceptives may be ineffective.	Hepatotoxicity, hyperuricemia, arthralgia, GI tract disturbances, pruritus, rash.	Optic neuritis (usually reversible), decreased red-green color discrimination, GI tract disturbances, hypersensitivity.

Note: GI = gastrointestinal; PO = oral(ly); TB = tuberculosis. Detailed information on TB treatment regimens and guidance can be found in the Official American Thoracic Society/Centers for Disease Control and Prevention/Infectious Diseases Society of America Clinical Practice Guidelines at: https://www.idsociety.org/practice-guideline/treatment-of-drug-susceptible-tb. As TB treatment guidelines are frequently updated, it is always best to consult the most current versions.

10. Prevention—

1) Primary prevention:

- Prompt diagnosis and treatment: render smear-positive active pulmonary and extrapulmonary TB noninfectious within 4 to 7 days by using an effective management regimen. Active case-finding by investigation of close contacts of infectious patients and among high-risk populations and provision of adequate treatment for all cases are key to reducing transmission. This normally requires a well-functioning TB program at the lowest health authority level coordinated with primary care facilities, using national best practice, training, supervision, and performance monitoring. Required are clinical, laboratory, and radiology facilities; physical examination of patients and contacts; provision of a regimen based on 4 essential anti-TB drugs; and support to patients through completion of treatment.

- Public education: inform the public regarding mode of spread, symptoms, methods of control, and importance of early diagnosis and continued adherence to treatment. Actively reduce stigma of TB disease and address incorrect beliefs about the incurability of TB.

- Infection control measures: establish and maintain effective TB infection control measures in institutional settings where health care is provided, especially where immunocompromised patients congregate, including hospitals, drug treatment programs, prisons, nursing homes, and homeless shelters.

- BCG vaccination: BCG is protective against TB disease in children with some benefit extending into adulthood. When given to newborns, it significantly reduces the risk of extrapulmonary TB (TB meningitis and disseminated disease) in children younger than 5 years and reduces the risk of pulmonary TB well into adulthood. Because the risk of infection is low in high-income countries, BCG is not used routinely in these settings. In countries with high TB prevalence, WHO recommends BCG vaccination for newborns as part of the routine immunization program. As it is a live attenuated vaccine, BCG is contraindicated in persons with immunodeficiency disorders, including infants and children with symptomatic HIV infection, because of the risk of disseminated BCG disease. There are ongoing efforts to develop a vaccine more effective than BCG and several promising candidate vaccines are currently in human clinical trials.

- Eliminate bovine TB among dairy cattle: tuberculin testing and slaughtering of positive reactors; pasteurize or boil milk and dairy products for human consumption.

- Address social determinants: reduce or eliminate social and economic conditions that increase the risk of infection and progression to disease, including poor living conditions, malnutrition, indoor air pollution, smoking, and alcohol and substance use disorder.

2) Secondary prevention:

- Treatment of latent TB infections: treatment for latent TB may be warranted for persons with a positive TST or IGRA. Previously known as preventive chemotherapy or chemoprophylaxis, it previously consisted of the administration of isoniazid for 6 to 9 months. This has been effective in preventing the progression of latent TB infection to TB disease in up to 70% of adherent individuals. Updated guidelines now recommend use of shorter regimens: 4 months of daily rifampin, 3 months of weekly rifapentine/isoniazid combination therapy, or 3 months of daily isoniazid and rifampin—all of which have been shown to be at least as effective.

  It is essential to rule out active pulmonary and extrapulmonary TB before starting treatment for latent TB infection in order to avoid inadvertently treating active disease with a 1- or 2-drug regimen that would engender the development of drug resistance.

  Persons started on preventive treatment for latent TB must be informed of possible adverse reactions and should be educated on how to recognize them. Active monitoring through health care visits or laboratory tests is not indicated. Rather, patients should be advised to discontinue treatment and seek medical advice if symptoms suggestive of adverse reactions or active TB develop. Checking liver function tests is important in patients with signs, symptoms, or a history of liver disease and in those who abuse alcohol.

  During pregnancy, it may be wise to postpone treatment for latent TB infection until after delivery, except in high-risk individuals, in whom it should be administered with caution. If isoniazid treatment is prescribed for pregnant women or in the immediate postpartum period, monthly routine hepatic transaminases should be monitored. Breastfeeding is not contraindicated.

  WHO recommends latent TB treatment for all people with HIV. In high–TB- and high–HIV-prevalence settings with a high rate of transmission and reinfection risk, 36 months of treatment with isoniazid is more effective in this group than 6 months, regardless of TST (or IGRA) status.

- Screening for active pulmonary and extrapulmonary TB: people living with HIV need to be screened for symptomatic TB at any clinical checkup using a simple symptom-based screening algorithm based on 4 symptoms (presence of cough of any duration, weight loss, fever, and night sweats). They should be investigated for active pulmonary or extrapulmonary TB disease if any 1 of the symptoms is reported through proper medical history and examination, including Xpert MTB/RIF and chest X-ray. In the absence of symptoms and if patients have tested positive with TST or IGRA, they should be offered treatment for latent TB.

11. Special considerations—

1) Reporting: report active pulmonary or extrapulmonary TB to local public health authorities when diagnosis is suspected; case reports are obligatory in most countries. They should state whether the case is bacteriologically confirmed (AFB smear–positive, culture-positive, or positive by molecular detection) or the diagnosis is based on clinical and/or radiographic findings and whether the patient was previously treated. Public health authorities should maintain a register of patients requiring treatment and must be actively involved with planning and monitoring the course of treatment.

2) TB and air travel: several incidents of potential transmission of TB related to international air travel have been reported since the early 1990s. More recently, the emergence of MDR-TB and XDR-TB has raised the concern of air travel and TB transmission. The 2007 International Health Regulations, which provide a legal framework for a more effective and coordinated international response to public health emergencies and risks, including those caused by outbreaks of communicable diseases such as XDR-TB, have important provisions for the detection and control of TB during air travel. Available evidence indicates that the risk of transmission of TB on board aircraft is low and limited to persons in close proximity to an infectious person for 8 hours or longer. Passenger-to-passenger transmission of *M. tuberculosis* has been documented only among passengers seated in the same section as the index case. The risk of TB among cabin crew members is similar to that of the general population. Therefore, mandatory routine or periodic screening is not indicated for cabin crew. There is no evidence that recirculation of cabin air facilitates the transmission of infectious disease agents on board.

3) Further information can be found at:

- https://www.who.int/tb/en
- https://www.cdc.gov/tb/default.htm
- http://www.stoptb.org.

II. DISEASES DUE TO OTHER MYCOBACTERIA
(mycobacterioses, nontuberculous mycobacterial disease)

1. Clinical features—Clinical syndromes associated with the non-tuberculous mycobacteria (NTM or mycobacteria other than *M. tuberculosis* complex organisms and *Mycobacterium leprae*) can be classified broadly as follows:

1) Disseminated disease—often in the presence of severe immunodeficiency such as HIV/acquired immunodeficiency syndrome or medical immunosuppression—can be caused by *Mycobacterium avium* complex (MAC), *Mycobacterium kansasii*, *Mycobacterium haemophilum*, *Mycobacterium genavense*, and the rapidly growing mycobacteria (RGM). Symptoms often include fever with night sweats, inadvertent weight loss, anemia, and fatigue. Diagnosis can be achieved through culture from blood, liver, or bone marrow.

2) Pulmonary disease resembling TB: MAC, *M. kansasii*, *Mycobacterium abscessus* (MAB), *Mycobacterium xenopi*, *Mycobacterium simiae*, and *Mycobacterium malmoense*. NTM pulmonary disease should be suspected in cases of prolonged cough with sputum production, especially in patients with underlying chronic pulmonary disease with AFB-positive sputum for whom *M. tuberculosis* has been ruled out.

3) Lymphadenitis (primarily cervical): MAC and *M. kansasii.*

4) Skin ulcers: *Mycobacterium ulcerans* (see "Buruli Ulcer"), *Mycobacterium marinum*, and the RGM. These infections may appear nodular or ulcerating; at times, they spread proximally along the lymphatics (i.e., sporotrichoid spread).

5) Posttraumatic wound infections: *Mycobacterium fortuitum*, *Mycobacterium chelonae*, *M. abscessus*, *M. marinum*, and MAC.

6) Nosocomial disease: RGM associated with surgical wound infections, catheter-related infections (bacteremia and peritonitis), post-injection abscesses, and infections introduced by contaminated bronchoscopes.

2. Risk groups—Immunocompromised persons are at risk for NTM infections. Patients with advanced HIV are susceptible to disseminated NTM but not pulmonary disease. Patients with rheumatologic and autoimmune diseases taking TNF-α inhibitors are uniquely susceptible to pulmonary and extrapulmonary NTM infections. Patients with abnormal lung architecture such as those with cystic fibrosis and chronic obstructive pulmonary disease are also at increased risk for pulmonary NTM infections such as MAC and MAB.

3. Causative agents—From 41 valid species in 1980, currently the genus *Mycobacterium* encompasses more than 200 recognized species. Some species also are further classified as subspecies. For example, MAC includes *Mycobacterium avium* subsp. *avium*, *Mycobacterium avium* subsp. *intracellulare*, *Mycobacterium avium* subsp. *paratuberculosis*, *Mycobacterium avium* subsp. *chimaera*, and others, whereas MAB includes *Mycobacterium abscessus* subsp. *abscessus*, *Mycobacterium abscessus* subsp. *massiliense*, and *Mycobacterium abscessus* subsp.

bolletti. One group of NTM are classified together based on their rapid growth (within 7 days) after subculture on a solid medium. The so-called RGM include the MAB complex, *M. chelonae*, *M. fortuitum*, and *Mycobacterium peregrinum*.

4. Diagnosis—Guidance regarding diagnosis of NTM infections can be found at: https://www.thoracic.org/statements/resources/mtpi/non-tuberculous-mycobacterial-diseases.pdf. An update to this document is anticipated but currently this is a useful source for distinguishing colonization, laboratory contamination, and clinically important infections. For example, a symptomatic patient suspected of NTM pulmonary disease should meet radiographic (e.g., nodular or cavitary opacities on chest X-ray or multifocal bronchiectasis with multiple small nodules on a high-resolution computed tomography scan) and microbiologic criteria:

1) Positive culture results from at least 2 separate expectorated sputum samples OR
2) Positive culture results from at least 1 bronchial wash or lavage OR
3) Transbronchial or other lung biopsy with mycobacterial histopathologic features (granulomatous inflammation or AFB) and positive culture for NTM or biopsy showing mycobacterial histopathologic features (granulomatous inflammation or AFB) and 1 or more sputum or bronchial washing that is culture-positive for NTM.

Consistent with this, it should be noted that a single isolation of NTM from sputum may be evidence of simple pulmonary or oropharyngeal colonization or laboratory contamination. This is especially true of certain NTM (e.g., *Mycobacterium gordonae*) but a single isolate of other NTM may be sufficient to consider treatment (e.g., *M. kansasii*).

Unlike for pulmonary NTM disease, a single positive culture from blood, a wound, or tissue is generally considered diagnostic.

5. Occurrence—Currently, there is no mandate to report individual NTM cases to public health authorities, so reliable surveillance data are not available. Most authorities believe, however, that the incidence of these infections is increasing. Clusters of diseases should be reported to public health authorities because these may represent widespread outbreaks such as have been seen with RGM outbreaks following medical tourism (e.g., cosmetic surgery) to international health care settings. There have been other nosocomial outbreaks related to contaminated medical devices, such as contaminated bronchoscopes, and a global outbreak with *M. chimaera* linked conclusively to the heater-cooler units used during cardiac surgery.

6. Reservoirs—NTM are ubiquitous environmental microorganisms that can be recovered from soil, freshwater, and seawater.

7. Incubation period—Unknown for each NTM species.

8. Transmission—Because NTM may be found in both natural and man-made reservoirs, most human infections are suspected to be acquired from environmental sources such as aerosolized hot water (e.g., hot tubs), dirt, or contaminated medical devices. Human-to-human transmission of NTM has only been documented for *M. abscessus* among patients with cystic fibrosis.

9. Treatment—Treatment of NTM infections is also reviewed in the American Thoracic Society statement (http://www.thoracic.org/sections/publications/statements/pages/mtpi/nontuberculous-mycobacterial-diseases.html). In brief, traditional anti-TB drugs may not be effective for NTM. Treatment is reliably effective against *M. kansasii* pulmonary disease (rifamycin and ethambutol with either a macrolide or isoniazid) and *M. marinum* cutaneous disease (2- or 3-drug combinations of a macrolide, sulfonamides, ethambutol, and tetracyclines appear effective, usually for 3-4 months) but other NTM may be more difficult to treat. Drug susceptibility tests are increasingly available in Europe and the USA but in vivo correlations of most results and treatment success are limited. For example, when drug susceptibility testing shows a MAC isolate to be sensitive to a macrolide, noncavitary pulmonary MAC disease can usually be treated successfully with approximately 18 months of ethambutol, rifamycin (rifampin or rifabutin), plus a macrolide (clarithromycin or azithromycin). Pulmonary MAB disease is extremely difficult to treat, often requiring an induction with both oral and intravenous antimycobacterials (especially when an active *erm*-resistant gene is present), followed by a prolonged oral continuation phase. In such cases, surgical resection or debulking may improve outcomes.

10. Prevention—NTM commonly contaminate environmental sources. Available information does not support specific recommendations regarding avoidance of exposure. HIV-infected adults and adolescents should receive chemoprophylaxis with a macrolide against disseminated MAC disease if their cluster of differentiation (CD4+) count is lower than 50 cells/μl, unless they are promptly started on antiretroviral therapy with the expectation that their CD4+ count improves rapidly.

11. Special considerations—Exposure to or infection with many NTM species may cause false-positive TST results. By contrast, *M. kansasii*, *M. marinum*, *Mycobacterium riyadhense*, and *Mycobacterium szulgai* are the only NTM that may cause false-positive IGRA results.

[L. Adams, D. de Gijsel, E. Talbot]

TULAREMIA

(rabbit fever, deer-fly fever, water-rat trapper's disease, wild hare disease [yato-byo], Ohara's disease, Francis disease)

DISEASE	ICD-10 CODE
TULAREMIA	ICD-10 A21

1. Clinical features—Tularemia is a bacterial zoonotic infection that produces 1 of 6 clinical syndromes depending on the site of inoculation and the virulence of the infecting organism. The most common syndrome is ulceroglandular tularemia, characterized by fever, a skin ulcer—often with a central eschar—and regional lymphadenopathy following tick or animal exposure. Occasionally more than 1 skin lesion may be present. Glandular tularemia has a similar presentation but lacks an obvious skin ulcer. Oropharyngeal tularemia presents following the ingestion of contaminated food or water. Signs and symptoms include fever and painful pharyngitis (with or without exudate or ulceration) and marked cervical lymphadenopathy, which may be unilateral. Pneumonic tularemia may be primary, following inhalation of the organism, or secondary, owing to hematogenous spread to the lungs from other parts of the body, especially in the setting of ulceroglandular or typhoidal disease. Patients typically present with fever, constitutional symptoms, and a minimally productive cough. Substernal or pleuritic chest pain may occur. Although not readily distinguished from other forms of community-acquired pneumonia, pneumonic tularemia is often accompanied by an exudative pleural effusion with lymphocytic predominance that yields the organism if cultured. Secondary pneumonic tularemia often presents with bilateral infiltrates. Pneumonic tularemia can be life-threatening; however the overall case-fatality rate is less than 5% with proper treatment. In addition to community-acquired pneumonia, the differential diagnosis includes anthrax, brucellosis, plague, staphylococcal and streptococcal infections, and tuberculosis. Oculoglandular tularemia is characterized by conjunctivitis, which may be purulent, punctate palpebral ulcers, and periauricular, posterior auricular, submandibular, or cervical lymphadenopathy. The sixth syndrome, typhoidal tularemia, presents as a nonspecific and nonlocalizing febrile illness accompanied by constitutional symptoms such as arthralgias, myalgias, headache, malaise, cough, sore throat, abdominal pain, and diarrhea. The presentation may range from an acute septic syndrome to a chronic febrile illness. Fever may subside after a few days but then return. Associated laboratory findings may include hyponatremia, renal insufficiency, and an elevated categorycreatine phosphokinase. The white blood count may be low, normal, or high. Thrombocytopenia and transaminase elevation are occasionally present.

2. Risk groups—As with other zoonotic diseases, the risk of acquiring tularemia is closely linked to occupational and recreational activities. Hunters, trappers, sheepshearers, veterinarians, forest rangers, game wardens, hikers, campers, and others with frequent animal or arthropod exposure are at increased risk of infection. In some areas, farmers and landscapers appear to be at increased risk of pneumonic tularemia as a consequence of exposure to contaminated dust and aerosols. *Francisella tularensis* is highly infectious when grown in culture and numerous cases have been documented among laboratory workers. A few recent cases have been linked to commercially traded pets, suggesting that persons in the pet industry may also be at increased risk.

3. Causative agents—*F. tularensis* is a highly infectious, small, faintly staining, pleomorphic Gram-negative coccobacillus. The majority of human infections are caused by 2 subspecies that differ in distribution and virulence: *Francisella tularensis* subsp. *tularensis* (Jellison type A, generally the more virulent) and *Francisella tularensis* subsp. *holarctica* (Jellison type B). A third subspecies, *Francisella tularensis* subsp. *mediasiatica*, has been isolated from animals in Central Asia but has not been linked to human illness. Related species, including *Francisella novicida*, *Francisella philomiragia*, and *Francisella hispaniensis*, are rare causes of human illness.

4. Diagnosis—Tularemia should be suspected in those presenting with a compatible clinical syndrome and a risk of exposure. The diagnosis is generally established serologically by demonstrating a 4-fold rise in specific antibody titers between acute and convalescent sera using tube agglutination or microagglutination. Cross-reactions with *Brucella* or *Legionella* spp. have been observed when using tube agglutination. In some instances a sufficiently high titer in a single specimen is considered positive. Enzyme-linked immunosorbent assays for tularemia have also been used, especially in Europe. Culture can provide a conclusive diagnosis but must be attempted only with appropriate biosafety conditions. Appropriate specimens include swabs or scrapings of skin lesions, lymph node aspirates or biopsies, pharyngeal swabs, sputum, bronchial/tracheal washings, sputum, or pleural fluid, depending on the form of illness. Blood cultures should also be collected, although the yield is low.

When tularemia is suspected, it should be communicated to laboratory personnel beforehand because of the need to select the most appropriate specimens and the requirement for using special isolation procedures. A presumptive diagnosis of tularemia may be made through the testing of suspected isolates using direct fluorescent antibody testing, immunohistochemical staining, or polymerase chain reaction assays. In some jurisdictions *F. tularensis* has been identified as a select agent and therefore only registered laboratories are allowed to work with the organism.

5. Occurrence—Tularemia occurs regionally throughout the Northern Hemisphere. It has been reported in Scandinavia, continental Europe, Central Asia, the Middle East, Russia, northern regions of China, and Japan but not north of the Arctic Circle or in the British Isles. In North America,

F. tularensis has been found from northern Mexico to the Arctic Circle in Alaska. Whereas type B infections occur throughout the Northern Hemisphere, the more virulent type A infections are limited to North America. Seasonality depends on the predominant mode of transmission and can be bimodal, with arthropod-associated infections occurring in the warmer months and rabbit-associated infections occurring in the winter. Outbreaks of human tularemia usually occur in association with animal epizootics, although these may not be recognized without a careful environmental investigation. Epidemics among humans may also be triggered by war and social disruption.

   6. Reservoirs—Reservoirs for the infection include wild animals, especially rabbits, hares, voles, muskrats, water rats, beavers, and some domestic animals, as well as various hard ticks. A rodent-mosquito cycle has been described for *F. tularensis* subsp. *holarctica* in the Scandinavian countries and Russia. Recent studies have suggested a possible role for free-living amoeba as a reservoir for type B strains.

   7. Incubation period—The incubation period for the development of symptoms is related to the size of the inoculum and is usually 3 to 5 days (range, 1-21 days).

   8. Transmission—Humans become infected through arthropod bites, handling infected animal tissues, ingestion of contaminated food or water, or inhalation of contaminated aerosols. Symptoms vary according to the route of exposure (see Clinical Features in this chapter). Principal tick vectors in North America include *Dermacentor variabilis*, *Dermacentor andersoni*, and *Amblyomma americanum*; Eurasian tick vectors include *Ixodes ricinus*, *Dermacentor reticulatus*, and *Dermacentor marginatus*. Tabanid flies (*Chrysops* spp.) are mechanical vectors that can transmit infection to a wide range of hosts. Mosquitoes have been implicated as vectors in Eurasia but not in North America. Hunting-associated cases are usually associated with rabbits, hares, muskrats, or voles; a small outbreak in Spain was linked to collecting freshwater crayfish. Waterborne transmission has been reported as a result of unchlorinated wells and municipal systems and of natural bodies of water. Inhalational exposures can occur during agricultural activities, including sorting contaminated hay and mowing. The average infectious dose for humans is estimated at 10 organisms by subcutaneous inoculation and 25 organisms by aerosol. All ages are susceptible and long-term immunity follows recovery. Reinfection is extremely rare but has been reported in laboratory staff. Person-to-person transmission has never been reported.

9. Treatment—

Preferred therapy	Mild disease:
	<ul><li>Ciprofloxacin 500 mg PO BID for 14 days OR</li><li>Doxycycline 100 mg PO BID for 14 days</li></ul>
	Moderate-to-serious disease:
	<ul><li>Streptomycin 7.5–10 mg/kg IM every 12 hours for 7–14 days</li></ul>
	Meningitis:
	<ul><li>Streptomycin (7.5–10 mg/kg IM every 12 hours for 7–14 days) OR gentamicin (adults: 5 mg/kg IM or IV daily divided every 8 hours for 14–21 days) PLUS</li><li>Chloramphenicol 15–25 mg/kg IV every 6 hours for 14–21 days OR doxycycline 100 mg IV every 12 hours for 14–21 days</li></ul>
Alternative therapy options	Moderate-to-serious disease:
	<ul><li>Streptomycin 15 mg/kg IM every 12 hours for 3 days, THEN 7.5 mg/kg every 12 hours through day 7 or day 10 OR</li><li>Gentamicin 5 mg/kg/day IM or IV divided every 8 hours for 7–10 days</li></ul>
Special considerations and comments	<ul><li>Doxycycline should be used in patients < 8 years only if the risks are outweighed by the benefits.</li><li>Doses > 2 g/day of streptomycin in adults do not increase efficacy and should not be given.</li><li>Streptomycin is the drug of choice for adults and gentamicin is the drug of choice for children. Dosing must be adjusted according to serum concentrations for individuals with renal insufficiency and for pediatric patients. Target serum streptomycin concentrations for IM administration are trough < 10 μg/mL and peak ≤ 20–25 μg/mL. Streptomycin is ototoxic and warrants audiometric testing for situations in which serum concentration monitoring is warranted. For obese patients dosing should be determined based on adjusted weight.</li></ul>

Note: BID = twice daily; IM = intramuscular(ly); IV = intravenous(ly); PO = oral(ly).

10. Prevention—

1) Educate the public to avoid bites of ticks, flies, and mosquitoes, for example by using long sleeves and repellents, and to avoid contact with untreated water where infection is endemic among wild animals.

2) Use impervious gloves when skinning or handling animals, especially rabbits. Cook the meat of wild rabbits and rodents thoroughly. Avoid handling such meat together with vegetables.

3) Use universal precautions in direct handling of small animals (especially pets) that are exhibiting signs and symptoms of illness.

4) Live attenuated vaccines applied intradermally by scarification are used extensively in Russia and to a limited extent for occupational risk groups in some other countries such as Sweden.

5) Take appropriate precautions (using face masks, gowns, and impervious gloves and carrying out work under class II biosafety cabinets) when handling cultures of *F. tularensis*.

11. Special considerations—

1) Reporting: reporting of documented cases to local health authorities may be required in some endemic areas.

2) In epidemics search for sources of infection related to arthropods, animal hosts, water, and environments soiled by small mammals, including hay. Control measures should be employed as outlined under Prevention in this chapter.

3) *F. tularensis* is a category A bioterrorism agent that could be weaponized in aerosol form and would produce pneumonia in affected hosts several days after exposure. Such cases require prompt identification and specific treatment to prevent a fatal outcome. All diagnosed cases, and especially clusters of pneumonia due to *F. tularensis*, must be reported immediately to the health department for appropriate investigation.

[D. Longworth, A. Davis]

TYPHOID FEVER AND PARATYPHOID FEVER

DISEASE	ICD-10 CODE
TYPHOID FEVER	ICD-10 A01.0
PARATYPHOID FEVER	ICD-10 A01.1–A01.4

1. Clinical features—A systemic bacterial disease characterized by the insidious onset of sustained fever, marked headache, and malaise. Other symptoms and signs present in some patients include anorexia, relative bradycardia, splenomegaly, nonproductive cough in the early stage of the illness, rose spots on the trunk (visible in 25% of light-skinned patients), and constipation more often than diarrhea in adults. The clinical picture varies from mild illness with low-grade fever to severe clinical disease with abdominal discomfort and multiple complications. Severity is influenced by factors such as strain virulence, quantity of inoculum ingested, duration of illness before adequate treatment, age, and, for typhoid fever, typhoid vaccination. Inapparent or mild illnesses occur, especially in endemic areas; 60% to 90% of patients with typhoid fever do not receive medical attention or are treated as outpatients. Mild cases show no systemic involvement; the clinical picture is that of gastroenteritis (see "Salmonellosis"). Fevers without sweating, delirium or coma, hearing loss, and parotitis may occur. Peyer patches in the ileum can ulcerate, with intestinal hemorrhage or perforation (3% of cases in the developing world) occurring most commonly in the absence of timely, appropriate antimicrobial therapy. Severe forms with altered mental status and other neurologic complications have been associated with high case-fatality rates. The case-fatality rate of 10% to 20% observed in the pre-antibiotic era can fall to less than 1% with prompt appropriate antimicrobial therapy. Ten to twenty percent of patients experience relapses (generally milder than the initial clinical illness).

Paratyphoid fever presents with a similar clinical picture. The ratio of typhoid fever to paratyphoid fever is estimated to be about 4:1; this may decrease as typhoid vaccination becomes more common. Relapses occur in 3% to 4% of cases.

2. Risk groups—In endemic areas, typhoid fever is most common in children; in epidemic areas, cases of typhoid fever have a broad age distribution. Travelers to endemic areas are also at risk, as are individuals with gastric achlorhydria. Partial immunity follows recovery from clinical disease, inapparent infection, and active immunization.

3. Causative agents—*Salmonella enterica* serotype Typhi is the etiologic agent of typhoid fever. Paratyphoid fever may be caused by *S. enterica* serotypes Paratyphi A, Paratyphi B, or Paratyphi C. The term "enteric fever" is sometimes used to describe invasive febrile infections caused by serotypes Typhi, Paratyphi A, Paratyphi B, and Paratyphi C. Paratyphi B is differentiated into 2 distinct pathotypes: one is unable to ferment tartrate and is associated with paratyphoid fever (referred to as Paratyphi B) and the other ferments tartrate and is associated with uncomplicated gastroenteritis—referred to as Paratyphi B subsp. L(+) tartrate(+). Although some nontyphoidal *Salmonella* serotypes (e.g., serotypes Dublin and Choleraesuis) may also commonly cause invasive infections, the term "enteric fever" is limited to disease caused by the Typhi and Paratyphi serotypes (not including serotype Paratyphi B subsp. L (+) tartarate(+)).

4. Diagnosis—The causal organisms can be isolated from blood early in the disease and from urine and feces after the first week. Blood culture is the diagnostic mainstay for typhoid fever but bone marrow culture provides the most sensitive method for bacteriologic confirmation even in patients who have already received antimicrobial agents. Because of limited sensitivity and specificity, serologic tests based on agglutinating antibodies (Widal) are generally of little diagnostic value. Although rapid serodiagnostic tests (such as TUBEX TF) based on the detection of specific antibodies have better sensitivity and specificity than the Widal test, these culture-independent diagnostic tests (CIDTs) are still poorly suited for individual patient diagnosis. Bacterial isolation from culture is necessary for determining serotype and performing antimicrobial susceptibility testing to inform clinical management. CIDTs, in contrast, are more useful for rapid identification of the cause of an outbreak of febrile illness.

5. Occurrence—Worldwide, the annual estimated incidence of typhoid fever is 11 million to 21 million cases and 128,000 to 161,000 deaths. Most of the disease burden occurs in the developing world. Most cases in industrialized countries are sporadic and are acquired during travel in endemic areas. Paratyphoid fever occurs sporadically or in limited outbreaks, probably more frequently than reports suggest. Of the 3 serotypes, Paratyphi A is the most common, Paratyphi B is less frequent, and Paratyphi C is extremely rare.

6. Reservoirs—Exclusively humans for serotypes Typhi and Paratyphi A; humans and possibly domestic animals for other serotypes. A carrier state may follow acute or mild illness or even subclinical infections. Short-term fecal carriers are more common than urinary carriers. The chronic carrier state, with organism excretion lasting more than 12 months, is most common (2%–5%) among persons infected during middle age, especially women; serotype Typhi colonizes the gallbladder and carriers frequently have biliary tract abnormalities including gallstones. The chronic urinary carrier state is rare and has been associated with schistosome infections, urinary tract abnormalities, or kidney stones.

7. Incubation period—Depends on inoculum size and on host factors; for typhoid fever, usually 8 to 14 days but with a range of 3 to 60 days; for paratyphoid fever, the incubation period is usually 1 to 10 days.

8. Transmission—Through ingestion of food and water contaminated by feces or urine of patients and carriers. Important vehicles include shellfish (particularly oysters) from sewage-contaminated beds, raw fruit and vegetables, frozen fruit, contaminated milk or milk products (usually contaminated through hands of carriers), and untreated drinking water. Flies may contaminate foods in which the organism then multiplies to infective doses (those are reportedly lower for typhoid than for paratyphoid bacteria). Epidemiologic data suggest that, whereas waterborne transmission of *S. enterica* serotype Typhi usually involves small inocula, foodborne transmission is associated with large inocula and high attack rates over short periods. Sexual transmission of typhoid fever from an asymptomatic carrier has been documented. Patients are infectious for as long as bacilli appear in excreta—usually from the first week throughout convalescence; variable thereafter (commonly 1-2 weeks for paratyphoid bacteria). About 10% of untreated typhoid fever patients discharge bacilli for 3 months after onset of symptoms. Both treated and untreated patients can become chronic carriers; fewer persons infected with paratyphoid organisms become chronic carriers.

9. Treatment—The selection of appropriate empiric therapy depends on the severity of disease, risk of infection with an antibiotic-resistant strain, and age of the patient. Appropriate antibiotic therapy reduces mortality and morbidity. Supportive care (e.g., hydration and nutrition) and monitoring for complications are important aspects of management. Complications include organ system dysfunction, encephalopathy, and septic shock.

A complete travel history and culture and antimicrobial susceptibility testing are important in the management of suspected cases. Antibiotic therapy should be tailored to susceptibility results when feasible. Although fluoroquinolones (e.g., ciprofloxacin) and traditional antibiotics (ampicillin, chloramphenicol, and trimethoprim-sulfamethoxazole) are effective against susceptible strains, nonsusceptibility to these agents is now widespread globally. Fluoroquinolone nonsusceptibility (defined as intermediate or full resistance) is high among Typhi and Paratyphi A isolates in the USA ($\geq$ 66% in 2015); this is even higher among isolates from travelers returning from South Asia ($\geq$ 90% during 2008–2012). Infections with fluoroquinolone-non-susceptible strains have been associated with treatment failure and delayed clinical response. Therefore, fluoroquinolones are not recommended as empiric therapy, particularly for infections in travelers from South Asia and other regions where rates of fluoroquinolone nonsusceptibility are high. Third-generation cephalosporins (e.g., ceftriaxone) are recommended for empiric treatment of severe or complicated disease. Azithromycin is used for the empiric management of uncomplicated disease, particularly in areas or settings where fluoroquinolone-nonsusceptible and multidrug-resistant strains are common. Third-generation cephalosporin resistance and azithromycin resistance remain rare in the USA. However, a large outbreak of *Salmonella* Typhi infections resistant to ceftriaxone and nonsusceptible to fluoroquinolones emerged in Pakistan in 2016 and was ongoing in late 2019. Azithromycin and selected carbapenems have been used for treatment. Sporadic cases of azithromycin-resistant infections have been reported outside the USA.

1) Empiric therapy:

Empiric Treatment of Severe or Complicated Disease

Drug	Ceftriaxone (third-generation cephalosporins)
Dose	• Adults: 2 g once or twice daily ($\leq$ 4 g/day) • Children: 50–100 mg/kg/day in 1 or 2 divided doses ($\leq$ 2 g/day)
Route	IV
Duration	10–14 days

Alternative drug	• Cefotaxime:
	  ○ Adults: 1–2 g IV every 6 or 8 hours for 10–14 days
	  ○ Children: 150–200 mg/kg/day IV in 3–4 divided doses for 10–14 days ($\leq$ 8 g/day)

Special considerations and comments	• In 2016–2019, a large outbreak of XDR typhoid fever—defined as infections resistant to third-generation cephalosporins, nonsusceptible to fluoroquinolones, and resistant to traditional first-line antibiotics ampicillin, chloramphenicol, and TMP/SMX—was reported in Pakistan, with cases documented in global travelers. For severe or complicated XDR infections, a carbapenem is recommended. • Adjunctive therapy with high-dose corticosteroid can decrease mortality. • In patients with intestinal perforation, prompt surgical intervention improves survival.

Note: IV = intravenous(ly); TMP/SMX = trimethoprim-sulfamethoxazole; XDR = extensively drug-resistant.

2) Directed therapy:

Empiric Treatment of Uncomplicated Disease

Drug	Azithromycin
Dose	• Adults: 1 g once, THEN 500 mg or 1 g once daily • Children: 10–20 mg/kg once daily ($\leq$ 1 g/day)
Route	PO
Duration	5–7 days

Alternative drug	• Cefixime:
	  ○ Adults: 200 mg PO BID for 10–14 days
	  ○ Children: 20 mg/kg PO in 2 divided doses for 10–14 days ($\leq$ 400 mg/day)

Special considerations and comments	• Azithromycin is recommended for empiric therapy of uncomplicated infections, particularly those acquired in South Asia or other areas where fluoroquinolone-nonsusceptible strains are common. It is also recommended for uncomplicated XDR infections. • There have been sporadic reports of azithromycin-resistant infections outside the USA.

Note: BID = twice daily; PO = oral(ly); XDR = extensively drug-resistant.

Treatment of Fluoroquinolone-Susceptible Infection

Drug	Ciprofloxacin (fluoroquinolones)
Dose	• Adults: 500 mg BID • Children: 30 mg/kg/day in 2 divided doses (≤ 1 g/day)
Route	PO
Duration	7–10 days

Alternative drug	• Azithromycin[a]
	• Cefixime[a]
	• Ofloxacin:
	  ○ Adults: 400 mg PO BID for 7–10 days
	  ○ Children: 15–30 mg/kg/day PO in 2 divided doses (≤ 800 mg/day) for 7–10 days[b]

Special considerations and comments	• Fluoroquinolones are not recommended for routine use in children < 18 years but can be used in severe infection or when no alternative agent is available. • For pregnant women, routine fluoroquinolone use is not recommended given concerns of possible teratogenicity; azithromycin is generally considered safe. • Most Typhi and Paratyphi A infections in the USA are acquired during international travel and are caused by fluoroquinolone-nonsusceptible strains.

Note: BID = twice daily; PO = oral(ly).
[a]See earlier table for doses.
[b]Limited data available to inform pediatric dosing.

Treatment of Fluoroquinolone-Nonsusceptible Infection

Drug	Azithromycin
Dose	• Adults: 1 g once, THEN 500 mg or 1 g once daily • Children: 10–20 mg/kg once daily (≤ 1 g/day)
Route	PO
Duration	5–7 days
Alternative drug	• Ceftriaxone[a] • Cefixime[a]
Special considerations and comments	• Azithromycin is recommended for uncomplicated infections. • When azithromycin cannot be used, other options, depending on antimicrobial susceptibility and severity of disease, include third-generation cephalosporins (e.g., ceftriaxone, cefixime), amoxicillin, TMP/SMX, chloramphenicol.

Note: PO = oral(ly); TMP/SMX = trimethoprim-sulfamethoxazole.
[a]See earlier table for doses.

10. Prevention—Prevention is based on access to safe water and proper sanitation and on adherence to safe food-handling practices.

1) Instruct the community, patients, convalescents, and carriers in personal hygiene. Emphasize handwashing as a routine practice after defecation and before preparing, serving, or eating food. Provide suitable handwashing facilities, particularly for food handlers and attendants involved in the care of patients and children.

2) Dispose of human feces safely and maintain fly-proof latrines. Where culturally appropriate, encourage use of sufficient toilet paper to minimize hand contamination. Under field conditions, dispose of feces by burial at a site distant and downstream from the source of drinking water. Discourage the use of human feces as fertilizer.

3) Protect, purify, and chlorinate public water supplies, provide safe private supplies, and avoid possible backflow connections between water and sewer systems. For individual and small-group protection and during travel or in the field, consume boiled, chemically treated, or bottled water.

4) Use scrupulous cleanliness in food preparation and handling; refrigerate as appropriate. Pay particular attention to the storage of salads and other foods served cold. These provisions apply to home and public eating places. If uncertain about sanitary practices, select foods that are cooked and served hot and fruit that is peeled by the consumer.

5) Pasteurize or boil all milk and dairy products. Supervise the sanitary aspects of commercial milk production, storage, and delivery.

6) Enforce suitable quality-control procedures in industries that prepare food and drink for human consumption. Use chlorinated water for cooling during canned food processing.

7) Limit the collection and marketing of shellfish to supplies from approved sources. Boil or steam (10 minutes) before serving.

8) Encourage breastfeeding throughout infancy; boil all milk and water used for infant feeding in developing countries or where there may be breaches in pasteurization.

9) Typhoid carriers should be excluded from handling food and from providing patient care. Identify, treat, and follow up typhoid carriers to ensure eradication of carriage. Chronic carriers should not be released from follow-up and restriction of occupation until local or state regulations are met—often not until 3 consecutive negative cultures are obtained from fecal specimens (and urine in areas endemic for schistosomiasis) over the course of several days

to 2 months and at least 48 hours after antimicrobial therapy has stopped. Fresh stool specimens are preferred to rectal swabs. It has been suggested that at least 1 of the 3 consecutive negative stool specimens should be obtained by purging, though this is rarely practical. Administration of ciprofloxacin or norfloxacin twice daily for 28 days provides successful treatment of chronic carriers in 80% to 90% of cases. Several studies have suggested 14 to 21 days of treatment to be equally efficacious. However, treatment regimens can also be complicated by antimicrobial resistance; multidrug- and ceftriaxone-resistant strains have been isolated from chronic carriers in India. Antimicrobial susceptibility testing is helpful to ensure appropriate therapy and follow-up cultures are necessary to confirm cure.

10) Control flies by screening and use of insecticidal baits and traps or, where appropriate, spraying with insecticides. Control fly breeding through frequent garbage collection and disposal and through fly control measures in latrine construction and maintenance.

11) Immunization for typhoid fever is not routinely recommended in nonendemic areas except for those subject to unusual occupational exposure to enteric infections (e.g., clinical microbiology technicians) and household members of known carriers. WHO recommends vaccination for people who travel to endemic high-risk areas and children living in endemic areas where typhoid fever control is a priority (see: http://www.who.int/immunization/policy/position_papers/typhoid/en). Vaccination of high-risk populations is considered a promising strategy for the control of endemic typhoid fever; this approach has rarely been used as a control measure for ongoing outbreaks. An oral, live multidose vaccine using *S. enterica* serotype Typhi strain Ty21a and a single-dose parenteral vaccine containing the polysaccharide Vi antigen are widely available. However, Ty21a should not be used in pregnant women, immunocompromised persons, or in persons receiving antibiotics until 24 hours or more after the last antibiotic dose. Booster doses every 2 to 5 years, according to vaccine type, are desirable for those at continuing risk of infection. Neither vaccine is licensed for children younger than 2 years; Ty21a is only licensed for children aged 6 years and older in the USA but is licensed for younger children in other countries. In 2018, WHO prequalified a new typhoid conjugate vaccine (TCV), with longer-lasting immune responses, for use in children aged 6 months or older. TCV is recommended for routine vaccination of infants and children aged 6 months or older in

endemic countries; it is not available in the USA. No vaccines for paratyphoid fever are available. Ty21a offers only limited cross-reacting humoral intestinal immune response for partial protection against Paratyphi B antigens.

11. Special considerations—

1) Reporting: case report to local health authorities is obligatory in most countries.

2) Epidemic measures: search intensively for the case/carrier who is the source of infection and for the vehicle (water or food) through which infection was transmitted. Selectively eliminate suspected contaminated food. Pasteurize or boil milk, or exclude milk supplies and other foods suspected on epidemiologic evidence, until safety is ensured. Chlorinate suspected water supplies adequately under competent supervision or avoid use. All drinking water must be chlorinated, treated with iodine, or boiled before use. Preemptive vaccination before seasonal outbreaks, or in areas at risk of an outbreak, may be considered.

3) Disaster implications: with disruption of usual water supply and sewage disposal and of controls on food and water, transmission and large-scale outbreaks of typhoid fever may occur if there are active cases or carriers in a displaced population. Efforts should be made to restore safe drinking-water supplies and excreta disposal facilities. Selective immunization of stabilized groups such as schoolchildren, prisoners, and utility, municipal, or hospital personnel may be helpful.

4) International measures: for typhoid fever, immunization is advised for international travelers to endemic areas, especially if travel is likely to involve exposure to unsafe food and water or close contact in rural areas with local residents. Vaccination is not a legal requirement for entry into any country.

WHO Collaborating Centres provide support as required. Further information can be found at: https://www.who.int/about/who-we-are/structure/collaborating-centres.

[G. Appiah, K. Chatham-Stephens, M. Hughes, F. Medalla]

TYPHUS

DISEASE	ICD-10 CODE
TYPHUS FEVER	ICD-10 A75
EPIDEMIC LOUSE-BORNE TYPHUS FEVER	ICD-10 A75.0
BRILL-ZINSSER DISEASE	ICD-10 A75.1
ENDEMIC FLEA-BORNE TYPHUS FEVER	ICD-10 A75.2
SCRUB TYPHUS	ICD-10 A75.3
Queensland tick typhus (see "Rickettsioses")	

I. EPIDEMIC LOUSE-BORNE TYPHUS FEVER; SYLVATIC TYPHUS (louse-borne typhus, typhus exanthematicus, classic typhus fever, Brill-Zinsser disease)

1. Clinical features—A rickettsial disease with variable presentation and time of onset but often with abrupt onset of fever, severe headache, chills, malaise, and general pains. A macular rash appears 4 to 7 days after illness onset—initially on the upper trunk, followed by spread to the entire body, but usually not to the face, palms, or soles. The rash can be difficult to observe on patients with darkly pigmented skin and is absent in up to 40% of patients. Cough and tachypnea may be present and neurologic signs are common; these can include confusion, drowsiness, coma, seizures, and hearing loss. The case-fatality rate increases with patient age and can be as high as 30% in the absence of treatment. Mild infections may occur without rash, especially in children. Recrudescence can occur years after the primary attack (Brill-Zinsser disease); this form of the disease is often milder, with fewer complications, and has a lower case-fatality rate but can be severe in some cases. Sylvatic typhus appears to be a milder disease, although this may reflect the typical better health and nutritional status of the affected individuals.

2. Risk groups—Outbreaks of louse-borne epidemic typhus are most often associated with the clustering of large populations in unhygienic circumstances such as those resulting from war or famine, when body-louse infestation is common. It occurs in refugee camp settings and prisons and within homeless populations. It can also occur by aerosol exposure to infected louse feces in contaminated clothing. Individuals living in arboreal habitats in the eastern USA (Florida to Massachusetts), where the southern flying squirrel is common, are at risk of sylvatic typhus.

3. Causative agents—*Rickettsia prowazekii.*

4. Diagnosis—As with many rickettsial diseases, thrombocytopenia and elevated serum liver enzymes are typical, so their presence may aid in determining the diagnosis. Laboratory confirmation of a diagnosis by serology typically occurs late in the disease process and is therefore not useful for treatment decisions. The indirect immunofluorescence assay (IFA) is the most widely available method for laboratory confirmation and requires paired sera with a 4-fold increase in antibody titers between a patient's acute and convalescent serum specimens. An acute serum sample should be obtained in the first week of symptoms and a convalescent serum sample should be obtained 2 to 4 weeks later. Antibody tests usually become positive in the second to third week of illness. An acute titer taken in the first week of illness should be used as a baseline for comparison with the convalescent sample; a negative acute result does not rule out active infection nor does a single positive acute serologic result confirm the diagnosis. Common serologic tests do not always discriminate between louse-borne and murine typhus unless the sera are differentially absorbed with the respective rickettsial antigen prior to testing or microagglutination is employed. Other diagnostic methods with varying degrees of sensitivity and specificity are enzyme immunoassay, polymerase chain reaction (PCR), immunohistochemical (IHC) staining of tissues, microagglutination with intact rickettsial antigens, and the toxin neutralization test in mice. The Weil-Felix agglutination assays may be used in international settings; however, they lack sensitivity and specificity and are not generally used in the USA. Skin biopsy samples of rash sites can be tested by IHC (chromatic specific antibody staining or with agent-specific fluorescent molecular probes) or PCR, but only PCR with sequence analysis or use of specific probes provides definitive agent identification. Sending lice from clothes or the environment to a reference laboratory for PCR testing can be useful during an outbreak of epidemic louse-borne typhus fever to detect the causative agent. Fleas, lice, and mites, from flying squirrels and their nests, may also be analyzed by PCR.

5. Occurrence—Worldwide distribution, commonly seen where people live under unhygienic conditions and where infestation with body lice is prevalent. Explosive epidemics may occur in conditions that prevent regular bathing and washing of clothes, such as during war, famine, drought, and other natural disasters. Endemic foci exist in the mountainous regions of Mexico, in Central and South America, in central and eastern Africa, and numerous countries in Asia. Large late-20th-century outbreaks have been observed in Burundi and Rwanda. In the eastern USA, cases of sylvatic typhus associated with contact with flying squirrels and their ectoparasites have been reported; occasionally in familial clusters.

6. Reservoirs—Humans are the reservoir for louse-associated epidemic typhus and are responsible for maintaining the infection during interepidemic periods. Although not a major source of human disease, sporadic sylvatic typhus cases may be associated with flying squirrels, possibly via aerosols generated from the feces of squirrel fleas and lice.

7. Incubation period—From 1 to 2 weeks.

8. Transmission—The human body louse, *Pediculus humanus corporis*, is infected by feeding on the blood of a patient with acute typhus fever. Patients with Brill-Zinsser disease can infect lice and serve as sources of new outbreaks in louse-infested communities. Infected lice excrete rickettsiae in their feces and usually defecate at the time of feeding. People are infected by rubbing feces or crushed lice into the bite or into superficial abrasions. Inhalation of infective louse feces in dust may account for some infections. Transmission from the flying squirrel is presumed to be through the bite of the squirrel flea, but squirrel louse or flea feces may also be infectious. One attack usually confers long-lasting immunity. *Amblyomma* ticks from northeast Mexico and Ethiopia have also been implicated as minor vectors of epidemic typhus.

The disease is not directly transmitted from person to person; however, incidence can be epidemic when conditions favor person-to-person transmission of the human body louse. Patients are infective for lice during the febrile illness and possibly for 2 to 3 days after defervescence. Infected lice pass rickettsiae in their feces within 2 to 6 days after the blood meal; they are infective earlier if crushed. The louse invariably dies within 2 weeks after infection; rickettsiae may remain viable in the dead louse for weeks under arid conditions.

9. Treatment—

Drug	Doxycycline
Dose	• Adults: 100 mg BID • Children < 45 kg: 2.2 mg/kg BID
Route	IV or PO
Alternative drug	Chloramphenicol 50 mg/kg/day IV every 6 hours[a]
Duration	≥ 3 days after defervescence, usually 7–10 days, although large single-dose regimens can be employed during large-scale epidemic conditions.
Special considerations and comments	Doxycycline has not been demonstrated to cause cosmetic staining of developing permanent teeth when used in the dose and duration recommended to treat rickettsial diseases (≤ 10 days). Follow appropriate and updated local clinical guidance with use.

Note: BID = twice daily; IV = intravenous(ly); PO = oral(ly).
[a]If alternative drug used, this is one possible dosing regimen or consult local expert opinion.

10. Prevention—Primary prevention of louse-borne typhus relies on measures to avoid infestation with body lice.

  1) Because body lice are found on clothing close to human skin, discarding infected clothes can be an effective measure in controlling infestation.

2) Apply an effective residual insecticide powder at appropriate intervals by hand or power blower to clothes and skin of persons of populations living under conditions favoring louse infestation. The insecticide used should be effective on local lice and used according to safety labeling and instructions. Lice eggs are resistant to most insecticides, so several applications may be necessary. Removal of flying squirrels from domestic habitats (e.g., walls, attics) should be accompanied by aerosol protection (masks) and ectoparasite control measures with pesticides to prevent flea bites.

3) Improve living conditions with provisions for bathing and washing clothes in hot water.

4) Treat prophylactically those who are subject to risk by applying residual insecticide to clothing (dusting or impregnation) and, in the case of an epidemic, directly to the skin as well (see Special Considerations for appropriate insecticides).

11. Special considerations—

1) Reporting: reporting of louse-borne typhus fever is required as a disease under surveillance by WHO. Further information can be found at: http://www.who.int/collaboratingcentres/database/en.

2) Epidemic measures: the best measure for rapid control of louse-borne typhus is to apply an insecticide with residual effect to all contacts. Where louse infestation is known to be widespread, systematic application of residual insecticide to all people in the community is indicated. Single high-dose oral doxycycline treatment of cases in an epidemic has also been used to reduce the spread of disease. In epidemics, individuals may protect themselves by wearing silk or plastic clothing tightly fastened around wrists, ankles, and neck and impregnating clothes with repellents or permethrin.

3) Disaster implications: typhus can be expected to be a significant problem in louse-infested populations in endemic areas concurrent with social upheavals and crowding.

4) International measures: notification by governments to WHO and to adjacent countries of the occurrence of a case or an outbreak of louse-borne typhus fever in an area previously free of the disease.

5) Measures in cases of deliberate use: *R. prowazekii* has been produced as a possible bioweapon and was used before World War II. It is infectious by aerosol, with a high case-fatality rate. The initial reference treatment of any suspected case is a single dose of 200 mg doxycycline in situations where doxycycline is limited in supply, although a small proportion of patients may relapse if not treated for the full 7 to 10 days.

II. ENDEMIC FLEA-BORNE TYPHUS FEVER (murine typhus, shop typhus, flea-borne rickettsiosis)

1. Clinical features—The clinical course of flea-borne rickettsial diseases resembles that of louse-borne typhus but is frequently milder, with a less abrupt onset of fever, headache, and myalgia. Macular or maculopapular rash occurs in approximately 50% of patients, typically appearing at the end of the first week of illness and lasting 1 to 4 days. Abdominal symptoms such as nausea, vomiting, and abdominal pain may occur and are more common in children. Complications such as acute renal failure and respiratory failure can occur but are not common. Illness seldom lasts longer than 2 weeks. The case-fatality rate for all ages is less than 5% but increases with age. The presence of fleas, absence of louse infestation, geographic and seasonal distribution of illness, and presence of rats or other hosts differentiate flea-borne from louse-borne typhus.

2. Risk groups—No specific risk factors.

3. Causative agents—*Rickettsia typhi*.

4. Diagnosis—See Epidemic Louse-Borne Typhus Fever in this chapter.

5. Occurrence—Worldwide. Found in areas where people and rats occupy the same buildings. Multiple cases may occur in the same household owing to common exposure to the source of infection.

6. Reservoirs—Rats, mice, and possibly other small and medium-sized mammals in which infection is inapparent. Infection is maintained in nature by a host-flea-host cycle (commonly *Xenopsylla cheopis* on *Rattus rattus* and *Rattus norvegicus*). A complex of bacteria related to *Rickettsia felis* is found worldwide in diverse flea species, particularly *Ctenocephalides felis*, and maintained transovarially. However, these agents cause a presentation of flea-borne rickettsiosis that is different from murine typhus.

7. Incubation period—From 6 to 14 days, commonly reported at 12 days.

8. Transmission—Infective fleas defecate bacteria while taking a blood meal; this contaminates the bite site and other fresh skin wounds. Occasionally, a case may follow inhalation of dried infective flea feces. Not directly transmitted from person to person. Once infected, fleas remain so for life (up to 1 year) and transfer infection to their progeny. Endemic typhus infection confers lasting immunity.

9. Treatment—

Drug	Doxycycline
Dose	• Adults: 100 mg BID • Children < 45 kg: 2.2 mg/kg BID
Route	IV or PO
Alternative drug	Chloramphenicol (50 mg/kg/day IV every 6 hours) but may not be as effective[a]
Duration	$\geq$ 3 days after defervescence, usually 7–10 days
Special considerations and comments	Doxycycline has not been demonstrated to cause cosmetic staining of developing permanent teeth when used in the dose and duration recommended to treat rickettsial diseases ($\leq$ 10 days).

Note: BID = twice daily; IV = intravenous(ly); PO = oral(ly).
[a]If alternative drug used, this is one possible dosing regimen or consult local expert opinion.

10. Prevention—

1) To avoid increased exposure of humans, wait until flea populations have first been reduced by insecticides before instituting rodent control measures because fleas will seek other hosts, including humans (see "Plague").
2) Apply insecticide powders with residual action to rat runs, burrows, and harborages.

11. Special considerations—

1) Reporting: case report to local health authority is obligatory in many countries and some states.
2) Epidemic measures: in endemic areas with numerous cases, use of a residual insecticide effective against rat or cat fleas will reduce the flea index and the incidence of infection in humans.
3) Disaster implications: cases can be expected when people, rats, and fleas are forced to coexist in close proximity, such as occurs with reduced sanitation, in temporary shelters or in refugee settings, or floods, but murine typhus has not been a major contributor to elevated disease rates in such situations. Most common in urban areas and port cities and along rivers.

WHO Collaborating Centres provide support as required. Further information can be found at: http://www.who.int/collaboratingcentres/database/en.

III. SCRUB TYPHUS (tsutsugamushi disease, mite-borne typhus fever)

1. Clinical features—A rickettsial disease often characterized by 1 or more primary skin ulcers (eschars) corresponding to the sites of attachment of infected mites (chiggers). Not all patients with scrub typhus have an eschar and the frequency of this symptom varies by region. A systemic acute febrile onset follows within several days, along with headache, profuse sweating, conjunctival injection, and lymphadenopathy. A transient maculopapular rash appears on the trunk in up to half of patients around day 7 of fever. Cough and radiographic evidence of pneumonitis are common and may progress to acute respiratory distress syndrome and respiratory failure. Neurologic findings ranging from slight confusion to delirium or hearing loss may occur. Hepatomegaly and splenomegaly are sometimes observed. This disease may cause spontaneous abortions in pregnant women. Without appropriate antibiotic therapy, fever lasts for about 14 days. The case-fatality rate in untreated cases varies from 1% to 60% according to geographic area, strain of infectious agent, and previous exposure to disease; it is higher among older people but can occur at all ages.

2. Risk groups—Military troops and agricultural workers in endemic areas. Occupational infection occurs mainly in adult workers (males more than females) who frequent overgrown agricultural habitats or other mite-infested areas, such as forest clearings, reforested areas, new settlements, mountainous and tropical environments, and even newly irrigated desert regions. An attack confers short-term protection—but not long-lasting immunity—against the homologous strain of *Orientia tsutsugamushi* but only weak and transient immunity against heterologous strains. Heterologous infection results in mild disease within the first few months after primary infection but produces typical illness after a year or so as immunity wanes quickly. Second and even third attacks of naturally acquired scrub typhus (usually benign or inapparent) occur among people who spend their lives in endemic areas or who have not been adequately treated.

3. Causative agents—*O. tsutsugamushi* with multiple, serologically distinct strains present both focally and between different sites and countries.

4. Diagnosis—See Epidemic Louse-Borne Typhus Fever in this chapter. While IFA detection of a 4-fold rise in titer and/or an immunoglobulin class M titer greater than 1:32 remain the gold standard, enzyme-linked immunosorbent assay and rapid dipstick and chromatographic flow assays are available that detect either antibodies or antigen in a patient's serum. Reinfections with different strains may occur and serologic diagnosis may need to include testing for multiple *O. tsutsugamushi* strains to improve assay sensitivity and specificity. The commercial rapid diagnostic kits provide results within 1 hour, although the cost of these kits may be prohibitive in some areas. PCR of blood, eschar, and swabs of subeschar lesions is often clinically diagnostic. Mites are rarely collected and technically challenging to test by PCR.

5. Occurrence—Central, eastern, and southeastern Asia; from southeastern Siberia and northern Japan to northern Australia and Vanuatu, as far west as Pakistan, to as high as 3,000 m (10,000 ft) above sea level in the Himalaya Mountains. Often acquired by humans in the innumerable small typhus islands (some covering an area of only a few square feet) where the causative agent, infected vectors, and suitable rodent hosts exist simultaneously. Epidemics occur when susceptible individuals are brought into endemic areas with highly virulent strains, especially in military operations in which 20% to 50% of troops have been infected within weeks or months. Other species of *Orientia* that cause scrub typhus have been reported from Africa and South America and related agents may exist in Europe.

6. Reservoirs—Infected larval stage of trombiculid mites (chiggers); *Leptotrombidium deliense* and related species (varying with area) are the most common vectors for humans, although a number of other trombiculid mite genera are also infected. *Orientia* is maintained by transovarial and transstadial passage in mites.

7. Incubation period—From 6 to 21 days, usually 10 to 12 days.

8. Transmission—Through the bite of infected larval mites; nymphs and adults do not feed on vertebrate hosts. No direct person-to-person transmission.

9. Treatment—

Drug	Doxycycline
Dose	• Adults: 100 mg BID • Children < 45 kg: 2.2 mg/kg BID
Route	IV or PO
Duration	≥ 3 days after defervescence
Special considerations and comments	Doxycycline has not been demonstrated to cause cosmetic staining of developing permanent teeth when used in the dose and duration recommended to treat rickettsial diseases (≤ 10 days).

Note: BID = twice daily; IV = intravenous(ly); PO = oral(ly).

10. Prevention—

1) Prevent contact with infected mites through personal prophylaxis by impregnating clothes and blankets with miticidal chemicals (permethrin and benzyl benzoate) and applying mite repellents (diethyltoluamide) to exposed skin surfaces.
2) Eliminate mites from the specific sites through the application of chlorinated hydrocarbons, such as lindane, dieldrin, or

chlordane, to ground and vegetation in environs of camps, mine buildings, and other populated zones in endemic areas.

3) In a small group of volunteers, the administration of weekly doses of doxycycline was found to be an effective prophylactic regimen.

11. Special considerations—

1) Reporting: report to local health authority may be required in some endemic areas.

2) Epidemic measures: rigorously employ procedures in the affected area as described in Prevention in sections I and II of this chapter; carry out daily observation of all people at risk for fever and appearance of primary lesions; institute treatment on first indication of illness.

3) Disaster implications: only if refugee centers or new habitations are sited in or near typhus islands.

WHO Collaborating Centres provide support as required. Further information can be found at: http://www.who.int/collaboratingcentres/database/en.

[A. E. Peterson, D. Cherry-Brown, G. A. Dasch]

VARICELLA AND HERPES ZOSTER

DISEASE	ICD-10 CODE
VARICELLA	ICD-10 B01
HERPES ZOSTER	ICD-10 B02

1. Clinical features—Varicella-zoster virus (VZV) causes 2 distinct diseases: varicella, or chickenpox, which is the primary infection, and later, if VZV reactivates, herpes zoster, or shingles. Varicella is characterized by fever and generalized, pruritic, maculopapulo-vesicular rash. The lesions are maculopapular for a few hours, vesicular and pustular for 3 to 4 days, then crust, leaving granular scabs. The vesicles are superficial, unilocular, and collapse on puncture. Lesions commonly occur in successive crops for 3 to 7 days with several stages of maturity present at the same time; they tend to be centrally distributed and are more abundant on the trunk and proximal extremities. Lesions may appear on the scalp, high in the axilla, on mucous membranes of the mouth and upper respiratory tract, and on the conjunctivae.

Breakthrough varicella is defined as varicella that develops more than 42 days after vaccination; most (~70%) breakthrough disease is mild with mildly elevated or no fever and with papules that do not generally progress to vesicles.

Occasionally, especially in adults and in persons with cellular immune deficiencies, such as malignancies and human immunodeficiency virus (HIV)/acquired immunodeficiency syndrome, fever and constitutional manifestations of varicella may be severe. Serious complications of varicella include pneumonia, secondary bacterial infections, hemorrhagic complications, and encephalitis. Secondary bacterial infections of the vesicles may leave disfiguring scars or result in necrotizing fasciitis or septicemia. Rarely, complications may result in death; the case-fatality rate is lower for children (1:100,000 varicella cases in the 5–9 age group) than for adults (1:5,000).

Herpes zoster is a local manifestation of reactivation of latent VZV in the dorsal root ganglia. Vesicles with an erythematous base are restricted to skin areas supplied by sensory nerves of a single or associated group of dorsal root ganglia. Rash is typically unilateral and most commonly affects thoracic, cervical, and ophthalmic dermatomes. Small numbers of lesions may appear outside the primary dermatome. In immunosuppressed persons and those with malignancies, but sometimes in otherwise healthy individuals, extensive varicella-like lesions may appear outside the dermatome. Lesions are histologically identical to those of varicella but are deeper seated and more closely aggregated. The rash lasts about 7 to 10 days and heals within 2 to 4 weeks. The most common complication of herpes zoster is chronic severe pain, also called postherpetic neuralgia, which can last for months or even years; about 10% to 15% of shingles patients have pain for at least 90 days after shingles onset. Nonpain complications may occur in about 10% of cases. Herpes zoster occasionally results in permanent neurologic damage, such as cranial nerve palsy and contralateral hemiplegia, or visual impairment following herpes zoster ophthalmicus.

2. Risk groups—Infants, adolescents, adults, immunocompromised persons, and pregnant women are at higher risk for severe varicella and complications. Neonates whose mothers are not immune and patients with leukemia may suffer severe, prolonged, or fatal varicella. Among neonates whose mothers develop varicella 5 days prior to, or within 2 days after, delivery and who do not receive varicella-zoster immunoglobulin (discussed later) or antiviral therapy, the case-fatality rate can reach 30%.

Infection during the first trimester of pregnancy may lead to congenital varicella syndrome in 1% of cases; at 13 to 20 weeks' gestation, the risk for congenital varicella syndrome is 2%. Few cases consistent with congenital varicella syndrome have been reported after 20 weeks' gestation. Intrauterine infection and varicella in the first year of life are associated with herpes zoster in childhood.

Deficiencies in cell-mediated immunity are risk factors for both herpes zoster and its severe manifestations. The incidence of both herpes zoster and postherpetic neuralgia increases with age. Cancer and HIV patients have a higher risk of herpes zoster, with highest rates among children. Herpes zoster is also more common following hematopoietic stem cell and solid organ transplants, especially in the first year and among patients on immunosuppressive medications. Additionally, persons with cancer (especially of lymphoid tissue), immunodeficient patients, and those on immunosuppressive therapy have an increased frequency of severe herpes zoster.

Varicella infection usually confers immunity for life; second attacks of varicella are rare in immunocompetent persons but have been documented; subclinical reinfection is common.

3. Causative agents—Human (alpha) herpesvirus 3 (VZV), a member of the Herpesviridae family.

4. Diagnosis—Laboratory tests are not routinely required for diagnosis but are useful in complicated cases. Viral strain identification may be needed (e.g., to document whether rash in a vaccine recipient is due to vaccine or wild virus). Several antibody assays are now commercially available but they are not sensitive enough to be used for postimmunization testing of immunity.

5. Occurrence—Worldwide. Infection is nearly universal. In temperate climates, at least 90% of the population has had varicella by age 15 and at least 95% by young adulthood. In temperate zones, varicella occurs most frequently in winter and early spring. In tropical countries, a higher proportion of cases occur among adults. In developed countries, herpes zoster occurs in up to 30% of the population, mostly in adults older than 50 years.

6. Reservoirs—Humans.

7. Incubation period—10 to 21 days; commonly 14 to 16 days; may be prolonged to 28 days after passive immunization against varicella and may be shorter in immunodeficient persons.

8. Transmission—Person-to-person by direct contact, airborne spread of vesicle fluid of skin lesions of acute varicella and herpes zoster, or infected secretions of the respiratory tract of varicella cases that also might be aerosolized; indirectly through articles freshly soiled by discharges from vesicles and mucous membranes of infected people. In contrast to vaccinia and variola, scabs from varicella lesions are not infective.

Varicella is communicable from 1 to 2 days before onset of rash until all lesions are crusted (usually ~ 5 days) after rash onset. Infectiousness may be prolonged in patients with altered immunity. Herpes zoster patients are infectious while they have active (vesiculopustular) lesions (usually 7-10 days). Susceptible exposed individuals should be considered potentially infectious for 8 to 21 days following exposure (or 28 days if they received passive immunization).

Varicella in unvaccinated persons is one of the most readily communicable diseases; secondary attack rates in susceptible household contacts range from 61% to 100%. Herpes zoster has a lower rate of transmission: data from a household study showed that approximately 20% of those who were varicella-susceptible developed varicella when they were in contact with persons who had herpes zoster.

9. Treatment—

Preferred therapy	Acyclovir:
	• Varicella zoster: 800 mg PO every 6 hours for 5 days • Herpes zoster: 800 mg PO every 4 hours for 7–10 days
	Acyclovir for immunocompromised patients:
	• Varicella zoster: 10–15 mg/kg IV every 8 hours for 7–10 days • Herpes zoster: 10 mg/kg IV every 8 hours for 7 days
Alternative drug	Immunocompetent patients with varicella or herpes zoster:
	• Valacyclovir 1,000 mg PO every 8 hours for 7 days • Famciclovir 500 mg PO every 8 hours for 7 days
Special considerations and comments	Not applicable

Note: IV = intravenous(ly); PO = oral(ly).

10. Prevention—

1) Varicella vaccination: live attenuated varicella vaccines are available throughout the world. They are licensed for use in healthy persons aged 12 months and older, except for the GSK vaccine, which can be administered as early as 9 months old in some countries. A quadrivalent vaccine (measles, mumps, rubella, and varicella) has been licensed for use in healthy children aged between 9 to 12 months and 12 years. One dose of varicella vaccine has an effectiveness estimated at 70% to 90% (median 84%) for prevention of all varicella and at greater than 95% for prevention of combined moderate and severe disease in children followed for up to 10 years. Two doses of varicella vaccine produce an improved immune response that correlates with improved protection against disease. Routine varicella vaccination programs for children have been introduced primarily in industrialized countries. Countries that adopted varicella vaccination programs have recommended either 1 or 2 doses among children; while the first dose is usually

recommended at the minimum age, the age for the second dose is variable, with some countries recommending it at age 4 to 6 years and others at 4 to 6 weeks after the first dose. In the USA, for example, the recommendations are for the first dose at age 12 to 15 months and the second dose at 4 to 6 years—and second-dose catch-up vaccination for persons who previously received only 1 dose. Routine childhood immunization may be considered in countries where the disease is a public health and socioeconomic problem, where immunization is affordable, and where sustained high vaccine coverage (85%-90%) can be achieved.

For persons aged 13 years and older, 2 doses of vaccine 4 to 8 weeks apart are recommended for susceptible persons. Vaccination is generally offered based on a negative history of varicella and without confirmation of seronegativity. Some countries have vaccination programs targeted at populations considered at high risk. Priority groups for adult immunization include close contacts (e.g., health care workers and household contacts of immunocompromised persons or persons at high risk for serious complications); persons who live or work in environments where transmission of varicella is likely (e.g., teachers of young children, day care employees, residents, staff in institutional settings) or can occur (e.g., college students, inmates, staff members of correctional institutions, military personnel); nonpregnant women of childbearing age; adolescents and adults; and international travelers.

Duration of immunity after 1 dose is unknown but antibody persistence for more than 10 years has been documented in settings in which wild virus continues to circulate. Large-scale vaccination of children with varicella vaccine and older adults with herpes zoster vaccine may have an important impact on the incidence of herpes zoster and postherpetic neuralgia. Postlicensure data indicate that children (both immunocompetent and immunocompromised) immunized against varicella have a lower risk for herpes zoster and the clinical presentations of herpes zoster seem to be milder varicella. Rare occasions of herpes zoster following varicella vaccination and confirmed to be due to vaccine strain VZV show that the currently used vaccine strains may induce latency with the subsequent risk of reactivation, although in children the rate is lower than after natural disease.

A mild varicella-like rash at the site of vaccine injection or at distant sites has been observed in 2% to 4% of children and about 5% of adults. Contraindications to varicella vaccination are as follows:

- Immunocompromised persons, including those with:

  o Blood discrasias, leukemia, lymphoma of any type, or malignant neoplasms affecting the bone marrow or lymphatic systems

  o HIV infection; single-antigen varicella vaccine can be considered, however, for HIV-infected children with cluster of differentiation 4 (CD4+) glycoprotein T-lymphocyte counts greater than or equal to 200 cells/mL ($\leq$ 15%) and for HIV-infected adolescents and adults with CD4+ counts greater than or equal to 200 cells/mL

  o Immunosuppressive therapy (including systemic steroids within the previous month)

- History of anaphylactic reactions to any component of the vaccine (including neomycin)
- Pregnancy (theoretical risk to the fetus—pregnancy should be avoided for 4 weeks following vaccination)
- Acute severe illness
- History of congenital immune disorders in first-degree relatives unless the immune competence of potential vaccine recipient has been demonstrated

2) A herpes zoster vaccine for older adults has been approved and recommended for use in some countries for healthy persons aged 50 years and older (in the USA the vaccine is recommended for persons $\leq$ 60 years). The herpes zoster vaccine contains the same VZV strain used in the varicella vaccine but with a higher potency.

11. Special considerations—

1) Reporting: deaths may be reportable to health authorities.
2) Epidemic measures: outbreaks of varicella are common in schools and other institutional settings, such as emergency housing situations; they may be protracted, disruptive, and associated with complications. Infectious cases should be isolated and susceptible contacts immunized promptly. Persons ineligible for immunization should be evaluated immediately for administration of varicella-zoster immunoglobulin.

[H. Badaruddin]

WEST NILE VIRUS DISEASE

DISEASE	ICD-10 CODE
WEST NILE FEVER	ICD-10 A92.3
WEST NILE VIRUS ENCEPHALITIS	ICD-10 A83.8
WEST NILE VIRUS MENINGITIS	ICD-10 A87.8
WEST NILE VIRUS ACUTE FLACCID PARALYSIS	ICD-10 A88.8
KUNJIN	ICD-10 A83.4

1. Clinical features—Approximately 70% to 80% of human West Nile virus (WNV) infections are asymptomatic. Most symptomatic people experience an acute systemic febrile illness (West Nile fever) that often includes headache, myalgia, or arthralgia; gastrointestinal tract symptoms and a transient maculopapular rash are also commonly reported. Fewer than 1% of infected people develop neuroinvasive disease, which typically manifests as meningitis, encephalitis, or acute flaccid paralysis. WNV meningitis is indistinguishable clinically from aseptic meningitis caused by most other viruses. Patients with WNV encephalitis usually present with seizures, mental status changes, focal neurologic deficits, or movement disorders (features of Parkinsonism). WNV acute flaccid paralysis is often clinically and pathologically identical to poliovirus-associated acute flaccid paralysis, with damage to anterior horn cells, and may progress to respiratory paralysis requiring mechanical ventilation. WNV-associated Guillain-Barré syndrome has also been reported and can be distinguished from WNV acute flaccid paralysis by clinical manifestations and electrophysiologic testing. Cardiac dysrhythmias, myocarditis, rhabdomyolysis, optic neuritis, uveitis, chorioretinitis, orchitis, pancreatitis, and hepatitis have been described rarely after WNV infection. Most patients with WNV nonneuroinvasive disease (i.e., West Nile fever) or meningitis recover completely but fatigue, malaise, and weakness can linger for weeks or months. Patients who recover from WNV encephalitis or acute flaccid paralysis often have residual neurologic deficits. Among patients with neuroinvasive disease, the overall case-fatality rate is approximately 10% but is significantly higher in WNV encephalitis and acute flaccid paralysis than in WNV meningitis.

WNV disease should be considered in the differential diagnosis of acute neurologic or febrile illnesses associated with recent exposure to mosquitoes, blood transfusion, or organ transplantation and of illnesses in neonates whose mothers were infected with WNV during pregnancy or while breastfeeding. In addition to other more common causes of aseptic meningitis and encephalitis (e.g., herpes simplex virus and enteroviruses), other arboviruses should also be considered in the differential diagnosis (see Arboviral Encephalitides in "Arboviral Diseases").

2. Risk groups—Risk of WNV infection is generally determined by exposure to infected vectors and is dependent on many factors, including environmental conditions, season, and human activities. Once infected, older age, chronic renal disease, immune suppression, those who acquired the disease through a transplanted organ, history of alcohol abuse, diabetes, and hypertension have been associated with higher risk of neuroinvasive or severe disease (e.g., hospitalization or death). Infection generally results in lifelong immunity.

3. Causative agents—WNV, of the family Flaviviridae and genus *Flavivirus*.

4. Diagnosis—Identifying anti-WNV immunoglobulin class M (IgM) antibodies in serum or cerebrospinal fluid (CSF) is the most common way to diagnose WNV infection. The presence of anti-WNV IgM is usually good evidence of recent WNV infection but may indicate infection with another closely related flavivirus. Because anti-WNV IgM can persist in some patients for more than 1 year, a positive test result may occasionally reflect past infection. IgM antibody to WNV develops in a majority of WNV-infected patients by the fourth day of symptom onset; 95% of infected patients develop IgM antibody within 7 days of symptom onset. Detection of WNV IgM in CSF is diagnostic of neuroinvasive disease. For patients in whom serum collected within 10 days of illness lacks detectable IgM, testing should be repeated on a convalescent-phase sample. Immunoglobulin class G (IgG) antibody is generally detectable shortly after IgM and can persist for years. Plaque-reduction neutralization tests can be performed to measure virus-specific neutralizing antibodies and to discriminate between cross-reacting antibodies in primary flavivirus infections. A 4-fold or greater increase in virus-specific neutralizing antibodies between acute- and convalescent-phase serum specimens collected 2 to 3 weeks apart may be used to confirm recent WNV infection. In patients who have been immunized against, or infected with, another flavivirus in the past (i.e., who have secondary flavivirus infections), cross-reactive antibodies in IgM, IgG, and neutralization assays may make it difficult to identify which flavivirus is causing the patient's illness. WNV has been well-known to have significant serologic cross-reactivity with multiple flaviviruses (most notably Zika virus, St Louis encephalitis [SLEV], and Japanese encephalitis virus [JEV]). Immunization history (past yellow fever or JEV vaccine), date of symptom onset, and information regarding other flaviviruses known to circulate in the geographic area (e.g., dengue, SLEV) that may cross-react in serologic assays should be considered when interpreting results.

Viral culture and WNV nucleic acid amplification tests (including reverse transcription polymerase chain reaction [RT-PCR]) can be performed on acute-phase serum, CSF, or tissue specimens. However, by the time most immunocompetent patients present with clinical symptoms, WNV ribonucleic acid is usually no longer detectable owing to low-level and short-lived viremia generated by the virus; thus, RT-PCR is not recommended for diagnosis in immunocompetent patients. The sensitivity of these tests is likely higher in immunocompromised patients. Immunohistochemical staining can detect WNV antigens in fixed tissue but negative results are not definitive.

5. Occurrence—WNV disease has been documented on every continent except Antarctica. In temperate and subtropical regions, most human WNV infections occur in summer or early fall. Seasonal outbreaks often occur in local areas, with the location of outbreaks often varying from year to year.

Since the 1990s, the largest outbreaks of WNV neuroinvasive disease have occurred in the Middle East, Europe, and North America. WNV was first detected in the Western Hemisphere in New York City in 1999 and subsequently spread across the continental USA and Canada and into Central and South America. In recent years, several countries in Southern Europe (e.g., Italy, Greece, and Spain) have reported outbreaks of WNV neuroinvasive disease. In 2012, the largest outbreak of WNV in the USA occurred since its discovery, with 48 states reporting cases and 80% of cases occurring in 13 states.

6. Reservoirs—WNV is transmitted in an enzootic cycle between mosquitoes and amplifying vertebrate hosts, primarily birds. Birds infect feeding vector mosquitoes that then transmit the virus to humans and other mammals during subsequent feeding. Some birds (e.g., corvids) will become sick and may die because of WNV infection, while others (e.g., chickens) develop viremia but do not become unwell. Viremia in humans usually lasts less than 7 days in immunocompetent persons and concentrations of the virus in blood are generally too low to infect mosquitoes, making humans incidental or dead-end hosts. Several other mammals can be infected by WNV but most are incidental hosts. Some mammals, like horses, can become symptomatic following WNV infection.

7. Incubation period—Usually 2 to 6 days but ranges from 2 to 14 days and can be as long as 21 days in immunocompromised people. The incubation period tends to be longer in cases transmitted through an infected transplanted organ.

8. Transmission—WNV is transmitted to humans primarily through the bite of infected mosquitoes, predominantly *Culex* mosquitoes. These mosquitoes feed most avidly from dusk to dawn and breed mostly in peridomestic standing water with high organic content or in pools created by irrigation or rainfall. In the USA, the incidence of neuroinvasive disease fluctuates by region and is highest in the months of July to September. Humans usually do not develop a level or duration of viremia sufficient to infect mosquitoes. However, person-to-person WNV transmission can occur through blood transfusion and solid organ transplantation. Intrauterine transmission and probable transmission via human milk have also been described but appear to be uncommon. Transmission through percutaneous and mucosal exposure has occurred in laboratory workers and occupational settings.

9. Treatment—No definitive licensed therapy for humans is available at this time; however, several investigational inhibitor compounds and monoclonal antibodies are being tested against various flaviviruses.

10. Prevention—

1) Vector prevention measures (see Arboviral Encephalitides in "Arboviral Diseases").

2) Vaccine: WNV vaccines for horses are available in several countries. Human WNV vaccines are not yet available but several candidate vaccines have been evaluated in preclinical and clinical trials.

3) Other prevention measures:

- Screening of blood and organ donations is useful in certain settings. Since 2003, blood products have been routinely screened for WNV in the USA and Canada, leading to thousands of infected products being removed from the blood supply.
- To prevent laboratory infections, precautions should be taken when handling viruses in the laboratory at the appropriate biosafety level (https://www.cdc.gov/niosh/docs/2006-115/pdfs/2006-115.pdf?id=10.26616).
- WNV may also be transmitted through human milk but transmission appears rare. Because the benefits of breastfeeding likely outweigh the risk of illness in breastfeeding infants, mothers should be encouraged to breastfeed even in areas of ongoing WNV transmission.

11. Special considerations—

1) Reporting: local health authority may be required to report cases in selected endemic areas or in areas where WNV previously has not been reported.

2) Epidemic measures: use personal protective measures, including mosquito repellents. Eliminate or treat all potential mosquito breeding places. Consider adult mosquito control measures.

[S. L. Robinson, C. F. Decker]

❖

YAWS
(framboesia tropica)

DISEASE	ICD-10 CODE
YAWS	ICD-10 A66

1. Clinical features—Yaws is a chronic, relapsing nonvenereal treponematosis. It is characterized by highly contagious early stages manifesting in primary and secondary cutaneous lesions (early yaws) and a noncontagious later stage that may involve tertiary destructive lesions (late yaws).

The typical initial lesion (mother yaw) is a papilloma on the face or extremities—typically the leg—that persists for weeks or months and is painless unless secondarily infected. This proliferates slowly and may form a framboesial (raspberry-like) lesion or ulcerate (ulcero-papilloma).

Secondary disseminated or satellite papillomata and/or papules (daughter yaws) and squamous macules appear before, or shortly after, healing of the initial lesion. These appear in successive crops, often accompanied by periostitis of the long bones (saber shin) and fingers (polydactylitis) and mild constitutional symptoms. In the dry season, papillomatous crops are attenuated, with more typical lesions restricted to the moist skinfolds and with papules or macular lesions predominating. Painful, and usually disabling, papillomata and hyperkeratosis on palms and soles may appear in both early and late stages. Lesions heal spontaneously but relapses after periods of latency are not uncommon. Early yaws can last up to 5 years after initial infection.

In late yaws, destructive lesions of skin, cartilage, and/or bone occur in about 10% to 20% of untreated patients, usually 5 or more years after infection. Yaws is rarely fatal but can be very disfiguring and disabling, resulting in social stigma and economic impact.

The differential diagnosis includes impetigo, ecthyma, tinea versicolor, molluscum contagiosum, lichen planus, psoriasis, tropical ulcers, plantar warts, scabies, tungiasis (jiggers infestation), sarcoidosis, leprosy, and cutaneous leishmaniasis. Bony lesions in late yaws can resemble lesions of syphilis, bejel, tuberculosis, African histoplasmosis, bacterial osteomyelitis, and sickle cell anemia.

2. Risk groups—Almost all cases of yaws occur in children younger than 15 years, with the peak incidence in children aged 6 to 10 years. Yaws occurs in rural communities located in tropical (hot and humid) climates with heavy rainfall and is promoted by overcrowding and poor hygiene. The incidence is similar in males and females. There is no evidence of natural resistance. Infection produces immunity to reinfection and may offer some protection against infection by other pathogenic treponemes.

3. Causative agents—*Treponema pallidum* subsp. *pertenue*, a spirochete bacterium in the genus *Treponema* that is genetically almost identical to *Treponema pallidum* subsp. *pallidum* (the causative agent for syphilis) and is morphologically identical to other *T. pallidum* subsp. The organism multiplies very slowly in humans, does not grow in culture, and is easily killed by drying, elevated temperatures, or exposure to oxygen.

4. Diagnosis—Usually based on clinical and epidemiologic findings along with direct detection (definitive) or serologic (presumptive) tests. Dark-field microscopic examination of exudates from primary or secondary lesions allows direct detection of spirochetes. Additionally, molecular methods using polymerase chain reaction and deoxyribonucleic acid (DNA) sequencing have been developed to detect *T. pallidum* subsp. *pertenue*-specific sequences in lesion exudate, although these are typically available only in research laboratories. Many clinically suspicious lesions have no detectable treponemal DNA but may have an alternative organism, most commonly *Haemophilus ducreyi*, detected.

Laboratory-based nontreponemal and treponemal tests are often available and both tests should be done for a presumptive diagnosis. Nontreponemal serologic tests (e.g., venereal disease research laboratory and rapid plasma reagin tests), which become reactive during the initial stage, remain so during the early infection and tend to become nonreactive after many years of latency, even in the absence of specific treatment; in some patients, they remain reactive at a low titer for life. Treponemal serologic tests (e.g., *T. pallidum* particle agglutination and fluorescent treponemal antibody absorption) usually remain reactive for life despite adequate treatment. Rapid point-of-care treponemal syphilis tests that can be used in rural or remote settings with minimal or no laboratory capacity are increasingly available. However, these treponemal tests are unable to distinguish between past and active infection. At least 1 dual treponemal and non-treponemal rapid test is available that can be used in field settings.

In the laboratory, endemic treponematoses (yaws, bejel, pinta) and venereal syphilis are distinguishable with molecular testing of early lesion material but cannot be differentiated by other direct detection tests or serologic assays.

5. Occurrence—Predominantly a disease of children living under crowded, lower socioeconomic conditions in rural, humid tropical areas of Africa, Central and South America, the Caribbean, and the equatorial islands of Southeast Asia and the Pacific, all regions where wet and dry seasons alternate. The prevalence of infectious yaws lesions increases during the rainy season. Mass penicillin treatment campaigns in the 1950s and 1960s dramatically decreased worldwide prevalence but yaws has reemerged in parts of equatorial and western Africa, with scattered foci of infection persisting in Latin America, the Caribbean islands, southeastern Asia, and some South Pacific islands. In September 2006, India declared yaws eliminated, with no cases reported since 2004. In 2007, WHO launched a new global program to eradicate yaws, initially focusing on selected endemic districts in 7 countries

(Cameroon, Ghana, Indonesia, Papua New Guinea, the Solomon Islands, Timor Leste, and Vanuatu). Yaws should be considered in the evaluation of a reactive syphilis serology in any person who has emigrated from an endemic area.

6. Reservoirs—Humans and possibly higher primates.

7. Incubation period—From 10 to 90 days (average 21 days).

8. Transmission—Transmissibility is high in the early stages. Yaws is principally transmitted by direct, nonsexual contact with the exudate of primary and secondary skin lesions of infected people. Indirect transmission through contamination from scratching, skin-piercing articles, and flies on open wounds is possible but of unknown importance. The period of communicability varies and may extend intermittently over several years when moist lesions are present. Late yaws lesions are not infectious. The spread of yaws is facilitated by crowding and poor community sanitation (i.e., lack of soap and water for bathing and washing clothing).

It is often reported that yaws is unlike syphilis in that it does not affect the cardiovascular or central nervous system or cross the placenta. However, many case reports of yaws-associated aortitis, ophthalmic involvement, and fetal infection exist, although these are presumed to be rare.

9. Treatment—

Preferred treatment	• Adults: benzathine penicillin 1.2 MU IM as a single dose • Children: 600,000 units IM as a single dose
Alternative drug	• Azithromycin 20 mg/kg ($\leq$ 2 g) PO as a single dose[a] • For patients allergic to penicillin and azithromycin, doxycycline 100 mg PO BID for 7 days
Special considerations and comments	• Cases should be reported to the health authority. • In 2018, results from a yaws elimination campaign in Papua New Guinea were published documenting macrolide resistance in *Treponema pallidum* subsp. *pertenue* infections.

Note: BID = twice daily; IM = intramuscular(ly); MU = million units; PO = oral(ly).
[a]Yaws eradication campaigns using mass treatment strategies have promoted azithromycin owing to its easier administration and logistical considerations (see Special Considerations in this chapter).

10. Prevention—The following apply to yaws and other nonvenereal treponematoses:

1) Educate the public about the value of better sanitation, including liberal use of soap and water and the importance of improving social and economic conditions over a period of years to reduce incidence. Improve access to health services.

2) Organize intensive control activities on a community level suitable to the local problem. Examine entire populations and treat patients with active or latent disease. Treatment of asymptomatic contacts is beneficial. WHO recommends treating the entire population when the prevalence rate for active disease is greater than 10%; if prevalence is 5% to 10%, treat patients, contacts, and all children younger than 15 years; if prevalence is less than 5%, treat active cases plus household and other contacts. Periodic clinical resurveys and continuous surveillance are essential for success.

3) Conduct serologic surveys for latent cases, particularly in children. This is to prevent relapses and development of infective lesions that maintain the disease in the community and to detect ongoing community transmission, if any.

4) Provide facilities for early diagnosis and treatment as part of a plan in which mass control campaigns are eventually consolidated into permanent local health services.

11. Special considerations—

1) Reporting: yaws should be reported to the local health authority. Differentiation of venereal and nonvenereal treponematoses, with proper reporting of each, has particular importance in the evaluation and consolidation of mass campaigns.

2) Disaster implications have not been observed but there is a potential risk in refugee or displaced populations in endemic areas with crowding and/or without hygiene facilities.

3) International measures: to protect countries from reinfection where active mass treatment programs are in progress, adjacent countries in the endemic area should institute measures against yaws. Movement of infected people across frontiers may require supervision (see "Syphilis").

[M. Kamb, A. Pillay]

YELLOW FEVER

DISEASE	ICD-10 CODE
YELLOW FEVER	ICD-10 A95

Yellow fever virus, a mosquito-borne flavivirus, is present in tropical areas of Africa and South America. In humans, the majority of yellow fever virus infections are asymptomatic. Clinical disease varies from a mild, undifferentiated febrile illness to severe disease with jaundice and hemorrhage. Because no treatment exists and there is the potential for explosive outbreaks, maintaining high population-level immunity through vaccination, surveillance, and mosquito control is critical to reduce transmission risk and mortality. A live attenuated yellow fever vaccine is recommended for those aged 9 months and older who are traveling to, or living in, areas of South America and Africa with a risk of yellow fever virus transmission. Because of the risk of serious adverse events following yellow fever vaccination, health care providers should only vaccinate persons who are at risk for exposure to yellow fever virus or who require proof of vaccination for country entry.

1. Clinical features—Majority ($\sim$ 55%) of infected persons are asymptomatic. Clinical disease varies from mild febrile illness to severe disease with jaundice and hemorrhage. Initial symptoms include sudden onset of fever, chills, headache, backache, general muscle pain, prostration, nausea, and vomiting. The pulse may be slow and weak, out of proportion to the elevated temperature (Faget sign). Leukopenia appears early and is most pronounced about the fifth day; however, leukocytosis is often seen in the second week of the disease. Most symptoms resolve at this stage.

In approximately 12% of patients, there is a brief remission of hours to days, followed by recurrence of initial symptoms with progression to more severe symptoms that can include jaundice or hemorrhage. Elevated liver enzymes, abnormal clotting factors, albuminuria, and anuria may occur as a result of liver and renal failure. An estimated 2% to 12% of all infections result in death. However, for patients with severe disease involving hepatorenal dysfunction, the case-fatality ratio is 30% to 60%. Recovery from yellow fever results in lifelong immunity.

2. Risk groups—Risk groups include unvaccinated travelers to endemic areas, forest workers in endemic areas, and those living near forest areas or in *Aedes aegypti*-infested areas who do not have vaccine- or naturally acquired immunity. The disease is highly communicable where many susceptible people and abundant vector mosquitoes coexist. Transient passive immunity in infants born to immune mothers may persist for up to 6 months.

3. Causative agents—Yellow fever virus is a ribonucleic acid (RNA) virus of the family Flaviviridae and genus *Flavivirus.*

4. Diagnosis—In acute disease, laboratory diagnosis can often be made through demonstration of viral RNA in blood or tissue by reverse transcription polymerase chain reaction (RT-PCR) or isolation of virus from blood. RT-PCR and sequencing can aid in distinguishing acute infections from recent vaccination. Immunohistochemical staining can detect viral antigen in tissues, especially liver, and is often used in postmortem diagnosis. Serologic diagnosis includes demonstrating virus-specific immunoglobulin class M (IgM) antibodies in early sera or a 4-fold or greater rise in titer of virus-specific antibodies in paired acute and convalescent sera. Serologic cross-reactions occur with other flaviviruses, and IgM antibodies against wild-type yellow fever virus cannot be differentiated from those derived through vaccination. Therefore, the patient's epidemiologic situation, clinical signs and symptoms, and vaccination status should be considered when interpreting results.

5. Occurrence—According to WHO, 47 countries, comprising 34 in Africa and 13 in Central and South America, are endemic for, or have regions that are endemic for, yellow fever. (See Figure 1 in this chapter.) Sub-Saharan West African countries have traditionally reported the most yellow fever infections on an annual basis. However, owing to recent vaccination campaigns, the number of infections reported from West Africa has decreased substantially. More recently, large outbreaks have been documented in Angola, the Democratic Republic of the Congo, Ethiopia, Sudan (Darfur), and Uganda. In South America, most yellow fever infections have been reported from the Orinoco, Amazon, and Araguaia river basins and contiguous grasslands in Bolivia, Brazil, Colombia, and Peru. However, from 2007 to 2009, human and epizootic disease was documented in many areas and countries that had not seen activity for several decades, such as Argentina, southern Brazil, Paraguay, and Trinidad and Tobago. Starting in late 2016, yellow fever infections were documented for the first time in 20 to 70 years in coastal areas of Brazil as well as French Guiana and Suriname.

Yellow fever outbreaks occurred in Europe and North America until the early 1900s but autochthonous transmission has not been reported for more than 100 years. There is no evidence that yellow fever has ever been present in Asia.

6. Reservoirs—In urban areas, in humans and *Ae. aegypti* mosquitoes; in forest and savanna areas, in vertebrates other than humans, mainly nonhuman primates and tree-hole–breeding mosquitoes (e.g., *Aedes africanus*, *Aedes bromeliae*, *Aedes luteocephalus*, and *Haemagogus* spp.).

7. Incubation period—Typically 3 to 6 days.

8. Transmission—There are 3 transmission cycles for yellow fever virus: sylvatic (jungle), savanna (intermediate), and urban. (See Figure 2 in this chapter.) Disease occurrence is influenced by the specific transmission cycle present in an area.

Sylvatic transmission is restricted to tropical regions of Africa and Latin America, most often among occupationally exposed young adult males in forested or transitional areas. The intermediate cycle involves humans in humid or semihumid areas of Africa where infected mosquitoes feed on both monkeys and humans, resulting in small-scale outbreaks. Urban transmission can lead to large epidemics affecting all age groups.

(a)

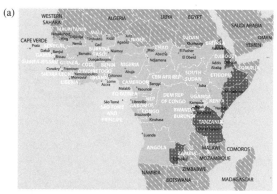

(b)

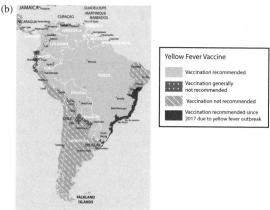

Yellow Fever Vaccine

Vaccination recommended

Vaccination generally
not recommended

Vaccination not recommended

Vaccination recommended since
2017 due to yellow fever outbreak

Source: Adapted from CDC.[1]

Note: Areas where vaccine is recommended (in light gray) are considered to have yellow fever transmission. Areas where vaccine has been recommended since 2017 (in dark gray) are in response to a recent yellow fever outbreak impacting areas not previously considered at risk for transmission. Areas where vaccine is generally not recommended (in darker gray with white dots) are considered to have a low potential for transmission. Areas where vaccine is not recommended (in light gray with stripes) are areas considered not at risk for yellow fever virus transmission. For the most up-to-date information, see: https://wwwnc.cdc.gov/travel/notices.

Figure 1. Areas at Risk for Yellow Fever Virus Transmission: (a) Africa and (b) South America.

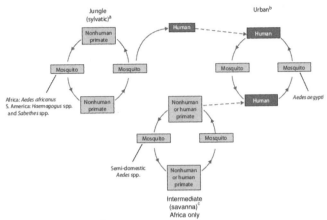

Source: Adapted from CDC.[2]

[a]The jungle (sylvatic) transmission cycle involves transmission of the virus between nonhuman primates and mosquito species found in the forest canopy. The virus is transmitted via mosquitoes from nonhuman primates to humans when the humans encroach into the jungle during occupational or recreational activities.

[b]The urban transmission cycle involves transmission of the virus between human and urban mosquitoes, primarily *Aedes aegypti*. Viremic humans traveling from one region to another can feed into and serve as a source of infection for mosquitoes in other transmission cycles (dotted line).

[c]In Africa, an intermediate (savanna) cycle involves transmission of yellow fever virus from tree-hole-breeding *Aedes* spp. to humans living or working in jungle border areas. In this cycle, the virus can be transmitted from nonhuman primate to human or from human to human via these mosquitoes.

Figure 2. Yellow Fever Virus Transmission Cycles.

Humans can transmit the virus to mosquitoes before onset of fever and for the first 3 to 5 days of illness. The extrinsic incubation period in *Ae. aegypti* is 9 to 12 days at the usual tropical temperatures. Once infected, mosquitoes remain so for life. Vertical transmission of the infection through the eggs in mosquitoes occurs but its contribution to maintaining transmission is unknown.

Since yellow fever vaccine virus has been documented to be transmitted through breastfeeding and blood transfusions, it is likely that wild-type yellow fever virus can be transmitted through breastfeeding or exposure to infected blood or organs. There is 1 case report of possible perinatal transmission of yellow fever virus. Laboratory infections occur, especially in unvaccinated workers.

The disease is not communicable through contact or fomites and there are no reports of congenital or sexual transmission, though yellow fever viral RNA was recently detected in semen.

9. Treatment—No specific antiviral therapies are available; treatment is supportive. Use blood and body fluid precautions. Prevent access of mosquitoes to the patient for at least 5 days after onset by screening the sick room, spraying quarters with residual insecticide, and using insecticide-treated bed nets. Spray homes of patients and all houses in the vicinity promptly with an effective insecticide. In endemic areas, family and other contacts and neighbors not previously immunized should be immunized promptly.

10. Prevention—Mechanisms to prevent yellow fever disease include vaccinating persons at risk and mosquito surveillance and control. Maintaining human and nonhuman primate disease surveillance with appropriate response mechanisms is essential.

1) Management of contacts and the immediate environment: when a disease case is identified, inquire about all contacts and all places (including forested areas) visited by the patient 3 to 10 days before onset to locate focus of yellow fever and observe all people visiting that focus. Search patient's premises and places of work or visits over the preceding several days for mosquitoes capable of transmitting infection and apply effective insecticide. Investigate febrile illnesses and unexplained deaths suggesting yellow fever.

2) Vaccination: recommended for all people aged 9 months or older who are at risk of acquiring infection due to residence, occupation, or travel. WHO provides yellow fever vaccination requirements and recommendations by country (http://www.who.int/ith/en). Many countries require proof of yellow fever vaccination (yellow fever certificate) for entry.

A single subcutaneous injection of attenuated yellow fever 17D vaccine is effective in more than 95% of recipients with antibodies appearing 7 to 10 days after immunization. WHO no longer recommends a booster dose as a single dose is sufficient to provide lifelong immunity. Booster doses may be recommended for certain travelers who are immunosuppressed or with higher-risk travel and for laboratory workers who routinely handle wild-type virus; recommendations vary by country.

Yellow fever vaccine can be safely administered simultaneously with other vaccines such as inactivated vaccines and measles vaccine. However, recent studies have documented a reduced immunologic response to yellow fever, mumps, and rubella viruses when yellow fever vaccine is coadministered with measles, mumps, and rubella vaccine(s). Additional studies are ongoing to determine whether yellow fever vaccine should be separated from measles, mumps, and rubella vaccines in infant immunization schedules in endemic areas.

Serious adverse events have been observed following yellow fever vaccination, including anaphylaxis, neurologic disease, and viscerotropic disease. With the latter 2 conditions, the vaccine virus replicates in either the brain or other organs, such as the liver, to cause disease or incite an autoimmune event (e.g., Guillain-Barré syndrome or acute disseminating encephalomyelitis). Two possible risk factors for developing a serious reaction, in particular viscerotropic disease, are advanced age and diseases of the thymus gland. Proper surveillance and support for adverse events following immunization should be part of any standard vaccine program or large vaccination campaign.

Yellow fever vaccine is contraindicated in children younger than 6 months and should be considered for those aged 6–8 months only if the risk of exposure is judged to exceed the risk of vaccine-associated encephalitis—the main complication in this age group. Because of the documented or theoretical risk of serious adverse events following immunization, the vaccine is also contraindicated in persons who have primary immunodeficiencies, are taking medicines that suppress their immune system, are allergic to vaccine components, have symptomatic human immunodeficiency virus (HIV) or HIV with severe immunosuppression (cluster of differentiation 4 [CD4+] glycoprotein T-lymphocyte counts $< 200/\text{mm}^3$), or have thymus disorder associated with abnormal immune function.

Specific recommendations for use of vaccine in individuals with asymptomatic HIV infection with no-to-moderate immunosuppression will depend on their CD4+ counts. Limited data suggest immunity wanes more rapidly in individuals with asymptomatic HIV infection than in persons without HIV. Age 60 years or older is a precaution to yellow fever vaccination because of the increased risk of serious adverse events. The vaccine is also not recommended during pregnancy or breastfeeding unless the risk of disease is believed to be higher than the theoretical risk to the fetus or infant. There is no evidence of major malformations occurring in the fetus secondary to the vaccine. However, one study observed lower rates of maternal seroconversion; checking antibody titers or reimmunizing women after the end of the pregnancy may therefore be warranted. At least 3 cases of breastfeeding-associated transmission of vaccine virus to infants, resulting in neurotropic disease in the child, have been documented. All infants were younger than 1 month at the time of exposure, suggesting that age of the infant may affect whether or not an adverse event might occur.

In 2016, in response to large outbreaks in Africa that depleted vaccine stocks, WHO approved the use of fractional dosing of yellow fever vaccine in emergency situations when there is a shortage of vaccine. Determining the appropriate volume (one-half or one-fifth of a standard dose) should be done in conjunction with WHO. Fractional dosing should not be used for routine immunization and does not meet the requirements to obtain yellow fever certificates.

The Yellow Fever Initiative, targeting 47 endemic countries, was launched in 2006 to introduce yellow fever vaccination into routine childhood immunization programs and to conduct preventive mass vaccination campaigns in at-risk areas. The initiative substantially reduced the number of yellow fever outbreaks in targeted countries in West Africa. However, in 2016, large outbreaks in Angola and in the Democratic Republic of the Congo highlighted the need for a new strategy to extend beyond the current known high-risk areas in Africa and the Americas and to include, along with vaccination strategies, emphasis on strengthening surveillance and laboratory capacity, application of the International Health Regulations (IHR), and the involvement of the private sector. The new strategy, Eliminate Yellow Fever Epidemics, was launched in 2017 and has a goal of eliminating yellow fever epidemics by vaccinating 1.4 billion persons by 2026.

3) Mosquito bite prevention measures:

- For urban yellow fever, eliminate or control the vector through disposal of standing water–holding containers (reducing breeding sites) and the use of larvicides and insecticides (see "Arboviral Encephalitides").
- For jungle or sylvan yellow fever, environmental vector control measures are typically not successful. Protective clothing, bed nets, and repellents are advised for those not immunized.
- For travelers who cannot be immunized and travel is unavoidable, using protective clothing; staying in locations with air-conditioning, screens, or bed nets; and using repellents may help lower the risk of disease (see "Arboviral Encephalitides").

11. Special considerations—

1) Reporting: IHR require events involving yellow fever infections to be assessed at the national level for potential notification to WHO.
2) Epidemic measures:

- Urban or *Ae. aegypti*-transmitted yellow fever: mass immunization, beginning with people most exposed and those living in *Ae. aegypti*-infested areas who have not been vaccinated against yellow fever. Eliminate or treat all potential breeding places. Spraying the inside of all houses in the community with insecticides has shown promise for controlling urban epidemics.

- Jungle or sylvan yellow fever: immediately immunize all people living in or near forested areas or entering such areas. Ensure that nonimmunized individuals avoid those tracts of forest where infection has been localized and that those just immunized avoid those areas for 7 to 10 days after immunization.

- In regions where yellow fever may occur, a diagnostic postmortem examination service should be organized to collect small specimens of tissues, especially liver, from fatal febrile illnesses, provided biologic safety can be ensured. Facilities for molecular or serologic confirmation are necessary to establish diagnosis.

- In Central and South America, confirmed deaths of howler and spider monkeys in the forest are presumptive evidence of the presence of yellow fever virus. Confirmation by the histopathologic examination of livers of moribund or recently dead monkeys, by virus isolation or molecular assays, is highly desirable. In Africa, monkeys are rarely symptomatic and rarely die from infections with yellow fever virus and thus cannot be used to indicate the presence of yellow fever virus circulation.

- Serosurveys through neutralization tests of wild primates captured in forested areas are useful in defining enzootic areas. Serologic surveys of human populations are not useful where yellow fever vaccine has been widely used and can be difficult to interpret in places with other endemic flaviviruses (e.g., dengue, Zika, West Nile viruses).

3) Disaster implications: consider mass vaccination if an epidemic is feared.

4) International measures:

- Measures applicable to ships, aircraft, and land transport arriving from areas with ongoing yellow fever virus transmission are no longer specified in the IHR. There are, however, applicable guidelines listed in the IHR for any areas with ongoing disease transmission.

- Animal quarantine: owing to the risk of nonhuman primates carrying zoonotic pathogens such as yellow fever, the World Organisation for Animal Health recommends—in the Terrestrial Animal Health Code (2010)—that captive-bred nonhuman primates be held in quarantine for 30 days and nonhuman primates captured from the wild be held in quarantine for 12 weeks.

- International travel: a valid International Certificate of Vaccination or Prophylaxis (yellow card) against yellow fever is required by many countries for entry of travelers coming from, or going to, recognized yellow fever zones of Africa and South America; otherwise, quarantine measures are applicable for up to 6 days. Immunizing practitioners and travelers should consult country-specific requirements and recommendations for yellow fever vaccination to determine whether vaccine administration should be considered (http://www.who.int/ith/en). The International Certificate of Vaccination against yellow fever is valid from 10 days after the date of immunization.

References

1. CDC. Yellow fever maps. Available at: https://www.cdc.gov/yellowfever/maps/index.html. Accessed May 13, 2020.
2. CDC. Transmission of yellow fever virus. Available at: https://www.cdc.gov/yellowfever/transmission/index.html. Accessed May 13, 2020.

[E. Staples, S. Martin]

YERSINIOSIS

DISEASE	ICD-10 CODE
INTESTINAL YERSINIOSIS	ICD-10 A04.6
EXTRAINTESTINAL YERSINIOSIS	ICD-10 A28.2

This chapter is about illness caused by *Yersinia enterocolitica* and other non–*Yersinia pestis* spp. associated with gastrointestinal symptoms. Illness caused by *Y. pestis*, the causative agent of plague, is described in "Plague."

1. Clinical features—Typically manifested by acute febrile diarrhea with abdominal pain (especially in young children). Bloody diarrhea can also occur. Other manifestations include acute mesenteric lymphadenitis mimicking appendicitis (especially in older children and adults), exudative pharyngitis, and systemic infection. The most common postinfectious complications are erythema nodosum and reactive arthritis. Ileitis is the characteristic lesion of *Y. enterocolitica* infection but diarrhea may be absent in up to a third of patients. *Yersinia pseudotuberculosis* causes acute mesenteric lymphadenitis, characterized by an appendicitis-like syndrome, sometimes with diarrhea. Because infections in older children and adolescents can mimic acute appendicitis, outbreaks can rarely be recognized by a local increase in appendectomies.

2. Risk groups—Diarrhea is more prominent in children. Postinfectious arthritis is more severe in adolescents and older adults. *Y. enterocolitica* equally affects men and women. Reactive arthritis and Reiter syndrome occur more often in people with the HLA-B27 genetic type. Septicemia occurs most often among people with iron overload (hemochromatosis) or immunosuppression.

3. Causative agents—Gram-negative bacilli. Globally, *Y. enterocolitica* is the species most commonly associated with human infection, causing up to 1% to 3% of acute enteritis in some areas. *Y. enterocolitica* has more than 60 serotypes and 6 biotypes, many nonpathogenic. *Y. pseudotuberculosis* has 6 serotypes with 4 subtypes.

4. Diagnosis—Usually made through stool culture. Cefsulodin–irgasan–novobiocin medium is highly selective and should be used if infection with *Yersinia* is suspected; at 28°C (78.4°F), it permits identification in 24 hours. The organisms may be recovered on usual enteric media if precautions are taken to prevent overgrowth of fecal flora. Cold enrichment in buffered saline at 4°C (39°F) for 2 to 3 weeks can be used but this procedure usually enhances the isolation of nonpathogenic species. *Yersinia* can be isolated from blood with standard commercial blood culture media. Yersiniosis is increasingly diagnosed by culture-independent diagnostic tests (CIDTs). In 2017, more than half of all *Yersinia* cases reported by US FoodNet sites were detected by CIDTs. Of note, CIDT panels typically target only *Y. enterocolitica* and panels detect antigen rather than live bacteria, so false-positives could occur. Prospective studies to evaluate the specificity and sensitivity of CIDT platforms have not been published and may be difficult to conduct in settings where yersiniosis is uncommon. Culture is required to determine species and antibiotic susceptibility. Serologic diagnosis is possible (agglutination test or enzyme-linked immunosorbent assay) but availability is generally limited to research settings.

5. Occurrence—The distribution of pathogenic *Y. enterocolitica* varies by geographic region. Serotypes O:3 and O:9 account for most cases in

Europe. In the USA and Canada, most isolates are serotypes O:3 and O:8. The highest isolation rates have been reported during the cold season in temperate climates, including northern Europe (especially Scandinavia), North America, and temperate regions of South America. Approximately two-thirds of *Y. enterocolitica* illness occurs among infants and children. Similarly, three-quarters of those with *Y. pseudotuberculosis* illness are aged 5 to 20 years. In some countries, such as Japan and Russia, *Y. pseudotuberculosis* is the main cause of yersiniosis. Specific *Y. pseudotuberculosis* syndromes (Izumi fever, Far East scarlet-like fever) have been reported in Japan and Russia.

6. Reservoirs—Animals. Pigs are the main reservoir for *Y. enterocolitica* serotype O:3. Asymptomatic pharyngeal carriage is common in swine, especially in winter, and serotype O:9 has been isolated from ovine, bovine, and caprine origins. *Y. pseudotuberculosis* is widespread among many avian and mammalian hosts, particularly rodents and other small mammals.

7. Incubation period—Usually 3 to 7 days; generally less than 10 days.

8. Transmission—Fecal-oral transmission through consumption of contaminated food or water or through contact with infected people or animals. *Y. enterocolitica* has been isolated from many foods; pathogenic strains are associated most commonly with raw pork or pork products. Vehicles implicated in *Y. enterocolitica* outbreaks include soybean cake (tofu), pork chitterlings (large intestines), and milk. *Y. enterocolitica* can multiply under refrigeration and microaerophilic conditions. Nosocomial transmission has occurred as has transmission by transfusion of stored blood products, most commonly reported with transfusion of red blood cells, from donors who were asymptomatic or had mild gastrointestinal illness.

Human illness with *Y. pseudotuberculosis* has been reported in association with infections in household pets, particularly puppies and kittens. Outbreaks of *Y. pseudotuberculosis* have been reported from northern Europe, Japan, and Canada; vehicles implicated include produce, pasteurized milk, and vegetable juice.

Secondary transmission appears rare. There is fecal shedding at least as long as symptoms exist, usually for 2 to 3 weeks. Untreated persons may excrete the organism for 2 to 3 months. Prolonged asymptomatic carriage has been reported in both children and adults.

9. Treatment—Optimal antibiotic treatment is not clearly established. Most cases of uncomplicated yersiniosis are self-limited; antibiotics have not been shown to reduce the duration or severity of illness. Antibiotic treatment is recommended for septicemia. Therefore, antibiotic treatment of most infections (i.e., uncomplicated gastrointestinal infections) is not recommended. Antibiotics might result in faster clearance of the pathogen from stool, which could potentially affect public health response in outbreak situations for example.

Patients With Septicemia

Preferred therapy	• Ceftriaxone 2 g IV daily (100 mg/kg/day in 1 or 2 divided doses, ≤ 4 g/day in children) PLUS • Gentamicin 5 mg/kg IV once daily
Alternative therapy options	Ciprofloxacin 400 mg IV BID[a]
Special considerations and comments	• Therapy lasts 3 weeks (may convert to oral therapy after initial response). • There are no controlled trials establishing optimal antibiotic choice or duration of treatment for *Yersinia* septicemia. • Most strains of *Yersinia enterocolitica* harbor β-lactamases and are resistant to ampicillin and first-generation cephalosporins; clinical failures have been reported with cefuroxime, ceftazidime, and cefopera-zone. Most strains are susceptible to aminoglycosides, ciprofloxacin, doxycycline, and TMP/SMX. • *Yersinia pseudotuberculosis* is typically susceptible to ampicillin. Patients with septicemia should receive ampicillin 100 mg/kg/day IV in divided doses. • There are no clinical trials supporting treatment benefit in gastroenteritis. For high-risk patients such as those with immunosuppression or iron overload disorders, consider consultation with an infectious disease specialist. Ciprofloxacin (adults) or TMP/SMX (children) may be used in select cases pending susceptibility testing, if available.

Note: BID = twice daily; IV = intravenous(ly); TMP/SMX = trimethoprim-sulfamethoxazole.
[a]Ciprofloxacin is not FDA-approved for use in children and has a black box warning regarding tendon rupture.

10. Prevention—

1) Use separate cutting boards for meat and other foods and carefully clean all cutting boards, countertops, and utensils with soap and hot water after preparing raw meat.

2) Avoid eating raw pork and unpasteurized milk or milk products. Irradiation of meat kills *Yersinia*.

3) Wash hands before handling food and eating, after handling raw pork, and after contact with animals.

4) Prevent cross-contamination of food preparation areas, particularly when preparing high-risk foods like chitlins (chitterlings, pig intestines). Keep young children out of the kitchen while high-risk foods are prepared.

5) Wash hands after contact with animals or animal feces. Protect water supplies from animal and human feces; purify appropriately.

6) Control rodents and birds (for *Y. pseudotuberculosis*).

7) During the slaughtering of pigs, the head and neck should be removed from the body to avoid contaminating meat with tissue from the pharynx (including tonsils), which may be heavily colonized.

8) Defer prospective blood donors with recent history of gastro-enteritis and implement blood-handling practices aimed at reducing rates of transfusion-transmitted bacterial infections.

Detailed guidance on the prevention of yersiniosis can be found at: https://www.cdc.gov/yersinia/prevention.html.

11. Special considerations—Reporting: any group of cases of acute gastroenteritis or a cluster of suspected appendicitis should be reported to the local health authority, even before a pathogen is identified.

[C. Friedman, L. K. Francois Watkins]

ZIKA
(Zika virus disease, Zika virus infection, Zika fever)

DISEASE	ICD-10 CODE
ZIKA	ICD-10 A92.8

1. Clinical features—Zika virus infection is often asymptomatic but in a proportion of patients (thought to be ~20%) infection manifests as self-limited disease characterized by slight elevation of temperature (often short-term and low-grade), rash, pruritus, nonpurulent conjunctivitis, arthralgia (small joints of hands and feet), myalgia, fatigue, headache, and occasionally prostatitis. Exanthema, with or without fever, is the most common presentation. Other symptoms reported less frequently include retro-orbital pain, edema of the hands and feet, dysuria, and hematospermia. Severe disease has been observed in very few individuals with immunologic disorders. Hospitalization is uncommon and death is rare.

The main differential diagnosis for Zika virus disease includes other arboviral diseases such as dengue and chikungunya; bacterial infections including leptospirosis and rickettsial, and group A streptococcal infections; and infections due to non–arthropod-borne viruses (e.g., parvovirus, rubella virus, measles virus, adenovirus, and enteroviruses). Symptoms and signs of Zika virus infection, dengue, and chikungunya, as well as the main differences in their clinical presentations, are shown in Table 1 in this chapter, but frequently they are indistinguishable. The virus genome can be detected by polymerase chain reaction (PCR) in serum but the amount of virus is low and the duration of the viremia is short (usually < 5 days). However, there are reports that the virus is detectable in whole blood for longer and that the amount can fluctuate during pregnancy. The virus can also be detected by PCR in urine, semen, cerebrospinal fluid (CSF), and other body fluids for several weeks after symptoms disappear.

Table 1. Differential Diagnosis Among Dengue-, Zika-, and Chikungunya-Infected Individuals

Clinical and Laboratory Findings	Dengue	Zika	Chikungunya
Fever	> 38°C (100.4°F) Intense (several times daily)	A febrile or mild fever of ≤ 38.5°C (101.3°F)	> 38°C (100.4°F) Intense (once or twice daily)
		Sporadic fever (once or twice daily)	
Fever duration	4–7 days	1–2 days	2–3 days
Exanthema	Starts on day 4	Starts on day 1 or 2	Starts on day 2 or 5
Exanthema frequency	30%–50% of cases	90%–100% of cases	50% of cases
Myalgia frequency	High	Medium	Low
Arthralgia frequency	Low	Medium	High
Joint pain intensity	Light	Light/moderate	Moderate/intense
Joint edema	Rare	Frequent and of light intensity	Frequent and moderate to intense
Conjunctivitis	Rare	50%–90% of cases	30% of cases
Headache intensity	High	Medium	Medium
Ganglionar hypertrophy	Low	High	Medium
Hemorrhagic dyscrasia	Medium	Absent	Low
Risk of death	High	Not known	Low
Neurologic damage	Medium	High	Low (mostly in neonates)
Lymphopenia	Variable	Not common	Frequent
Risk of thrombocytopenia	High	Absent	Low
Risk of leukopenia	High	High	High

Neurologic manifestations associated with infection are rare, occurring in fewer than 0.1% of cases, but there are serious complications of Zika virus infection; these typically appear as acute flaccid paralysis a few days (1–15 days, with an average of 6 days) after the onset of acute symptoms of Zika infection. Symptoms are varied and can be similar to demyelinating syndromes of the central and peripheral nervous system such as Guillain-Barré syndrome, acute disseminated encephalomyelitis, or optic neuritis. Acute motor axonal neuropathy is the typical electrophysiologic pattern found in patients with Guillain-Barré–type syndrome associated with Zika and about 20% to 35% of patients require respiratory support.

Electrophysiologic studies are more frequently compatible with acute inflammatory demyelinating polyradiculoneuropathy or acute motor axonal neuropathy, although other variants, such as acute motor-sensory axonal neuropathy and Miller Fisher syndrome, have been reported. Despite rapid progression of disease, clinical outcome is generally favorable. Neurologic symptoms can last for weeks and may not fully disappear in a significant proportion of patients. Other reported neurologic complications of Zika virus infection include meningoencephalitis and acute myelitis.

Congenital malformation may result from Zika virus infection during the first, and possibly into the second, trimester of gestation when there is intrauterine transmission of Zika virus from the mother to the fetus. However, maternal-fetal transmission seems to be less frequent and less severe when it occurs late in pregnancy. The typical malformation is microcephaly, often associated with facial disproportionality and with the appearance of cutis girata.

A wide spectrum of malformations associated with Zika infection is recognized and is now named congenital Zika syndrome. The risk of congenital brain abnormalities associated with Zika virus infection is not yet clearly defined; some initial data suggest that it could be up to 50 times greater than the usual baseline rates of these abnormalities in the general population. Neonates with congenital Zika are typically born with a high Apgar score (≥ 8) and no symptoms of distress. Neurologic examination shows normal primitive (newborn) reflexes, but spasticity, hyperreflexia, tremors, and convulsions may occur.

Radiologic examination often shows ventriculomegaly, abnormalities of the corpus callosum, and cortical disorders (lissencephaly). Retinal lesions are very frequent and it is important to perform retinal examination and begin treating those with lesions using visual stimulations. Auditory problems have also been reported. Intracranial calcifications at the gray matter–white matter junction are frequent and calcifications in the basal ganglia and/or thalamus are common. These findings are often present in infants with microcephaly but also may be present in infants with normal skull diameter.

2. Risk groups—The entire nonimmune population living in areas where Zika virus and mosquito vectors are known to be present and where transmission is known to occur should be considered at risk. In general, lower socioeconomic groups living in low-rise areas with high population density and with poor public services such as unreliable trash collection and intermittent water supply might be at increased risk because of increased mosquito breeding and exposure. The fact that Zika virus can also be transmitted sexually means that travelers returning from endemic areas can transmit the Zika virus to their sexual partners in their home countries. Because most infections are mild and neurologic complications rare, the main risk group of concern is pregnant women. However, the risk for congenital infection following maternal infection and the spectrum of outcomes associated with Zika virus infection during pregnancy are not well understood at this time.

Anecdotally, individuals with autoimmune disease and other immunologic disturbances present more severe disease, but unusually complicated human immunodeficiency virus and Zika coinfections have not been reported. Immunologic memory to other flaviviruses (especially dengue) could potentially modulate the clinical outcome of the Zika virus infection but the epidemiologic significance of cross-reactivity is still under investigation. Most flavivirus infections result in long-term immunity, so it is possible that a Zika virus infection confers lifelong immunity. However, this has not yet been confirmed.

3. Causative agents—The Zika virus was first isolated in Entebbe, Uganda, in 1947 from the blood of a sentinel rhesus monkey in the Zika Forest. It is a member of the Flaviviridae family, along with yellow fever, dengue, and West Nile viruses. The Zika virus has a lipid membrane envelope and is a positive single-stranded ribonucleic acid (RNA) virus with a genome of approximately 11 kilobases. The virus envelope glycoprotein mediates the binding to host cell receptors. The formation of nonneutralizing viral immune complexes may facilitate the infection of cells expressing antibody and complement receptors with a mechanism similar to that of the dengue antibody-dependent enhancement. There are 2 main Zika virus genotypes—African and Asian. The Asian genotype has been associated with congenital Zika virus infection, but it is not apparent whether this association also occurs with the African genotype; study is currently underway.

4. Diagnosis—Case definitions and laboratory diagnostics for Zika virus are rapidly evolving; clinical diagnosis in symptomatic cases is therefore important. A conclusive diagnosis is often difficult with current diagnostic tools and most often the diagnosis is presumptive in many countries.

Laboratory confirmation is based on virus detection using molecular techniques such as reverse transcription–polymerase chain reaction (RT-PCR), which has high specificity and, when positive, is considered a definitive diagnosis. Serum specimens can also be tested for virus-specific immuno-globulin class M (IgM) antibody using an enzyme immunoassay. IgM is usually detectable within the first week after onset of illness; based on experience with other flaviviral infections, it is likely to persist for several months.

Virus isolation can be attempted but is often difficult because viremia is generally low level. Other specimens in which viral RNA has been detected include CSF, urine, saliva, amniotic fluid, semen, breast milk, placenta, and neurologic tissues. Viral RNA has been detected for periods of longer duration in urine and semen than in blood. The current serologic tests for Zika virus antibody are often difficult to interpret because of cross-reactivity among flaviviruses, which leads to nonspecific positive results following dengue infection. Ideally, dengue and Zika serologic testing should be done in parallel, but frequently both are positive and the diagnosis is that of a flavivirus infection (e.g., following acute dengue virus infection, both dengue and Zika IgM might be positive). Viral neutralization antibody testing may help distinguish among flaviviruses, but these tests can usually only be performed in specialized laboratories. New and more specific diagnostics for Zika and dengue are being developed, using specific monoclonals and tests based on detection of anti-Zika IgG3 subclass.

Confirmation of Zika virus infection with neurologic complications may be difficult because medical assistance is usually sought when viral RNA is no longer present in the blood. To be certain of neurologic complications of Zika virus infection requires confirmed diagnosis of a peripheral or central demyelinating syndrome associated with a recent history of confirmed or suspected clinical Zika infection. A presumptive diagnosis of neurologic complications of Zika infection can be made if other common causes of demyelinating diseases in a region where Zika virus transmission is occurring are excluded.

The presence of IgM or detection of virus by PCR in the CSF, with negative IgM for dengue virus, suggests a primary Zika virus infection of the central nervous system (CNS). However, the presence of Zika RNA in the urine confirms the diagnosis.

Confirmation of congenital Zika virus infection is challenging because of the time relationship between the maternal infection, fetal death, and/or neurologic disorder at birth. Confirmation of congenital infection may be by the detection of viral RNA in amniotic fluid, at the time of delivery when infant serum is collected from the umbilical cord, or directly from the infant; amniotic fluid is tested for viral RNA, Zika IgM, and neutralizing antibodies. RT-PCR and immunohistochemical staining to detect specific viral antigen can also be used for placenta or other tissue. Confirmation can also be made by identification of virus RNA or IgM in the CSF of a neonate. Negative laboratory tests do not exclude the possibility of congenital Zika virus infection. Congenital malformations identified in an area where there has been a preceding Zika outbreak or ongoing transmission must be investigated thoroughly. A case with a history of confirmed or suspected Zika virus infection during gestation and exclusion of other probable causes can be considered a presumptive congenital Zika virus infection.

5. Occurrence—Zika virus transmission has been documented in countries in Africa, Asia, the Pacific, the Americas, and the Caribbean. Between 1947—when the Zika virus was discovered—and 2007, human infections were reported sporadically, with no major outbreaks. The recent series of Zika outbreaks first occurred in Yap island (the Federated States of Micronesia) in 2007. This was followed by a 2013–2014 outbreak in French Polynesia and subsequently an outbreak commencing in 2015 in the northeast region of Brazil. Fifty-eight countries reported outbreaks after 2015.

At the time of writing, these outbreaks had thus far resulted in an estimated 1 million Zika virus infections. More than 25,000 cases of microcephaly and/ or CNS malformation suggestive of congenital Zika virus infections, or potentially associated with a Zika virus infection, have been reported in the area of the Zika outbreaks. The two best-documented outbreaks of Zika are those in French Polynesia and Brazil. The attack rate of Zika virus in the Pacific Islands is thought to have been high, but precise measurements are hindered by a lack of specific serologic tools for determining incidence and seroprevalence. It is assumed that the outbreak resulted in high levels of herd immunity in these Island populations. It is estimated that attack rates in Brazil could be as high as 50% or more, and the outbreak is spreading throughout the country. Attack rates appear higher than those previously observed for dengue and chikungunya in the same population, which have usually varied between 5% and 15%.

Zika outbreaks are now occurring throughout Latin America and in some of the Caribbean island nations; limited outbreaks have also occurred in North America. Recent outbreaks in some Asian countries appear to be associated with increases in microcephaly and study continues in these areas.

6. Reservoirs—The ecology of the Zika virus is not well-defined and is highly speculative. The natural Zika virus reservoir is thought by some to be African and Asian monkeys, though this is an unconfirmed hypothesis. Rodents have been shown to be susceptible to virus infection and replication in the laboratory, but there is no evidence of rodent infections in nature. Some scientists have postulated that transmission patterns of Zika virus may have changed sometime before the 2007 outbreak in Yap island, with hypotheses ranging from reservoir adaptation to mutation that has resulted in a virus highly adapted to human transmission in urban settings. Studies are being designed to provide more information.

7. Incubation period—Although the exact incubation period for Zika virus disease has not yet been fully determined, evidence from case reports and experience from related flavivirus infections indicates it is likely 3 to 14 days. It is difficult to determine the exact incubation period because symptoms are mild. Based on a few recent case reports, there is some suggestion that the incubation period for sexual transmission could be longer than for mosquito-mediated transmission, but this is based on preliminary data only and must be confirmed.

8. Transmission—Zika infection is predominantly mosquito-borne and transmission patterns show associations with mosquito levels and seasonality. The main mosquito vector in the Americas is assumed to be the day-biting *Aedes aegypti*. Vector competence studies have been limited, however, and roles for other mosquito species have not been ruled out, although recent studies suggest low vector competence of *Culex* spp.

Zika virus has been isolated from several other species of *Aedes* mosquitoes, including *Aedes africanus* and *Aedes albopictus*. It has also been isolated from *Anopheles coustani* and viral RNA was found in *Culex* saliva, but these are not thought likely to be important vectors for human-mosquito-human transmission. In the outbreaks in Yap island and French Polynesia, *Aedes hensilli* and *Aedes polynesiensis* were thought to be the primary vectors.

The extrinsic incubation period in the mosquito is thought to be approximately 10 days. In humans, intrauterine and sexual transmission are other important modes of transmission. The frequency and risk factors for intrauterine transmission and the extent to which sexual transmission contributes to spread of infection are unknown. Infectious Zika virus has also been detected in saliva, and this may suggest other possible mechanisms of viral transmission.

Other documented routes of transmission include perinatal transmission, blood transfusion, and laboratory exposure. The potential for transmission by blood transfusion is a significant concern because it appears the virus can remain in the blood, undetectable by currently available PCR techniques. This is especially important because conventional triage questionnaires may not be able to exclude donors with recent asymptomatic infection. Based on experience with other flaviviruses, organ and tissue transplantation are also possible modes of transmission. Zika virus RNA has been detected in breast milk, although transmission by breast milk has not been documented.

9. Treatment—No definitive treatment is available. Supportive care is usually considered.

10. Prevention—There are no available vaccines or chemoprophylaxis to prevent Zika virus disease. The main means of prevention are avoidance of mosquito bites, especially during daytime; measures to reduce indoor and outdoor exposure to mosquitoes; and measures to reduce the likelihood of sexual transmission of Zika virus. Personal protective measures include using mosquito repellents, treating clothes with permethrin, reducing amount of exposed skin surface area by wearing long sleeves and trousers, using air-conditioning, installing window and door screens, and sleeping under a bed net.

Vector control measures include source reduction, larval control, and adult mosquito control. Source reduction includes removing discarded, unused, and unmaintained containers, which can collect water and become ideal larval habitats. Larval control includes application of biologic or chemical larvicides to potential larval habitats. Adult mosquito control is generally only used in outbreak situations. Indoor residual spraying has been shown to be effective in some settings.

Public vector control programs are very important to reduce transmission of all arboviral diseases, with a goal to decrease mosquito populations to a minimum, possibly targeting vector eradication. Partial reduction of transmission may paradoxically increase the risk of congenital Zika virus infection, as suggested by epidemiologic modeling; for girls living in areas where vector control is partially effective in decreasing mosquito populations, those living in areas with high Zika virus transmission could reach reproductive age already immune and therefore at low risk of congenital Zika virus transmission, while those girls living in low-transmission areas could reach reproductive age susceptible to Zika virus infection and hence have a higher risk of congenital transmission. It is therefore important for the vector control programs to take into consideration these nonlinear epidemiologic dynamics.

Pregnant women living outside areas of Zika virus transmission should postpone travel to those areas until after delivery and avoid unprotected sexual contact with male partners returning from endemic areas for up to 6 months, as recommended by WHO. For women living in areas with Zika virus transmission and considering conception, factors including level of risk for Zika virus exposure and reproductive life plans might influence the decision. In general, however, women who live in areas where Zika outbreaks are occurring should consider postponing pregnancy until after the outbreak is over—or time the conception to begin the pregnancy at low mosquito season.

11. Special considerations—Reporting of Zika virus infection is mandatory in some countries, including notification of all suspected cases and immediate notification of pregnant women with suspected infection. The Pan American Health Organization has developed guidelines for the surveillance of microcephaly in newborns in settings with risk of Zika virus circulation (http://iris.paho.org/xmlui/handle/123456789/28229).

[L. Yee-Sin]

INDEX

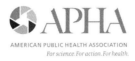

The American Public Health Association (APHA) champions the health of all people and communities. Our members represent all public health disciplines and more than 40 countries. APHA is the only organization that combines 140-plus years of perspective, a broad-based constituency, and the ability to influence federal policy to advocate for and improve the public's health.

APHA builds a collective voice for public health, working to ensure access to health care, protect funding for core public health services, and eliminate health disparities, among a myriad of other issues. Through its strong flagship publishing program that produces *Control of Communicable Diseases Manual,* the peer-reviewed *American Journal of Public Health,* the award-winning newspaper *The Nation's Health,* along with its e-newsletter Inside Public Health. APHA also leads public health awareness through its Get Ready campaigns and National Public Health Week. Together, we are creating the Healthiest Nation in One Generation.

To join APHA, visit www.apha.org or contact Membership Services at membership.mail@apha.org.